Recent Developments in Comparative Endocrinology and Neurobiology

Recent Developments in Comparative Endocrinology and Neurobiology

Editor: Cooper Grant

MURPHY & MOORE
www.murphy-moorepublishing.com

www.murphy-moorepublishing.com

MURPHY & MOORE

Cataloging-in-Publication Data

Recent developments in comparative endocrinology and neurobiology / edited by Cooper Grant.
p. cm.
Includes bibliographical references and index.
ISBN 978-1-63987-480-4
1. Endocrinology, Comparative. 2. Comparative neurobiology. 3. Medicine, Comparative.
4. Physiology, Comparative. 5. Endocrinology. 6. Neurobiology. I. Grant, Cooper.
QP187 .R43 2022
612.4--dc23

Murphy & Moore Publishing,
1 Rockefeller Plaza,
New York City, NY 10020, USA

ISBN 978-1-63987-480-4 (Hardback)

Contents

Preface

Every book is initially just a concept; it takes months of research and hard work to give it the final shape in which the readers receive it. In its early stages, this book also went through rigorous reviewing. The notable contributions made by experts from across the globe were first molded into patterned chapters and then arranged in a sensibly sequential manner to bring out the best results.

The field of study which deals with the different complexities of the endocrine systems of vertebrate and invertebrate systems is termed as comparative endocrinology. It conducts analysis at the sub-molecular, cellular, molecular and organismal level. Comparative endocrinology mainly focuses on the morphological and functional aspects. The field of science which studies the nervous system is termed as neurobiology. It combines concepts from a variety of disciplines such as anatomy, physiology, molecular biology, cytology and developmental biology. The major areas of study within this discipline are the emergent and basic properties of neural circuits and neurons. Some of its prominent branches are affective neuroscience, cellular neuroscience, cultural neuroscience and molecular neuroscience. This book unravels the recent studies in the field of comparative endocrinology and neurobiology. It traces the progress of this field and highlights some of its key concepts and applications. Those in search of information to further their knowledge will be greatly assisted by this book.

It has been my immense pleasure to be a part of this project and to contribute my years of learning in such a meaningful form. I would like to take this opportunity to thank all the people who have been associated with the completion of this book at any step.

Editor

1

Endocrine FGFs: Evolution, physiology, pathophysiology and pharmacotherapy

Nobuyuki Itoh[1]*, Hiroya Ohta[2] and Morichika Konishi[2]

[1] Medical Innovation Center, Kyoto University Graduate School of Medicine, Kyoto, Japan, [2] Department of Microbial Chemistry, Kobe Pharmaceutical University, Kobe, Japan

Edited by:
Peter Blume-Jensen, Metamark Genetics, Inc., USA

Reviewed by:
Wendong Huang, Beckman Research Institute of City of Hope, USA
Mikhail Karganov, Russian Academy of Medical Sciences, Russia

****Correspondence:***
Nobuyuki Itoh, Medical Innovation Center, Kyoto University Graduate School of Medicine, Shogoin-Kawara-cho, Sakyo, Kyoto 606-8507, Japan
nobuyuki.itoh.56c@st.kyoto-u.ac.jp

The human fibroblast growth factor (FGF) family comprises 22 structurally related polypeptides that play crucial roles in neuronal functions, development, and metabolism. FGFs are classified as intracrine, paracrine, and endocrine FGFs based on their action mechanisms. Paracrine and endocrine FGFs are secreted signaling molecules by acting via cell-surface FGF receptors (FGFRs). Paracrine FGFs require heparan sulfate as a cofactor for FGFRs. In contrast, endocrine FGFs, comprising FGF19, FGF21, and FGF23, require α-Klotho or β-Klotho as a cofactor for FGFRs. Endocrine FGFs, which are specific to vertebrates, lost heparan sulfate-binding affinity and acquired a systemic signaling system with α-Klotho or β-Klotho during early vertebrate evolution. The phenotypes of endocrine *FGF* knockout mice indicate that they play roles in metabolism including bile acid, energy, and phosphate/active vitamin D metabolism. Accumulated evidence for the involvement of endocrine FGFs in human genetic and metabolic diseases also indicates their pathophysiological roles in metabolic diseases, potential risk factors for metabolic diseases, and useful biomarkers for metabolic diseases. The therapeutic utility of endocrine FGFs is currently being developed. These findings provide new insights into the physiological and pathophysiological roles of endocrine FGFs and potential diagnostic and therapeutic strategies for metabolic diseases.

Keywords: biomarker, disease, endocrine, FGF, Klotho, metabolism, mutation, polymorphism

Introduction

Cell–cell communication with secreted signaling molecules ensures proper development and metabolism. Most fibroblast growth factors (FGFs) are well-established secreted signaling proteins that play critical roles in development and metabolism. The FGF family comprises 22 structurally and evolutionarily related proteins including FGF1–FGF23 in humans and mice (1). The human and mouse FGF families do not include FGF15 and FGF19, respectively, as they are orthologs. FGFs are classified as intracrine, paracrine, and endocrine FGFs by their action mechanisms (**Figure 1A**). Paracrine and endocrine FGFs, which comprise 15 and 3 FGFs, respectively, are secreted signaling proteins. In contrast, intracrine FGFs, which comprise four FGFs, are intracellular proteins that are not functionally related to paracrine or endocrine FGFs (1).

Endocrine FGFs comprise FGF19, FGF21, and FGF23. The mouse is a mammalian model that is useful for investigating gene functions through gene targeting. All endocrine *FGF* knockout mice have been generated and extensively analyzed, with their phenotypes indicating important roles in

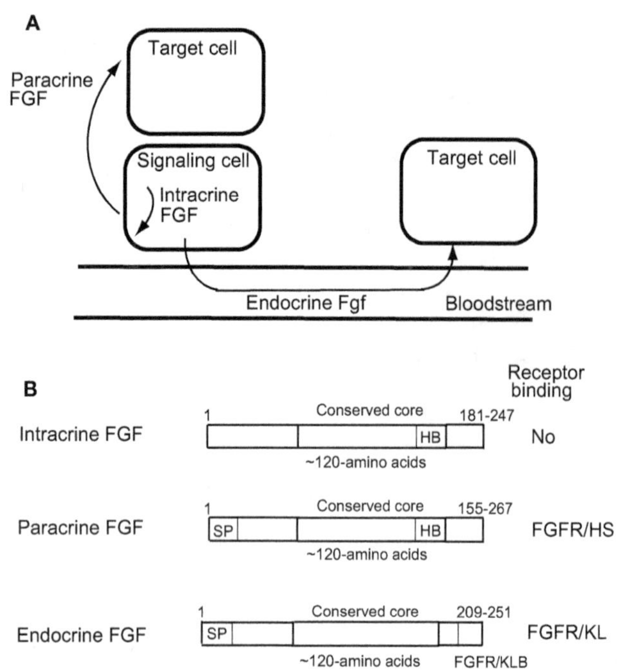

FIGURE 1 | (A) Action mechanisms of FGFs. FGFs act on target cells in an intracrine, paracrine, or endocrine manner. **(B)** Schematic representations of FGF structures. SP, HB, and FGFR/KB indicate a secreted signal sequence, heparan sulfate-binding site, and FGFR/Klotho complex-binding site, respectively.

metabolism (1). Evidence to support the involvement of endocrine FGFs in human inherited and metabolic diseases has also been accumulated. We herein have reviewed the physiological/pathophysiological roles and diagnostic/therapeutic utility of endocrine FGFs.

Identification of Endocrine FGFS

FGF15 was originally identified as a downstream target of the chimeric homeodomain oncoprotein E2A-Pbx1 in mice (2). *FGF19* was also originally identified by a homology-based DNA database search in humans (3, 4). However, *FGF19* was later found to be the human ortholog of mouse *FGF15* (5). Only rodent orthologs were named *FGF15*. Other vertebrate orthologs were named *FGF19*.

FGF21 was originally identified by a homology-based polymerase chain reaction in mice and humans (6). FGF21 was later found to be a stimulator of glucose uptake in cultured mouse adipocytes (7). *FGF21* was also identified as a hepatic gene inducible by fasting or a ketogenic diet in mice (8, 9).

FGF23 was originally identified by a homology-based DNA database search in mice and humans (10). Human *FGF23* was simultaneously identified as a gene responsible for autosomal dominant hypophosphatemic rickets (ADHR) characterized by low serum phosphate levels, rickets, osteomalacia, lower extremity deformities, a short stature, bone pain, and dental abscesses (11). Human *FGF23* was subsequently found to be a causative humoral protein for human tumor-induced osteomalacia characterized by hypophosphatemia caused by renal phosphate wasting (12).

Unique Actions of Endocrine FGFS with FGF Receptors and Klotho Coreceptors

Paracrine and endocrine FGFs, which are extracellular signaling molecules, bind to and activate cell-surface FGF receptors (FGFRs). The human *FGFR* gene family comprises four members, *FGFR1–FGFR4*, that encode single-pass transmembrane proteins of ~800 amino acids with three extracellular immunoglobulin-like domains I, II, and III and a split intracellular tyrosine kinase domain. *FGFR1*, *FGFR2*, and *FGFR3* genes encode two alternative splicing variants (b and c) of immunoglobulin-like domain III, which is a determinant of ligand-binding specificities (1). Thus, there are seven FGFR proteins, FGFRs 1b, 1c, 2b, 2c, 3b, 3c, and 4, with distinct ligand-binding specificity. The functional dimerization and transphosphorylation of FGFRs induced by FGF binding result in the activation of FGFRs, followed by the activation of intracellular FGF signaling pathways including RAS–RAF–MAPK, PI3K–AKT, STAT, and PLCγ pathways (1).

Paracrine FGFs bind to heparan sulfate proteoglycans, which extracellularly localize at neighboring cells as cofactors for FGFRs. Binding to heparan sulfate proteoglycans is essential for FGF signaling in a paracrine manner (**Figure 1B**) (1). In contrast, endocrine FGFs with reduced heparan sulfate-binding affinity are unable to function in a paracrine manner. Endocrine FGFs require α-Klotho or β-Klotho as a cofactor for FGFRs to function in an endocrine manner (1). α-Klotho and β-Klotho, which share structural similarities and characteristics with each other, are single-pass transmembrane proteins of ~1,000 amino acids with a short cytoplasmic domain (13). However, endocrine FGFs cannot efficiently bind to FGFR, α-Klotho, or β-Klotho alone; they efficiently bind to the FGFR–Klotho complex. The binding site for the FGFR–Klotho complex is localized in the C-terminal tail of endocrine FGF (**Figure 1B**) (14). FGF19 activates FGFR4 with β-Klotho and FGF21 activates FGFR1c with β-Klotho, whereas FGF23 activates FGFR1c with α-Klotho (1). FGF19 and FGF23 exhibit metabolic and proliferative activities. However, FGF21 is a unique FGF with metabolic activity, but no proliferative activity (15).

The Evolutionary History of Vertebrate-Specific Endocrine *FGF* Genes

The FGF signaling system has been conserved throughout metazoan evolution. The evolutionary history of the *FGF* gene family has already been proposed (5). The founder of the *FGF* family is an intracrine *FGF*. Intracrine FGFs, which are not secreted proteins, possess heparan sulfate-binding sites, but no secreted signal sequences. The prototype of the paracrine *FGF* subfamily was generated from the founder by gene duplication events early in metazoan evolution. During this evolution, paracrine FGFs acquired secreted signal sequences, thereby allowing them to function as extracellular FGFs in a paracrine manner. Intracrine and paracrine *FGF*s have been identified in invertebrates and vertebrates. In contrast, endocrine *FGF*s have been detected in vertebrates, but not invertebrates, indicating that they are specific to vertebrates (**Figure 2**). The prototypic endocrine *FGF* was generated from the prototype of paracrine *FGF* by local gene duplication early in vertebrate evolution. *FGF19*, *FGF21*, and *FGF23* were subsequently generated from the prototype by two large-scale genome duplication events early in vertebrate evolution (5). Endocrine FGFs lost heparan sulfate-binding affinity and acquired FGFR/Klotho complex-binding affinity for a systemic signaling system in an endocrine manner during their evolution (5). *FGF19* and *FGF23* have been identified in all vertebrates examined, including teleosts, amphibians, reptiles, birds, and mammals. However, *FGF21* was not detected in any birds examined, indicating that *FGF21* was lost in the avian lineage (16, 17). The avian genome is principally characterized by its constrained size with the loss of many genes in the avian lineage, indicating that pan-avian genomic diversity covaries with adaptations to different lifestyles and the convergent evolution of traits (18).

Roles of Endocrine FGFs Indicated by Their Knockout Mouse Phenotypes

The mouse is a mammalian model that is useful for investigating gene functions. All endocrine *FGF* knockout mice have been extensively analyzed, indicating their important physiological roles in metabolism (**Table 1**).

FGF15

FGF15 knockout mice survive until E10.5, but then gradually die due to defects in the cardiac outflow tract, indicating that FGF15 is required for proper morphogenesis of the cardiac outflow tract during embryonic development in the heart (2, 19). *FGF15* is selectively expressed in the ileum at postnatal stages, and a small number of *FGF15* knockout mice survive until postnatal stages, which suggests that FGF15 plays crucial roles in regulating hepatic bile acid synthesis and gallbladder filling in an endocrine manner (20, 21). Surviving *FGF15* knockout mice also fail to properly maintain blood concentrations of glucose and normal postprandial amounts of liver glycogen, indicating that FGF15 is a postprandial, insulin-independent activator of hepatic protein and glycogen synthesis (22). Surviving hepatectomized *FGF15* knockout mice exhibit severe defects in liver regeneration, indicating that FGF15 also plays a role in liver regeneration (23, 24). Ileal *FGF15* expression is increased in mice undergoing carcinogenesis. Fibrosis-induced hepatocellular carcinogenesis results in fewer and smaller tumors in surviving *FGF15* knockout mice than in wild-type mice, suggesting that ileal FGF15 enhances the development of carcinoma (25).

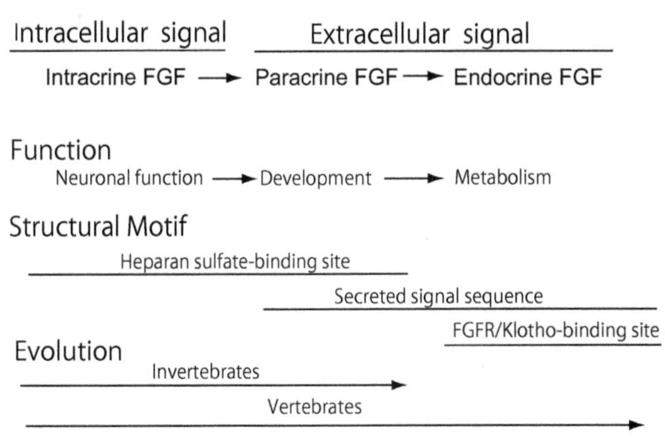

FIGURE 2 | The functional evolutionary history of the FGF family.

FGF21

FGF21 is expressed in the liver, pancreas, white adipose tissue, and muscle of mice (6, 26, 27). The phenotypes of *FGF21* knockout mice, which are viable and fertile, indicate that FGF21 stimulates lipolysis in the white adipose tissue during feeding, but inhibits it during fasting (28). *FGF21* knockout mice fed a ketogenic diet also indicate that FGF21 plays a role in the adaptation to a ketogenic diet and impairs adipocyte insulin sensitivity (29, 30). *FGF21* knockout mice also indicate that FGF21 is an upstream effector of adiponectin in white adipocytes and that adiponectin also mediates many of the systemic effects of FGF21 on energy metabolism and insulin sensitivity in the liver and skeletal muscle (31, 32). Glucagon, an essential regulator of glucose homeostasis, modulates lipid metabolism and promotes weight loss. Glucagon receptor activation increases hepatic *FGF21* expression in mice. *FGF21* knockout mice indicate that FGF21 contributes, at least in part, to glucose, energy, and lipid metabolism controlled by glucagon (33). *FGF21* knockout mice also exhibit insulin resistance, while being normoglycemic, and this is associated with increases in pancreatic beta-cell proliferation and insulin synthesis, which act as compensatory responses. This resistance results from enhanced growth hormone sensitivity in *FGF21* knockout pancreatic islets, indicating that FGF21 is important in the regulation of pancreatic beta-cell proliferation and insulin synthesis, possibly via the modulation of growth hormone signaling (34). Endoplasmic reticulum (ER) stress leads to the development and progression of various diseases such as obesity and diabetes. ER stress induces hepatic *FGF21* expression. ER stress and hepatic lipid accumulation are increased in *FGF21* knockout mice, indicating that FGF21 plays a role in the adaptive responses to ER stress (35). *FGF21* knockout mice also have an increased relative heart weight and develop enhanced

TABLE 1 | Roles of endocrine FGFs indicated by their knockout mouse phenotypes.

FGF15	Morphogenesis of the cardiac outflow tract (2, 19), hepatic bile acid metabolism (20), gallbladder filling (21), hepatic protein and glycogen metabolism (22), liver regeneration (23, 24), and fibrosis-induced hepatocellular carcinogenesis (25)
FGF21	Lipolysis in white adipose tissue (28), adaptation to a ketogenic diet (29, 30), upstream effector of adiponectin (31, 32), glucagon action (33), pancreatic beta-cell proliferation and insulin synthesis (34), adaptation to ER stress (35), cardiac hypertrophy (36, 37), pancreatitis (38), diabetic cardiomyopathy (39), and aortic remodeling (40)
FGF23	Renal phosphate and active vitamin D metabolism (41) and ear development and function (42)

signs of dilatation. FGF21 is markedly secreted by cardiac cells in response to cardiac stress. Thus, the heart appears to be a target of locally generated FGF21, indicating that FGF21 acts on cardiomyocytes, possibly in a paracrine manner (36). FGF21 prevents the production of reactive oxygen species in cardiac cells by acting as an antioxidant factor in the heart, thereby preventing pro-oxidative pathways under inflammatory or hypertrophic conditions (37). The expression of *FGF21* in pancreatic acinar cells is markedly increased during cerulein-induced pancreatitis. *FGF21* knockout mice have higher serum amylase levels and more tissue damage, suggesting a novel function for FGF21 as an immediate response gene protecting pancreatic acini from overt damage (38). *FGF21* knockout mice with streptozotocin-induced diabetes exhibit severe cardiac dysfunction, increased cardiac lipid accumulation, and severe aortic remodeling, indicating that FGF21 plays roles in the development and progression of diabetic cardiomyopathy and aortic remodeling (39, 40).

FGF23

FGF23 is mainly expressed in osteocytes in mice. *FGF23* knockout mice survive until birth, but then gradually die by 11 weeks after birth. The phenotypes of *FGF23* knockout mice indicate that osteocytic FGF23 is a regulator for phosphate and active vitamin D metabolism in the kidney (41). FGF23 is also ubiquitously expressed throughout the cochlea. *FGF23* heterozygous knockout mice are profoundly deaf with moderate hearing loss and a near-normal morphology. However, *FGF23* homozygous knockout mice have dysplastic bulla and ossicles. These findings indicate that FGF23 is critical for normal development of the middle ear as well as the functions of the middle and inner ear (42).

Roles of Endocrine FGFs Indicated by Human Diseases

Evidence has been accumulated to support the involvement of FGF19 and FGF23 in human diseases and also indicates their crucial pathophysiological roles in diseases (**Table 2**).

FGF19

Paraneoplastic Diseases with Gain-of-Function

Extrahepatic cholestasis is a condition in which the release of bile acid is blocked in the bile ducts. Cholestasis is caused by a pancreatic tumor. Markedly increased serum FGF19 levels and the abundant expression of hepatic *FGF19* are observed in cholestatic patients, indicating that FGF19 signaling is involved in some of the adaptations that protect the liver against bile acid toxicity (43).

FGF23

Inherited Disease with Loss-of-Function Mutations

Hyperphosphatemic familial tumoral calcinosis (HFTC) is a rare autosomal recessive metabolic disorder characterized by the deposition of calcium phosphate crystals. HFTC was initially attributed to loss-of function mutations in *GLANT3* encoding a glycosyltransferase (44). Loss-of-function mutations in *FGF23* are also associated with HFTC (45, 46).

TABLE 2 | Roles of endocrine FGFs indicated by human diseases.

Inherited disease with loss-of-function mutations	
FGF23	Hyperphosphatemic familial tumoral calcinosis (45, 46)
Inherited disease with gain-of-function mutations	
FGF23	Autosomal dominant hypophosphatemic rickets (11, 47)
Paraneoplastic diseases with gain-of-function	
FGF19	Extrahepatic cholestasis (43)
FGF23	Osteomalacia (12)
SNPS as potential risk factors for diseases	
FGF21	Intake of dietary macronutrients (48), metabolic syndrome, obesity, and diabetes (49)
FGF23	Cardiac abnormalities in Kawasaki disease (50) and prostate cancer (51)
Serum levels as biomarkers for diseases	
FGF19	Renal failure (52, 53), coronary artery disease (54), intestinal failure-associated liver disease (55), diabetes (56), Crohn's disease (57, 58), and prostate cancer (60)
FGF21	Renal failure (61), cardiovascular disease (62–64), mitochondrial disease (65, 66), obesity and diabetes (56, 67–70), anorexia nervosa (71), Cushing's syndrome (72), Brown adipose tissue activity (73), non-alcoholic fatty liver disease (74, 75), chronic hepatitis C with steatosis (76), systemic inflammatory response syndrome (77), and rheumatoid arthritis (78)
FGF23	Renal failure (79–81), cardiovascular failure (82–86), and stroke (87, 88)

Inherited Disease with Gain-of-Function Mutations

Autosomal dominant hypophosphatemic rickets is characterized by isolated renal phosphate wasting, hypophosphatemia, and inappropriately normal 1,25-dihydroxyvitamin D3 levels. Gain-of-function mutations in *FGF23* result in AHDR. Cleaved FGF23 forms due to intracellular proteolysis lose their biological activities. *FGF23* mutations in ADHR result in impaired proteolysis of FGF23, resulting in increased serum levels of active FGF23 (11, 47).

Paraneoplastic Diseases with Gain-of-Function

Osteomalacia is characterized by the softening of bones due to defective bone mineralization. Tumors that overexpress *FGF23* induce tumor-induced osteomalacia characterized by hypophosphatemia, which is caused by renal phosphate wasting (12).

Single-Nucleotide Polymorphisms in Endocrine *FGF* Genes as Potential Risk Factors for Diseases

Single-nucleotide polymorphisms (SNPs) are DNA sequence variations that commonly occur within a population (e.g., 1%) with a single nucleotide in the genome. These SNP variations underlie differences in the susceptibility of humans to diseases. The severity of illnesses and the responses of the human body to treatments are also manifestations of SNPs. SNPs in endocrine *FGFs* also suggest their potential roles in risk factors for diseases (**Table 2**).

FGF21

The intake of dietary macronutrients such as carbohydrates, protein, and fat is associated with the risk of obesity and diabetes. A SNP located in the exon of *FGF21* is significantly associated with the percentage of total caloric intake from protein and carbohydrates, indicating that *FGF21* is a potential susceptibility gene for obesity and diabetes (48). SNPs in the 3′ untranslated region of *FGF21* are also associated with metabolic syndrome, obesity, and diabetes (49). However, the mechanisms underlying these associations currently remain unclear.

FGF23

Kawasaki disease, which is a systemic panvasculitis that affects all medium/small-sized vessels, mainly occurs in early childhood and increases the risk of cardiac abnormalities. A SNP in the intron of *FGF23* is significantly associated with higher serum FGF23 levels and cardiac abnormalities in children with Kawasaki disease (50). Three distinct SNPs in *FGF23* are also associated with an increased risk of prostate cancer, indicating that *FGF23* genetic variations increase prostate cancer susceptibility (51).

Serum Endocrine FGF Levels as Biomarkers for Diseases

Endocrine FGFs mainly play roles in an endocrine manner via the blood circulation system. Serum endocrine FGFs levels are sometimes altered in patients with metabolic and other diseases, indicating that endocrine FGFs are biomarkers for these diseases (**Table 2**).

FGF19

Renal Failure

Renal failure is a condition in which the kidneys fail to adequately filter waste products from the blood. Serum FGF19 levels are significantly increased in end-stage renal failure patients with chronic hemodialysis (52). The postprandial FGF19 response in serum is blunted in chronic kidney disease and is also associated with impaired insulin and C-peptide signaling (53).

Cardiovascular Disease

Coronary artery disease (CAD) is a group of diseases including stable angina, unstable angina, myocardial infarction, and sudden coronary death. Serum FGF19 levels are decreased in CAD in relation to its severity, suggesting that reductions in the expression of *FGF19* are involved in the development and progression of CAD (54).

Intestinal Failure-Associated Liver Disease

In pediatric intestinal failure (IF), serum FGF19 levels are decreased corresponding to IF-associated liver disease (IFALD). This suggests that FGF19 contributes to the pathogenesis of IFALD (55).

Energy Metabolism Disorder

Serum FGF19 levels are decreased in patients with type 2 diabetes, indicating that the FGF19 pathway is significantly perturbed in severe diabetes (56).

Bile Acid Metabolism Disorder

Bile acids are reabsorbed by the terminal ileum. However, their reabsorption is frequently impaired in Crohn's disease, resulting in secretory diarrhea. Serum FGF19 levels are decreased in Crohn's disease associated with diarrhea and disease activity, indicating that FGF19 has potential as a biomarker for the functioning ileum in Crohn's disease (57, 58). However, serum FGF19 levels are not affected in gallstone carriers (59).

Cancer

Serum FGF19 levels in the high Gleason grade of prostate cancer are higher than those in the low Gleason grade group, indicating that FGF19 promotes the progression of prostate cancer (60).

FGF21

Renal Failure

Serum FGF21 levels are increased in chronic kidney disease and acute kidney dysfunction, suggesting that renal excretion is a major route for the elimination of FGF21 (61).

Cardiovascular Disease

Coronary heart disease (CHD) is characterized by the narrowing of small blood vessels in the heart, which may lead to heart attacks. Serum FGF21 levels are significantly increased in CHD. Serum FGF21 levels in CHD patients with diabetes, hypertension, or both are higher than those in patients without these comorbidities. High serum FGF21 levels are associated with adverse lipid profiles in CHD patients, indicating that the paradoxical increase in serum FGF21 levels in CHD patients is a compensatory response or resistance to FGF21 (62). Serum FGF21 levels are positively correlated with carotid intima-media thickness (IMT) in women, but not in men, indicating that elevated serum FGF21 levels in women are an independent risk factor for increased carotid IMT (63). Preeclampsia, a serious cardiovascular complication in pregnancy, is associated with an increased future metabolic and cardiovascular risk. Serum FGF21 levels are significantly increased in patients with preeclampsia during pregnancy (64).

Mitochondrial Disease

Mitochondrial disease caused by dysfunctional mitochondria is a group of disorders with highly variable phenotypes including mitochondrial myopathy, diabetes mellitus, deafness, optic neuropathy, and multiple sclerosis-type disease. Serum FGF21 levels are significantly increased in human mitochondrial disease and the best predictor of mitochondrial disease among classical indicators including creatine kinase, lactate, and pyruvate (65, 66).

Energy Metabolism Disorder

Serum FGF21 levels are significantly increased in patients with obese and type 2 diabetes, suggesting the direct positive metabolic effects of FGF21 (56, 67–70). Anorexia nervosa (AN) is an eating disorder that is characterized by a low weight and food restriction. Serum FGF21 levels are significantly decreased in AN, suggesting that FGF21 is involved in the pathophysiology of or a complex adaptive response to AN (71). Cushing's syndrome is caused by prolonged exposure to inappropriately high levels of glucocorticoids. Serum FGF21 levels are increased in patients with Cushing's syndrome. Increased serum FGF21 levels are attributed to their excessive fat accumulation and related metabolic abnormalities, but not to the direct effects of cortisol on the production of FGF21 (72). Brown adipose tissue, which contains a markedly higher number of mitochondria, generates body heat in animals without shivering. Since brown adipose tissue is expected to markedly contribute to energy homeostasis in humans, it may represent a therapeutic target of obesity. Serum FGF21 levels are associated with brown adipose tissue activity, indicating a novel mechanism by which brown adipose tissue activity may be enhanced (73).

Lipid Metabolism Disorder

Serum FGF21 levels are increased in patients with non-alcoholic fatty liver disease (NAFLD), which supports the role of FGF21 as a key regulator of hepatic lipid metabolism (74). In contrast to adults with NAFLD, serum FGF19 and FGF21 levels are inversely associated with hepatic damage in children with NAFLD, providing insights for a better understanding of the progression of NAFLD (75).

Infection and Inflammation

Hepatitis C (HC) is an infectious disease that is caused by the HC virus. Serum FGF21 levels are increased in chronic HC (CHC) patients with steatosis and are associated with the steatosis grade, which may be a useful diagnostic marker for determining hepatic steatosis in CHC (76). Sepsis is an illness in which the body has a severe response to infection. Systemic inflammatory response syndrome (SIRS) is an inflammatory state in the whole body due to the response of the immune system to infection. SIRS is also closely related to sepsis. Serum FGF21 levels are significantly increased in patients with sepsis and SIRS, suggesting a role for FGF21 in inflammation (77). Rheumatoid arthritis (RA) is a chronic inflammatory disease in small hand and foot joints. Serum FGF21 levels are significantly increased in patients with RA, indicating the compensatory response of FGF21 to inflammation and immune response (78).

FGF23

Renal Failure

Serum FGF23 levels are significantly increased in chronic kidney disease, indicating the important role of FGF23 in maintaining a neutral phosphate balance as the glomerular filtration rate decreases (79–81).

Cardiovascular Disease

Serum FGF23 levels are positively correlated with the risk of heart failure (82). Serum FGF23 levels are increased in children with heart failure (83). These findings indicate that increased serum FGF23 levels are a risk factor for heart failure. Serum FGF23 levels are also increased in association with angiographic severity and the extent of CAD (84). Increased serum FGF23 levels are also a risk factor for myocardial infraction and hemorrhagic stroke (85). Serum FGF23 levels are strongly associated with left ventricular hypertrophy (86). These findings provide additional evidence for the role of FGF23 in cardiovascular disease.

Stroke

Stroke is a disease that is caused by cutting off the blood supply to part of the brain (ischemic) or by bleeding into the surrounding brain tissue from a weakened vessel (hemorrhagic). Serum FGF23 levels are increased in patients with stroke (87, 88).

Therapeutic Utility of Endocrine FGFs in Humans or Monkeys

FGF19

FGF19 is expected to prevent bile acid-induced liver damage by reducing hepatic bile acid levels through the modulation of bile acid synthesis. However, since FGF19 also stimulates the proliferation of hepatocytes, the potential risk associated with prolonged exposure to supraphysiological levels of FGF19 represents a major hurdle in the development of an FGF19-based therapy in hepatocellular carcinogenesis. A manufactured FGF19 variant, M70, which carries three amino acid substitutions and a five-amino acid deletion, regulates bile acid metabolism without tumorigenicity (89). The administration of M70 to healthy human volunteers potently reduces serum levels of 7α-hydroxy-4-cholesten-3-one, a surrogate marker for the hepatic activity of cholesterol 7α-hydroxylase (CYP7A1), which catalyzes the rate-limiting step in the bile acid synthetic pathway. These findings indicate that the development of non-tumorigenic FGF19 variants represents an effective approach for the prevention and treatment of cholestatic liver diseases and other disorders associated with bile acid dysregulation (89) (**Table 3**).

FGF21

The daily administration of FGF21 to diabetic rhesus monkeys for 6 weeks induces marked reductions in fasting serum glucose, triglyceride, insulin, and glucagon levels, significant improvements in lipoprotein profiles, and significant weight loss, thereby supporting the development of FGF21 for the treatment of diabetes and other metabolic diseases in humans (90). LY2405319 (LY) is a manufactured FGF21 variant with significantly improved biopharmaceutical properties (91). The administration of LY to patients with obesity and type 2 diabetes for 28 days produces significant improvements in dyslipidemia, a shift to a potentially less atherogenic apolipoprotein concentration profile, and favorable effects on body weight. These findings indicate that FGF21-based therapies may be effective for the treatment of selected metabolic disorders (92).

FGF21 has a short half-life (1–2 h). Fc-FGF21 is a long-acting FGF21 variant that is generated by fusing with an Fc fragment. In obese rhesus monkeys treated with FGF21 (once a day) or Fc-FGF21

TABLE 3 | Therapeutic utility of endocrine FGFs in humans or monkeys.

FGF19	Cholestatic liver disease and bile acid dysregulation (89)
FGF21	Diabetes and metabolic disease (90)
FGF21 variant (LY2405319)	Obesity and metabolic disease (91, 92)
FGF21 variant (Fc-FGF21)	Diabetes (93)
FGF21 variant (PF-05231023)	Diabetes (94)
FGF21 Avimer	Obesity (95)
Anti-FGF23 (KRN23)	X-linked hypophosphatemia (96, 97)

(once a week), serum glucose, insulin, cholesterol, and triglyceride levels and body weight are markedly lower with Fc-FGF21 than with FGF21, indicating that the administration of Fc-FGF21 once a week leads to similar or greater efficacy than FGF21 administered daily (93). PF-05231023 is also a long-acting FGF21 variant generated by covalently conjugating FGF21 molecules to a non-targeting human IgG1 κ scaffold. Single intravenous injection of PF-05231023 to type 2 diabetes mellitus patients decreases serum triglyceride, total cholesterol, and low-density lipoprotein cholesterol levels and increases high-density lipoprotein cholesterol levels, but have no apparent effect on glucose levels (94).

As an alternative to FGF21, bispecific Avimer polypeptides that bind with high affinity and specificity to one of the receptor and coreceptor pairs used by FGF21, FGFR1c, and β-Klotho have been generated. These Avimers exhibit FGF21-like activity with greater potency than FGF21 *in vitro*. In obese male cynomolgus monkeys, a bispecific Avimer exhibits improved metabolic parameters and leads to greater reductions in body weight than those with FGF21, thereby supporting a novel therapeutic approach to target this potentially important pathway in the treatment of diabetes and obesity (95).

FGF23

X-linked hypophosphatemia (XLH) with elevated serum FGF23 levels is the most common heritable form of rickets and osteomalacia. KRN23 is a human anti-FGF23 antibody that has been developed as a potential treatment for XLH patients. KRN23 significantly increases the maximum renal tubular threshold for phosphate reabsorption, serum phosphate, and 1,25-dihydroxyvitamin D in XLH patients, suggesting utility for KRN23 in XLH patients (96, 97).

Conclusion

Endocrine FGFs comprising FGF19, FGF21, and FGF23 require FGFR and α-Klotho or β-Klotho as a cofactor for FGFR for their signaling in an endocrine manner. Endocrine FGFs lost heparan sulfate-binding affinity and acquired systemic signaling system with α-Klotho or β-Klotho during their evolution. The phenotypes of endocrine *FGF* knockout mice indicate that endocrine FGFs play important physiological roles in metabolism including bile acid metabolism, energy metabolism, and phosphate/active vitamin D metabolism. Evidence for the involvement of endocrine FGFs in human inherited and metabolic diseases has also been increasing, indicating their crucial pathophysiological roles in metabolic diseases, their SNPs as potential risk factors for diseases, and their serum levels as useful biomarkers for metabolic diseases. Furthermore, the therapeutic utility of endocrine FGFs is currently being developed. These findings provide new insights into the physiological and pathophysiological roles of endocrine FGFs and may provide potential diagnostic and therapeutic strategies for metabolic diseases.

References

1. Ornitz DM, Itoh N. The fibroblast growth factor signaling pathway. *Wiley Interdiscip Rev Dev Biol* (2005) **4**:215–66. doi:10.1002/wdev.176
2. McWhirter JR, Goulding M, Weiner JA, Chun J, Murre C. A novel fibroblast growth factor gene expressed in the developing nervous system is a downstream target of the chimeric homeodomain oncoprotein E2A-Pbx1. *Development* (1997) **124**:3221–32.
3. Nishimura T, Utsunomiya Y, Hoshikawa M, Ohuchi H, Itoh N. Structure and expression of a novel human FGF, FGF-19, expressed in the fetal brain. *Biochim Biophys Acta* (1999) **1444**:148–51. doi:10.1016/S0167-4781(98)00255-3
4. Xie MH, Holcomb I, Deuel B, Dowd P, Huang A, Vagts A, et al. FGF-19, a novel fibroblast growth factor with unique specificity for FGFR4. *Cytokine* (1999) **11**:729–35. doi:10.1006/cyto.1999.0485
5. Itoh N, Ornitz DM. Functional evolutionary history of the mouse Fgf gene family. *Dev Dyn* (2008) **237**:18–27. doi:10.1002/dvdy.21388
6. Nishimura T, Nakatake Y, Konishi M, Itoh N. Identification of a novel FGF, FGF-21, preferentially expressed in the liver. *Biochim Biophys Acta* (2000) **1492**:203–6. doi:10.1016/S0167-4781(00)00067-1
7. Kharitonenkov A, Shiyanova TL, Koester A, Ford AM, Micanovic R, Galbreath EJ, et al. FGF-21 as a novel metabolic regulator. *J Clin Invest* (2005) **115**:1627–35. doi:10.1172/JCI23606
8. Inagaki T, Dutchak P, Zhao G, Ding X, Gautron L, Parameswara V, et al. Endocrine regulation of the fasting response by PPARalpha-mediated induction of fibroblast growth factor 21. *Cell Metab* (2007) **25**:415–25. doi:10.1016/j.cmet.2007.05.003
9. Badman MK, Pissios P, Kennedy AR, Koukos G, Flier JS, Maratos-Flier E. Hepatic fibroblast growth factor 21 is regulated by PPARalpha and is a key mediator of hepatic lipid metabolism in ketotic states. *Cell Metab* (2007) **5**:426–37. doi:10.1016/j.cmet.2007.05.002
10. Yamashita T, Yoshioka M, Itoh N. Identification of a novel fibroblast growth factor, FGF-23, preferentially expressed in the ventrolateral thalamic nucleus of the brain. *Biochem Biophys Res Commun* (2000) **277**:494–8. doi:10.1006/bbrc.2000.3696
11. Consortium ADHR. Autosomal dominant hypophosphataemic rickets is associated with mutations in FGF23. *Nat Genet* (2000) **26**:345–8. doi:10.1038/81664
12. Shimada T, Mizutani S, Muto T, Yoneya T, Hino R, Takeda S, et al. Cloning and characterization of FGF23 as a causative factor of tumor-induced osteomalacia. *Proc Natl Acad Sci U S A* (2001) **98**:6500–5. doi:10.1073/pnas.101545198
13. Kuro-o M. Klotho and βKlotho. *Adv Exp Med Biol* (2012) **728**:25–40. doi:10.1007/978-1-4614-0887-1_2
14. Beenken A, Mohammadi M. The structural biology of the FGF19 subfamily. *Adv Exp Med Biol* (2012) **728**:1–24. doi:10.1007/978-1-4614-0887-1_1
15. Wu X, Ge H, Lemon B, Vonderfecht S, Weiszmann J, Hecht R. FGF19-induced hepatocyte proliferation is mediated through FGFR4 activation. *J Biol Chem* (2010) **285**:5165–70. doi:10.1074/jbc.M109.068783
16. Itoh N. Hormone-like (endocrine) Fgfs: their evolutionary history and roles in development, metabolism, and disease. *Cell Tissue Res* (2010) **342**:1–11. doi:10.1007/s00441-010-1024-2
17. Oulion S, Bertrand S, Escriva H. Evolution of the FGF gene family. *Int J Evol Biol* (2012) **2012**:298147. doi:10.1155/2012/298147
18. Zhang G, Li C, Li Q, Li B, Larkin DM, Lee C, et al. Comparative genomics reveals insights into avian genome evolution and adaptation. *Science* (2014) **346**:1311–20. doi:10.1126/science.1251385
19. Vincentz JW, McWhirter JR, Murre C, Baldini A, Furuta Y. Fgf15 is required for proper morphogenesis of the mouse cardiac outflow tract. *Genesis* (2005) **41**:192–201. doi:10.1002/gene.20114
20. Inagaki T, Choi M, Moschetta A, Peng L, Cummins CL, McDonald JG, et al. Fibroblast growth factor 15 functions as an enterohepatic signal to regulate bile acid homeostasis. *Cell Metab* (2005) **2**:217–25. doi:10.1016/j.cmet.2005.09.001
21. Choi M, Moschetta A, Bookout AL, Peng L, Umetani M, Holmstrom SR, et al. Identification of a hormonal basis for gallbladder filling. *Nat Med* (2006) **12**:1253–5. doi:10.1038/nm1501
22. Kir S, Beddow SA, Samuel VT, Miller P, Previs SF, Suino-Powell K, et al. FGF19 as a postprandial, insulin-independent activator of hepatic protein and glycogen synthesis. *Science* (2011) **331**:1621–4. doi:10.1126/science.1198363
23. Uriarte I, Fernandez-Barrena MG, Monte MJ, Latasa MU, Chang HC, Carotti S, et al. Identification of fibroblast growth factor 15 as a novel mediator of

liver regeneration and its application in the prevention of post-resection liver failure in mice. *Gut* (2013) **62**:899–910. doi:10.1136/gutjnl-2012-302945

24. Kong B, Huang J, Zhu Y, Li G, Williams J, Shen S, et al. Fibroblast growth factor 15 deficiency impairs liver regeneration in mice. *Am J Physiol Gastrointest Liver Physiol* (2014) **306**:G893–902. doi:10.1152/ajpgi.00337.2013
25. Uriarte I, Latasa MU, Carotti S, Fernandez-Barrena MG, Garcia-Irigoyen O, Elizalde M, et al. Ileal FGF15 contributes to fibrosis-associated hepatocellular carcinoma development. *Int J Cancer* (2015) **136**:2469–75. doi:10.1002/ijc.29287
26. Kharitonenkov A, Shanafelt AB. FGF21: a novel prospect for the treatment of metabolic diseases. *Curr Opin Investig Drugs* (2009) **10**:359–64.
27. Fon Tacer K, Bookout AL, Ding X, Kurosu H, John GB, Wang L, et al. Research resource: comprehensive expression atlas of the fibroblast growth factor system in adult mouse. *Mol Endocrinol* (2010) **24**:2050–64. doi:10.1210/me.2010-0142
28. Hotta Y, Nakamura H, Konishi M, Murata Y, Takagi H, Matsumura S, et al. Fibroblast growth factor 21 regulates lipolysis in white adipose tissue but is not required for ketogenesis and triglyceride clearance in liver. *Endocrinology* (2009) **150**:4625–33. doi:10.1210/en.2009-0119
29. Badman MK, Koester A, Flier JS, Kharitonenkov A, Maratos-Flier E. Fibroblast growth factor 21-deficient mice demonstrate impaired adaptation to ketosis. *Endocrinology* (2009) **150**:4931–40. doi:10.1210/en.2009-0532
30. Murata Y, Nishio K, Mochiyama T, Konishi M, Shimada M, Ohta H, et al. Fgf21 impairs adipocyte insulin sensitivity in mice fed a low-carbohydrate, high-fat ketogenic diet. *PLoS One* (2013) **8**:e69330. doi:10.1371/journal.pone.0069330
31. Lin Z, Tian H, Lam KS, Lin S, Hoo RC, Konishi M, et al. Adiponectin mediates the metabolic effects of FGF21 on glucose homeostasis and insulin sensitivity in mice. *Cell Metab* (2013) **17**:779–89. doi:10.1016/j.cmet.2013.04.005
32. Holland WL, Adams AC, Brozinick JT, Bui HH, Miyauchi Y, Kusminski CM, et al. An FGF21-adiponectin-ceramide axis controls energy expenditure and insulin action in mice. *Cell Metab* (2013) **17**:790–7. doi:10.1016/j.cmet.2013.03.019
33. Habegger KM, Stemmer K, Cheng C, Müller TD, Heppner KM, Ottaway N, et al. Fibroblast growth factor 21 mediates specific glucagon actions. *Diabetes* (2013) **62**:1453–63. doi:10.2337/db12-1116
34. So WY, Cheng Q, Xu A, Lam KS, Leung PS. Loss of fibroblast growth factor 21 action induces insulin resistance, pancreatic islet hyperplasia and dysfunction in mice. *Cell Death Dis* (2015) **6**:e1707. doi:10.1038/cddis.2015.80
35. Kim SH, Kim KH, Kim HK, Kim MJ, Back SH, Konishi M, et al. Fibroblast growth factor 21 participates in adaptation to endoplasmic reticulum stress and attenuates obesity-induced hepatic metabolic stress. *Diabetologia* (2015) **58**:809–18. doi:10.1007/s00125-014-3475-6
36. Planavila A, Redondo I, Hondares E, Vinciguerra M, Munts C, Iglesias LA, et al. Fibroblast growth factor 21 protects against cardiac hypertrophy in mice. *Nat Commun* (2013) **4**:2019. doi:10.1038/ncomms3019
37. Planavila A, Redondo-Angulo I, Ribas F, Garrabou G, Casademont J, Giralt M, et al. Fibroblast growth factor 21 protects the heart from oxidative stress. *Cardiovasc Res* (2015) **106**:19–31. doi:10.1093/cvr/cvu263
38. Johnson CL, Weston JY, Chadi SA, Fazio EN, Huff MW, Kharitonenkov A, et al. Fibroblast growth factor 21 reduces the severity of cerulein-induced pancreatitis in mice. *Gastroenterology* (2009) **137**:1795–804. doi:10.1053/j.gastro.2009.07.064
39. Yan X, Chen J, Zhang C, Zhou S, Zhang Z, Chen J, et al. FGF21 deletion exacerbates diabetic cardiomyopathy by aggravating cardiac lipid accumulation. *J Cell Mol Med* (2015) **19**:1557–68. doi:10.1111/jcmm.12530
40. Yan X, Chen J, Zhang C, Zeng J, Zhou S, Zhang Z, et al. Fibroblast growth factor 21 deletion aggravates diabetes-induced pathogenic changes in the aorta in type 1 diabetic mice. *Cardiovasc Diabetol* (2015) **14**:77. doi:10.1186/s12933-015-0241-0
41. Shimada T, Kakitani M, Yamazaki Y, Hasegawa H, Takeuchi Y, Fujita T, et al. Targeted ablation of Fgf23 demonstrates an essential physiological role of FGF23 in phosphate and vitamin D metabolism. *J Clin Invest* (2004) **113**:561–8. doi:10.1172/JCI200419081
42. Lysaght AC, Yuan Q, Fan Y, Kalwani N, Caruso P, Cunnane M, et al. FGF23 deficiency leads to mixed hearing loss and middle ear malformation in mice. *PLoS One* (2014) **9**:e107681. doi:10.1371/journal.pone.0107681
43. Schaap FG, van der Gaag NA, Gouma DJ, Jansen PL. High expression of the bile salt-homeostatic hormone fibroblast growth factor 19 in the liver of patients with extrahepatic cholestasis. *Hepatology* (2009) **49**:1228–35. doi:10.1002/hep.22771
44. Topaz O, Shurman DL, Bergman R, Indelman M, Ratajczak P, Mizrachi M, et al. Mutations in GALNT3, encoding a protein involved in O-linked glycosylation, cause familial tumoral calcinosis. *Nat Genet* (2004) **36**:579–81. doi:10.1038/ng1358
45. Chefetz I, Heller R, Galli-Tsinopoulou A, Richard G, Wollnik B, Indelman MA, et al. Novel homozygous missense mutation in FGF23 causes familial tumoral calcinosis associated with disseminated visceral calcification. *Hum Genet* (2005) **118**:261–6. doi:10.1007/s00439-005-0026-8
46. Garringer HJ, Malekpour M, Esteghamat F, Mortazavi SM, Davis SI, Farrow EG, et al. Molecular genetic and biochemical analyses of FGF23 mutations in familial tumoral calcinosis. *Am J Physiol Endocrinol Metab* (2008) **295**:E929–37. doi:10.1152/ajpendo.90456.2008
47. White KE, Carn G, Lorenz-Depiereux B, Benet-Pages A, Strom TM, Econs MJ. Autosomal-dominant hypophosphatemic rickets (ADHR) mutations stabilize FGF-23. *Kidney Int* (2001) **60**:2079–86. doi:10.1046/j.1523-1755.2001.00064.x
48. Chu AY, Workalemahu T, Paynter NP, Rose LM, Giulianini F, Tanaka T, et al. Novel locus including FGF21 is associated with dietary macronutrient intake. *Hum Mol Genet* (2013) **22**:1895–902. doi:10.1093/hmg/ddt032
49. Zhang M, Zeng L, Wang YJ, An ZM, Ying BW. Associations of fibroblast growth factor 21 gene 3′ untranslated region single-nucleotide polymorphisms with metabolic syndrome, obesity, and diabetes in a Han Chinese population. *DNA Cell Biol* (2012) **31**:547–52. doi:10.1089/dna.2011.1302
50. Falcini F, Rigante D, Masi L, Covino M, Franceschelli F, Leoncini G, et al. Fibroblast growth factor 23 (FGF23) gene polymorphism in children with Kawasaki syndrome (KS) and susceptibility to cardiac abnormalities. *Ital J Pediatr* (2013) **39**:69. doi:10.1186/1824-7288-39-69
51. Kim HJ, Kim KH, Lee J, Oh JJ, Cheong HS, Wong EL, et al. Single nucleotide polymorphisms in fibroblast growth factor 23 gene, FGF23, are associated with prostate cancer risk. *BJU Int* (2014) **114**:303–10. doi:10.1111/bju.12396
52. Reiche M, Bachmann A, Lössner U, Blüher M, Stumvoll M, Fasshauer M. Fibroblast growth factor 19 serum levels: relation to renal function and metabolic parameters. *Horm Metab Res* (2010) **42**:178–81. doi:10.1055/s-0029-1243249
53. Li M, Qureshi AR, Ellis E, Axelsson J. Impaired postprandial fibroblast growth factor (FGF)-19 response in patients with stage 5 chronic kidney diseases is ameliorated following antioxidative therapy. *Nephrol Dial Transplant* (2013) **28**(Suppl 4):iv212–9. doi:10.1093/ndt/gft337
54. Hao Y, Zhou J, Zhou M, Ma X, Lu Z, Gao M, et al. Serum levels of fibroblast growth factor 19 are inversely associated with coronary artery disease in Chinese individuals. *PLoS One* (2013) **8**:e72345. doi:10.1371/journal.pone.0072345
55. Mutanen A, Lohi J, Heikkilä P, Jalanko H, Pakarinen MP. Loss of ileum decreases serum fibroblast growth factor 19 in relation to liver inflammation and fibrosis in pediatric onset intestinal failure. *J Hepatol* (2015) **62**:1391–7. doi:10.1016/j.jhep.2015.01.004
56. Roesch SL, Styer AM, Wood GC, Kosak Z, Seiler J, Benotti P, et al. Perturbations of fibroblast growth factors 19 and 21 in type 2 diabetes. *PLoS One* (2015) **10**:e0116928. doi:10.1371/journal.pone.0116928
57. Pattni SS, Brydon WG, Dew T, Johnston IM, Nolan JD, Srinivas M. Fibroblast growth factor 19 in patients with bile acid diarrhoea: a prospective comparison of FGF19 serum assay and SeHCAT retention. *Aliment Pharmacol Ther* (2013) **38**:967–76. doi:10.1111/apt.12466
58. Nolan JD, Johnston IM, Pattni SS, Dew T, Orchard TR, Walters JR. Diarrhea in Crohn's disease: investigating the role of the ileal hormone fibroblast growth factor 19. *J Crohns Colitis* (2015) **9**:125–31. doi:10.1093/ecco-jcc/jju022
59. Renner O, Harsch S, Matysik S, Lütjohann D, Schmitz G, Stange EF. Upregulation of hepatic bile acid synthesis via fibroblast growth factor 19 is defective in gallstone disease but functional in overweight individuals. *United European Gastroenterol J* (2014) **2**:216–25. doi:10.1177/2050640614527938
60. Nagamatsu H, Teishima J, Goto K, Shikuma H, Kitano H, Shoji K, et al. FGF19 promotes progression of prostate cancer. *Prostate* (2015) **75**:1092–101. doi:10.1002/pros.22994
61. Hindricks J, Ebert T, Bachmann A, Kralisch S, Lössner U, Kratzsch J, et al. Serum levels of fibroblast growth factor-21 are increased in chronic and acute renal dysfunction. *Clin Endocrinol (Oxf)* (2014) **80**:918–24. doi:10.1111/cen.12380
62. Lin Z, Wu Z, Yin X, Liu Y, Yan X, Lin S, et al. Serum levels of FGF-21 are increased in coronary heart disease patients and are independently associated with adverse lipid profile. *PLoS One* (2010) **5**:e15534. doi:10.1371/journal.pone.0015534

63. Chow WS, Xu A, Woo YC, Tso AW, Cheung SC, Fong CH, et al. Serum fibroblast growth factor-21 levels are associated with carotid atherosclerosis independent of established cardiovascular risk factors. *Arterioscler Thromb Vasc Biol* (2013) **33**:2454–9. doi:10.1161/ATVBAHA.113.301599
64. Stepan H, Kley K, Hindricks J, Kralisch S, Jank A, Schaarschmidt W, et al. Serum levels of the adipokine fibroblast growth factor-21 are increased in preeclampsia. *Cytokine* (2013) **62**:322–6. doi:10.1016/j.cyto.2013.02.019
65. Salehi MH, Kamalidehghan B, Houshmand M, Aryani O, Sadeghizadeh M, Mossalaeie MM. Association of fibroblast growth factor (FGF-21) as a biomarker with primary mitochondrial disorders, but not with secondary mitochondrial disorders (Friedreich ataxia). *Mol Biol Rep* (2013) **40**:6495–9. doi:10.1007/s11033-013-2767-0
66. Davis RL, Liang C, Edema-Hildebrand F, Riley C, Needham M, Sue CM. Fibroblast growth factor 21 is a sensitive biomarker of mitochondrial disease. *Neurology* (2013) **81**:1819–26. doi:10.1212/01.wnl.0000436068.43384.ef
67. Mraz M, Bartlova M, Lacinova Z, Michalsky D, Kasalicky M, Haluzikova D, et al. Serum concentrations and tissue expression of a novel endocrine regulator fibroblast growth factor-21 in patients with type 2 diabetes and obesity. *Clin Endocrinol (Oxf)* (2009) **71**:369–75. doi:10.1111/j.1365-2265.2008.03502.x
68. Lin Y, Xiao YC, Zhu H, Xu QY, Qi L, Wang YB, et al. Serum fibroblast growth factor 21 levels are correlated with the severity of diabetic retinopathy. *J Diabetes Res* (2014) **2014**:929756. doi:10.1155/2014/929756
69. Korwutthikulrangsri M, Mahachoklertwattana P, Chanprasertyothin S, Pongratanakul S, Poomthavorn P. Serum fibroblast growth factor 21 in overweight and obese Thai children and adolescents: its relation to glucose metabolism and its change after glucose loading. *Clin Endocrinol (Oxf)* (2015). doi:10.1111/cen.12808
70. Reinehr T, Karges B, Meissner T, Wiegand S, Fritsch M, Holl RW, et al. Fibroblast growth factor 21 and fetuin-A in obese adolescents with and without type 2 diabetes. *J Clin Endocrinol Metab* (2015) **100**:3004–10. doi:10.1210/jc.2015-2192
71. Dostálová I, Kaválková P, Haluzíková D, Lacinová Z, Mráz M, Papezová H, et al. Plasma concentrations of fibroblast growth factors 19 and 21 in patients with anorexia nervosa. *J Clin Endocrinol Metab* (2008) **93**:3627–32. doi:10.1210/jc.2008-0746
72. Durovcová V, Marek J, Hána V, Matoulek M, Zikán V, Haluzíková D, et al. Plasma concentrations of fibroblast growth factors 21 and 19 in patients with Cushing's syndrome. *Physiol Res* (2010) **59**:415–22.
73. Hanssen MJ, Broeders E, Samms RJ, Vosselman MJ, van der Lans AA, Cheng CC, et al. Serum FGF21 levels are associated with brown adipose tissue activity in humans. *Sci Rep* (2015) **5**:10275. doi:10.1038/srep10275
74. Li H, Fang Q, Gao F, Fan J, Zhou J, Wang X, et al. Fibroblast growth factor 21 levels are increased in nonalcoholic fatty liver disease patients and are correlated with hepatic triglyceride. *J Hepatol* (2010) **53**:934–40. doi:10.1016/j.jhep.2010.05.018
75. Alisi A, Ceccarelli S, Panera N, Prono F, Petrini S, De Stefanis C, et al. Association between serum atypical fibroblast growth factors 21 and 19 and pediatric nonalcoholic fatty liver disease. *PLoS One* (2013) **8**:e67160. doi:10.1371/journal.pone.0067160
76. Kukla M, Berdowska A, Stygar D, Gabriel A, Mazur W, Łogiewa-Bazger B, et al. Serum FGF21 and RBP4 levels in patients with chronic hepatitis C. *Scand J Gastroenterol* (2012) **47**:1037–47. doi:10.3109/00365521.2012.694901
77. Gariani K, Drifte G, Dunn-Siegrist I, Pugin J, Jornayvaz FR. Increased FGF21 plasma levels in humans with sepsis and SIRS. *Endocr Connect* (2013) **2**:146–53. doi:10.1530/EC-13-0040
78. Hulejová H, Andrés Cerezo L, Kuklová M, Pecha O, Vondráček T, Pavelka K, et al. Novel adipokine fibroblast growth factor 21 is increased in rheumatoid arthritis. *Physiol Res* (2012) **61**:489–94.
79. Ozeki M, Fujita S, Kizawa S, Morita H, Sohmiya K, Hoshiga M, et al. Association of serum levels of FGF23 and α-Klotho with glomerular filtration rate and proteinuria among cardiac patients. *BMC Nephrol* (2014) **15**:147. doi:10.1186/1471-2369-15-147
80. Portale AA, Wolf M, Jüppner H, Messinger S, Kumar J, Wesseling-Perry K, et al. Disordered FGF23 and mineral metabolism in children with CKD. *Clin J Am Soc Nephrol* (2014) **9**:344–53. doi:10.2215/CJN.05840513
81. Taal MW, Thurston V, McIntyre NJ, Fluck RJ, McIntyre CW. The impact of vitamin D status on the relative increase in fibroblast growth factor 23 and parathyroid hormone in chronic kidney disease. *Kidney Int* (2014) **86**:407–13. doi:10.1038/ki.2013.537
82. di Giuseppe R, Buijsse B, Hirche F, Wirth J, Arregui M, Westphal S, et al. Plasma fibroblast growth factor 23, parathyroid hormone, 25-hydroxyvitamin D3, and risk of heart failure: a prospective, case-cohort study. *J Clin Endocrinol Metab* (2014) **99**:947–55. doi:10.1210/jc.2013-2963
83. Isakova T, Houston J, Santacruz L, Schiavenato E, Somarriba G, Harmon WG, et al. Associations between fibroblast growth factor 23 and cardiac characteristics in pediatric heart failure. *Pediatr Nephrol* (2013) **28**:2035–42. doi:10.1007/s00467-013-2515-7
84. Xiao Y, Peng C, Huang W, Zhang J, Xia M, Zhang Y, et al. Circulating fibroblast growth factor 23 is associated with angiographic severity and extent of coronary artery disease. *PLoS One* (2013) **8**:e72545. doi:10.1371/journal.pone.0072545
85. di Giuseppe R, Kühn T, Hirche F, Buijsse B, Dierkes J, Fritsche A, et al. Plasma fibroblast growth factor 23 and risk of cardiovascular disease: results from the EPIC-Germany case-cohort study. *Eur J Epidemiol* (2015) **30**:131–41. doi:10.1007/s10654-014-9982-4
86. Jovanovich A, Ix JH, Gottdiener J, McFann K, Katz R, Kestenbaum B, et al. Fibroblast growth factor 23, left ventricular mass, and left ventricular hypertrophy in community-dwelling older adults. *Atherosclerosis* (2013) **231**:114–9. doi:10.1016/j.atherosclerosis.2013.09.002
87. Wright CB, Dong C, Stark M, Silverberg S, Rundek T, Elkind MS, et al. Plasma FGF23 and the risk of stroke: the Northern Manhattan study (NOMAS). *Neurology* (2014) **82**:1700–6. doi:10.1212/WNL.0000000000000410
88. Panwar B, Jenny NS, Howard VJ, Wadley VG, Muntner P, Kissela BM, et al. Fibroblast growth factor 23 and risk of incident stroke in community-living adults. *Stroke* (2015) **46**:322–8. doi:10.1161/STROKEAHA.114.007489
89. Luo J, Ko B, Elliott M, Zhou M, Lindhout DA, Phung V, et al. A nontumorigenic variant of FGF19 treats cholestatic liver diseases. *Sci Transl Med* (2014) **6**:247ra100. doi:10.1126/scitranslmed.3009098
90. Kharitonenkov A, Wroblewski VJ, Koester A, Chen YF, Clutinger CK, Tigno XT, et al. The metabolic state of diabetic monkeys is regulated by fibroblast growth factor-21. *Endocrinology* (2007) **148**:774–81. doi:10.1210/en.2006-1168
91. Adams AC, Halstead CA, Hansen BC, Irizarry AR, Martin JA, Myers SR, et al. LY2405319, an engineered FGF21 variant, improves the metabolic status of diabetic monkeys. *PLoS One* (2013) **8**:e65763. doi:10.1371/journal.pone.0065763
92. Gaich G, Chien JY, Fu H, Glass LC, Deeg MA, Holland WL, et al. The effects of LY2405319, an FGF21 analog, in obese human subjects with type 2 diabetes. *Cell Metab* (2013) **18**:333–40. doi:10.1016/j.cmet.2013.08.005
93. Véniant MM, Komorowski R, Chen P, Stanislaus S, Winters K, Hager T, et al. Long-acting FGF21 has enhanced efficacy in diet-induced obese mice and in obese rhesus monkeys. *Endocrinology* (2012) **153**:4192–203. doi:10.1210/en.2012-1211
94. Dong JQ, Rossulek M, Somayaji VR, Baltrukonis D, Liang Y, Hudson K, et al. Pharmacokinetics and pharmacodynamics of PF-05231023, a novel long-acting FGF21 mimetic, in a first-in-human study. *Br J Clin Pharmacol* (2015). doi:10.1111/bcp.12676
95. Smith R, Duguay A, Bakker A, Li P, Weiszmann J, Thomas MR, et al. FGF21 can be mimicked in vitro and in vivo by a novel anti-FGFR1c/β-Klotho bispecific protein. *PLoS One* (2013) **8**:e61432. doi:10.1371/journal.pone.0061432
96. Carpenter TO, Imel EA, Ruppe MD, Weber TJ, Klausner MA, Wooddell MM, et al. Randomized trial of the anti-FGF23 antibody KRN23 in X-linked hypophosphatemia. *J Clin Invest* (2014) **124**:1587–97. doi:10.1172/JCI72829
97. Imel EA, Zhang X, Ruppe MD, Weber TJ, Klausner MA, Ito T, et al. Prolonged correction of serum phosphorus in adults with X-linked hypophosphatemia using monthly doses of KRN23. *J Clin Endocrinol Metab* (2015) **100**:2565–73. doi:10.1210/jc.2015-1551

2

Divergent cardio-ventilatory and locomotor effects of centrally and peripherally administered urotensin II and urotensin II-related peptides in trout

Gilmer Vanegas[1], **Jérôme Leprince**[2], **Frédéric Lancien**[1], **Nagi Mimassi**[1], **Hubert Vaudry**[2] **and Jean-Claude Le Mével**[1]*

[1] Institut National de la Santé et de la Recherche Médicale UMR1101, Laboratoire de Neurophysiologie, SFR ScInBioS, Université de Brest, Brest, France, [2] Institut National de la Santé et de la Recherche Médicale U982, UA Centre National de la Recherche Scientifique, Différenciation et Communication Neuronale et Neuroendocrine, Université de Rouen, Mont-Saint-Aignan, France

Edited by:
Stephane Gasman,
Centre National de la Recherche Scientifique, France

Reviewed by:
Lixin Wang,
University of California, Los Angeles, USA
Leo T. O. Lee,
The University of Hong Kong, China

***Correspondence:**
Jean-Claude Le Mével,
Laboratoire de Neurophysiologie, Faculté de Médecine, LaTIM UMR 1101, Université de Brest, 22 Rue Camille Desmoulins, 29200 Brest, France
jean-claude.lemevel@univ-brest.fr

The urotensin II (UII) gene family consists of four paralogous genes called UII, UII-related peptide (URP), URP1 and URP2. UII and URP peptides exhibit the same cyclic hexapeptide core sequence (CFWKYC) while the N- and C-terminal regions are variable. UII, URP1, and URP2 mRNAs are differentially expressed within the central nervous system of teleost fishes, suggesting that they may exert distinct functions. Although the cardiovascular, ventilatory and locomotor effects of UII have been described in teleosts, much less is known regarding the physiological actions of URPs. The goal of the present study was to compare the central and peripheral actions of picomolar doses (5–500 pmol) of trout UII, URP1, and URP2 on cardio-ventilatory variables and locomotor activity in the unanesthetized trout. Compared to vehicle, intracerebroventricular injection of UII, URP1 and URP2 evoked a gradual increase in total ventilation (V_{TOT}) reaching statistical significance for doses of 50 and 500 pmol of UII and URP1 but for only 500 pmol of URP2. In addition, UII, URP1 and URP2 provoked an elevation of dorsal aortic blood pressure (P_{DA}) accompanied with tachycardia. All peptides caused an increase in locomotor activity (A_{CT}), at a threshold dose of 5 pmol for UII and URP1, and 50 pmol for URP2. After intra-arterial (IA) injection, and in contrast to their central effects, only the highest dose of UII and URP1 significantly elevated V_{TOT} and A_{CT}. UII produced a dose-dependent hypertensive effect with concomitant bradycardia while URP1 increased P_{DA} and heart rate after injection of only the highest dose of peptide. URP2 did not evoke any cardio-ventilatory or locomotor effect after IA injection. Collectively, these findings support the hypothesis that endogenous UII, URP1 and URP2 in the trout brain may act as neurotransmitters and/or neuromodulators acting synergistically or differentially to control the cardio-respiratory and locomotor systems. In the periphery, the only physiological actions of these peptides might be those related to the well-known cardiovascular regulatory actions of UII. It remains to determine whether the observed divergent physiological effects of UII and

URPs are due to differential interaction with the UT receptor or binding to distinct UT subtypes.

Keywords: urotensin II, urotensin II-related peptides, ventilatory variables, heart rate, blood pressure, locomotor activity, brain, trout

Introduction

Urotensin II (UII) is a cyclic neuropeptide that was originally isolated and purified from the caudal neurosecretory system of the teleost fish *Gillichthys mirabilis* (longjaw mudsucker) on the basis of its smooth muscle-stimulating activity (Bern and Lederis, 1969; Pearson et al., 1980). Recently, it has been demonstrated that UII belongs to a family of structurally related peptides that include UII and UII-related peptides (URPs) called URP, URP1, and URP2 (Lihrmann et al., 2013). UII, URP, URP1, and URP2 exhibit the same cyclic hexapeptide core sequence (CFWKYC) while the N- and C-terminal regions are variable (Conlon, 2008; Lihrmann et al., 2013). In the teleost lineage, all four paralog genes are present but only two of them, UII and URP, are found in tetrapods (Quan et al., 2012; Tostivint et al., 2013). In mammals, UII and URP genes are mostly expressed in cholinergic neurons of the brainstem and spinal cord but variable levels of expression occur in most brainstem nuclei (Vaudry et al., 2015) suggesting that the peptides may exert distinct biological functions. UII and URP mRNAs are also differentially expressed in peripheral tissues, including notably the cardiovascular, renal and endocrine systems (Sugo et al., 2003; Dubessy et al., 2008; Vaudry et al., 2015). UII and URP both activate the UT receptor with the same potency (Sugo et al., 2003) but the two peptides may exert differential modulatory effects due to recruitment of different intracellular signaling pathways (Vaudry et al., 2010). The UT receptor is present in several areas of the brain and spinal cord but also in various peripheral organs including the cardiovascular system, endocrine tissues and kidney (Vaudry et al., 2015). UII exerts a large array of biological effects including regulation of various behaviors, motor and neuroendocrine activities, as well as central and peripheral control of blood pressure and heart rate but much less is known about the biological actions of URPs (Vaudry et al., 2010, 2015). In fish, UII, URPs and the UT receptor are also present in the brain and spinal cord. Pioneer studies have demonstrated that UII-like immunoreactivity is primarily found in cerebrospinal fluid (CSF)-contacting neurons located within the ventral ependyma lining the central canal along the entire length of the spinal cord and the medulla oblongata (Yulis and Lederis, 1986, 1988). These CSF-contacting neurons containing UII-like immunorecativity project their axons toward the external surface of the spinal cord and ascending fibers innervate various regions of the brain (Yulis and Lederis, 1986, 1988). UII has been purified and characterized from extracts of the brains of an elasmobranch, the skate *Raja rhina*, and a teleost, the rainbow trout *Oncorhynchus mykiss* (Waugh and Conlon, 1993). The expression of UII mRNA in fish brain has been confirmed by RT-PCR in the European flounder *Platichthys flesus* (Lu et al., 2006), in the zebrafish *Danio rerio* (Parmentier et al., 2008) and in the orange-spotted grouper *Epinephelus coioides* (Sun et al., 2014). Extensive studies on the differential expression of URP, URP1 and URP2 in the central nervous system (CNS) have been conducted in the Japanese eel *Anguilla japonica* (Nobata et al., 2011) and in the zebrafish (Parmentier et al., 2011; Quan et al., 2015). In zebrafish, URP mRNA is present in motoneurons (cited in Quan et al., 2015). In both species, URP1 is mainly expressed in motoneurons of the medulla oblongata. In zebrafish, URP2 mRNA is found in cells located along the ventral edge of the fourth ventricle, probably in CSF-contacting neurons, and in the spinal cord, URP1 and URP2 mRNAs colocalize in same cells that are also CSF-contacting neurons (Quan et al., 2015). In the flounder (Lu et al., 2006), the killifish *Fundulus heteroclitus* (Evans et al., 2011) and the orange-spotted grouper (Sun et al., 2014), the UT receptor is strongly expressed in the caudal neurosecretory system, the CNS (brain and spinal cord) but also in various peripheral tissues including the heart, gill, kidney and ovary. UII is known to be involved in osmoregulation in fish (Marshall and Bern, 1979; Lu et al., 2006; Evans et al., 2011) and a few studies have examined the cardiovascular effects of UII and URP1 in teleosts. In the rainbow trout, centrally administered UII evokes an increase in dorsal aortic blood pressure (P_{DA}) with variable action on the heart (Le Mével et al., 1996), while intra-arterial (IA) injection of UII provokes a dose-dependent elevation in P_{DA} with a concomitant bradycardia (Le Mével et al., 1996). In the Japanese eel, the cardiovascular effects of centrally and peripherally injected UII and URP1 are quite similar. Both peptides preferentially elevate blood pressure in the ventral aorta than in the dorsal aorta and evoke tachycardia (Nobata et al., 2011). In addition, in the rainbow trout, central injection of UII produces a hyperventilatory response and a long-lasting increase in locomotor activity (Lancien et al., 2004). Nonetheless, due to the relatively recent discovery of UPRs, nothing is known about the potential actions of URP1 on ventilatory and locomotor functions and those of URP2 on cardio-ventilatory and locomotor functions. The differential although similar expression of UII, URP1, and URP2 in the CNS of teleosts suggests that these peptides may have synergistic or divergent biological effects. It is thus important to determine the *in vivo* integrative actions of these peptides on physiological functions and behavior in the same animal. Therefore, the main goal of the present study was to analyze the central effects of trout UII, URP1, and URP2 on ventilatory and cardiovascular functions and on locomotor activity in our established trout model. To this end, we have analyzed the effects of intracerebroventricular (ICV) administration of synthetic replicates of these peptides on ventilatory amplitude (V_{AMP}), ventilatory frequency (f_V), total ventilation (V_{TOT}), P_{DA},

Abbreviations: A_{CT}, locomotor activity; a.u., arbitrary unit; CNS, central nervous system; ECG, electrocardiographic; f_H, heart rate; f_V, ventilatory rate; IA, intra-arterial; ICV, intracerebroventricular; P_{DA}, dorsal aortic blood pressure; UII, urotensin II; URP, urotensin II-related peptide; URP1, urotensin II-related peptide 1; URP2, urotensin II-related peptide 2; V_{AMP}, ventilatory amplitude; V_{TOT}, total ventilation.

heart rate (f_H), and locomotor activity (A_{CT}). Additionally, the central actions of the peptides were also compared with their effects after IA injection.

Material and Methods

Peptides and Chemicals

The primary sequence of the urotensin peptides examined in this study is shown in **Table 1**. Trout UII, URP1, and URP2 (Waugh and Conlon, 1993; Tostivint et al., 2013) were synthesized as previously described (Chatenet et al., 2004; Lancien et al., 2004). The peptides were dissolved in Ringer's solution (vehicle) and stored in stock solutions at $-25°C$. Immediately before use, UII, URP1, or URP2 were diluted to the desired concentration with Ringer's solution. The composition of the Ringer's solution was (in mM): NaCl 124, KCl 3, $CaCl_2$ 0.75, $MgSO_4$ 1.30, $KH_2PO_4$1.24, $NaHCO_3$ 12, glucose 10 (pH 7.8). All solutions were sterilized by filtration through 0.22 μm filters (Millipore, Molsheim, France) before injection.

Animals

Adult rainbow trout *Oncorhynchus mykiss* (247 $\pm$ 24 g body wt, mean $\pm$ SEM, $n = 95$) of both sexes were purchased locally and transferred in a well-oxygenated and thermostatically controlled water tank to the laboratory. All fish were kept in a 1000-liter tank containing circulating dechlorinated and aerated tap water (11–12°C), under a standard photoperiod (lights on 09:00–20:00). The fish were allowed at least 3 weeks to acclimate under these conditions before the experiments were started. Experimental protocols were approved by the Regional Ethics Committee in Animal Experiments of Brittany, France.

Experimental Procedures

All surgical procedures were made under tricaine methanesulfonate (3-aminobenzoic acid ethyl ester methanesulfonate; 60 mg/L in tap water buffered with $NaHCO_3$ to pH 7.3–7.5) anesthesia. The techniques used for placement of the electrocardiographic (ECG) electrodes, placement of the buccal catheter, cannulation of the dorsal aorta and insertion of the ICV microguide have previously been described in detail (Le Mével et al., 1993; Lancien et al., 2004). Briefly, two ECG AgCl electrodes (Comepa, Bagnolet, France) were subcutaneously implanted ventrally and longitudinally at the level of the pectoral fins. The incision was sutured across the electrodes and the leads were sutured to the skin. The dorsal aorta was cannulated with a PE-50 catheter (Clay Adams, Le Pont De Claix, France). A flared cannula (PE-160) was inserted into a hole drilled between the nares such that its flared end was resting against the roof of the mouth. This cannula was used to record any changes in buccal ventilatory pressure. The absence of a neocortex in fish allows the accurate placement of the ICV microguide under stereomicroscopic guidance. A 25-gauge needle fitted with a PE-10 polyethylene catheter was inserted between the two habenular ganglia and descended into the third ventricle until its tip lay between the two preoptic nuclei (Le Mével et al., 2009). An obturator was placed at the end of the PE-10 tubing and the cranial surface was covered with hemostatic tissue followed by light quick-curing resin. After surgery, the animals were force-ventilated with dechlorinated tap water until recovery of opercular movements and transferred to a 6-liter blackened chamber supplied with dechlorinated and aerated tap water (10–11°C) that was both re-circulating and through-flowing. Oxygen partial pressure within the water tank (PwO_2) and pH were continuously recorded and maintained at constant levels (PwO_2 = 20 kPa; pH = 7.4–7.6). A small horizontal aperture was made along the upper edge of the chamber in order to connect the ECG leads to an amplifier and to connect the dorsal aorta and the buccal cannula to pressure transducers. This aperture also permitted ICV and IA injections of peptides without disturbing the animals.

Trout were allowed to recover from surgery and to become accustomed to their new environment for 48–72 h. Each day, the general condition of the animals was assessed by observing their behavior, checking the ventilatory and the cardiovascular variables, and measuring their hematocrit. Animals that did not appear healthy, according to the range of values detailed in our previous studies, were discarded. After stable V_{AMP}, f_V, P_{DA}, and f_H were maintained for at least 90 min, parameters were recorded for 30 min without any manipulation in control experiments. To minimize the use of experimental animals, some trout received both ICV and IA injections. In this later case, the delay between the two injections was 1 day, and the order of the injections was randomized among animals. No single fish was studied for more than 2 days and control experiments revealed that there was no significant change in performance over this period.

TABLE 1 | Amino-acid sequence of trout urotensin II (Waugh and Conlon, 1993) and teleost URP1 and URP2 (Tostivint et al., 2013) examined for their cardio-ventilatory effects and locomotor activity following central and peripheral injection in the unanesthetized rainbow trout *Oncorhynchus mykiss*.

Urotensin II peptides	Amino-acid sequence
UII	H-Gly-Gly-Asn-Ser-Glu-**Cys-Phe-Trp-Lys-Tyr-Cys**-Val-OH
URP1	H-Ala-**Cys-Phe-Trp-Lys-Tyr-Cys**-Val-Thr-Asn-OH
URP2	H-Val-**Cys-Phe-Trp-Lys-Tyr-Cys**-Ser-Gln-Asn-OH

The conserved cyclic hexapeptide core sequence (Cys-Phe-Trp-Lys-Tyr-Cys or CFWKYC) of each peptide is in bold characters.

Intracerebroventricular Administration of Peptides

The injector was introduced within the ICV guide prior to the beginning of a recording session which lasted 30 min. All injections were made at the fifth minute of the test but the injector was left in place for a further 5 min to allow for complete diffusion of the agent and to minimize the spread of substances upwards in the cannula tract. The fish received first an ICV injection of vehicle (0.5 μl) and 30 min later, an ICV injection of UII, URP1, or URP2 (5, 50, and 500 pmol in 0.5 μl). The rationale for using these doses was that they were in the same range as those previously used for studies on the cardiovascular effects of UII in trout and for comparison of effects between peptides (Le Mével et al., 1996, 2012). Previous control experiments using two ICV injections 30 min apart have shown no time-dependent changes in the measured variables using this protocol (Le Mével et al., 2009). The animals received no more than two ICV injections of peptide per day with a delay of at least 5 h between the injections.

Intra-Arterial Administration of Peptides

Five minutes after the beginning of the recording session, 50 μl of vehicle, UII, URP1, or URP2 at doses of 5, 50, and 500 pmol was injected through the dorsal aorta and immediately flushed by 150 μl of vehicle.

Data Acquisition and Analysis of Cardio-Ventilatory Variables and Motor Activity

The ECG electrodes were connected to a differential amplifier (band pass: 5–50 Hz; Bioelectric amplifier, Gould & Nicolet, Courtaboeuf, France) and a stainless steel bar was immersed in the water of the tank to act as a reference electrode. The aortic cannula and the buccal catheter were connected to P23XL pressure transducers (band pass: 0–15 Hz; Gould & Nicolet). These pressure transducers were calibrated each day using a static water column. At the beginning of the experiments, the zero-buccal pressure level was set electronically. The output signals from the devices were digitalized at 1000 Hz and visualized on the screen of a PC using PowerLab 4/30 data acquisition system (ADInstruments, Oxford, England) and LabChart Pro software (v.7.0; ADInstruments, Oxford, England) during the 30-min recording period and the data were stored on a disk. The time-series related to the ventilatory, the pulsatile P_{DA} and the ECG signals were then processed off-line with custom-made programs written in LabView 6.1 (Laboratory Virtual Instrument Engineering Workbench, National Instruments, Austin, USA). Motor activity, ventilatory and cardiovascular variables were calculated as previously described (Lancien et al., 2004; Le Mével et al., 2007). Motor activity was detected as artifacts on the ventilatory signal (Lancien et al., 2004) and the total duration of locomotor activity (A_{CT}, in seconds) was determined from ventilatory signal (Lancien et al., 2004). Thereafter, segments free of any movement artifacts on the ventilatory signal were selected and f_V (breaths min^{-1}) and V_{AMP} (arbitrary units, a.u.) were determined. The f_V was calculated from the first harmonic of the power spectrum of the ventilatory signal using the fast Fourier transformation. V_{AMP} was calculated from the difference between the maximal abduction phase and the maximal adduction phase for each ventilatory cycle. Spontaneous coughings, which correspond to rapid and robust changes in the abduction/adduction phases of the ventilatory cycle, were excluded from this analysis. The net effect of the changes in f_V and V_{AMP} on ventilation was estimated according to the formula $V_{TOT} = f_V \times V_{AMP}$, where V_{TOT} (a.u.)is total ventilation. Mean P_{DA} (kPa) was calculated from the pulsatile P_{DA} as the arithmetic mean between systolic blood pressure and diastolic blood pressure, and the f_H (beats min^{-1}) was determined from the ECG signal. All calculations for mean f_V, V_{AMP}, V_{TOT}, P_{DA}, f_H, and A_{CT} were made for the pre-injection period (0–5 min) and for five post-injection periods of 5 min for each trout. To reduce the amount of data, only the maximal effects of the various treatments in the above parameters were analyzed and the results were averaged for trout subjected to the same protocol. One-Way ANOVA analysis of baseline values of f_V, V_{AMP}, V_{TOT}, P_{DA}, f_H, and A_{CT} during the pre-injection period revealed that there was no statistical difference between groups prior ICV or IA injection of vehicle or the various peptides (not shown).

Statistical Analysis

Data are expressed as means + SEM (standard error of the mean). The data were analyzed by One-Way ANOVA test followed by the multiple comparison tests of Dunnett or Tukey. The criterion for statistical difference between groups was $P < 0.05$. The statistical tests were performed using GraphPad Prism 5.0 (GraphPad, San Diego, USA).

Results

Ventilatory, Cardiovascular and Locomotor Activity Responses to Central UII, URP1, and URP2

The effects of ICV injections of vehicle, UII, URP1, and URP2 on ventilatory and cardiovascular variables, and on locomotor activity are summarized in **Figures 1–3**, respectively. Compared with ICV injection of vehicle, all peptides evoked quite similar increase in V_{AMP} (**Figures 1A, 2A, 3A**) and f_V (**Figures 1B,2B,3B**). However, the threshold dose of UII inducing a significant effect on V_{AMP} was only 5 pmol while a 10-fold higher dose was required for URP1 and URP2. All peptides provoked an elevation of f_V for a threshold dose of 50 pmol with minor differences between peptides at the higher dose (**Figures 1B,2B,3B**). The net effect of the ICV administration of the peptides was a hyperventilatory response involving a gradual and significant increase in V_{TOT} for doses of 50 and 500 pmol of UII and URP1 but for only 500 pmol of URP2 (**Figures 1C,2C,3C**). In addition, UII, URP1, and URP2 provoked a non-dose-dependent increase in P_{DA} (**Figures 1D,2D,3D**). However, the threshold dose for this effect was only 5 pmol for UII and URP1 (**Figures 1D, 2D**) but 500 pmol for URP2 (**Figure 3D**). During this hypertensive effect of the peptides, there was no bradycardia but instead, a significant tachycardia occurred at the 50 and 500 pmol doses for most of the peptides (**Figures 1F,2F,3F**). UII, URP1, and URP2 also caused a potent increase in A_{CT} for a threshold dose of 5 pmol for UII and URP1 but 50 pmol for URP2.

Ventilatory, Cardiovascular and Locomotor Activity Responses to Peripheral UII, URP1, and URP2

Figures 4–6 depict the results obtained after IA administration of the different peptides on ventilatory and cardiovascular variables and on motor activity. In contrast to their central effects, only the highest dose of UII and URP1 (500 pmol) significantly elevated V_{AMP} and the net effect of these peptides was a hyperventilatory response since V_{TOT} significantly increased (**Figures 4C,5C**). Contrary to its ICV effects, IA injection of UII produced a significant dose-dependent increase in P_{DA} (**Figure 4D**) accompanied with a f_H decrease, a bradycardia statistically significant for the 5 and 50 pmol doses of peptide (**Figure 4E**). Only the highest dose of URP1 (500 pmol) provoked

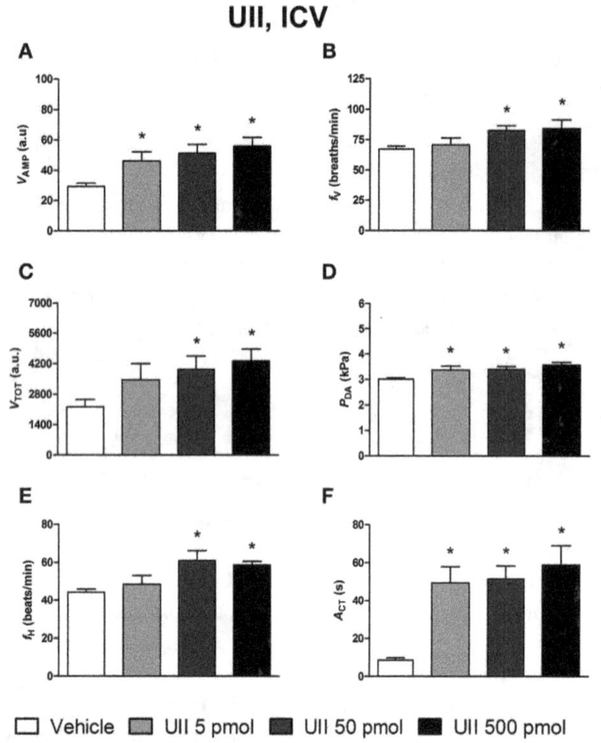

FIGURE 1 | Histograms showing the maximal effects of ICV injection of 0.5 μl of vehicle ($n = 34$), 5 pmol UII ($n = 11$), 50 pmol UII ($n = 14$) and 500 pmol UII ($n = 12$) on ventilatory amplitude (V_{AMP}, A), ventilatory frequency (f_V, B), total ventilation (V_{TOT}, C), dorsal aortic blood pressure (P_{DA}, D), heart rate (f_H, E), and motor activity (A_{CT}, F).
*$P < 0.05$ vs. vehicle injection.

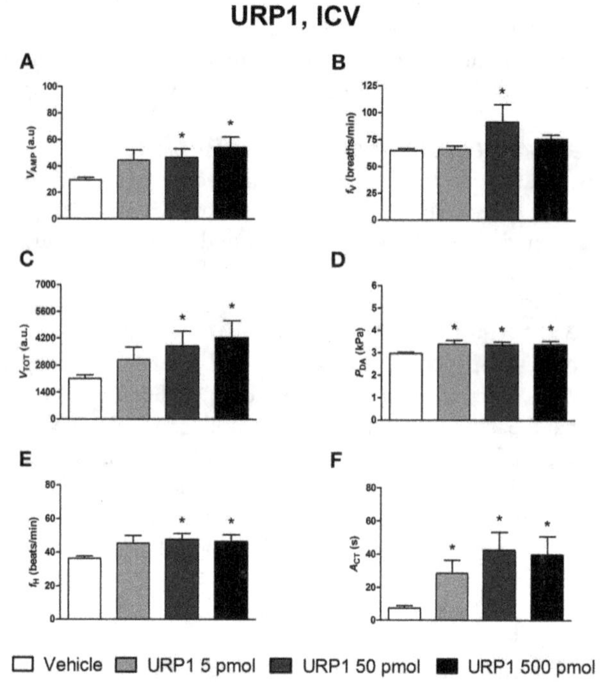

FIGURE 2 | Histograms showing the maximal effects of ICV injection of 0.5 μl vehicle ($n = 31$), 5 pmol URP1 ($n = 11$), 50 pmol URP1 ($n = 12$) and 500 pmol URP1 ($n = 10$) on ventilatory amplitude (V_{AMP}, A), ventilatory frequency (f_V, B), total ventilation (V_{TOT}, C), dorsal aortic blood pressure (P_{DA}, D), heart rate (f_H, E), and motor activity (A_{CT}, F).
*$P < 0.05$ vs. vehicle injection.

an elevation in P_{DA} accompagnied by a significant tachycardia (**Figures 5D,E**). IA injection of the highest dose of UII and URP1 caused an increase in A_{CT} (**Figures 4F,5F**). Peripheral administration of URP2 at any dose did not produce any effect on the cardio-ventilatory variables and locomotor activity (**Figures 6A–F**).

Discussion

This is the first functional study evaluating the integrative effects of UII, URP1, and URP2 on physiological variables including ventilation, blood pressure and locomotor activity in fish. The most important outcome of this study is that ICV or IA administration of picomolar doses of these peptides exert both common and specific biological activities depending on the route of administration. The demonstration that ICV injection of UII and URPs evoked a stimulatory action on ventilation, cardiovascular variables and locomotion for doses that did not produce any effect or evoked differential action after peripheral administration, supports the assumption that following ICV injection, central neuronal sites are involved in the action of the peptides. In addition, after IA injection, the exclusive effect of low picomolar doses of UII on P_{DA} and f_H, confirms that this peptide may act also to peripheral sites.

Ventilatory, Cardiovascular and Locomotor Actions of Centrally Administered UII, URP1, and URP2

The central actions of UII, URP1, and URP2 on cardio-ventilatory and motor functions may be compared to those reported in previous studies conducted with UII or URP1 in fish or in other vertebrates species. The present results on UII are consistent with our previous data demonstrating that, in trout, UII administered through the ICV route causes a non-dose-dependent elevation of P_{DA} without bradycardia (Le Mével et al., 1996). In the eel, central administration of UII and URP1 preferentially elevates blood pressure of the branchial circulation higher than that of the systemic circulation (Nobata et al., 2011). Consequently, the hypertensive effect of eel UII on ventral aortic blood pressure (P_{VA}) is significant for doses higher than 0.15 nmol while doses higher than 0.5 nmol are required to increase P_{DA}. URP1 (0.3–0.5 nmol) provokes a significant dose-dependent increase in P_{VA}, but does not affect P_{DA} at any dose(Nobata et al., 2011). The effect of URP1 was longer lasting than that of UII and the two peptides evoked tachycardia (Nobata et al., 2011). The absence of bradycardia in response to an increase in blood pressure following ICV injection of UII and URP1 in trout and eel, and URP2 in trout suggests that the cardio-inhibitory baroreceptor reflex is altered following central injection of these peptides. In normotensive and hypertensive unanesthetized rats (Lin et al., 2003a,b) and in unanesthetized sheep (Watson and May,

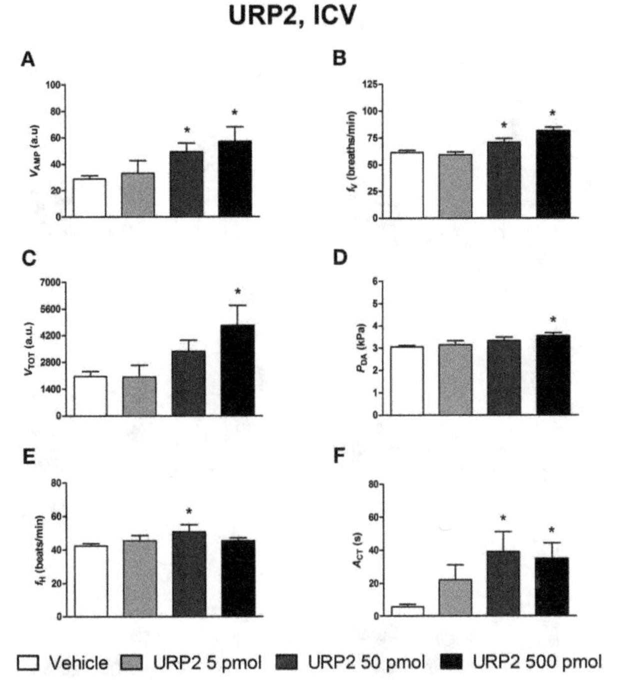

FIGURE 3 | Histograms showing the maximal effects of ICV injection of 0.5 μl vehicle ($n = 25$), 5 pmol URP2 ($n = 9$), 50 pmol URP2 ($n = 12$) and 500 pmol URP2 ($n = 9$) on ventilatory amplitude (V_{AMP}, A), ventilatory frequency (f_V, B), total ventilation (V_{TOT}, C), dorsal aortic blood pressure (P_{DA}, D), heart rate (f_H, E), and motor activity (A_{CT}, F).
*$P < 0.05$ vs. vehicle injection.

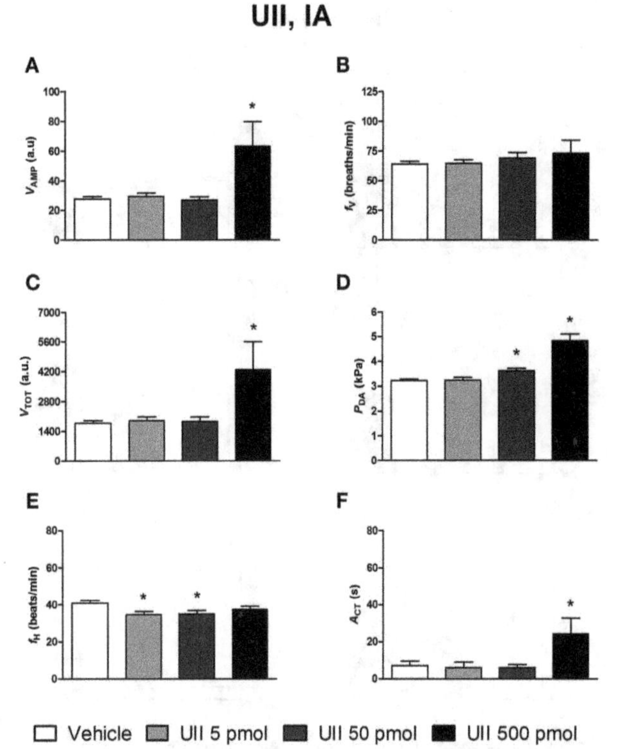

FIGURE 4 | Histograms showing the maximal effects of IA injection of 50 μl vehicle ($n = 29$), 5 pmol UII ($n = 10$), 50 pmol UII ($n = 16$) and 500 pmol UII ($n = 7$) on ventilatory amplitude (V_{AMP}, A), ventilatory frequency (f_V, B), total ventilation (V_{TOT}, C), dorsal aortic blood pressure (P_{DA}, D), heart rate (f_H, E), and motor activity (A_{CT}, F).
*$P < 0.05$ vs. vehicle injection.

2004), ICV administration of UII causes pressor and tachycardic responses through activation of the sympathetic system indicating that, in these species, also the cardiac baroreflex response is impaired. Studies conducted on unanesthetized sheep to test this hypothesis demonstrated that, after ICV infusion of UII (0.2 nmol/kg for 1 h), the cardiac baroreflex response is effectively blunted since no changes occur in the cardiac sympathetic nerve activity in spite of an increase in blood pressure (Hood et al., 2005). In rats, the central cardiovascular action of UII is site-dependent and local administration of UII in discrete brain nuclei produces differential cardiovascular responses (Lu et al., 2002). To our knowledge, the central action of URP in mammals has never been explored.

We have previously demonstrated that, in addition to its central cardiovascular effects, UII produces a hyperventilatory response and a stimulatory effect on locomotion (Lancien et al., 2004, 2005). In the present study, UII-induced hyperventilation was mimicked by URP1 and to a lesser extent by URP2. Furthermore, at the low dose of 5 pmol, UII, URP1 but not URP2 provoked an increase in locomotion. Nonetheless, at this picomole dose, UII and URP1 did not induced any change in V_{TOT}. These observations suggest that UII and URP1 act preferentially on central neuronal networks controlling locomotion than ventilation. This stimulatory effect of UII on locomotor activity in fish is in accord with results obtained in rats (Gartlon et al., 2001) and mice (Do-Rego et al., 2005) showing that ICV injection of human UII (hURP, ACFWKYCV) and mouse UII, respectively, elicit motor activity in a familiar environment. It should be noted, however, that the threshold doses eliciting locomotor effects in rats and mice are in the nanomole range. Because UII and URPs induced a marked increased in locomotor activity in trout, we cannot exclude that the changes observed in cardio-ventilatory parameters may be secondary effects of the peptides. Finally, in our study and after ICV injection, a trend in the potency order of UII, URP1, and URP2 emerged being UII ≥ URP1 > URP2 notably for the hyperventilatory, hypertensive and locomotor actions of these peptides.

The receptor site(s) and the multisynaptic pathways involved in initiating cardio-ventilatory and locomotor responses after UII, URP1, and URP2 injection within the brain are matter of speculation and require further studies. Nevertheless, as previously mentioned for the central actions of other neuropeptides, some neuroanatomical prerequisites and some neurophysiological data exist that may support some working hypothesis (Le Mével et al., 2012). Because the peptides were injected within the third ventricle in close proximity to the preoptic nucleus (NPO), they can activate these preoptic neurons leading to hyperventilatory and hypertensive responses through neuroendocrine and/or neurogenic pathways. Preoptic neurons synthesize the nonapeptides vasotocin (AVT) and isotocin (IT). AVT and IT

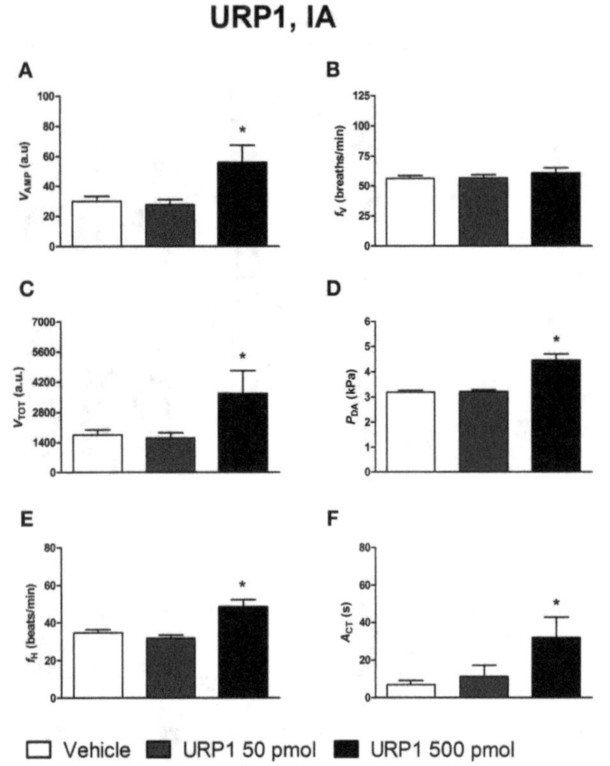

FIGURE 5 | Histograms showing the maximal effects of IA injection of 50 μl vehicle ($n = 20$), 50 pmol URP1 ($n = 15$) and 500 pmol URP1 ($n = 11$), on ventilatory amplitude (V_{AMP}, A), ventilatory frequency (f_V, B), total ventilation (V_{TOT}, C), dorsal aortic blood pressure (P_{DA}, D), heart rate (f_H, E), and motor activity (A_{CT}, F). *$P < 0.05$ vs. vehicle injection.

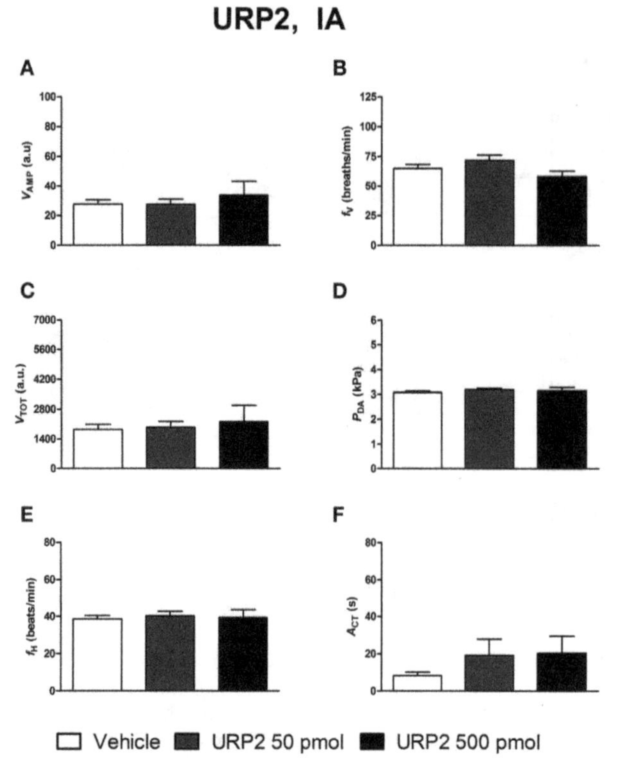

FIGURE 6 | Histograms showing the maximal effects of IA injection of 50 μl vehicle ($n = 19$), 50 pmol URP2 ($n = 11$) and 500 pmol URP2 ($n = 9$) on ventilatory amplitude (V_{AMP}, A), ventilatory frequency (f_V, B), total ventilation (V_{TOT}, C), dorsal aortic blood pressure (P_{DA}, D), heart rate (f_H, E), and motor activity (A_{CT}, F).

neurons project not only to the neurohypophysis, but also to the brainstem cardiovascular and ventilatory nuclei (Batten et al., 1990; Saito et al., 2004). It should be emphasized that in trout, AVT produces a hypertensive response acting both centrally and peripherally (Le Mével et al., 1993). UII and URPs injected within the third ventricle may also stimulate locomotion through the direct or indirect projection of neurons from the NPO to midbrain locomotor nuclei (Lancien et al., 2004) or spinal motor neurons as previously suggested for the control of sexual behavior (Demski and Sloan, 1985; Gregory and Tweedle, 1985). In addition, since the peptides are injected within the CSF, they can diffuse to the mid- and hindbrain to affect motor nuclei involved in cardio-ventilatory functions and swimming behavior (see also 23). Interestingly, the presence of immunoreactive UII, and URP2 gene expression, in CSF-contacting neurons in regions surrounding notably the fourth ventricular wall, has already been documented in various teleosts (Yulis and Lederis, 1988; Parmentier et al., 2011; Quan et al., 2015), suggesting that these cells may sense the composition of the CSF and/or release their products within the ventricular system. Furthermore, in the eel brainstem, the URP1 gene is detected within neurons of the commissural nucleus of Cajal, a nucleus homologous to the nucleus tractus solitary, the first central relay in the cardiovascular baroreflex loop (Nobata et al., 2011). Concurrently, in the zebrafish, URP1-expressing cells are located in the reticular formation and the glosso-pharyngeal-vagal-motor nuclei (Quan et al., 2015). Collectively, our functional study and these neuroanatomical data support a role of endogenous UII, URP1 and URP2 as neurotransmitters or neuromodulators involved in the central command of autonomic cardio-ventilatory and locomotor functions.

Ventilatory, Cardiovascular and Locomotor Actions of Peripherally Administered UII, URP1, and URP2

The peripheral actions of UII, URP1, and URP2 on cardio-ventilatory and locomotor functions may be compared with those reported in previous studies that explored the peripheral effects of UII, URP, or URP1 in fish or in other vertebrate species but also with their central actions. The present results on UII are in line with our previous data obtained in trout demonstrating that low picomole doses of UII cause a dose-dependent hypertensive response and a bradycardia (Le Mével et al., 1996). In addition, we previously investigated the cardiovascular actions of peripherally injected trout UII (50 pmol) and hURP (50 and 500 pmol) in trout (Le Mével et al., 2008). It appears that hURP is about ten times less potent than trout UII in evoking a hypertensive response since hURP (50 pmol, about 0.2 nmol/kg) had no significant effect on cardiovascular variables and only the highest dose of hURP (500 pmol, about 2 nmol/kg) produced a similar peak increase in P_{DA}. Furthermore, the hypertensive response observed following the IA injection of hURP was of shorter duration than after IA injection of UII and there was no concomitant bradycardia. The cardiovascular effects of UII/URPs in trout are quite different to those obtained in eel, suggesting that the cardiovascular actions of UII/URPs may be species dependent. Indeed, at an equimolar dose of 0.1 nmol/kg in eel, the vasopressor effects of native UII and URP1 are similar, but as for the ICV injection, the effect of UII is longer lasting than the action of URP1. However, in eel, both eel UII and URP1 evoke a tachycardia (Nobata et al., 2011). In addition, after peripheral injections, both hUII and URP are also less potent than the homologous peptides in eel. Thus, the results obtained with heterologous peptides in trout and in eel, emphasize the importance of the amino-acid residues flanking the N-terminus of the cyclic core of the fish UII-molecule in interacting with the fish UT receptor. In trout, the hypertensive effect of UII is mediated through an increase in the systemic vascular resistance since cardiac output decreases (Le Mével et al., 1996). In mammals including humans, a great amount of heterogeneity of vasoactive responses to UII has been observed among vascular beds from species, as well as different regions within the same species (Douglas et al., 2000). The physiological relevance of our experiments may be questioned since the concentration of the injected peptides within the circulation might be more pharmacological than physiological. Consequently, it remains to be determined if physiological plasma concentration of UII may have a role in the cardiovascular regulation in teleosts. In the present study, the highest doses of UII and URP1 but not URP2 evoked cardio-ventilatory and locomotor effects similar to those observed after ICV injection of these peptides. We make the assumption that these effects were mediated through a neurogenic pathway after diffusion of these peptides to critical target sites in the brain that lack the blood-brain barrier (BBB). Some neuroanatomical and functional data favor this hypothesis. At the level of the medulla oblongata, the area postrema is devoid of BBB and acts as a circumventricular organ in the goldfish *Carassius auratus* (Morita and Finger, 1987) and in the eel *Anguilla japonica* (Tsukada et al., 2007). In eel, the organum vasculosum of the lamina terminalis is another circumventricular organ without BBB that may serve as a window for a central action of peripherally injected regulatory peptides (Mukuda et al., 2013). Of interest, this latter organ projects to the NPO. Collectively, these neuro-anatomical data in fish and mammals are consistent with the view that circulating UII, and eventually URP1 but not URP2, may act also as signaling molecules to command some neurally-mediated regulatory mechanisms and notably cardio-ventilatory but also locomotor outputs.

In mammals, the UT receptor is the only high affinity receptor for UII/URP known so far (Vaudry et al., 2015). The UT receptor in teleosts shares about 60% identity with the human UT receptor and, as previously mentioned, is strongly expressed in the caudal neurosecretory system, the CNS and in various peripheral tissues (Lu et al., 2006; Evans et al., 2011; Sun et al., 2014). However, recent data provide evidence for the existence of a vertebrate ancestral UT gene that possessed five distinct UT subtypes in teleosts (Tostivint et al., 2014). The functional role of these receptor subtypes in physiological regulations is currently unknown. It might be questioned whether the divergent physiological effects of UII and URPs after central and peripheral injection observed in the present study may be due to differential interaction with the UT receptor or binding to distinct UT receptor subtypes.

In conclusion, we have examined for the first time in fish the integrative central and peripheral physiological effects of UII, URP1 and URP2 on cardio-ventilatory and locomotor functions. The principal and novel findings of this study are that all peptides produce a central stimulatory effect on ventilation, blood pressure, heart rate and locomotion but with variable potency among peptides. Since the UII, URP1, and URP2 genes are expressed in the CNS, our results suggest that the endogenous peptides may be implicated as neurotransmitters or neuromodulators in the regulation of cardio-ventilatory and locomotor functions in trout. After systemic administration of low picomole doses, none of the UII and URP peptides affect ventilation or locomotion, but only UII evokes hypertension and bradycardia, indicating that endogenous UII may have a role as circulating hormone involved in cardiovascular regulation in trout. Further studies are clearly required to determine under which circumstances the different neuroendocrine and neuronal pathways that mediate the integrative effects of the urotensinergic system are recruited to participate in cardio-ventilatory and locomotor regulations.

Acknowledgments

We thank Stéphanie Deshayes for her excellent technical assistance and care in the maintenance of the animals. This work was supported by the European Regional Development Fund (ERDF) for the Peptide Research Network of Excellence (PeReNE).

References

Batten, T. F., Cambre, M. L., Moons, L., and Vandesande, F. (1990). Comparative distribution of neuropeptide-immunoreactive systems in the brain of the green molly, *Poecilia latipinna*. *J. Comp. Neurol.* 302, 893–919. doi: 10.1002/cne.903020416

Bern, H. A., and Lederis, K. (1969). A reference preparation for the study of active substances in the caudal neurosecretory system of teleosts. *J. Endocrinol.* 45(Suppl.), xi–xii.

Chatenet, D., Dubessy, C., Leprince, J., Boularan, C., Carlier, L., Ségalas-Milazzo, I., et al. (2004). Structure-activity relationships and structural conformation of a novel urotensin II-related peptide. *Peptides* 25, 1819–1830. doi: 10.1016/j.peptides.2004.04.019

Conlon, J. M. (2008). Liberation of urotensin II from the teleost urophysis: an historical overview. *Peptides* 29, 651–657. doi: 10.1016/j.peptides.2007.04.021

Demski, L. S., and Sloan, H. E. (1985). A direct magnocellular-preopticospinal pathway in goldfish: implications for control of sex behavior. *Neurosci. Lett.* 55, 283–288. doi: 10.1016/0304-3940(85)90449-5

Do-Rego, J. C., Chatenet, D., Orta, M. H., Naudin, B., Le Cudennec, C., Leprince, J., et al. (2005). Behavioral effects of urotensin-II centrally administered in mice. *Psychopharmacology (Berl.)* 183, 103–117. doi: 10.1007/s00213-005-0140-2

Douglas, S. A., Sulpizio, A. C., Piercy, V., Sarau, H. M., Ames, R. S., Aiyar, N. V., et al. (2000). Differential vasoconstrictor activity of human urotensin-II in vascular tissue isolated from the rat, mouse, dog, pig, marmoset and cynomolgus monkey. *Br. J. Pharmacol.* 131, 1262–1274. doi: 10.1038/sj.bjp.0703690

Dubessy, C., Cartier, D., Lectez, B., Bucharles, C., Chartrel, N., Montero-Hadjadje, M., et al. (2008). Characterization of urotensin II, distribution of urotensin II, urotensin II-related peptide and UT receptor mRNAs in mouse: evidence of urotensin II at the neuromuscular junction. *J. Neurochem.* 107, 361–374. doi: 10.1111/j.1471-4159.2008.05624.x

Evans, D. H., Hyndman, K. A., Cornwell, E., and Buchanan, P. (2011). Urotensin II and its receptor in the killifish gill: regulators of NaCl extrusion. *J. Exp. Biol.* 214(Pt 23), 3985–3991. doi: 10.1242/jeb.065243

Gartlon, J., Parker, F., Harrison, D. C., Douglas, S. A., Ashmeade, T. E., Riley, G. J., et al. (2001). Central effects of urotensin-II following ICV administration in rats. *Psychopharmacology (Berl.)* 155, 426–433. doi: 10.1007/s002130100715

Gregory, W. A., and Tweedle, C. D. (1985). Horseradish peroxidase evidence for a spinal projection from the preoptic area of the goldfish, a light and electron microscopic study. *Brain Res.* 341, 82–91. doi: 10.1016/0006-8993(85)91475-1

Hood, S. G., Watson, A. M., and May, C. N. (2005). Cardiac actions of central but not peripheral urotensin II are prevented by beta-adrenoceptor blockade. *Peptides* 26, 1248–1256. doi: 10.1016/j.peptides.2005.01.005

Lancien, F., Leprince, J., Mimassi, N., Mabin, D., Vaudry, H., and Le Mével, J. C. (2004). Central effects of native urotensin II on motor activity, ventilatory movements, and heart rate in the trout *Oncorhynchus mykiss*. *Brain Res.* 1023, 167–174. doi: 10.1016/j.brainres.2004.07.008

Lancien, F., Leprince, J., Mimassi, N., Mabin, D., Vaudry, H., and Le Mével, J. C. (2005). Time-course effects of centrally administered native urotensin-II on motor and cardioventilatory activity in trout. *Ann. N.Y. Acad. Sci.* 1040, 371–374. doi: 10.1196/annals.1327.065

Le Mével, J. C., Lancien, F., Mimassi, N., and Conlon, J. M. (2007). Ventilatory and cardiovascular actions of centrally administered trout tachykinins in the unanesthetized trout. *J. Exp. Biol.* 210(Pt 18), 3301–3310. doi: 10.1242/jeb.006106

Le Mével, J. C., Lancien, F., Mimassi, N., and Conlon, J. M. (2009). Central hyperventilatory action of the stress-related neurohormonal peptides, corticotropin-releasing factor and urotensin-I in the trout *Oncorhynchus mykiss*. *Gen. Comp. Endocrinol.* 164, 51–60. doi: 10.1016/j.ygcen.2009.03.019

Le Mével, J. C., Lancien, F., Mimassi, N., and Conlon, J. M. (2012). Brain neuropeptides in central ventilatory and cardiovascular regulation in trout. *Front. Endocrinol.* 3:124. doi: 10.3389/fendo.2012.00124

Le Mével, J. C., Lancien, F., Mimassi, N., Leprince, J., Conlon, J. M., and Vaudry, H. (2008). Central and peripheral cardiovascular, ventilatory, and motor effects of trout urotensin-II in the trout. *Peptides* 29, 830–837. doi: 10.1016/j.peptides.2007.06.020

Le Mével, J. C., Olson, K. R., Conklin, D., Waugh, D., Smith, D. D., Vaudry, H., et al. (1996). Cardiovascular actions of trout urotensin II in the conscious trout, *Oncorhynchus mykiss*. *Am. J. Physiol.* 271, R1335–R1343.

Le Mével, J. C., Pamantung, T. F., Mabin, D., and Vaudry, H. (1993). Effects of central and peripheral administration of arginine vasotocin and related neuropeptides on blood pressure and heart rate in the conscious trout. *Brain Res.* 610, 82–89. doi: 10.1016/0006-8993(93)91220-M

Lihrmann, I., Tostivint, H., Bern, H., and Vaudry, H. (2013). "Urotensin II peptides," in *Handbook of Biologically Active Peptides, 2nd Edn.*, eds A. J. Kastin (New York, NY: Academic Press), 957–965.

Lin, Y., Tsuchihashi, T., Matsumura, K., Abe, I., and Iida, M. (2003a). Central cardiovascular action of urotensin II in conscious rats. *J. Hypertens.* 21, 159–165. doi: 10.1097/00004872-200301000-00026

Lin, Y., Tsuchihashi, T., Matsumura, K., Fukuhara, M., Ohya, Y., Fujii, K., et al. (2003b). Central cardiovascular action of urotensin II in spontaneously hypertensive rats. *Hypertens. Res.* 26, 839–845. doi: 10.1291/hypres.26.839

Lu, W., Greenwood, M., Dow, L., Yuill, J., Worthington, J., Brierley, M. J., et al. (2006). Molecular characterization and expression of urotensin II and its receptor in the flounder (*Platichthys flesus*): a hormone system supporting body fluid homeostasis in euryhaline fish. *Endocrinology* 147, 3692–3708. doi: 10.1210/en.2005-1457

Lu, Y., Zou, C. J., Huang, D. W., and Tang, C. S. (2002). Cardiovascular effects of urotensin II in different brain areas. *Peptides* 23, 1631–1635. doi: 10.1016/S0196-9781(02)00104-3

Marshall, W. S., and Bern, H. A. (1979). Teleostean urophysis: urotensin II and ion transport across the isolated skin of a marine teleost. *Science* 204, 519–521. doi: 10.1126/science.432657

Morita, Y., and Finger, T. E. (1987). Area postrema of the goldfish, *Carassius auratus*: ultrastructure, fiber connections, and immunocytochemistry. *J. Comp. Neurol.* 256, 104–116. doi: 10.1002/cne.902560109

Mukuda, T., Hamasaki, S., Koyama, Y., Takei, Y., Kaidoh, T., and Inoue, T. (2013). A candidate of organum vasculosum of the lamina terminalis with neuronal connections to neurosecretory preoptic nucleus in eels. *Cell Tissue Res.* 353, 525–538. doi: 10.1007/s00441-013-1663-1

Nobata, S., Donald, J. A., Balment, R. J., and Takei, Y. (2011). Potent cardiovascular effects of homologous urotensin II (UII)-related peptide and UII in unanesthetized eels after peripheral and central injections. *Am. J. Physiol. Regul. Integr. Comp. Physiol.* 300, R437–R446. doi: 10.1152/ajpregu.00629.2010

Parmentier, C., Hameury, E., Dubessy, C., Quan, F. B., Habert, D., Calas, A., et al. (2011). Occurrence of two distinct urotensin II-related peptides in zebrafish provides new insight into the evolutionary history of the urotensin II gene family. *Endocrinology* 152, 2330–2341. doi: 10.1210/en.2010-1500

Parmentier, C., Hameury, E., Lihrmann, I., Taxi, J., Hardin-Pouzet, H., Vaudry, H., et al. (2008). Comparative distribution of the mRNAs encoding urotensin I and urotensin II in zebrafish. *Peptides* 29, 820–829. doi: 10.1016/j.peptides.2008.01.023

Pearson, D., Shively, J. E., Clark, B. R., Geschwind, I. I., Barkley, M., Nishioka, R. S., et al. (1980). Urotensin II: a somatostatin-like peptide in the caudal neurosecretory system of fishes. *Proc. Natl. Acad. Sci. U.S.A.* 77, 5021–5024. doi: 10.1073/pnas.77.8.5021

Quan, F. B., Bougerol, M., Rigour, F., Kenigfest, N. B., and Tostivint, H. (2012). Characterization of the true ortholog of the urotensin II-related peptide (URP) gene in teleosts. *Gen. Comp. Endocrinol.* 177, 205–212. doi: 10.1016/j.ygcen.2012.02.018

Quan, F. B., Dubessy, C., Galant, S., Kenigfest, N. B., Djenoune, L., Leprince, L., et al. (2015). Comparative distribution and *in vitro* activities of the urotensin II-related peptides URP1 and URP2 in zebrafish: evidence for their colocalization in spinal cerebrospinal fluid-contacting neurons. *PLoS ONE* 10:e0119290. doi: 10.1371/journal.pone.0119290

Saito, D., Komatsuda, M., and Urano, A. (2004). Functional organization of preoptic vasotocin and isotocin neurons in the brain of rainbow trout: central and neurohypophysial projections of single neurons. *Neuroscience* 124, 973–984. doi: 10.1016/j.neuroscience.2003.12.038

Sugo, T., Murakami, Y., Shimomura, Y., Harada, M., Abe, M., Ishibashi, Y., et al. (2003). Identification of urotensin II-related peptide as the urotensin II-immunoreactive molecule in the rat brain. *Biochem. Biophys. Res. Commun.* 310, 860–868. doi: 10.1016/j.bbrc.2003.09.102

Sun, C., Duan, D., Li, B., Qin, C., Jia, J., Wang, B., et al. (2014). UII and UT in grouper: cloning and effects on the transcription of hormones related to growth control. *J. Endocrinol.* 220, 35–48. doi: 10.1530/JOE-13-0282

Tostivint, H., Ocampo Daza, D., Bergqvist, C. A., Quan, F. B., Bougerol, M., Lihrmann, I., et al. (2014). Molecular evolution of GPCRs: somatostatin/urotensin II receptors. *J. Mol. Endocrinol.* 52, T61–T86. doi: 10.1530/JME-13-0274

Tostivint, H., Quan, F. B., Bougerol, M., Kenigfest, N. B., and Lihrmann, I. (2013). Impact of gene/genome duplications on the evolution of the urotensin II and somatostatin families. *Gen. Comp. Endocrinol.* 188, 110–117. doi: 10.1016/j.ygcen.2012.12.015

Tsukada, T., Nobata, S., Hyodo, S., and Takei, Y. (2007). Area postrema, a brain circumventricular organ, is the site of antidipsogenic action of circulating atrial natriuretic peptide in eels. *J. Exp. Biol.* 210(Pt 22), 3970–3978. doi: 10.1242/jeb.010645

Vaudry, H., Do Rego, J. C., Le Mével, J. C., Chatenet, D., Tostivint, H., Fournier, A., et al. (2010). Urotensin II, from fish to human. *Ann. N.Y. Acad. Sci.* 1200, 53–66. doi: 10.1111/j.1749-6632.2010.05514.x

Vaudry, H., Leprince, J., Chatenet, D., Fournier, A., Lambert, D. G., Le Mével, J. C., et al. (2015). International Union of Basic and Clinical Pharmacology. XCII. Urotensin II, Urotensin II–related peptide and their receptor: from structure to function. *Pharmacol. Rev.* 67, 214–258. doi: 10.1124/pr.114.009480

Watson, A. M., and May, C. N. (2004). Urotensin II, a novel peptide in central and peripheral cardiovascular control. *Peptides* 25, 1759–1766. doi: 10.1016/j.peptides.2004.04.016

Waugh, D., and Conlon, J. M. (1993). Purification and characterization of urotensin II from the brain of a teleost (trout, *Oncorhynchus mykiss*) and an elasmobranch (skate, *Raja rhina*). *Gen. Comp. Endocrinol.* 92, 419–427. doi: 10.1006/gcen.1993.1178

Yulis, C. R., and Lederis, K. (1986). Extraurophyseal distribution of urotensin II immunoreactive neuronal perikarya and their processes. *Proc. Natl. Acad. Sci. U.S.A.* 83, 7079–7083. doi: 10.1073/pnas.83.18.7079

Yulis, C. R., and Lederis, K. (1988). Occurrence of an anterior spinal, cerebrospinal fluid-contacting, urotensin II neuronal system in various fish species. *Gen. Comp. Endocrinol.* 70, 301–311. doi: 10.1016/0016-6480(88)90150-5

3

Endocrine disrupting chemicals: Effects on endocrine glands

Rosa Lauretta[1], *Andrea Sansone*[2], *Massimiliano Sansone*[2], *Francesco Romanelli*[2] *and Marialuisa Appetecchia*[1*]

[1] Endocrinology Unit, IRCCS Regina Elena National Cancer Institute, Rome, Italy, [2] Section of Medical Pathophysiology, Food Science and Endocrinology, Department of Experimental Medicine, Sapienza Università di Roma, Rome, Italy

Edited by:
Justo P. Castaño,
Instituto Maimonides de Investigación Biomédica de Cordoba (IMIBIC), Spain

Reviewed by:
James M. Olcese,
Florida State University, United States
Csaba Fekete,
Institute of Experimental Medicine (MTA), Hungary

***Correspondence:**
Marialuisa Appetecchia
marialuisa.appetecchia@ifo.gov.it

In recent years, endocrine disrupting chemicals have gained interest in human physiopathology and more and more studies aimed to explain how these chemicals compounds affect endocrine system. In human populations, the majority of the studies point toward an association between exposure to endocrine disrupting chemicals and the disorders affecting endocrine axis. A great number of endocrine disrupting chemicals seem to be able to interfere with the physiology of hypothalamus-pituitary-gonadal axis; however, every endocrine axis may be a target for each EDCs and their action is not limited to a single axis or organ. Several compounds may also have a negative impact on energy metabolic homeostasis altering adipose tissue and promoting obesity, metabolic syndrome, and diabetes. Different mechanism have been proposed to explain these associations but their complexity together with the degree of occupational or environmental exposure, the low standardization of the studies, and the presence of confounding factors have prevented to establish causal relationship between the endocrine disorders and exposure to specific toxicants so far. This manuscript aims to review the state of art of scientific literature regarding the effects of endocrine-disrupting chemicals (EDCs) on endocrine system.

Keywords: endocrine disruptors, hormones, endocrine system, thyroid, ovary, testis, adrenal gland, pituitary gland

BACKGROUND

In the last years, scientific literature has ever-increasingly focused on the role of endocrine-disrupting chemicals (EDCs) in human pathophysiology. A growing body of evidence, including reviews, clinical trials, and reports highlight new roles and effects of EDCs. EDCs are defined as "exogenous chemicals or mixture of chemicals that interfere with any aspect of hormone action" (1, 2). According to US Environmental Protection Agency (EPA), an EDC is an exogenous compound that may interfere with synthesis, secretion, transport, metabolism, receptor binding or elimination of endogenous hormones, altering the endocrine and homeostatic systems (3–8). In the process of defining EDCs criteria proposed by European Commission, it seems clear that EDCs should exhibit three actions: (1) endocrine activity; (2) deleterious and/or pathologic endocrine mediated-activity; (3) cause-effect relationship between substance and endocrine activity in exposed subjects (9, 10). Furthermore, European Food Safety Authority (EFSA) suggests that the most of EDCs are artificial substances that interfere with endocrine system binding hormonal receptors and/or regulating genomic expression (11). Indeed, epigenetic changes, such as DNA methylation and/or acetylation and histone modifications, appear to be involved in mechanisms related to endocrine disruption (2, 11, 12).

According to their origin, EDCs can be grouped as follows: industrial [i.e., dioxins, polychlorinated biphenyls (PCBs), and alkylphenols], agricultural (i.e., pesticides, insecticide, herbicides, phytoestrogens, fungicides), residential (phthalates, polybrominated biphenyls, bisphenol A), pharmaceutical (parabens) (5, 7, 13). Even heavy metals such as cadmium, lead, mercury, and arsenic may be included in the long list of EDCs (5, 14).

EDCs may display different routes to contaminate human body. Generally, inhalation, food intake and direct contact represent the most common exposure pathways (2, 7, 15). According to these pathways, EDCs may enter the food chain and accumulate in animal tissues up to humans (15). Most EDCs appear to be highly lipophilic, therefore accumulating in the adipose tissue—hence their generally long half-life (2, 16, 17). These two features explain the reasons why EDCs are able to accumulate for years in the adipose tissue of any animal, making co-contamination very frequent (18). Humans and other big mammals and top predators are at the top of food chain, therefore they may store larger doses of EDCs according to the process of bioaccumulation and bioamplification. These processes may generate a "cocktail" of effects with unknown consequences (19). Indeed, lifelong exposure to multiple compounds may bring about cumulative, additive and/or synergic effects. Dose-effect relationships can be complex for many EDCs causing diverging effects at different concentrations; moreover, different EDCs exert non-traditional responses to the dose due to the different action they can have in the binding of hormone receptors (1, 2, 4, 7, 18). Last but not least, the complexity of the hazardous effects of EDCs includes the concept of windows of vulnerability; indeed, evidence shows that the timing of exposure is of primary importance in the assessment of the effects on the endocrine system (1, 4, 7, 14, 18, 20).

Professional workers using pesticides, fungicides, and chemicals are at high risk of exposure to EDCs. Since 1996, the EPA has been constantly developing and promoting the Endocrine Disruption Screening Program (EDSP), which aims to: (1) develop protocols to research accurate, efficient and reproducible detection methods; (2) establish a priority regarding the substances to be studied; (3) assess practical guidelines in order to discriminate the correct detection test for any exposure condition (1, 2, 21).

ENDOCRINE ASPECTS OF EDCs

The most documented mechanism in which EDCs act is represented by their ability to bind endocrine nuclear receptors (NRs) acting as total, partial, or inverted agonists or as antagonists (2–5). In particular, EDCs can bind to and activate various hormone receptors (androgen receptor, estrogen receptor, aryl hydrocarbon receptor, pregnane X receptor, constitutive androstane receptor, estrogen-related receptor, glucocorticoid receptor, thyroid hormone receptor, retinoid X receptor—AR, ER, AhR, PXR, CAR, ERR, GR, TR, RXR) and then mimic the natural hormone's action (3, 4, 13, 15). In some cases the same substance may activate certain receptor isoforms (i.e., agonist) and block other isoforms (i.e., antagonist), similarly to selective estrogen receptor modulators (SERM) behavior (14). Finally, EDCs may also interfere with the synthesis, transport, metabolism, and elimination of hormones, thereby decreasing the concentration of endogenous hormones (1, 3, 5). Furthermore, it should be considered that EDCs are able to affect endocrine system with addictive or synergistic effects as well. A specific EDCs may be innocuous *per se*, but its association with other EDCs may result in hazardous effects (i.e., cocktail effect) (6, 15, 18). The complexity of mixture toxicity, their interaction, and the presence of sensitive time windows make the risk assessment process extremely complex (7, 18, 22, 23). Every endocrine axis may be a target for each EDCs; their action is not limited to a single axis or organ but it is now clear that hypothalamus-pituitary gland-thyroid (HPT), hypothalamus-pituitary gland-gonads (HPG), hypothalamus-pituitary gland-adrenal (HPA) represent the main targets of EDCs (2, 7). Nevertheless, evidence shows that some EDCs may affect central nervous system (CNS) impairing hypothalamic and pituitary functions, therefore disrupting the proper actions of peripheral glands with unclear effects (2, 5, 7). Recent evidence shows that EDCs may disrupt energy metabolic homeostasis altering adipose tissue (increase in number and size of adipose cells), impairing endocrine regulation of adipose tissue and adipocytokine production, reducing basal metabolic rate and changing the regulation of appetite and satiety (24). This happens especially if the exposure occurs during early development. These chemicals, called "obesogens," could predispose some people to weight gain despite following a low caloric diet and increasing physical activity (4, 16, 25). For example, Diethylstilbestrol (DES) is an estrogenic chemical binding with high affinity to both ERα and ERβ which plays an important role in adiposity regulation as well as central and peripheral energy balance. Developmental exposure to DES in mice induces adipogenesis and causes mice to become obese or overweight (2, 16). Indeed, the onset of many chronic metabolic diseases, such as obesity, diabetes, hypertension, and dyslipidemia may be accelerated by chronic, low-dose exposures that characterize human contact with environmental toxicants and their interactions (2, 16, 17). Recent data point out that exposure to EDCs during development can not only cause direct damage to the exposed individual, but also to the individual's offspring and to future generations—a process that is called transgenerational inheritance. From these evidences a new paradigm for non-communicable disease has been postulated: the evolutionary origins of health and disease (DOHaD).

Recent evidence has shown in several mammals, including humans, how EDCs can influence behavior and how this interaction is different in both sexes. There were differences in males and females after exposure to BPA *in utero* and early postnatal life. Recent literature has shown that chromosomal sex is a fundamental variable in accounting for the effects of BPA on behavior. Several studies have confirmed the ability of BPA and other EDCs to influence rodent brain development in a gender-specific way, even at very low doses, altering the normal steroidegenesis programmed in the two sexes through epigenetic alterations that can lead to differential gene expression (26).

Even in human epidemiological studies, it appears that BPA has specific effects on both sexes. Prenatal BPA levels are positively associated with an increase in externalizing behaviors in girls, against greater internalizing behavior, anxiety, and aggression in boys. Because several neuropsychiatric disorders show a gender-specific incidence, it is important to understand how hormones and other substances modify neurobehavioral dimorphisms.

PITUITARY GLAND

The diencephalic system represents a preferential target of EDCs, which may alter proper function of CNS mimicking neurotransmitter actions, beside their ability to bind endocrine receptors (27). Several EDCs act on the pituitary gland, therefore influencing the different endocrine axes: as a result, a wide spectrum of clinical manifestations has been associated with exposure to pollutants, such as precocious/delayed puberty (28) and circadian disruption (29).

REPRODUCTIVE SYSTEM

As the chemical structure of most of EDCs mimics sex gonadal hormones and has the ability to bind to endocrine receptors interfering with hormonal signals, reproductive system represents the most vulnerable endocrine axis to EDCs actions (13). The US EPA described five classes of EDCs endowed with anti-androgenic properties and, simultaneously, with weak estrogenic activity: (1) drugs or synthetic estrogens (i.e., 17 β estradiol, diethylstilbestrol), (2) phytoestrogens (i.e., isoflavonoids, cumestans, lignans, stilbens), (3) pesticides (i.e., organophosphates, carbamates, organochlorines, synthetic pyrethroids); (4) plasticizers and chemicals produced by incomplete combustion of polyvinyl chloride (PVC), paper and putrescible substances (i.e., dioxin); (5) industrial substances and their by-products (i.e., phenols, dioxins, heavy metals, perfluorooctanoic acid, flames retardants) (30, 31).

The timing of EDC exposure should be considered when assessing their effects on the organism; especially in the initial stages of development, when the mammalian organism is extremely sensitive to disturbing agents, exposure might have more pronounced and long-lasting effects (3, 14, 16, 20, 22, 32). It is therefore unsurprising that prenatal exposure may result in significant changes. The effects of EDC on ovarian development have mainly been investigated using animal models or *in vitro* systems. Collectively, the collected data in the literature have shown that some EDC exposures damage the developing ovary by interfering with germ cell nest destruction, meiosis, follicle formation and vitality (11, 16, 22, 32). Early postnatal exposure to EDCs may results in significant changes in genetic transcription of somatic cells, altering the proper timing of physiological process of puberty which may be delayed or anticipated (4). Furthermore, EDCs appears to have a consistent role in decreasing both male and female fertility; testicular hypotrophy and ovarian polycystic syndrome (PCOS) seems to be associated to EDCs exposure (4, 11). In particular, EDCs seems to have a causative role in the onset of testicular dysgenesis syndrome (TDS) (1, 4, 22). Impaired spermatogenesis, testicular cancer, undescedent testis and hypospadias may be considered the symptoms of a developmental disorder, TDS, an increasing disease due to adverse environmental influences. Experimental and epidemiological studies show that TDS is the result of an interruption of physiological embryonal programming and gonadal development during fetal life (33, 34). Generally, in the most severe forms low serum testosterone is observed (35) and an increased risk of testicular cancer compared to milder forms has been highlighted (4, 36). Phthalates, vinclozolin, acetaminophen, and polybrominated diphenyl ethers (PBDE) seem to play a significant etiopathogenetic role in the onset of TDS (4, 37, 38). In female, there is little evidence regarding the effects of EDCs on fertility. Nevertheless, this data seems to suggest that long-term exposure to EDCs may alter female fertility (39). In particular, EDCs appears to have an etiopathogenetic role in the onset of endometriosis and of ovarian pathology (40). Phthalates, diethylstilbestrol, bisphenol A (BPA), TCCD may be involved in the onset of endometriosis occurring in 10% of fertile women, causing infertility in 50% of affected subjects (5, 40). Ovarian pathology seems to be related to the exposure to: PCB, phtalates, atrazine, genistein, BPA, TCDD, parabens, triclosan, dichlorodiphenyltrichloroethane (DDT), and metoxychloride (MXC) (39, 41). Even in males, reproductive function may affected by pollutants and EDCs, but evidence is scarce; EDCs, such as phthalates, bisphenol A, biphenyls, and vinclozolin, widespread use of therapeutic drugs, obesity and sedentary life-style may play a crucial role in this supposed decrease of male fertility (3–5, 38, 42).

ADRENAL GLAND

Only a few studies have assessed the effects of EDC on the adrenal gland, especially concerning the risks related to exposure to chemicals. This paucity of evidence is not easily comprehensible, considering that the proper functionality of HPA axis is necessary for human life and it is a common target for many drugs and chemicals. Indeed, adrenal glands present some structural and biochemical features that make them ideal targets for EDCs, such as an elevated blood flow, lipophilic structure due to the high content in polyunsaturated fatty acids in cell membrane, and presence of CYP 450 enzymes producing toxic metabolites and free radicals (2, 43).

The most studied effect of EDCs on this axis is represented by their ability to interfere with the biosynthesis and metabolism of steroidal hormones through the modulation or the inhibition of enzymes involved in steroidogenesis. Aromatase, 5-α reductase, as well as 3-β, 11-β, 17-β hydroxysteroid dehydrogenases have a crucial role in metabolic pathways of adrenal steroidogenesis and their proper function is affected by EDCs, in particular xenoestrogens impair adrenal function inhibiting these enzymes (7, 17). Also, Steroid Acute Regulatory Protein (StAR), which regulates the first step of adrenal steroidogenesis, is a target of EDCs (44). Hundreds of chemicals and drugs may interact with HPA axis and every step of steroidogenesis may be affected by EDCs as well as each chemical disruptor may act altering different step of steroidogenesis (45). In evaluating the pathologic effects of EDCs on HPA axis, it should be considered that even a partial impairment of proper adrenal function may have severe effects on human health. In this perspective, bioaccumulation of these chemicals in adipose tissue might generate a "cocktail," with clinical effects that may be observed only after several years of constant, low-dose exposure (17). Hexachlorobenzene is among the chemicals which is able to disrupt corticoid hormone function in Wistar rats (5, 43).

THYROID GLAND

Several environmental chemical substances are known to alter iodine absorption by inhibiting the Sodium-Iodide symporter channel (NIS): in particular, perchlorate and thiocyanate are able to affect thyroidal metabolism inhibiting NIS (7). This channel transports iodine inside thyrocytes and, considering the pivotal role played by iodine in the biosynthesis of thyroid hormones, it is comprehensible that an alteration of NIS may impair thyroid function (2). High levels of perchlorate are present in explosives, fertilizers, and in air-bags (7). A survey performed by National Health and Nutrition Examination Survey (NHAMES) 2001–2008 suggests its presence also in foods, such as milk, vegetables, fruits, eggs in USA (2). Thiocyanate is present in cigarette smoke and in Brassicaceae. Braverman et al. observed 3,100 subjects exposed to perchlorate, thiocyanate, and nitrates; this exposure resulted in a significative decrease of free thyroxine levels, which was more marked in pubertal subjects and it was not associated to increase of TSH levels. Perchlorate, thiocyanate, and nitrates are widespread and their presence is not limited to industrial products, but many foods and potable water are contaminated by these EDCs. They are able to cause a loss of function of NIS binding to NIS and blocking iodide transporter. As a consequence, a lower iodine bioavailability may results in hypothyroidism, even more if the exposure to high doses is prolonged in certain area affected by iodine deficiency. No conclusive result can be drawn from current data, but iodine supplementation in pregnancy and in children may protect from the action of these EDCs. Further studies should investigate the dose-effects relationship in these regards (46).

EDCs AND ENDOCRINE GLANDS CANCER

Several scientific institutions (European Commission, European Environmental Agency, The Endocrine Society, WHO/UNEP, IARC) studied the association between EDCs and cancer affecting testis, prostate, thyroid and breast suggesting that the exposure to some EDCs may be a risk factor in the development of these tumors (2, 47–49). Fungicides, pesticides, PDBE, organochlorides, PCB, DDT, dichlorodiphenyldichloroethylene (DDE), arsenic, and cadmium have been proposed to play a role in testicular cancer with etiopathogenetic role in the onset of TDS. Otherwise, pesticides, TCDD, PCB, and solvents appears to be involved in thyroid cancer. Several other compounds are able to impair thyroid function; among the many EDCs, biocides are worth mentioning. "Biocide" is the definition applied to any substance or mixture in the form in which it is supplied to the user, consisting of, containing or capable of generating one or more active substances, for the purpose of destroying, eliminating and rendering harmless, preventing action or exercising other control effect on any harmful organism, by any means other than mere physical or mechanical action. Zeng et al. used data from a Connecticut case-control study and examined the association with occupational exposure to biocides and pesticides. Detailed information was collected on the name of the job, the tasks performed, the name of the company and the type of industry, starting and ending dates of the subjects during their life for at least 1 year. There was a significantly increased of thyroid cancer risk associated with exposure to pesticides and biocides (OR = 1.65; IC 95% 1.16–2.35) and this risk was more marked in male adults (OR = 3.11; IC 95% 1.25–7.72) (50). PCB, dioxins, cadmium, phytoestrogens, DES, furans, ethylene oxide may contribute in the development of breast cancer. Finally arsenic, cadmium, PCB, and pesticides seem to contribute importantly to prostate carcinogenesis (5). A recent study led by Benedetti et al. investigated the incidence of these tumors in certain polluted areas in Italy (the Italian National Priority Contaminated Sites (NPCSs). A significantly higher incidence of breast and prostate cancers was observed in these areas; nevertheless, incidence of breast cancer seems to be increased in each area, whereas incidence of prostate cancer appears to increase in certain areas and to decrease in others (51). This data suggests that a wide range of chemicals may contribute to development of breast cancer whereas specific chemical may affect prostate carcinogenesis. Otherwise, the scarce number of cases of testicular and thyroid cancer make impossible to draw conclusions regarding the role of EDCs in these pathologies.

A MODEL OF ENDOCRINE DISRUPTION: AHR

As aforementioned, EDCs may bind to and activate or block several endocrine receptors (5, 52), acting as total, partial or inverted agonist or antagonist. The ability to bind AhR with its consequent effects represents a well-known action of EDCs; AhR is a cell nuclear receptor and acts as ligand-activated transcription factor that senses the presence of foreign compounds such as Persistent Organic Pollutants (POPs) and leads to the activation of cytochrome P450 enzymes needed for their clearance from the body, being involved in modulating the response to xenobiotics (xenobiotic responsive elements, XREs) (53, 54). Besides the detoxification and bioactivation of XREs, AhR has been shown to regulate expression of enzymes necessary to the metabolism of endogenous substances (i.e., hormones) and to modulate a much wider range of cellular pathways involving proliferation, differentiation, apoptosis (5). Tetrachlorodibenzo-P-dioxin (TCDD), a well-known AhR ligand, has remarkable carcinogenic activity, suggesting that AhR activation may play a role in carcinogenesis (5, 14, 52). Furthermore, AhR may be activated by several EDCs, such as PCBs, dioxins, furans, and polycyclic aromatic hydrocarbons, albeit with different potency (18, 53, 55). In absence of its ligands, AhR lies in cytoplasm assisted by a complex of co-chaperone proteins (54, 56). In particular, AhR is assisted in cytoplasm by co-chaperone AhR-interacting protein (AIP). AIP plays a pivotal role in regulating the response to XREs; as a matter of fact, its mutation brings about the loss of its function and consequently an alteration of biological pathways controlled by AhR causing an impairment in the response to XREs (53). Otherwise, in the presence of its ligands, AhR enters the nucleus and binds to its nuclear translocator, known as AhR nuclear translocator (ARNT), and to its coactivators creating a molecular complex whose function is to bind XREs activating specific target-genes (38, 54, 57). Besides the detoxification and bioactivation of XREs, AhR has been shown to regulate expression of enzymes necessary to the metabolism of endogenous substances (i.e., hormones) and to modulate a much wider range of cellular pathways involving proliferation, differentiation, apoptosis (5). The loss of function of AIP caused by its mutation showed a marked association with Familiar Isolated Pituitary Adenomas (FIPAs); in particular it has been observed that FIPAs show unfavorable response to medical therapies, greater severity and earlier age of onset (58, 59). Some evidence showed the association between EDCs and the development of FIPA, highlighting that AhR may be targeted by EDCs with mutagenic properties (55); in particular, the association between a significant exposure to dioxins, able to bind AhR, and an increased incidence of FIPA has been investigated (60). Pesatori et al. showed that the massive exposure to dioxins caused by industrial pollution due to 2,4,5 trichlorophenol explosion in a chemical factory occurred at Seveso in 1976 was not accompanied by a significative increased incidence of FIPA (14). Nevertheless, Authors reported an increased number of cases of pituitary adenomas in exposed subjects, including not familiar pituitary adenomas and prolattinoma (61). Cannavò et al. focused their attention on the prevalence of GH-secreting adenomas observing an higher prevalence of acromegaly in the most polluted areas which could not be explained by familiar or genetic causes, and suggesting that chemicals may play a role in the pathogenesis of pituitary adenoma (62, 63).

CONCLUSION

In scientific literature the hazardous effects of environmental EDCs on endocrine system and their complex mechanisms of regulation have been reported with supporting evidence. However, further long-term studies performed on wide number of subjects are necessary to verify and assess the hypothesized causal relationship between EDCs and endocrine pathology. The aim should be represented by the detection of the substance, of its mechanism of action, the explanation of relationship dose-effect clarifying the causal link between the substance and pathology. Phenomena such as bio-accumulation and trans-generational inheritance are clear obstacles to research and new strategies in these regards should be pursued.

AUTHOR CONTRIBUTIONS

All authors listed have made a substantial, direct and intellectual contribution to the work, and approved it for publication.

REFERENCES

1. Zoeller RT, Brown TR, Doan LL, Gore AC, Skakkebaek NE, Soto AM, et al. Endocrine-disrupting chemicals and public health protection: a statement of principles from The Endocrine Society. *Endocrinology.* (2012) 153:4097–110. doi: 10.1210/en.2012-1422
2. Gore AC, Chappell VA, Fenton SE, Flaws JA, Nadal A, Prins GS, et al. EDC-2: The Endocrine Society's second scientific statement on endocrine-disrupting chemicals. *Endocr Rev.* (2015) 36:E1–150. doi: 10.1210/er.2015-1093
3. Mnif W, Hassine AI, Bouaziz A, Bartegi A, Thomas O, Roig B. Effect of endocrine disruptor pesticides: a review. *Int J Environ Res Public Health.* (2011) 8:2265–303. doi: 10.3390/ijerph8062265
4. Schug TT, Janesick A, Blumberg B, Heindel JJ. Endocrine disrupting chemicals and disease susceptibility. *J Steroid Biochem Mol Biol.* (2011) 127:204–15. doi: 10.1016/j.jsbmb.2011.08.007
5. De Coster S, van Larebeke N. Endocrine-disrupting chemicals: associated disorders and mechanisms of action. *J Environ Public Health.* (2012) 2012:713696. doi: 10.1155/2012/713696
6. Nohynek GJ, Borgert CJ, Dietrich D, Rozman KK. Endocrine disruption: fact or urban legend? *Toxicol Lett.* (2013) 223:295–305. doi: 10.1016/j.toxlet.2013.10.022
7. Kabir ER, Rahman MS, Rahman I. A review on endocrine disruptors and their possible impacts on human health. *Environ Toxicol Pharmacol.* (2015) 40:241–58. doi: 10.1016/j.etap.2015.06.009
8. Kiyama R, Wada-Kiyama Y. Estrogenic endocrine disruptors: molecular mechanisms of action. *Environ Int.* (2015) 83:11–40. doi: 10.1016/j.envint.2015.05.012
9. Committee ES. Scientific Opinion on the hazard assessment of endocrine disruptors: scientific criteria for identification of endocrine disruptors and appropriateness of existing test methods for assessing effects mediated by these substances on human health and the environment. *EFSA J.* (2013) 11:3132. doi: 10.2903/j.efsa.2013.3132
10. Slama R, Bourguignon JP, Demeneix B, Ivell R, Panzica G, Kortenkamp A, et al. Scientific issues relevant to setting regulatory criteria to identify endocrine-disrupting substances in the European Union. *Environ Health Perspect.* (2016) 124:1497–503. doi: 10.1289/EHP217
11. Zama AM, Uzumcu M. Epigenetic effects of endocrine-disrupting chemicals on female reproduction: an ovarian perspective. *Front Neuroendocrinol.* (2010) 31:420–39. doi: 10.1016/j.yfrne.2010.06.003
12. Baldi F, Mantovani A. A new database for food safety: EDID (Endocrine disrupting chemicals - Diet Interaction Database). *Ann Ist Super Sanita.* (2008) 44:57–63. doi: 10.1016/j.reprotox.2008.05.005
13. Monneret C. What is an endocrine disruptor? *C R Biol.* (2017) 340:403–5. doi: 10.1016/j.crvi.2017.07.004
14. Lubrano C, Genovesi G, Specchia P, Costantini D, Mariani S, Petrangeli E, et al. Obesity and metabolic comorbidities: environmental diseases? *Oxid Med Cell Longev.* (2013) 2013:640673. doi: 10.1155/2013/640673
15. Balaguer P, Delfosse V, Grimaldi M, Bourguet W. Structural and functional evidences for the interactions between nuclear hormone receptors and endocrine disruptors at low doses. *C R Biol.* (2017) 340:414–20. doi: 10.1016/j.crvi.2017.08.002
16. Heindel JJ, Newbold R, Schug TT. Endocrine disruptors and obesity. *Nat Rev Endocrinol.* (2015) 11:653–61. doi: 10.1038/nrendo.2015.163
17. Sargis RM. Metabolic disruption in context: clinical avenues for synergistic perturbations in energy homeostasis by endocrine disrupting chemicals. *Endocr Disruptors.* (2015) 3:e1080788. doi: 10.1080/23273747.2015.1080788
18. Barouki R. Endocrine disruptors: revisiting concepts and dogma in toxicology. *C R Biol.* (2017) 340:410–3. doi: 10.1016/j.crvi.2017.07.005
19. Zhang X, Ho SM. Epigenetics meets endocrinology. *J Mol Endocrinol.* (2011) 46:R11–32. doi: 10.1677/JME-10-0053

20. Unuvar T, Buyukgebiz A. Fetal and neonatal endocrine disruptors. *J Clin Res Pediatr Endocrinol.* (2012) 4:51–60. doi: 10.4274/Jcrpe.569
21. Marty S. Introduction to "screening for endocrine activity-experiences with the US EPA's endocrine disruptor screening program and future considerations". *Birth Defects Res B Dev Reprod Toxicol.* (2014) 101:1–2. doi: 10.1002/bdrb.21100
22. Campion S, Catlin N, Heger N, McDonnell EV, Pacheco SE, Saffarini C, et al. Male reprotoxicity and endocrine disruption. *Exp Suppl.* (2012) 101:315–60. doi: 10.1007/978-3-7643-8340-4_11
23. Fenichel P, Chevalier N. Environmental endocrine disruptors: new diabetogens? *C R Biol.* (2017) 340:446–52. doi: 10.1016/j.crvi.2017.07.003
24. Street ME, Angelini S. Current knowledge on Endocrine Disrupting Chemicals (EDCs) from animal biology to humans, from pregnancy to adulthood: highlights from a National Italian Meeting. *Int J Mol Sci.* (2018) 19:E1647. doi: 10.3390/ijms19061647
25. Janesick AS, Blumberg B. Obesogens: an emerging threat to public health. *Am J Obstet Gynecol.* (2016) 214:559–65. doi: 10.1016/j.ajog.2016.01.182
26. Masuo Y, Ishido M. Neurotoxicity of endocrine disruptors: possible involvement in brain development and neurodegeneration. *J Toxicol Environ Health B Crit Rev.* (2011) 14:346–69. doi: 10.1080/10937404.2011.578557
27. Gore AC. Neuroendocrine targets of endocrine disruptors. *Hormones.* (2010) 9:16–27. doi: 10.14310/horm.2002.1249
28. Soriano-Guillén L, Argente J. Central precocious puberty, functional and tumor-related. *Best Pract Res Clin Endocrinol Metab.* (2019) doi: 10.1016/j.beem.2019.01.003. [Epub ahead of print].
29. Sen A, Sellix MT. The circadian timing system and environmental circadian disruption: from follicles to fertility. *Endocrinology.* (2016) 157:3366–73. doi: 10.1210/en.2016-1450
30. Harding AK, Daston GP, Boyd GR, Lucier GW, Safe SH, Stewart J, et al. Endocrine disrupting chemicals research program of the U.S. Environmental Protection Agency: summary of a peer-review report. *Environ Health Perspect.* (2006) 114:1276–82. doi: 10.1289/ehp.8875
31. Browne P, Noyes PD, Casey WM, Dix DJ. Application of adverse outcome pathways to U.S. EPA's endocrine disruptor screening program. *Environ Health Perspect.* (2017) 125:096001. doi: 10.1289/EHP1304
32. Sweeney MF, Hasan N, Soto AM, Sonnenschein C. Environmental endocrine disruptors: effects on the human male reproductive system. *Rev Endocr Metab Disord.* (2015) 16:341–57. doi: 10.1007/s11154-016-9337-4
33. Skakkebaek NE, Rajpert-De Meyts E, Main KM. Testicular dysgenesis syndrome: an increasingly common developmental disorder with environmental aspects. *Hum Reprod.* (2001) 16:972–8. doi: 10.1093/humrep/16.5.972
34. Virtanen HE, Rajpert-De Meyts E, Main KM, Skakkebaek NE, Toppari J. Testicular dysgenesis syndrome and the development and occurrence of male reproductive disorders. *Toxicol Appl Pharmacol.* (2005) 207:501–5. doi: 10.1016/j.taap.2005.01.058
35. Wohlfahrt-Veje C, Main KM, Skakkebaek NE. Testicular dysgenesis syndrome: foetal origin of adult reproductive problems. *Clin Endocrinol.* (2009) 71:459–65. doi: 10.1111/j.1365-2265.2009.03545.x
36. Skakkebaek NE, Holm M, Hoei-Hansen C, Jorgensen N, Rajpert-De Meyts E. Association between testicular dysgenesis syndrome (TDS) and testicular neoplasia: evidence from 20 adult patients with signs of maldevelopment of the testis. *Apmis.* (2003) 111:1–9. doi: 10.1034/j.1600-0463.2003.11101031.x
37. Cook MB, Trabert B, McGlynn KA. Organochlorine compounds and testicular dysgenesis syndrome: human data. *Int J Androl.* (2011) 34(Pt. 2):e68–84. doi: 10.1111/j.1365-2605.2011.01171.x
38. Anawalt BD. The silent spermatozoon: are man-made endocrine disruptors killing male fertility? *Asian J Androl.* (2013) 15:165–8. doi: 10.1038/aja.2012.148
39. Minguez-Alarcon L, Gaskins AJ. Female exposure to endocrine disrupting chemicals and fecundity: a review. *Curr Opin Obstet Gynecol.* (2017) 29:202–11. doi: 10.1097/GCO.0000000000000373
40. Caserta D, Bordi G, Ciardo F, Marci R, La Rocca C, Tait S, et al. The influence of endocrine disruptors in a selected population of infertile women. *Gynecol Endocrinol.* (2013) 29:444–7. doi: 10.3109/09513590.2012.758702
41. Marques-Pinto A, Carvalho D. Human infertility: are endocrine disruptors to blame? *Endocr Connect.* (2013) 2:R15–29. doi: 10.1530/EC-13-0036
42. Handelsman DJ, Cooper TG. Falling sperm counts and global estrogenic pollution: what have we learned over 20 years? *Asian J Androl.* (2013) 15:159–61. doi: 10.1038/aja.2013.8
43. Harvey PW. Adrenocortical endocrine disruption. *J Steroid Biochem Mol Biol.* (2016) 155(Pt. B):199–206. doi: 10.1016/j.jsbmb.2014.10.009
44. Hampl R, Kubatova J, Starka L. Steroids and endocrine disruptors–history, recent state of art and open questions. *J Steroid Biochem Mol Biol.* (2016) 155(Pt. B):217–23. doi: 10.1016/j.jsbmb.2014.04.013
45. Martinez-Arguelles DB, Papadopoulos V. Mechanisms mediating environmental chemical-induced endocrine disruption in the adrenal gland. *Front Endocrinol.* (2015) 6:29. doi: 10.3389/fendo.2015.00029
46. Braverman LE, He X, Pino S, Cross M, Magnani B, Lamm SH, et al. The effect of perchlorate, thiocyanate, and nitrate on thyroid function in workers exposed to perchlorate long-term. *J Clin Endocrinol Metab.* (2005) 90:700–6. doi: 10.1210/jc.2004-1821
47. Lamb JC IV, Boffetta P, Foster WG, Goodman JE, Hentz KL, Rhomberg LR, et al. Critical comments on the WHO-UNEP State of the Science of Endocrine Disrupting Chemicals - 2012. *Regul Toxicol Pharmacol.* (2014) 69:22–40. doi: 10.1016/j.yrtph.2014.02.002
48. Trasande L, Zoeller RT, Hass U, Kortenkamp A, Grandjean P, Myers JP, et al. Burden of disease and costs of exposure to endocrine disrupting chemicals in the European Union: an updated analysis. *Andrology.* (2016) 4:565–72. doi: 10.1111/andr.12178
49. Watson R. European Commission tables scientific criteria for endocrine disruptors. *BMJ.* (2016) 353:i3459. doi: 10.1136/bmj.i3459
50. Zeng F, Lerro C, Lavoue J, Huang H, Siemiatycki J, Zhao N, et al. Occupational exposure to pesticides and other biocides and risk of thyroid cancer. *Occup Environ Med.* (2017) 74:502–10. doi: 10.1136/oemed-2016-103931
51. Benedetti M, Zona A, Beccaloni E, Carere M, Comba P. Incidence of breast, prostate, testicular, and thyroid cancer in Italian contaminated sites with presence of substances with endocrine disrupting properties. *Int J Environ Res Public Health.* (2017) 14:E355. doi: 10.3390/ijerph14040355
52. Kim JT, Lee HK. Childhood obesity and endocrine disrupting chemicals. *Ann Pediatr Endocrinol Metab.* (2017) 22:219–25. doi: 10.6065/apem.2017.22.4.219
53. Fujii-Kuriyama Y, Kawajiri K. Molecular mechanisms of the physiological functions of the aryl hydrocarbon (dioxin) receptor, a multifunctional regulator that senses and responds to environmental stimuli. *Proc Jpn Acad Ser B Phys Biol Sci.* (2010) 86:40–53. doi: 10.2183/pjab.86.40
54. Mackowiak B, Wang H. Mechanisms of xenobiotic receptor activation: direct vs. indirect. *Biochim Biophys Acta.* (2016) 1859:1130–40. doi: 10.1016/j.bbagrm.2016.02.006
55. Daly AF, Vanbellinghen JF, Khoo SK, Jaffrain-Rea ML, Naves LA, Guitelman MA, et al. Aryl hydrocarbon receptor-interacting protein gene mutations in familial isolated pituitary adenomas: analysis in 73 families. *J Clin Endocrinol Metab.* (2007) 92:1891–6. doi: 10.1210/jc.2006-2513
56. Swedenborg E, Ruegg J, Makela S, Pongratz I. Endocrine disruptive chemicals: mechanisms of action and involvement in metabolic disorders. *J Mol Endocrinol.* (2009) 43:1–10. doi: 10.1677/JME-08-0132
57. Cannavo S, Trimarchi F, Ferrau F. Acromegaly, genetic variants of the aryl hydrocarbon receptor pathway and environmental burden. *Mol Cell Endocrinol.* (2017) 457:81–8. doi: 10.1016/j.mce.2016.12.019
58. Jennings JE, Georgitsi M, Holdaway I, Daly AF, Tichomirowa M, Beckers A, et al. Aggressive pituitary adenomas occurring in young patients in a large Polynesian kindred with a germline R271W mutation in the AIP gene. *Eur J Endocrinol.* (2009) 161:799–804. doi: 10.1530/EJE-09-0406
59. Beckers A, Aaltonen LA, Daly AF, Karhu A. Familial isolated pituitary adenomas (FIPA) and the pituitary adenoma predisposition due to mutations in the aryl hydrocarbon receptor interacting protein (AIP) gene. *Endocr Rev.* (2013) 34:239–77. doi: 10.1210/er.2012-1013
60. Lloyd C, Grossman A. The AIP (aryl hydrocarbon receptor-interacting protein) gene and its relation to the pathogenesis of pituitary adenomas. *Endocrine.* (2014) 46:387–96. doi: 10.1007/s12020-013-0125-6
61. Pesatori AC, Baccarelli A, Consonni D, Lania A, Beck-Peccoz P, Bertazzi PA, et al. Aryl hydrocarbon receptor-interacting protein and pituitary adenomas:

a population-based study on subjects exposed to dioxin after the Seveso, Italy, accident. *Eur J Endocrinol.* (2008) 159:699–703. doi: 10.1530/EJE-08-0593
62. Cannavò S, Ferrau F, Ragonese M, Curto L, Torre ML, Magistri M, et al. Increased prevalence of acromegaly in a highly polluted area. *Eur J Endocrinol.* (2010) 163:509–13. doi: 10.1530/EJE-10-0465
63. Cannavò S, Ragonese M, Puglisi S, Romeo PD, Torre ML, Alibrandi A, et al. Acromegaly is more severe in patients with AHR or AIP gene variants living in highly polluted areas. *J Clin Endocrinol Metab.* (2016) 101:1872–9. doi: 10.1210/jc.2015-4191

4

Identification, functional characterization, and pharmacological profile of a serotonin type-2b receptor in the medically important insect, *Rhodnius prolixus*

Jean-Paul V. Paluzzi[1], Garima Bhatt[1,2], Chang-Hui J. Wang[2], Meet Zandawala[2], Angela B. Lange[2] and Ian Orchard[2]*

[1] Department of Biology, York University, Toronto, ON, Canada, [2] Department of Biology, University of Toronto Mississauga, Mississauga, ON, Canada

Edited by:
Hubert Vaudry,
University of Rouen, France

Reviewed by:
John Chang,
University of Alberta, Canada
Jozef Vanden Broeck,
Katholieke Universiteit Leuven,
Belgium

***Correspondence:**
Jean-Paul V. Paluzzi,
Department of Biology, York University,
4700 Keele Street, Toronto, ON M3J
1P3, Canada
paluzzi@yorku.ca;
www.yorku.ca/paluzzi

In the Chagas disease vector, *Rhodnius prolixus*, two diuretic hormones act synergistically to dramatically increase fluid secretion by the Malpighian tubules (MTs) during the rapid diuresis that is initiated upon engorgement of vertebrate blood. One of these diuretic hormones is the biogenic amine, serotonin (5-hydroxytryptamine, 5-HT), which controls a variety of additional activities including cuticle plasticization, salivary gland secretion, anterior midgut absorption, cardioacceleratory activity, and myotropic activities on a number of visceral tissues. To better understand the regulatory mechanisms linked to these various physiological actions of serotonin, we have isolated and characterized a serotonin type 2b receptor in *R. prolixus*, Rhopr5HTR2b, which shares sequence similarity to the vertebrate serotonin type 2 receptors. *Rhopr5HTR2b* transcript is enriched in well-recognized physiological targets of serotonin, including the MTs, salivary glands and dorsal vessel (i.e., insect heart). Notably, *Rhopr5HTR2b* was not enriched in the anterior midgut where serotonin stimulates absorption and elicits myotropic control. Using a heterologous functional receptor assay, we examined Rhopr5HTR2b activation characteristics and its sensitivity to potential agonists, antagonists, and other biogenic amines. Rhopr5HTR2b is dose-dependently activated by serotonin with an EC_{50} in the nanomolar range. Rhopr5HTR2b is sensitive to alpha-methyl serotonin and is inhibited by a variety of serotonin receptor antagonists, including propranolol, spiperone, ketanserin, mianserin, and cyproheptadine. In contrast, the cardioacceleratory activity of serotonin revealed a unique pharmacological profile, with no significant response induced by alpha-methyl serotonin and insensitivity to ketanserin and mianserin. This distinct agonist/antagonist profile indicates that a separate serotonin receptor type may mediate cardiomodulatory effects controlled by serotonin in *R. prolixus*.

Keywords: serotonin, 5-hydroxytryptamine (5-HT), G protein-coupled receptor (GPCR), diuresis, dorsal vessel, Malpighian tubules, serotonergic signaling, cardioacceleratory activity

Introduction

The widespread presence and diverse biological roles of the indoleamine, serotonin (5-hydroxytryptamine, 5-HT), spans protozoans, plants and the vast majority of metazoans, thus attesting to its evolutionary significance (see Turlejski, 1996). In mammals, and more specifically in humans, serotonin acts on many organ systems via 7 families of serotonin receptors (5-HTR_{1-7}) that constitute numerous receptor isoforms (see Pytliak et al., 2011; Verlinden et al., 2015). The serotonin receptor, 5-HTR_3, is a ligand-gated channel whereas all other serotonin receptor classes have been characterized as G-protein coupled receptors (GPCRs) (Millan et al., 2008). Released as both a neurotransmitter and a hormone, the functions of serotonin are extensive, ranging from regulating the mechanics of behaviors like learning, memory, perception, fear and appetite, to mediating a plethora of physiological processes (see Berger et al., 2009; Verlinden et al., 2015).

The similarity in serotonin's regulatory functions in vertebrates as well as invertebrates is noteworthy. To name a few, serotonin is associated with learning and memory in sea slugs (Rahn et al., 2013), social and anxiety-like behavior in crayfish (Momohara et al., 2013; Fossat et al., 2014) and aversive behavior in the nematode, *Caenorhabditis elegans* (Curran and Chalasani, 2012). Serotonin is also a key modulator of feeding-related behaviors, including salivation, bite-like movements, pharyngeal peristalsis, and control of blood meal ingestion in a blood-feeding aquatic invertebrate, the medicinal leech, *Hirudo medicinalis* (Lent and Dickinson, 1987, 1988; Lent et al., 1988).

In insects, serotonin influences feeding-associated behaviors in various species including the locust (Ali et al., 1993; Molaei and Lange, 2003), blowfly (Baumann and Walz, 2012), honeybee (French et al., 2014), cockroach (Troppmann et al., 2007), as well as an ant (Falibene et al., 2012). Studies in *Drosophila melanogaster* and *Apis mellifera* have linked serotonin to development and various behaviors associated with central pattern generators, such as olfaction, learning, memory and circadian rhythms (Blenau and Thamm, 2011; Johnson et al., 2011). The immunohistochemical mapping of serotonergic neurons in the nervous systems of several dipteran, orthopteran, lepidopteran, blattarian, and hemipteran species further emphasizes serotonin's role as a neurotransmitter and neurohormone in insects (Nassel, 1988; Bicker, 1999; Miggiani et al., 1999; Homberg, 2002; Siju et al., 2008).

Rhodnius prolixus, a chief vector of Chagas disease, depends on its serotonergic system to successfully complete blood meal engorgement and, even more importantly, to regulate haemolymph osmolarity after its dramatic feeding bout. On average, a fifth instar *R. prolixus* can consume blood meals that are 10 times its unfed body weight and then promptly eliminates excess water and ions via rapid hormone-controlled diuresis (Orchard, 2006, 2009). Serotonin is a principal diuretic hormone in *R. prolixus* and haemolymph titres of serotonin rise dramatically from low nanomolar ($<10\,nM$) to high nanomolar ($>100\,nM$) levels within 5 min of feeding (Lange et al., 1989; Maddrell et al., 1991). Upon its release via serotonergic neurohaemal sites, serotonin stimulates diuresis, muscle contractions of the dorsal vessel, salivary glands, esophagus (foregut), anterior midgut (i.e., crop), and hindgut (Orchard and Te Brugge, 2002; Orchard, 2006). In addition, serotonin is involved with the plasticization of the cuticle and the expulsion of waste (Orchard et al., 1988; Lange et al., 1989).

Along with a corticotropin-releasing factor (CRF)-like peptide, RhoprCRF/DH, serotonin is involved in the production of primary urine by stimulating secretion of excess water and ions by the Malpighian tubules (MTs) (see Martini et al., 2007). Unlike most other tissues where serotonin is known to play a role, the MTs lack innervation and are thus influenced by the rise in the haemolymph levels of serotonin, acting as a neurohormone (Lange et al., 1989). The presence of serotonin receptors on the epithelial cells of the MTs is therefore critical to the normal course of rapid post-feeding diuresis in *R. prolixus*. Interestingly, serotonin and RhoprCRF/DH have been shown to synergistically increase fluid secretion in the MTs, and both appear to be at least partially dependent on both intracellular calcium and cAMP-mediated signal transduction pathways (Paluzzi et al., 2013). A recent study corroborating the requirement of both intracellular calcium and cAMP revealed that serotonin triggers calcium signaling (derived specifically from intracellular stores), which is mediated by cAMP and cAMP-dependent kinase, protein kinase A (Gioino et al., 2014).

Based on similarity to the mammalian serotonin receptor families, research in insects has identified six serotonin receptor subtypes, including type 1a, type 1b, type 2a, type 2b, type 7, (Tierney, 2001; Vleugels et al., 2013, 2014; Verlinden et al., 2015) and a novel type 8, recently identified in the small white butterfly, *Pieris rapae* (Qi et al., 2014). In comparison to the vertebrate receptors, the insect serotonin receptors have different pharmacology and may utilize varying modes of signal transduction (Vleugels et al., 2014; Verlinden et al., 2015). Serotonin receptors have been predicted and/or cloned from several insects and their endogeneous roles are now being explored (Von Nickisch-Rosenegk et al., 1996; Pietrantonio et al., 2001; Dacks et al., 2006b; Hauser et al., 2006, 2008; Troppmann et al., 2010; Gasque et al., 2013; Thamm et al., 2013; Vleugels et al., 2013, 2014).

In spite of the wealth of knowledge on serotonin's physiological roles in *R. prolixus*, surprisingly little is known concerning their endogenous serotonin receptors. In addition, we were interested to see if there might be more than one serotonin receptor in the periphery mediating the physiological effects of serotonin. We chose a tissue that is not directly involved in the rapid post-feeding diuresis. Thus, we examined the effects of serotonin agonists and antagonists on serotonin-stimulated increases in heart beat frequency (see Orchard, 2006). The susceptibility of these serotonin receptors to agonists and antagonists could then be compared to the pharmacology of the cloned receptor. The overall aim of this study was to address this knowledge gap and to begin to identify the serotonin receptors that mediate the various functional activities of serotonin in *R. prolixus*.

Materials and Methods

Animals

Fifth instar *R. prolixus* were obtained from an established colony at the University of Toronto Mississauga. Insects were reared in incubators at 25°C under high humidity (~50%). Each post-embryonic developmental stage was blood fed through an artificial feeding membrane as described previously (Paluzzi et al., 2015) using defibrinated rabbit blood purchased from a local supplier (Cedarlane Laboratories Inc., Burlington, ON). During dissection of animals to retrieve RNA from different tissues, the insects were bathed in nuclease-free phosphate-buffered saline (PBS) (Sigma-Aldrich, Oakville, ON, Canada) and excised tissues were transferred directly into chilled RNA lysis buffer (see below).

Isolation of a *R. prolixus* Putative Serotonin Receptor cDNA

Based on the pharmacological sensitivity of serotonin-stimulated fluid secretion by isolated *R. prolixus* MTs to ketanserin (Maddrell et al., 1991; Te Brugge et al., 2001), a selective antagonist of serotonin type-2 receptors (Hedner and Persson, 1988), the *D. melanogaster* type-2A serotonin receptor (Colas et al., 1995) protein sequence (Genbank accession# CAA57429) was used in a local tblastn search of the *R. prolixus* preliminary genome using Geneious 6.1 software (Biomatters Ltd. Auckland, New Zealand) and genomic regions with high scoring matches were used to design several pairs of gene-specific primers (Sigma Aldrich, Oakville, ON, Canada). Using a previously prepared *R. prolixus* Malpighian tubule cDNA library (Paluzzi et al., 2010) as template, only one of these primer pairs (5htR2-forA and 5htR2-revA) was successful (see **Table 1**; unsuccessful primer pairs are not shown), which amplified an initial 263 bp cDNA product. PCR reactions used ThermoPol Taq Polymerase (New England Biolabs, Whitby, ON, Canada) following manufacturer recommendations and carried out on a PCR System 9700 thermal cycler (Perkin Elmer Applied Biosystems, Carlsbad, CA, USA) using the following settings: initial denaturation for 5 min at 95°C; 35 cycles of 1) denaturation for 1 min at 94°C, 2) annealing for 30 s at 58°C, and 3) extension for 30 s at 72°C; final extension for 10 min at 72°C. The amplified cDNA sequence was cloned into a sequencing vector, pGEM T-Easy (Promega Corporation, Madison, WI, USA) and bases identified by Sanger sequencing (Center for Applied Genomics, Hospital for Sick Children, Toronto, ON). The putative translation of this preliminary product was compared to the UniProt protein database using the ExPASy Bioinformatics Resource Portal (http://web.expasy.org/blast/) and found to be highly similar to several uncharacterized protein sequences including a *D. melanogaster* orphan receptor (Genbank accession#: AGP51353.1) having

TABLE 1 | Primer sequences used in this study.

Oligo name	Oligo sequence (5′-3′)	Description (cDNA nucleotide binding site)
5htR2-forA	TCGCGCACTTCATCTCG	Cloning initial partial cDNA (1969-1985)
5htR2-revA	TTCTTGAATGCTTGTCGAAAC	Cloning initial partial cDNA (2231-2211)
5htR2-for1	GCAGCTGGCAACATCC	Further cloning partial cDNA (250-265)
5htR2-for2	AGTTTACTGTTTGGCGTGG	Further cloning partial cDNA (417-435)
5htR2-for3	CAAATACTATAGTAACATGGGATTCC	Further cloning partial cDNA (1688-1713)
5htR2-rev1	CGATATCGACACAATAAGACTTTC	Further cloning partial cDNA (2252-2229)
5htR2-rev2	CTAAGTGGAAGACTCATAGCTATCG	Further cloning partial cDNA (614-590)
5htR2-rev3	GCATGACGAGTATGGCGAC	Further cloning partial cDNA (370-352)
5htR2_3raceF1	GAAGGAAAGCCAATGAAGAAGATAGG	3′ RACE PCR (1211-1236)
5htR2_3raceF2	GTATTCGATTTTGTCACATGGTTAGG	3′ RACE PCR (2134-2159)
5htR2_3raceF3	TAAAGTGTTTCGACAAGCATTCAAG	3′ RACE PCR (2205-2229)
5htR2_3raceR	TCTTGAATGCTTGTCGAAACAC	3′ RACE PCR positive control (2230-2209)
5htR2_5raceR1	TGCACCAAACTGTTGTAAAGC	5′ RACE PCR (1047-1027)
5htR2_5raceR2	CGCTCGCCCAACC	5′ RACE PCR (835-823)
5htR2_5raceR3	GCATGACGAGTATGGCGAC	5′ RACE PCR (370-352)
5htR2_5raceF	GCAGCTGGCAACATCC	5′ RACE PCR positive control (250-265)
5htR2-ORF-F1	GGCCAAGAAGAAGAGGATGTG	Amplification of complete open reading frame (153-173)
5htR2-ORF-R1	GTTATTGTTACATCTGCCTACGTTC	Amplification of complete open reading frame (2297-2273)
5htR2-ORF-kozak	GCCACCATGTGCAGTGATACAACAGG	Addition of Kozak translation initiation sequence into expression construct (169-188)
5htR2-ORF-R2	CTACGTTCTAGGTGTCCAGCG	Expression construct amplification (2280-2260)
5htR2-qPCR-F	GAACAACGGCAGAACTTGG	Sense primer for qPCR located on exon 4
5htR2-qPCR-R	AATGCCCTCCTCTTTGTATGG	Anti-sense primer for qPCR located on exon 5

Initial oligonucleotide sequences designed based on high-scoring hits from tBLASTn search of preliminary R. prolixus genome database using D. melanogaster serotonin receptor type-2 sequences as query. Oligonucleotide sequences used in screening of cDNA plasmid library and RACE PCR based on partial initial sequence obtained. Final primer sets for verification of complete open-reading frame (ORF) and mammalian expression contruct based on complete cDNA sequenced de novo and sequence comparisons with the preliminary R. prolixus genome assembly.

similarity to previously annotated serotonin receptors (Hauser et al., 2006) and recently classified as a serotonin receptor type-2B (Gasque et al., 2013). The *D. melanogaster* 5HTR-2B sequence was used for *in silico* screening of the *R. prolixus* genome (as described above) that yielded several high scoring matches. Similar to the *in silico* screen using the type 2A sequence as bait, many of the high-scoring candidate matches to the serotonin receptor type-2B localized to a single supercontig (GL563092) and so gene-specific primers (Sigma Aldrich, Oakville, ON, Canada) were designed to isolate a larger portion of this candidate *R. prolixus* 5HTR2 cDNA sequence (see **Table 1**) following PCR conditions similar to those described above using the ThermoPol Taq Polymerase (New England Biolabs, Whitby, ON, Canada). These efforts extended the partial cDNA sequence to a size of 2003 bp but which nonetheless remained incomplete on the 5′ and 3′ ends lacking start and stop codons, respectively.

In order to elucidate the entire open reading frame of the receptor, we screened a *R. prolixus* MT cDNA library implementing a PCR-based approach including *R. prolixus* 5HTR2b gene-specific primers (based on the incomplete 2003 bp partial cDNA sequence obtained above) and cDNA library plasmid-specific primers described previously (Paluzzi et al., 2010). In addition, to ensure we obtained the most complete cDNA encompassing both the coding sequence (i.e., open-reading frame) and the untranslated regions, we used a Rapid Amplification of cDNA Ends (RACE) approach following manufacturer suggestions (Roche Applied Science, Laval, QC, Canada) as described previously (Paluzzi et al., 2010). For 5′ and 3′ RACE, fresh cDNA was synthesized from 1 μg of total RNA isolated from a pool of fifth instar tissue samples including nervous, gastrointestinal tract and reproductive tissues. Finally, the complete open reading frame (ORF) sequence was amplified using Q5 high-fidelity DNA Polymerase (New England Biolabs, Whitby, ON) from freshly prepared fifth instar *R. prolixus* MT cDNA synthesized from 500 ng total RNA using iScript RT Supermix (Bio-Rad, Mississauga, ON) following manufacturer recommended conditions. Primers used to amplify the complete ORF are listed in **Table 1** and high-fidelity PCR cycling conditions were as follows: 98°C for 30 s for initial denaturation, 98°C for 8 s (denaturation), 65.5°C for 20 s (annealing) and 72°C for 60 s (extension) repeated for 35 cycles that was followed by a final extension at 72°C for 2 min. An aliquot of the PCR reaction was visualized using standard agarose-gel electrophoresis and the remaining PCR reactions were column-purified using the EZ-10 Spin Column PCR Products Purification Kit (Bio Basic, Markham, ON). Amplicons were A-tailed to facilitate T/A cloning into pGEM-T Easy (Promega, Madison, WI) sequencing vector as previously described (Paluzzi et al., 2015). Several independent clones were sequenced to ascertain base accuracy (Center for Applied Genomics, Hospital for Sick Children, Toronto, ON). Preparation of expression constructs in pcDNA3.1 mammalian expression vector was carried out similarly to that described previously (Paluzzi et al., 2010), using primers (see **Table 1**) incorporating the consensus Kozak translation initiation sequence (Kozak, 1986).

Receptor Functional Assay to Determine Ligand Specificity

The pcDNA3.1 Rhopr5HTR2b receptor construct was used for transient expression in a recombinant Chinese hamster ovary cell line (CHOK1-aeq) stably expressing the calcium-sensitive bioluminescent protein aequorin (Paluzzi et al., 2012). Controls using vector without the 5HTR2b insert were included to ensure the functional responses observed were specific to the transiently expressed *R. prolixus* 5HTR2b receptor. Approximately 24 h prior to transfection, CHOK1-aeq cells were seeded at high density into T-75 flasks and were subsequently transfected at either 90% confluence using XtremeGENE HP DNA transfection reagent (Roche Diagnostics, Laval, QC) or 70–80% confluence using Lipofectamine LTX (Life Technologies, Carlsbad, CA) following manufacturer recommendations. Approximately 36–48 h after transfection, cells were prepared for the luminescence assay as previously described (Paluzzi et al., 2010). Kinetic luminescent measurements were made using a VICTOR X Light luminescence plate reader (PerkinElmer, Woodbridge, ON) or a Synergy 2 multi-mode microplate reader (BioTek, Winooski, VT).

Putative ligands and other chemicals were purchased from local suppliers (Sigma-Aldrich, Oakville, ON) and included selected biogenic amines (serotonin, tyramine, octopamine, dopamine), agonists (α-methyl serotonin), and antagonists (ketanserin, mianserin, spiperone, cyproheptadine, gramine, propranolol), that were tested either in isolation or in combination as required for each particular experiment. Biogenic amines and agonists were made up in double distilled water at a stock concentration of 100 mM while antagonists were made up in ethanol at a stock concentration of 1 mM.

Sequence Analysis of the Rhopr5HTR-2b Receptor

The deduced protein sequence of the *R. prolixus* serotonin type-2b receptor was analyzed for predicted hydrophobic transmembrane domains using the HMMTOP transmembrane topology prediction server [http://www.enzim.hu/hmmtop/; (Tusnady and Simon, 2001)]. In addition, the deduced Rhopr5HTR-2b protein sequence was evaluated for potential phosphorylation sites using the kinase-specific phosphorylation prediction server, NetPhosK 1.0 (Blom et al., 2004).

The *R. prolixus* serotonin type-2b receptor identified here along with selected structurally related orthologous sequences previously identified in other organisms or predicted in genomic databases were used in a comparative investigation of their primary sequences using ClustalW in MEGA 6.0 (Tamura et al., 2013). To determine the relationship among the various serotonin receptors, including the sequence identified in the current study, phylogenetic analyses were performed using the neighbor-joining method (Saitou and Nei, 1987) and maximum-likelihood method based on the Jones-Thornton-Taylor matrix-based model (Jones et al., 1992), which produced trees that had nearly identical topologies. In order to verify the significance in the determined relationships between the serotonin receptor sequences examined in this analysis, we performed a bootstrap test with 1000 iterations (Felsenstein, 1985).

Rhopr5HTR-2b Tissue Expression Analysis Assessed by Quantitative PCR (qPCR)

Since we routinely use fifth instar *R. prolixus* as a model to study neuroendocrine-regulated physiological processes related to blood meal engorgement, tissues were dissected from this developmental stage under nuclease-free phosphate buffered saline prepared as previously described (Paluzzi et al., 2008). Specifically, total RNA was purified from tissues dissected from approximately an equal number of male and female fifth-instar *R. prolixus* fed between 4 and 5 weeks previously as fourth-instar nymphs. cDNA was synthesized for quantitative PCR (qPCR) using 500 ng total RNA isolated from a number of different pools of tissues as described previously (Paluzzi et al., 2015) and were subsequently diluted five-fold with nuclease-free water prior to their use as template. For time-course expression profiling related to blood feeding, MTs were isolated from four insects (4 whole tubules per insect totaling 16 tubules) and stored in RNAlater for subsequent RNA extraction. Time points included 0–30, 30–60 min, 2, 4, 6, and 24 h post-blood feeding (via artificial feeding strategy as described above) as well as unfed controls. Total RNA was isolated from each tissue sample using the Pure Link RNA extraction kit (Life Technologies, Carlsbad, CA) and cDNA was prepared as described previously (Paluzzi et al., 2015) using 250 ng total RNA as template. Since optimal primers over exon boundaries were not possible, primers were instead designed over different exons to facilitate amplification of only a 388 bp cDNA product. Specifically, we used a Rhopr5HTR2b sense primer that was located on the fourth exon while the anti-sense qPCR primer was located on the fifth exon (see **Table 1** for details), which span a genomic region of over 3.5 kb. SsoFast EvaGreen Supermix with low ROX (Bio-Rad, Mississauga, ON) was used in all qPCR experiments following recommended cycling conditions on an Mx4000 Quantitative PCR System (Stratagene, La Jolla, CA). *Rhopr5HTR-2b* transcript abundance was normalized to the geometric average expression of three reference genes, namely rp49, β-actin and α-tubulin, which were previously validated for transcript expression profiling in various tissues of fifth instar *R. prolixus* (Paluzzi and O'Donnell, 2012). Experiments were repeated in at least three biological replicates that each included no-template and no reverse transcriptase negative controls.

Dorsal Vessel Contraction Assay

Serotonin's effect on fifth instar *R. prolixus* dorsal vessel contractions was examined through an *ex vivo* bioassay described previously (Sarkar et al., 2003). Briefly, the insects were gently immobilized on soft dental wax dorsal-side down and the cuticle in the ventral abdominal region and gastrointestinal tract were removed to expose the dorsal vessel lying on the inner dorsal surface of the animal. The semi-isolated dorsal vessel preparations were placed into a Sylgard-lined glass petri dish with the inner dorsal surface facing upwards and were secured through the lateral margins of the dorsal cuticle using minuten pins. Electrodes were connected to an impedance converter (UFI model 2991, Morro Bay, CA, USA) and positioned on each side of the dorsal vessel just anterior to the alary muscles associated with the fifth and sixth abdominal segments. The preparations were maintained in 100 μL of physiological saline (pH 7.0; 150 mM NaCl, 8.6 mM KCl, 2 mM CaCl2, 4 mM NaHCO3, 34 mM glucose, 8.5 mM MgCl2, 5 mM HEPES [pH 7.2]) and different test compounds were applied by first removing 50 μL of the normal saline and replacing it with 50 μL of saline containing a two-fold concentration of the compound being tested. Each preparation served as its own control through monitoring dorsal

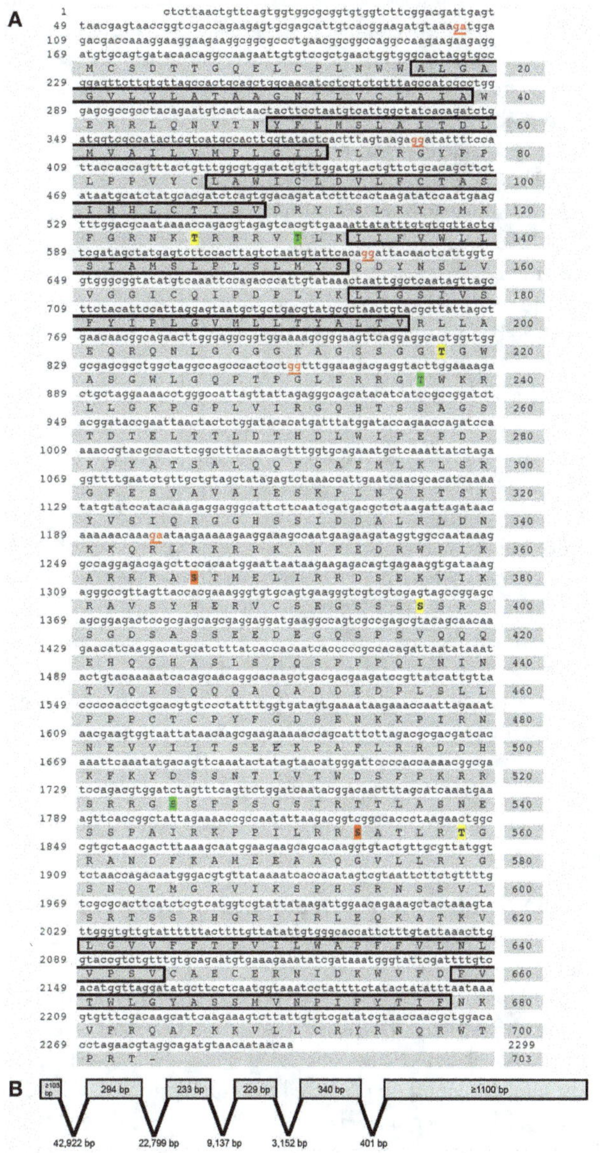

FIGURE 1 | *Rhodnius prolixus* cDNA, deduced protein sequence and predicted gene structure of the serotonin type 2b receptor, Rhopr5HTR2b. (A) Nucleotide and amino acid numbers are denoted on the left and right side of the sequences, respectively. Exon boundaries are denoted by nucleotides in red text. The predicted hydrophobic alpha-helices that form the seven transmembrane domains are outlined by black boxes. Residues predicted as phosphorylation sites exclusively by protein kinase C are highlighted in yellow (Thr_{126}, Thr_{218}, Ser_{397} and Ser_{559}) while exclusive sites for protein kinase A are highlighted in red (Ser_{366}, and Ser_{554}) and shared sites are highlighted in green (Thr_{131}, Thr_{237} and Ser_{525}). **(B)** The Rhopr5HTR2b cDNA identified is produced by six exons and five introns spanning a genomic region of over 80.7 kb.

vessel activity during an initial incubation with saline compared to a second treatment with a given test compound.

Results

Cloning and Gene Structure of a *R. prolixus* 5HTR2b Receptor

Using a combined approach involving homology-based *in silico* screening of the preliminary *R. prolixus* genome data and PCR-based strategy to confirm and obtain further sequence information over the 5′ and 3′ regions using RACE PCR, we have identified a *R. prolixus* 5HTR2b (Rhopr5HTR2b) cDNA (Genbank accession KP325472). The total length of the Rhopr5HTR2b cDNA amplified is 2299 bp (**Figure 1A**), with no additional splice variants identified. Using Geneious 6.1.2, the cloned 2299 bp *R. prolixus* 5HT2b cDNA was used for a local nucleotide BLAST search of the preliminary *R. prolixus* genome dataset to enable detection of exon-intron sites. The gene spans over 80.7 kb and includes six exons with lengths of ≥103 bp; 294, 233, 229, 340 bp and ≥1100 bp as well as five introns with lengths of 42,922, 22,799, 9137, 3152, and 401 bp (**Figure 1B**). The single open reading frame of 2109 bp produces a protein of 703 amino acid residues (**Figure 1A**) with an expected molecular mass of 78.7 kDa. In common with other members of the GPCR superfamily, the deduced protein sequence contains seven hydrophobic transmembrane domains. The amino-terminus (N-terminus) has a length of 16 amino acids while the carboxyl terminus (C-terminus) length is 25 amino acids. The open reading frame begins on the second exon, which also yields the first and second transmembrane domains. The third and fourth transmembrane domains are localized to the third exon while the fifth hydrophobic domain is found on the fourth exon. The fifth exon lacks any predicted transmembrane domains but yields the N-terminal region of the third intracellular loop while transmembrane domains six and seven are localized on the sixth and final exon.

Protein Sequence Analysis and Phylogenetics

Kinase specific phosphorylation sites were predicted using NetPhosK 1.0 (Blom et al., 2004) under a more stringent threshold cut-off (=0.75). A number of phosphorylation sites were predicted based on the deduced protein sequence (**Figure 1A**), although any functional significance awaits further study. Protein kinase A predicted phosphorylation sites include Thr_{131}, Thr_{237}, Ser_{366}, Ser_{525}, and Ser_{554}. Predicted protein kinase C phosphorylation sites in the Rhopr5HT2b sequence include Thr_{126}, Thr_{131}, Thr_{218}, Thr_{237}, Ser_{397}, Ser_{525}, and Ser_{559}. Within the third hydrophobic transmembrane region, a highly conserved aspartate residue (Asp_{93}) is present and is commonly found in aminergic neurotransmitter GPCRs as it is necessary for interaction with the positively charged amine moiety of aminergic ligands permitting receptor-ligand binding (Kristiansen and Dahl, 1996; Kristiansen et al., 2000). Additionally, vertebrate 5HTR type-2 receptors contain a highly conserved serine residue that is localized in close proximity to Asp_{93} (approximately one helical turn), which is a critical residue for interaction with the charged amine side chain of serotonin (Almaula et al., 1996). Notably, this serine residue facilitating receptor-ligand interaction is absent in Rhopr5HTR2b as well as orthologs from other insects.

Utilizing the ClustalW plugin in Geneious software, the *R. prolixus* 5HTR2b deduced protein sequence was compared to highly similar type 2b receptors from other insects including *Tribolium castaneum* [Genbank accession DAA64510; (Hauser et al., 2008)], *A. mellifera* [Genbank accession CBX90121; (Thamm et al., 2013)] and *D. melanogaster* [Genbank accession AGP51353; (Gasque et al., 2013)]. High sequence similarity or identity was observed largely over the predicted transmembrane domains (**Figure 2A**). In addition, regions of high similarity and identity were also observed over intracellular and extracellular loops, which may indicate regions essential for intracellular signaling and ligand recognition, respectively. In addition to the potential phosphorylation sites discussed above, the C-terminus contains a conserved cysteine residue (Cys_{692} in Rhopr5HTR2b) that may undergo post-translational palmitoylation (Thamm et al., 2013). The addition of palmitate groups could control multiple receptor functions (Gorinski and Ponimaskin, 2013) including receptor dimerization or G protein association (Zheng et al., 2012) since palmitoylation can create different intracellular loop arrangements with palmitate groups penetrating the lipid bilayer (Goddard and Watts, 2012). Phylogenetic analysis of the *R. prolixus* 5HTR2b receptor deduced protein sequence, which included a comparison to representative sequences from the three main families of insect serotonin receptors and structurally related vertebrate homologs, yielded a tree strongly supporting Rhopr5HTR2b as a member of the insect type-2b receptor subfamily (**Figure 2B**).

Transcript Expression Analyses of *Rhopr5HTR2b*

Quantitative PCR (qPCR) was used to examine the expression profile of the *Rhopr5HTR2b* receptor in fifth instar tissues. Highest transcript enrichment is found in the MTs and the salivary glands and lower levels, approximately three-fold less abundance, is found in the CNS, foregut, hindgut and dorsal vessel (**Figure 3A**). Expression was very low or absent in all other tissues examined which included midgut, reproductive tissues, prothoracic glands (with associated fat body) and a pool of tissue comprised of trachea, fat body, diaphragm, and abdominal nerves.

Considering the highest enrichment observed in MTs and the diuretic role of serotonin in the rapid post-feeding diuresis, we examined the expression profile between unfed and recently fed fifth-instar insects. We observed no changes in *Rhopr5HTR2b* transcript abundance between unfed and time points up to 6 h post-feeding (**Figure 3B**). Interestingly, expression is somewhat lower at 24 h post-feeding (by approximately 60%), but this was not significantly different from unfed insects (One-Way ANOVA, $p > 0.05$).

Cell Culture-based Receptor Functional Assay

In order to confirm this receptor as a *bona fide* target of serotonergic signaling, we utilized mammalian cell culture as a model to confirm the ligand and pharmacological sensitivity of this putative serotonin receptor. Recombinant CHOK1-aeq

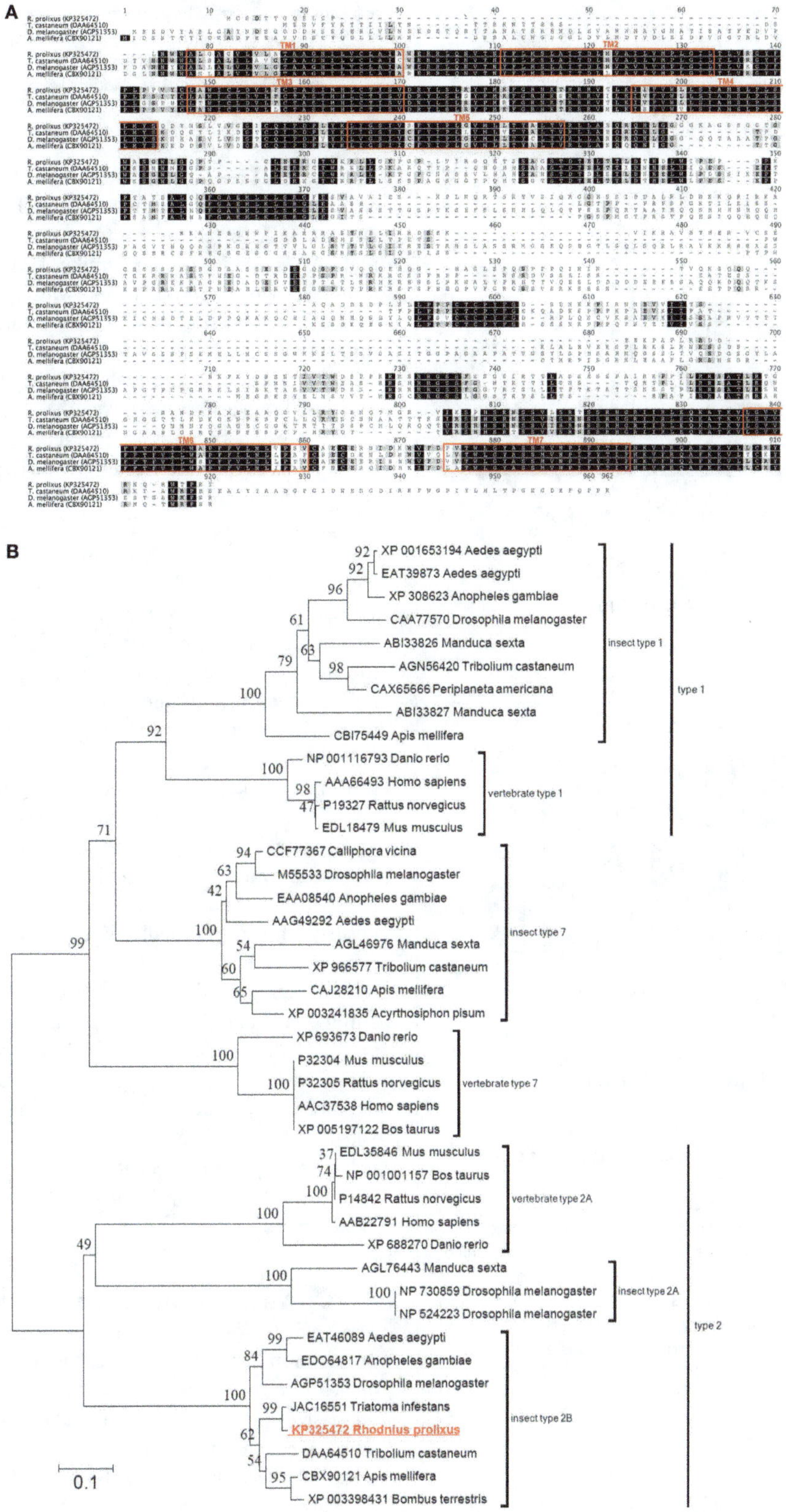

FIGURE 2 | Protein sequence alignment and phylogenetic analysis of selected serotonin receptors from insects and vertebrates. (A) ClustalW alignment of selected serotonin type 2b receptors, with regions of predicted transmembrane domains denoted by red outlined boxes. **(B)** Phylogenetic analysis using the neighbor-joining method of the deduced *(Continued)*

FIGURE 2 | Continued
Rhopr5HTR2b receptor protein sequence based on the cloned cDNA. Branch lengths on the tree are representative of the number of average number of amino acid substitutions per site. Percent bootstrap support for the clustering of the related sequences is indicated by the numbers adjacent to the nodes. Each protein sequence included in the analysis is identified by the GenBank accession number and the species name. The *R. prolixus* serotonin receptor identified in the current study (shown in red font) clusters within the clade including insect type 2b serotonin receptors.

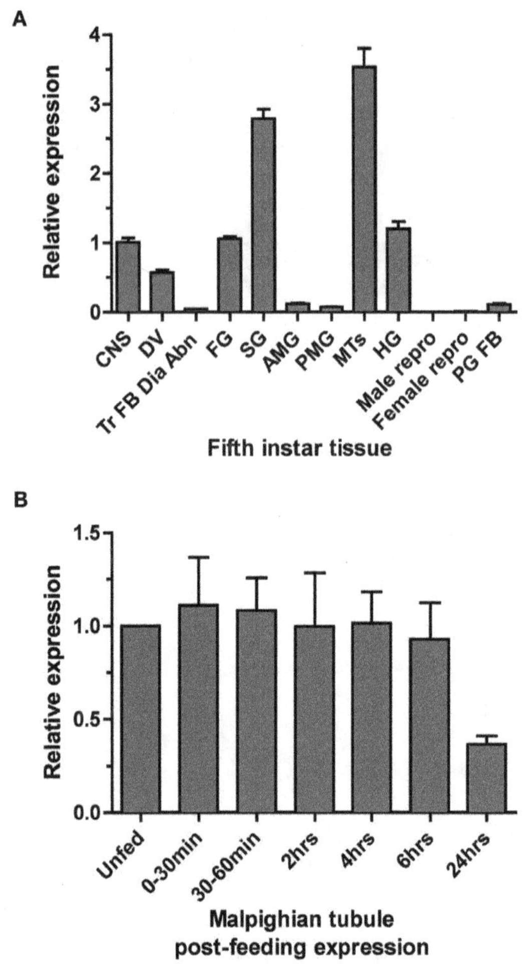

FIGURE 3 | *Rhodnius prolixus* serotonin receptor type 2b (*Rhopr5HTR2b*) transcript expression profile in fifth instar tissues determined by qPCR. (A) *Rhopr5HTR2b* transcript expression examined in fifth-instar tissues pooled from both male and female insects (except for sex-specific reproductive tissues). Relative expression is shown relative to levels in the CNS. **(B)** *Rhopr5HTR2b* transcript expression in MTs from unfed fifth instar and insects dissected at several time points up to 24 h post-blood meal engorgement. CNS, central nervous system; DV, dorsal vessel; Tr FB Dia Abn, trachea, fat body, dorsal/ventral diaphragm, and abdominal nerves; FG, foregut; SG, salivary gland; AMG, anterior midgut; PMG, posterior midgut; MTs, Malpighian tubule; HG, hindgut; PG FB, prothoracic gland and associated fat body; Male repro, male reproductive tissue; Female repro, female reproductive tissue.

cells stably expressing the jellyfish photoprotein apoaequorin (Paluzzi et al., 2012) were used for transient expression of the putative *R. prolixus* serotonin receptor (Rhopr5HT2b) using the pcDNA3.1 mammalian expression vector. CHOK1-aeq cells transiently expressing Rhopr5HTR2b yielded dose-dependent luminescence responses to serotonin (**Figure 4A**) with threshold activity in the low nanomolar range (EC_{50} = 201 nM). We also evaluated the vertebrate serotonin receptor type-2 agonist, alpha-methyl serotonin, which similarly yielded a dose-dependent luminescence response, albeit with lower potency (EC_{50} = 3.2 μM). Application of serotonin or alpha-methyl serotonin to untransfected cells or cells transfected with empty vector (lacking the *R. prolixus* 5HTR2b cDNA) did not exhibit a luminescence response (data not shown).

In order to more fully characterize and better classify the receptor subtype, we tested a variety of known serotonin receptor antagonists in the presence of a sub-maximal dose of serotonin (1 μM). All drugs were ineffective at a dose 100 nM as luminescence output was not different from controls (**Figure 4B**). Lower doses were also tested but similarly showed no inhibitory activity (data not shown). Increasing the concentration of the putative antagonists to 1 μM showed differential drug sensitivity. Specifically, no change in luminescence response was seen in the presence of gramine but variable levels of inhibition (30-5% inhibition) were observed with spiperone, mianserin, propranolol, ketanserin, and cyproheptadine. At the highest tested concentration of antagonists (10 μM), gramine still had no effect on the luminescence response induced by serotonin whereas all remaining antagonists caused a greater reduction in the luminescence response (~70–50% inhibition) observed for propranolol, spiperone, ketanserin, mianserin, and cyproheptadine (**Figure 4B**).

We examined the specificity of the 5HTR2 receptor for its aminergic ligand, 5-HT. Comparing to the luminescence output of 5HTR2b-transfected CHOK1-aeq cells treated with 1 μM 5HT, we tested other biogenic amines (**Figure 4C**) including dopamine, octopamine and tyramine at two doses (10 and 100 μM) expected to be saturating on their respective natural receptor targets. Our receptor yielded no response to any of the other amines tested with the exception of its confirmed natural ligand, 5-HT.

Dorsal Vessel Contraction Assay

The effects of serotonin on semi-isolated dorsal vessel preparations confirmed a stimulatory effect on the frequency of heart contractions (**Figure 5A**). Serotonin dose-dependently increased the rate of dorsal vessel contractions (**Figure 5B**) with threshold in the low nanomolar range (1–10 nM) and maximal effect observed in the mid micromolar range (10 μM). The average frequency of dorsal vessel contractions under physiological saline alone was 14.96 ± 0.7 beats/min and the most potent dose of serotonin (10 μM) led to an increase in contraction frequency by 24.5 ± 4.4 beats/min, which represents an approximate 165% increase relative to control.

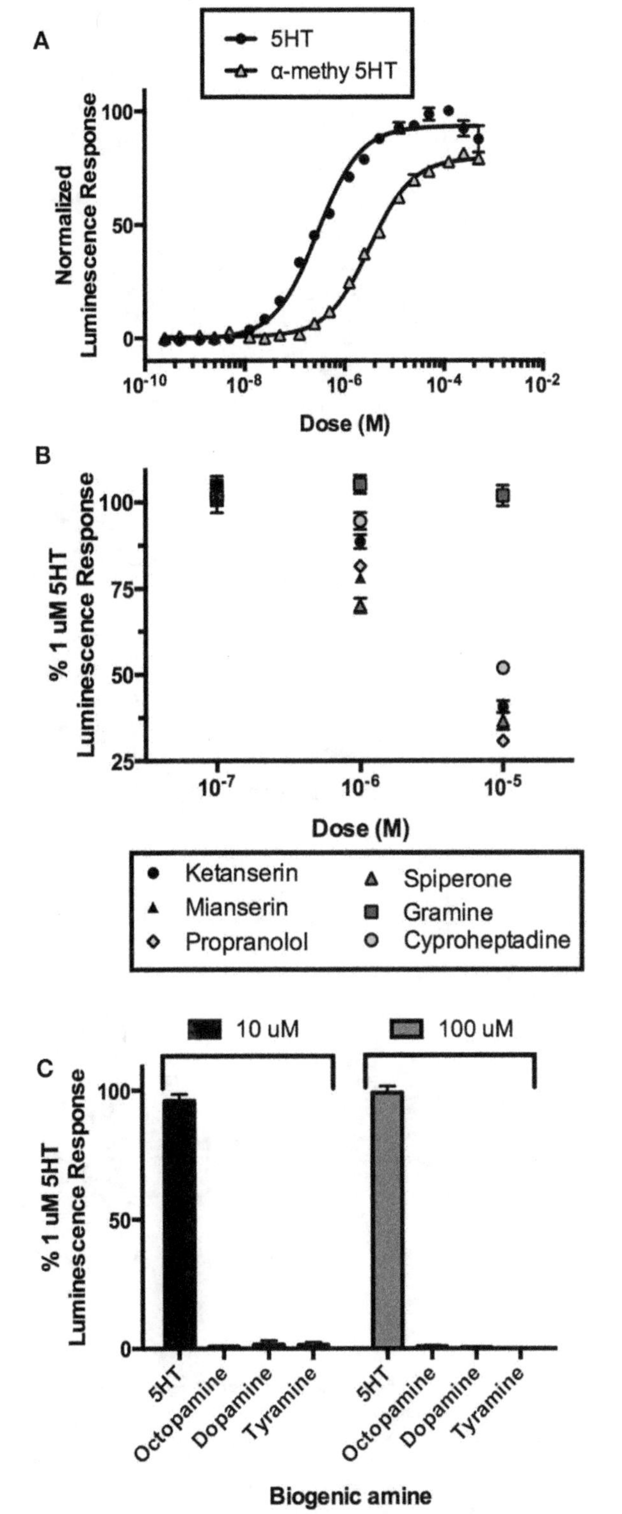

FIGURE 4 | Heterologous functional assay of the *R. prolixus* serotonin type 2b receptor (Rhopr5HTR2b) in CHOK1-aeq cells. (A) Dose-response curve demonstrating activity of serotonin and an agonist, alpha-methyl 5-HT, on the expressed Rhopr5HTR2b receptor. **(B)** Several serotonin receptor antagonists blocked the receptor-induced luminescent response, while gramine had no significant effect. **(C)** All other insect biogenic amines are inactive on the expressed Rhopr5HTR2b receptor.

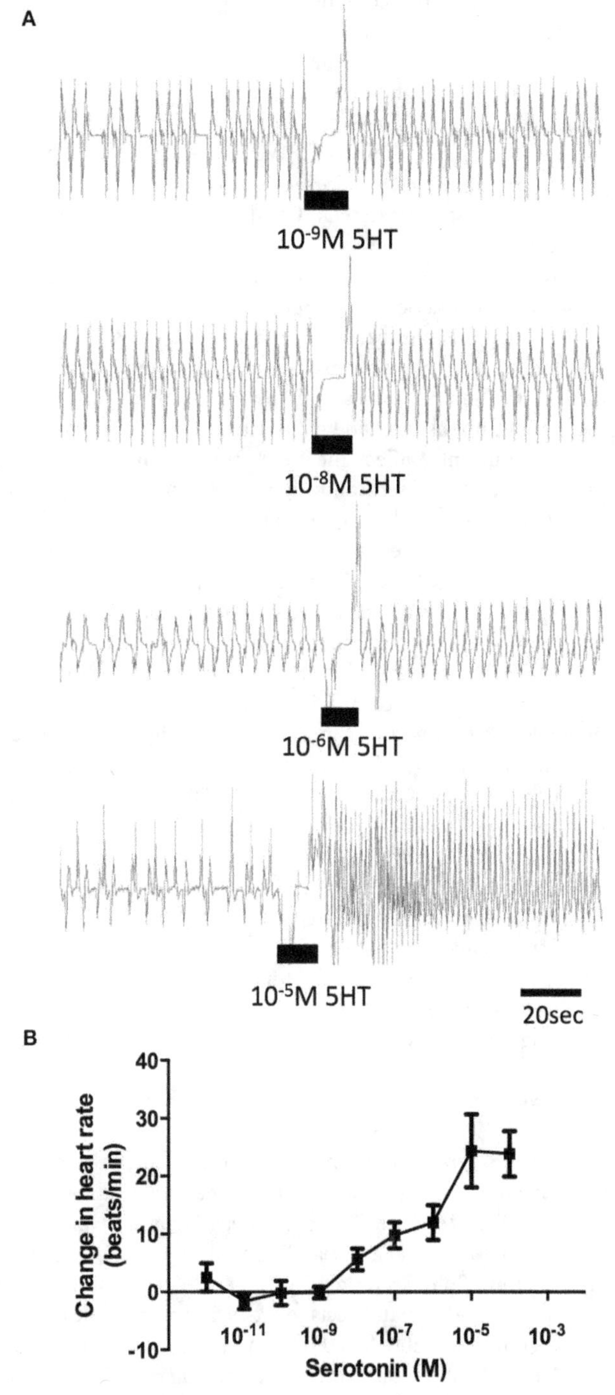

FIGURE 5 | Dose-dependent activity of serotonin on semi-isolated dorsal vessel preparations *in vitro*. (A) Sample traces of various concentrations of serotonin, where the black bar denotes time of application of serotonin to a preparation displaying spontaneous heart beats in saline. **(B)** Summary of dose-dependent effects of serotonin on the heart bioassay plotted as change in the heart rate (beats/min) from saline control. Data points are means ± standard error (n = 8–12 for each data point).

Given the sensitivity of the receptor isolated in this study to alpha-methyl serotonin (a serotonin type-2 receptor agonist) when examined in the cell culture-based receptor functional assay, we also tested this compound on the dorsal vessel bioassay. We selected an intermediate dose of serotonin (100 nM), which revealed a doubling in the frequency of dorsal vessel contractions (**Figures 5B, 6A**). As can be seen, alpha-methyl serotonin was not an effective agonist on the serotonin receptor type facilitating an increased heart rate (**Figure 6A**). We did observe some minor increases in the frequency of dorsal vessel contractions (i.e., heart rate) at the highest doses tested (10 μM); however, these were not significantly different from saline control treatments (**Figure 6B**).

In order to further elucidate the receptor type mediating the cardioacceleratory action in *R. prolixus*, we tested a subset of the receptor antagonists utilized in the cell culture-based receptor functional assay, namely mianserin, ketanserin and gramine. As shown in the sample traces and the summarizing bar graph, application of mianserin and ketanserin alone at a dose of 5 μM did not significantly affect the heart rate (**Figures 7A–C**). As shown earlier, 100 nM serotonin significantly increased the heart rate (**Figure 7C**) and also significantly increased the heart rate in the presence of the candidate antagonists mianserin and ketanserin (**Figures 7A–C**). Thus, unlike the result observed in the receptor functional assay, these two candidate antagonists were not effective at blocking serotonin's cardioacceleratory activity. We also examined the effects of gramine, which was not an effective antagonist on the isolated receptor when assessed using the cell culture-based functional assay (**Figure 4C**). When tested on its own, 50 μM gramine had no effect on heart rate. In the presence of 100 nM serotonin and 50 μM gramine, only a small increase to heart rate was observed (**Figure 7D**), which was not significantly different from the saline control. Upon wash off with saline, heart rate decreased and subsequent application of 100 nM serotonin alone led to an increased frequency of dorsal vessel contractions (i.e., elevated heart rate). Unlike our observations of the isolated receptor in the receptor functional assay, gramine appears to be a weak antagonist of the receptor controlling serotonin's chronotropic activity on the dorsal vessel.

Discussion

Diuresis in *R. prolixus* is under the control of at least two diuretic hormones, which includes the biogenic amine serotonin and RhoprCRF/DH (Lange et al., 1989; Maddrell et al., 1991; Te Brugge et al., 2011). In addition to its established role in stimulating fluid secretion by upper MTs, serotonin has a number of additional effects on a variety of tissues in *R. prolixus* (Orchard, 2006, 2009) as well as in other insects (Molaei and Lange, 2003; Dacks et al., 2006a; Wang et al., 2013; French et al., 2014; Majeed et al., 2014) that are mediated through a neurotransmitter, neuromodulator or neurohormone mechanism. We have identified a serotonin receptor that shares sequence characteristics most consistent with the insect type 2b serotonin receptors described previously (Hauser et al., 2008; Gasque et al., 2013; Thamm et al., 2013). The genomic organization is similar to that described in other insects, having either six (Thamm et al., 2013) or seven exons (Hauser et al., 2008; Gasque et al., 2013); however, the transmembrane domains in the *R. prolixus* 5HTR2b gene have different exon localizations (for comparison see Hauser et al., 2006; Thamm et al., 2013).

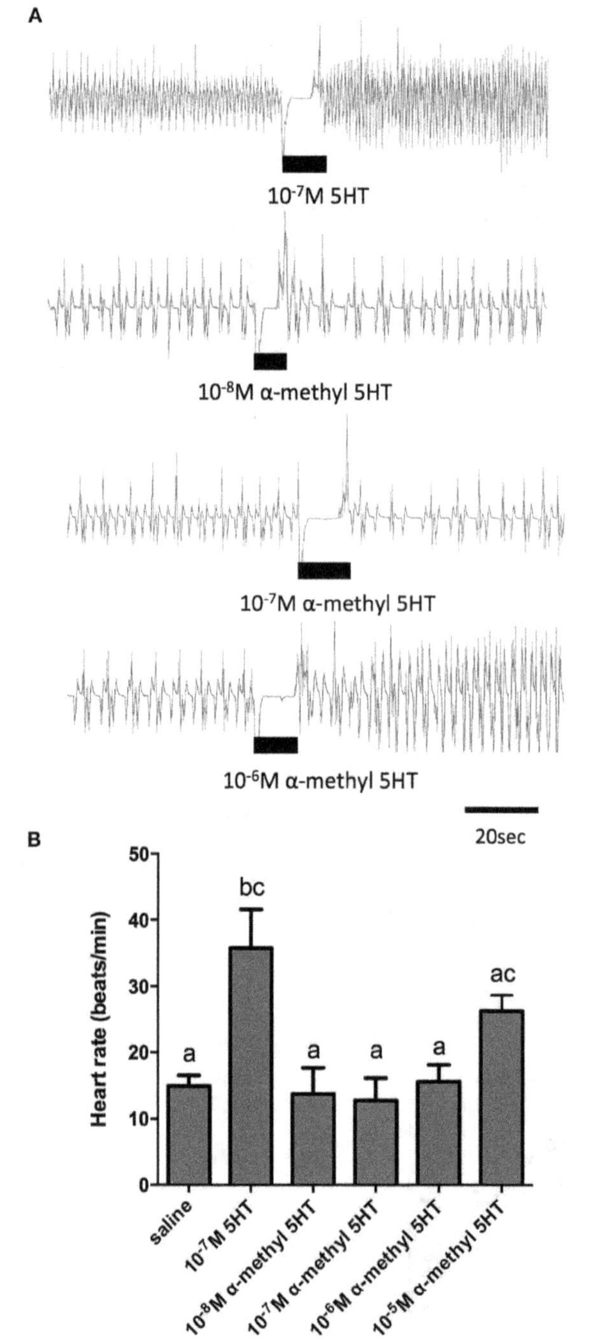

FIGURE 6 | The serotonin type 2 receptor agonist, α–methyl serotonin, is a weak cardioactive factor in *R. prolixus*. (A) Sample traces of 100 nM serotonin and selected concentrations of α–methyl serotonin. Black bars denotes application of serotonin or agonist at specified dose to preparations displaying spontaneous heart beats in saline. **(B)** Bar graph summary of the frequency of heart contractions (beats/min) under saline, serotonin or various concentrations of α–methyl serotonin. Columns marked with different letters are significantly different (ANOVA, Tukey-Kramer multiple comparison test, $P < 0.05$). Data points are means ± standard error ($n = 8$ for each data point).

Phylogenetic analysis also supports the notion that the receptor isolated here belongs to the insect serotonin receptor type-2b subfamily—a nomenclature used to differentiate members of this

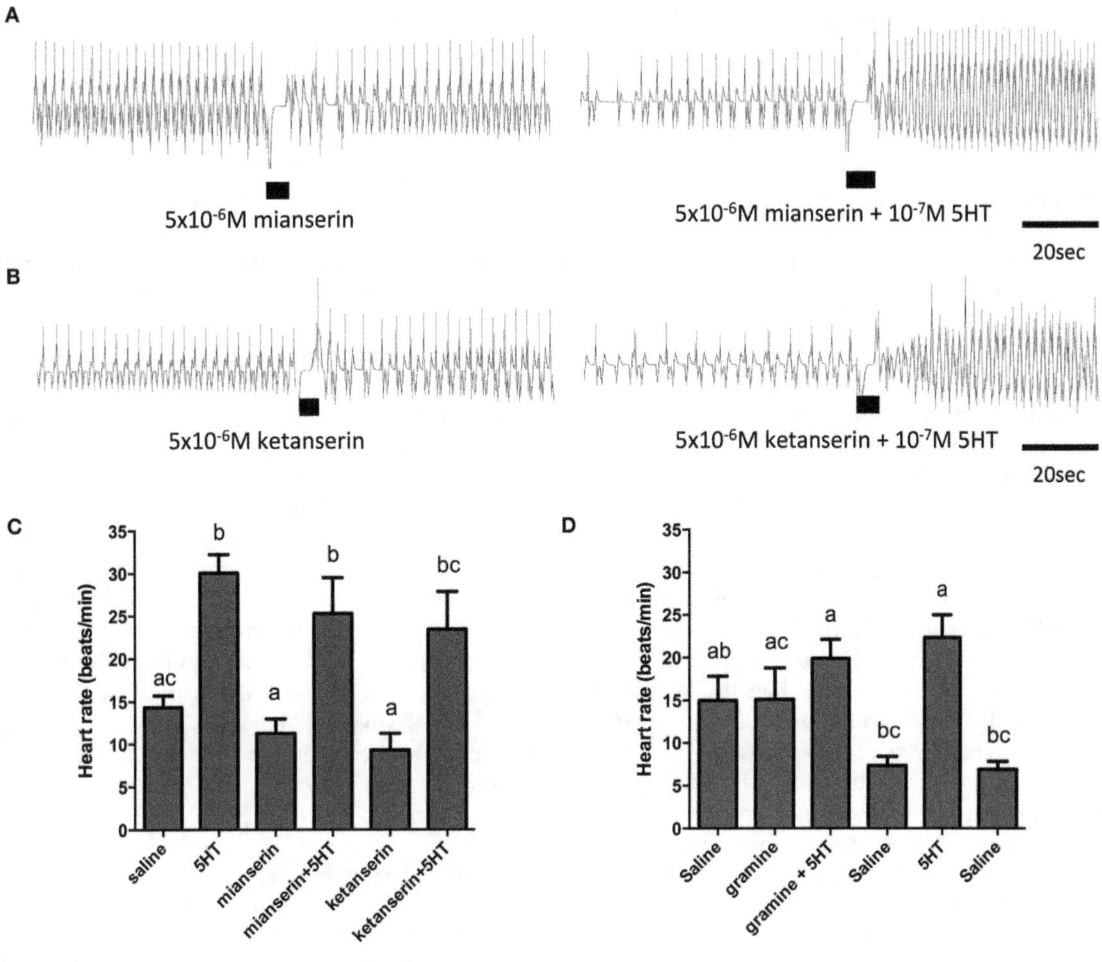

FIGURE 7 | The serotonin type 2 receptor antagonists, mianserin and ketanserin, are not effective inhibitors of serotonin-stimulated increases in heart rate. (A) Sample traces of 5 μM mianserin application in isolation and in the presence of 100 nM serotonin. **(B)** Sample traces of 5 μM ketanserin application in isolation and in the presence of 100 nM serotonin. Black bars denotes application of antagonist or antagonist with serotonin at specified concentrations, trace to the left of the black bar represents spontaneous myogenic contractions in saline and to the right of the black bar is the response to serotonin or agonist application. **(C,D)** Bar graph summary of the frequency of heart contractions (beats/min) under saline, serotonin alone, single antagonists alone or in combination with serotonin. Columns marked with different letters are significantly different (ANOVA, Tukey-Kramer multiple comparison test, $P < 0.05$). Data points are means ± standard error ($n = 6$ for each data point for assessments with mianserin and ketanserin; $n = 9$ for each data point for assessments with gramine).

subfamily from the insect serotonin receptor type-2a subfamily (Colas et al., 1995; Gasque et al., 2013).

Transcript expression profiling of *Rhopr5HTR2b* in various tissues of fifth instar stage *R. prolixus* revealed greatest enrichment in MTs and salivary glands. Pharmacological analyses in the heterologous system suggests this receptor could be the target of serotonin acting as a diuretic hormone enabling increased solute and water transport by the MTs following a blood meal. This notion is supported by previous studies that found ketanserin and spiperone are potent antagonists of serotonin-stimulated fluid secretion by MTs (Maddrell et al., 1991; Te Brugge et al., 2001), which were also the most active antagonists on the receptor we identified in this study. Interestingly, relative to the unfed animal, it appears there is no change in receptor transcript abundance over the first 24 h after blood meal engorgement, suggesting the Malpighian tubule serotonin receptor that responds to haemolymph-borne serotonin is available in advance of feeding to ensure a prompt response to initiate the rapid post-feeding diuresis.

The pharmacological characteristics of the serotonin receptor type on *R. prolixus* salivary glands are not known. In *Calliphora vicina* salivary glands, different serotonin receptor types may regulate salivation since ketanserin is not effective at blocking serotonin-stimulated fluid secretion by isolated salivary glands (Maddrell et al., 1991), although serotonin-stimulated salivation in *C. vicina* is significantly inhibited by gramine (Berridge, 1972; Trimmer, 1985). Gramine was not effective at inhibiting the activation of the Rhopr5HTR2b receptor functionally analyzed here. Two receptors have been recently identified in blowfly salivary glands belonging to the serotonin receptor type-2a and type-7 classes (Roser et al., 2012), although both receptors displayed sensitivity to ketanserin

(Roser et al., 2012). A different receptor subtype could be expressed in the *R. prolixus* salivary glands where serotonin is delivered in the nerve supply and induces a dose-dependent increase in the frequency and amplitude of phasic muscle contractions (Orchard and Te Brugge, 2002). Serotonin has also been reported to dose-dependently stimulate secretion of saliva (Orchard, 2006).

Rhopr5HTR2b transcript expression was also detected in the CNS, dorsal vessel, foregut and hindgut of fifth instar *R. prolixus*. In the nervous system of insects, serotonin is known to play a variety of roles that includes regulation of feeding (Falibene et al., 2012; French et al., 2014), motor output and locomotion (Claassen and Kammer, 1986; Silva et al., 2014), control of clock neurons (Hamasaka and Nassel, 2006; Kolodziejczyk and Nassel, 2011), and olfactory function (Mercer and Menzel, 1982; Kloppenburg et al., 1999; Dacks et al., 2006a; Tsuji et al., 2007; Kloppenburg and Mercer, 2008; Siju et al., 2008; Zhao and Berg, 2009; Watanabe et al., 2014). In *R. prolixus*, serotonin's distribution in the CNS is extensive, with approximately 150 neurons identified, whose projections and arborizations suggest that this neurochemical has a multitude of central as well as peripheral roles (Lange et al., 1988). A subset of the peripheral serotonin-like immunoreactive projections in *R. prolixus* are associated with regions of the gut including the foregut and hindgut (Orchard et al., 1988; Orchard, 2006), These regions of the gut also demonstrated *Rhopr5HTR2b* transcript enrichment, suggesting serotonin's roles could be mediated by this receptor in these tissues. In contrast, serotonin's action on the anterior midgut as a regulator of transepithelial transport (Farmer et al., 1981) and muscle contraction (Te Brugge et al., 2009) may not involve the identified receptor since no transcript was detected in this tissue. It is possible, however, that a closely related receptor (e.g., type 2a receptor class) may control these serotonergic actions in the anterior midgut since cAMP responsiveness to serotonin showed a similar pharmacological profile, including sensitivity to the agonist α-methyl serotonin and inhibition by antagonists including ketanserin, mianserin and cyproheptadine, while the serotonin-induced increase of cAMP in the anterior midgut was not affected by spiperone (Barrett et al., 1993), one of the more active antagonists effective on Rhopr5HTR2b. Spiperone may be useful in discriminating between these closely related receptor subtypes.

The dorsal vessel is the primary circulatory organ in insects and is regulated by a variety of cardioactive factors, such as serotonin (Chiang et al., 1992; Zornik et al., 1999; Koladich et al., 2002; Dasari and Cooper, 2006; Feliciano et al., 2011). As previously reported (Chiang et al., 1992; Orchard, 2006), serotonin stimulates increases in heart rate in the low nanomolar range (threshold between 1 and 10 nM). In contrast to the pharmacological sensitivity of Rhopr5HTR2b as determined through the heterologous functional assay, the cardioacceleratory activity of serotonin had a unique pharmacological profile. High doses of the type 2 agonist, alpha-methyl serotonin, were not effective in significantly modifying the frequency of heart contractions. In addition, the dorsal vessel bioassay revealed insensitivity to ketanserin and mianserin. Taken together, these results suggest that at least two distinct serotonin receptors control critical physiological functions in this blood-feeding insect, one of which is Rhopr5HTR2b, involved in fluid secretion by the MTs. Other serotonin receptors appear to be involved in absorption by the anterior midgut and cardioacceleratory effects on the dorsal vessel.

Acknowledgments

This research was supported through individual Natural Sciences and Engineering Research Council of Canada (NSERC) discovery grants to IO, AL, and JP.

References

Ali, D. W., Orchard, I., and Lange, A. B. (1993). The aminergic control of locust (Locusta-Migratoria) salivary-glands—evidence for dopaminergic and serotonergic innervation. *J. Insect Physiol.* 39, 623–632. doi: 10.1016/0022-1910(93)90067-2

Almaula, N., Ebersole, B. J., Zhang, D., Weinstein, H., and Sealfon, S. C. (1996). Mapping the binding site pocket of the serotonin 5-Hydroxytryptamine2A receptor. Ser3.36(159) provides a second interaction site for the protonated amine of serotonin but not of lysergic acid diethylamide or bufotenin. *J. Biol. Chem.* 271, 14672–14675. doi: 10.1074/jbc.271.25.14672

Barrett, F. M., Orchard, I., and Tebrugge, V. (1993). Characteristics of serotonin-induced cyclic-amp elevation in the integument and anterior midgut of the blood-feeding bug, rhodnius-prolixus. *J. Insect Physiol.* 39, 581–587. doi: 10.1016/0022-1910(93)90040-X

Baumann, O., and Walz, B. (2012). The blowfly salivary gland—a model system for analyzing the regulation of plasma membrane V-ATPase. *J. Insect Physiol.* 58, 450–458. doi: 10.1016/j.jinsphys.2011.11.015

Berger, M., Gray, J. A., and Roth, B. L. (2009). The expanded biology of serotonin. *Annu. Rev. Med.* 60, 355–366. doi: 10.1146/annurev.med.60.042307.110802

Berridge, M. J. (1972). The mode of action Of 5-Hydroxytryptamine. *J. Exp. Biol.* 56, 311–321.

Bicker, G. (1999). Biogenic amines in the brain of the honeybee: cellular distribution, development, and behavioral functions. *Microsc. Res. Tech.* 44, 166–178.

Blenau, W., and Thamm, M. (2011). Distribution of serotonin (5-HT) and its receptors in the insect brain with focus on the mushroom bodies: lessons from Drosophila melanogaster and Apis mellifera. *Arthropod Struct. Dev.* 40, 381–394. doi: 10.1016/j.asd.2011.01.004

Blom, N., Sicheritz-Ponten, T., Gupta, R., Gammeltoft, S., and Brunak, S. (2004). Prediction of post-translational glycosylation and phosphorylation of proteins from the amino acid sequence. *Proteomics* 4, 1633–1649. doi: 10.1002/pmic.200300771

Chiang, R. G., Chiang, J. A., and Davey, K. G. (1992). A sensorory input inhibiting heart rate in an insect, *Rhodnius prolixus*. *Experientia* 48, 1122–1125. doi: 10.1007/BF01948003

Claassen, D. E., and Kammer, A. E. (1986). Effects of octopamine, dopamine, and serotonin on production of flight motor output by thoracic ganglia of Manduca sexta. *J. Neurobiol.* 17, 1–14. doi: 10.1002/neu.480170102

Colas, J. F., Launay, J. M., Kellermann, O., Rosay, P., and Maroteaux, L. (1995). Drosophila 5-HT2 serotonin receptor: coexpression with fushi-tarazu during segmentation. *Proc. Natl. Acad. Sci. U.S.A.* 92, 5441–5445. doi: 10.1073/pnas.92.12.5441

Curran, K. P., and Chalasani, S. H. (2012). Serotonin circuits and anxiety: what can invertebrates teach us? *Inverteb. Neurosci.* 12, 81–92. doi: 10.1007/s10158-012-0140-y

Dacks, A. M., Christensen, T. A., and Hildebrand, J. G. (2006a). Phylogeny of a serotonin-immunoreactive neuron in the primary olfactory center of the insect brain. *J. Comp. Neurol.* 498, 727–746. doi: 10.1002/cne.21076

Dacks, A. M., Dacks, J. B., Christensen, T. A., and Nighorn, A. J. (2006b). The cloning of one putative octopamine receptor and two putative serotonin receptors from the tobacco hawkmoth, Manduca sexta. *Insect Biochem. Mol. Biol.* 36, 741–747. doi: 10.1016/j.ibmb.2006.07.002

Dasari, S., and Cooper, R. L. (2006). Direct influence of serotonin on the larval heart of Drosophila melanogaster. *J. Comp. Physiol. B* 176, 349–357. doi: 10.1007/s00360-005-0058-3

Falibene, A., Rossler, W., and Josens, R. (2012). Serotonin depresses feeding behaviour in ants. *J. Insect Physiol.* 58, 7–17. doi: 10.1016/j.jinsphys.2011.08.015

Farmer, J., Maddrell, S. H. P., and Spring, J. H. (1981). Absorption of fluid by the midgut of rhodnius. *J. Exp. Biol.* 94, 301–316.

Feliciano, D. F., Bassani, R. A., Oliveira, P. X., and Bassani, J. W. (2011). Pacemaker activity in the insect (T. molitor) heart: role of the sarcoplasmic reticulum. *Am. J. Physiol. Regul. Integr. Comp. Physiol.* 301, R1838–R1845. doi: 10.1152/ajpregu.00089.2011

Felsenstein, J. (1985). Confidence-limits on phylogenies—an approach using the bootstrap. *Evolution* 39, 783–791. doi: 10.2307/2408678

Fossat, P., Bacque-Cazenave, J., De Deurwaerdere, P., Delbecque, J. P., and Cattaert, D. (2014). Comparative behavior. Anxiety-like behavior in crayfish is controlled by serotonin. *Science* 344, 1293–1297. doi: 10.1126/science.1248811

French, A. S., Simcock, K. L., Rolke, D., Gartside, S. E., Blenau, W., and Wright, G. A. (2014). The role of serotonin in feeding and gut contractions in the honeybee. *J. Insect Physiol.* 61, 8–15. doi: 10.1016/j.jinsphys.2013.12.005

Gasque, G., Conway, S., Huang, J., Rao, Y., and Vosshall, L. B. (2013). Small molecule drug screening in Drosophila identifies the 5HT2A receptor as a feeding modulation target. *Sci. Rep.* 3:srep02120. doi: 10.1038/srep02120

Gioino, P., Murray, B. G., and Ianowski, J. P. (2014). Serotonin triggers cAMP and PKA-mediated intracellular calcium waves in Malpighian tubules of *Rhodnius prolixus*. *Am. J. Physiol. Regul. Integr. Comp. Physiol.* 307, R828–R836. doi: 10.1152/ajpregu.00561.2013

Goddard, A. D., and Watts, A. (2012). Regulation of G protein-coupled receptors by palmitoylation and cholesterol. *BMC Biol.* 10:27. doi: 10.1186/1741-7007-10-27

Gorinski, N., and Ponimaskin, E. (2013). Palmitoylation of serotonin receptors. *Biochem. Soc. Trans.* 41, 89–94. doi: 10.1042/BST20120235

Hamasaka, Y., and Nassel, D. R. (2006). Mapping of serotonin, dopamine, and histamine in relation to different clock neurons in the brain of Drosophila. *J. Comp. Neurol.* 494, 314–330. doi: 10.1002/cne.20807

Hauser, F., Cazzamali, G., Williamson, M., Blenau, W., and Grimmelikhuijzen, C. J. (2006). A review of neurohormone GPCRs present in the fruitfly Drosophila melanogaster and the honey bee Apis mellifera. *Prog. Neurobiol.* 80, 1–19. doi: 10.1016/j.pneurobio.2006.07.005

Hauser, F., Cazzamali, G., Williamson, M., Park, Y., Li, B., Tanaka, Y., et al. (2008). A genome-wide inventory of neurohormone GPCRs in the red flour beetle Tribolium castaneum. *Front. Neuroendocrinol.* 29:3. doi: 10.1016/j.yfrne.2007.10.003

Hedner, T., and Persson, B. (1988). Effects of a new serotonin antagonist, ketanserin, in experimental and clinical hypertension. *Am. J. Hypertens* 1, 317S–323S. doi: 10.1093/ajh/1.3.317S

Homberg, U. (2002). Neurotransmitters and neuropeptides in the brain of the locust. *Microsc. Res. Tech.* 56, 189–209. doi: 10.1002/jemt.10024

Johnson, O., Becnel, J., and Nichols, C. D. (2011). Serotonin receptor activity is necessary for olfactory learning and memory in Drosophila melanogaster. *Neuroscience* 192, 372–381. doi: 10.1016/j.neuroscience.2011.06.058

Jones, D. T., Taylor, W. R., and Thornton, J. M. (1992). The rapid generation of mutation data matrices from protein sequences. *Comput. Appl. Biosci.* 8, 275–282. doi: 10.1093/bioinformatics/8.3.275

Kloppenburg, P., Ferns, D., and Mercer, A. R. (1999). Serotonin enhances central olfactory neuron responses to female sex pheromone in the male sphinx moth manduca sexta. *J. Neurosci.* 19, 8172–8181.

Kloppenburg, P., and Mercer, A. R. (2008). Serotonin modulation of moth central olfactory neurons. *Annu. Rev. Entomol.* 53, 179–190. doi: 10.1146/annurev.ento.53.103106.093408

Koladich, P. M., Cusson, M., Bendena, W. G., Tobe, S. S., and McNeil, J. N. (2002). Cardioacceleratory effects of Manduca sexta allatotropin in the true armyworm moth, Pseudaletia unipuncta. *Peptides* 23, 645–651. doi: 10.1016/S0196-9781(01)00658-1

Kolodziejczyk, A., and Nassel, D. R. (2011). Myoinhibitory peptide (MIP) immunoreactivity in the visual system of the blowfly Calliphora vomitoria in relation to putative clock neurons and serotonergic neurons. *Cell Tissue Res.* 345, 125–135. doi: 10.1007/s00441-011-1198-2

Kozak, M. (1986). Point mutations define a sequence flanking the AUG initiator codon that modulates translation by eukaryotic ribosomes. *Cell* 44, 283–292. doi: 10.1016/0092-8674(86)90762-2

Kristiansen, K., and Dahl, S. G. (1996). Molecular modeling of serotonin, ketanserin, ritanserin and their 5-HT2C receptor interactions. *Eur. J. Pharmacol.* 306, 195–210. doi: 10.1016/0014-2999(96)00180-X

Kristiansen, K., Kroeze, W. K., Willins, D. L., Gelber, E. I., Savage, J. E., Glennon, R. A., et al. (2000). A highly conserved aspartic acid (Asp-155) anchors the terminal amine moiety of tryptamines and is involved in membrane targeting of the 5-HT(2A) serotonin receptor but does not participate in activation via a "salt-bridge disruption" mechanism. *J. Pharmacol. Exp. Ther.* 293, 735–746.

Lange, A. B., Orchard, I., and Barrett, F. M. (1989). Changes in hemolymph serotonin levels associated with feeding in the bloodsucking bug, *Rhodnius prolixus*. *J. Insect Physiol.* 35, 393–399. doi: 10.1016/0022-1910(89)90113-3

Lange, A. B., Orchard, I., and Lloyd, R. J. (1988). Immunohistochemical and electrochemical detection of serotonin in the nervous-system of the blood-feeding bug, rhodnius-prolixus. *Arch. Insect Biochem. Physiol.* 8, 187–201. doi: 10.1002/arch.940080305

Lent, C. M., and Dickinson, M. H. (1987). On the termination of ingestive behaviour by the medicinal leech. *J. Exp. Biol.* 131, 1–15.

Lent, C. M., and Dickinson, M. H. (1988). The neurobiology of feeding in leeches. *Sci. Am.* 258, 98–103. doi: 10.1038/scientificamerican0688-98

Lent, C. M., Fliegner, K. H., Freedman, E., and Dickinson, M. H. (1988). Ingestive behaviour and physiology of the medicinal leech. *J. Exp. Biol.* 137, 513–527.

Maddrell, S. H., Herman, W. S., Mooney, R. L., and Overton, J. A. (1991). 5-Hydroxytryptamine: a second diuretic hormone in *Rhodnius prolixus*. *J. Exp. Biol.* 156, 557–566.

Majeed, Z. R., Stacy, A., and Cooper, R. L. (2014). Pharmacological and genetic identification of serotonin receptor subtypes on Drosophila larval heart and aorta. *J. Comp. Physiol. B* 184, 205–219. doi: 10.1007/s00360-013-0795-7

Martini, S. V., Nascimento, S. B., and Morales, M. M. (2007). *Rhodnius prolixus* Malpighian tubules and control of diuresis by neurohormones. *Annu. Acad. Bras. Cienc.* 79, 87–95. doi: 10.1590/S0001-37652007000100011

Mercer, A., and Menzel, R. (1982). The effects of biogenic amines on conditioned and unconditioned responses to olfactory stimuli in the honeybee Apis mellifera. *J. Comp. Physiol. A* 145, 363–368. doi: 10.1007/BF00619340

Miggiani, L., Orchard, I., and Tebrugge, V. (1999). The distribution and function of serotonin in the large milkweed bug, Oncopeltus fasciatus. a comparative study with the blood-feeding bug, *Rhodnius prolixus*. *J. Insect Physiol.* 45, 1029–1036. doi: 10.1016/S0022-1910(99)00087-6

Millan, M. J., Marin, P., Bockaert, J., and Mannoury La Cour, C. (2008). Signaling at G-protein-coupled serotonin receptors: recent advances and future research directions. *Trends Pharmacol. Sci.* 29, 454–464. doi: 10.1016/j.tips.2008.06.007

Molaei, G., and Lange, A. B. (2003). The association of serotonin with the alimentary canal of the African migratory locust, Locusta migratoria:

distribution, physiology and pharmacological profile. *J. Insect Physiol.* 49, 1073–1082. doi: 10.1016/j.jinsphys.2003.08.004

Momohara, Y., Kanai, A., and Nagayama, T. (2013). Aminergic control of social status in crayfish agonistic encounters. *PLoS ONE* 8:e74489. doi: 10.1371/journal.pone.0074489

Nassel, D. R. (1988). Serotonin and serotonin-immunoreactive neurons in the nervous system of insects. *Prog. Neurobiol.* 30, 1–85. doi: 10.1016/0301-0082(88)90002-0

Orchard, I. (2006). Serotonin: a coordinator of feeding-related physiological events in the blood-gorging bug, *Rhodnius prolixus. Comp. Biochem. Physiol. A Mol. Integr. Physiol.* 144, 316–324. doi: 10.1016/j.cbpa.2005.11.010

Orchard, I. (2009). Peptides and serotonin control feeding-related events in *Rhodnius prolixus. Front. Biosci. (Elite. Ed).* 1, 250–262.

Orchard, I., Lange, A. B., and Barrett, F. M. (1988). Serotonergic supply to the epidermis of *Rhodnius prolixus*—evidence for serotonin as the plasticizing factor. *J. Insect Physiol.* 34, 873–879. doi: 10.1016/0022-1910(88)90121-7

Orchard, I., and Te Brugge, V. (2002). Contractions associated with the salivary glands of the blood-feeding bug, *Rhodnius prolixus*: evidence for both a neural and neurohormonal coordination. *Peptides* 23, 693–700. doi: 10.1016/S0196-9781(01)00663-5

Paluzzi, J. P., Haddad, A. S., Sedra, L., Orchard, I., and Lange, A. (2015). Functional characterization and expression analysis of the myoinhibiting peptide receptor in the Chagas disease vector, *Rhodnius prolixus. Mol. Cell. Endocrinol.* 399, 143–153. doi: 10.1016/j.mce.2014.09.004

Paluzzi, J. P., and O'Donnell, M. J. (2012). Identification, spatial expression analysis and functional characterization of a pyrokinin-1 receptor in the Chagas' disease vector, *Rhodnius prolixus. Mol. Cell. Endocrinol.* 363, 36–45. doi: 10.1016/j.mce.2012.07.007

Paluzzi, J. P., Park, Y., Nachman, R. J., and Orchard, I. (2010). Isolation, expression analysis, and functional characterization of the first antidiuretic hormone receptor in insects. *Proc. Natl. Acad. Sci. U.S.A.* 107, 10290–10295. doi: 10.1073/pnas.1003666107

Paluzzi, J. P., Russell, W. K., Nachman, R. J., and Orchard, I. (2008). Isolation, cloning, and expression mapping of a gene encoding an antidiuretic hormone and other CAPA-related peptides in the disease vector, *Rhodnius prolixus. Endocrinology* 149, 4638–4646. doi: 10.1210/en.2008-0353

Paluzzi, J. P., Yeung, C., and O'Donnell, M. J. (2013). Investigations of the signaling cascade involved in diuretic hormone stimulation of Malpighian tubule fluid secretion in *Rhodnius prolixus. J. Insect Physiol.* 59, 1179–1185. doi: 10.1016/j.jinsphys.2013.09.005

Paluzzi, J. P., Young, P., Defferrari, M. S., Orchard, I., Carlini, C. R., and O'Donnell, M. J. (2012). Investigation of the potential involvement of eicosanoid metabolites in anti-diuretic hormone signaling in *Rhodnius prolixus. Peptides* 34, 127–134. doi: 10.1016/j.peptides.2011.10.025

Pietrantonio, P. V., Jagge, C., and McDowell, C. (2001). Cloning and expression analysis of a 5HT7-like serotonin receptor cDNA from mosquito *Aedes aegypti* female excretory and respiratory systems. *Insect Mol. Biol.* 10, 357–369. doi: 10.1046/j.0962-1075.2001.00274.x

Pytliak, M., Vargova, V., Mechirova, V., and Felsoci, M. (2011). Serotonin receptors—from molecular biology to clinical applications. *Physiol. Res.* 60, 15–25. Available online at: http://www.biomed.cas.cz/physiolres/pdf/60/60_15.pdf

Qi, Y. X., Xia, R. Y., Wu, Y. S., Stanley, D., Huang, J., and Ye, G. Y. (2014). Larvae of the small white butterfly, Pieris rapae, express a novel serotonin receptor. *J. Neurochem.* 131, 767–777. doi: 10.1111/jnc.12940

Rahn, E. J., Guzman-Karlsson, M. C., and David Sweatt, J. (2013). Cellular, molecular, and epigenetic mechanisms in non-associative conditioning: implications for pain and memory. *Neurobiol. Learn. Mem.* 105, 133–150. doi: 10.1016/j.nlm.2013.06.008

Roser, C., Jordan, N., Balfanz, S., Baumann, A., Walz, B., Baumann, O., et al. (2012). Molecular and pharmacological characterization of serotonin 5-HT2alpha and 5-HT7 receptors in the salivary glands of the blowfly Calliphora vicina. *PLoS ONE* 7:e49459. doi: 10.1371/journal.pone.0049459

Saitou, N., and Nei, M. (1987). The neighbor-joining method: a new method for reconstructing phylogenetic trees. *Mol. Biol. Evol.* 4, 406–425.

Sarkar, N. R., Tobe, S. S., and Orchard, I. (2003). The distribution and effects of Dippu-allatostatin-like peptides in the blood-feeding bug, *Rhodnius prolixus. Peptides* 24, 1553–1562. doi: 10.1016/j.peptides.2003.07.015

Siju, K. P., Hansson, B. S., and Ignell, R. (2008). Immunocytochemical localization of serotonin in the central and peripheral chemosensory system of mosquitoes. *Arthropod Struct. Dev.* 37, 248–259. doi: 10.1016/j.asd.2007.12.001

Silva, B., Goles, N. I., Varas, R., and Campusano, J. M. (2014). Serotonin receptors expressed in Drosophila mushroom bodies differentially modulate larval locomotion. *PLoS ONE* 9:e89641. doi: 10.1371/journal.pone.0089641

Tamura, K., Stecher, G., Peterson, D., Filipski, A., and Kumar, S. (2013). MEGA6: molecular evolutionary genetics analysis version 6.0. *Mol. Biol. Evol.* 30, 2725–2729. doi: 10.1093/molbev/mst197

Te Brugge, V. A., Nassel, D. R., Coast, G. M., Schooley, D. A., and Orchard, I. (2001). The distribution of a kinin-like peptide and its co-localization with a CRF-like peptide in the blood-feeding bug, *Rhodnius prolixus. Peptides* 22, 161–173. doi: 10.1016/S0196-9781(00)00373-9

Te Brugge, V., Ianowski, J. P., and Orchard, I. (2009). Biological activity of diuretic factors on the anterior midgut of the blood-feeding bug, *Rhodnius prolixus. Gen. Comp. Endocrinol.* 162, 105–112. doi: 10.1016/j.ygcen.2009.01.025

Te Brugge, V., Paluzzi, J. P., Schooley, D. A., and Orchard, I. (2011). Identification of the elusive peptidergic diuretic hormone in the blood-feeding bug *Rhodnius prolixus*: a CRF-related peptide. *J. Exp. Biol.* 214, 371–381. doi: 10.1242/jeb.046292

Thamm, M., Rolke, D., Jordan, N., Balfanz, S., Schiffer, C., Baumann, A., et al. (2013). Function and distribution of 5-HT2 receptors in the honeybee (Apis mellifera). *PLoS ONE* 8:e82407. doi: 10.1371/journal.pone.0082407

Tierney, A. J. (2001). Structure and function of invertebrate 5-HT receptors: a review. *Comp. Biochem. Physiol. A Mol. Integr. Physiol.* 128, 791–804. doi: 10.1016/S1095-6433(00)00320-2

Trimmer, B. A. (1985). Serotonin and the Control of Salivation in the Blowfly Calliphora. *J. Exp. Biol.* 114, 307–328.

Troppmann, B., Balfanz, S., Baumann, A., and Blenau, W. (2010). Inverse agonist and neutral antagonist actions of synthetic compounds at an insect 5-HT1 receptor. *Br. J. Pharmacol.* 159, 1450–1462. doi: 10.1111/j.1476-5381.2010.00638.x

Troppmann, B., Walz, B., and Blenau, W. (2007). Pharmacology of serotonin-induced salivary secretion in Periplaneta americana. *J. Insect Physiol.* 53, 774–781. doi: 10.1016/j.jinsphys.2007.02.020

Tsuji, E., Aonuma, H., Yokohari, F., and Nishikawa, M. (2007). Serotonin-immunoreactive neurons in the antennal sensory system of the brain in the carpenter ant, Camponotus japonicus. *Zool. Sci.* 24, 836–849. doi: 10.2108/zsj.24.836

Turlejski, K. (1996). Evolutionary ancient roles of serotonin: long-lasting regulation of activity and development. *Acta Neurobiol. Exp. (Wars).* 56, 619–636.

Tusnady, G. E., and Simon, I. (2001). The HMMTOP transmembrane topology prediction server. *Bioinformatics* 17, 849–850. doi: 10.1093/bioinformatics/17.9.849

Verlinden, H., Vleugels, R., and Vanden Broeck, J. (2015). Serotonin, serotonin receptors and their actions in insects. *Neurotransmitter* 2:e314. doi: 10.14800/nt.314

Vleugels, R., Lenaerts, C., Baumann, A., Vanden Broeck, J., and Verlinden, H. (2013). Pharmacological characterization of a 5-HT1-type serotonin receptor in the red flour beetle, Tribolium castaneum. *PLoS ONE* 8:e65052. doi: 10.1371/journal.pone.0065052

Vleugels, R., Lenaerts, C., Vanden Broeck, J., and Verlinden, H. (2014). Signalling properties and pharmacology of a 5-HT7 -type serotonin receptor from Tribolium castaneum. *Insect Mol. Biol.* 23, 230–243. doi: 10.1111/imb.12076

Von Nickisch-Rosenegk, E., Krieger, J., Kubick, S., Laage, R., Strobel, J., Strotmann, J., et al. (1996). Cloning of biogenic amine receptors from moths (Bombyx mori and Heliothis virescens). *Insect Biochem. Mol. Biol.* 26, 817–827. doi: 10.1016/S0965-1748(96)00031-8

Wang, Q., Mohamed, A. A., and Takeda, M. (2013). Serotonin receptor B may lock the gate of PTTH release/synthesis in the Chinese silk moth, Antheraea pernyi; a diapause initiation/maintenance mechanism? *PLoS ONE* 8:e79381. doi: 10.1371/journal.pone.0079381

Watanabe, H., Shimohigashi, M., and Yokohari, F. (2014). Serotonin-immunoreactive sensory neurons in the antenna of the cockroach Periplaneta americana. *J. Comp. Neurol.* 522, 414–434. doi: 10.1002/cne.23419

Zhao, X. C., and Berg, B. G. (2009). Morphological and physiological characteristics of the serotonin-immunoreactive neuron in the antennal lobe of the male oriental tobacco budworm, Helicoverpa assulta. *Chem. Senses* 34, 363–372. doi: 10.1093/chemse/bjp013

Zheng, H., Pearsall, E. A., Hurst, D. P., Zhang, Y., Chu, J., Zhou, Y., et al. (2012). Palmitoylation and membrane cholesterol stabilize mu-opioid receptor homodimerization and G protein coupling. *BMC Cell Biol.* 13:6. doi: 10.1186/1471-2121-13-6

Zornik, E., Paisley, K., and Nichols, R. (1999). Neural transmitters and a peptide modulate Drosophila heart ate. *Peptides* 20, 45–51. doi: 10.1016/S0196-9781(98)00151-X

5

Populations collapses in marine invertebrates due to endocrine disruption

Marcos Antonio Fernandez*

Marine Ecotoxicology Laboratory, Chemical Oceanography Department, Faculty of Oceanography, Rio de Janeiro State University, Rio de Janeiro, Brazil

Edited by:
Leandro Miranda-Alves, Federal University of Rio de Janeiro, Brazil

Reviewed by:
Anna Di Cosmo, University of Naples Federico II, Italy
Sumonto Mitra, Karolinska Institute (KI), Sweden

*Correspondence:
Marcos Antonio Fernandez
hallfz@gmail.com

In the beginning of the twenty first century, the International Program on Chemical Safety published a document entitled *Global Assessment of the State-Of-The-Science of Endocrine Disruptors*. The work indicated only weak evidence of endocrine-related effects in human populations, and in wild animal populations. This document was revised in 2012 (*State of the Science of Endocrine Disrupting Chemicals–2012*) (1). The new document and the extensive scientific evidence it provided showed clearly that ED effects could be a risk to human and wildlife health. These works, however, were focused in human health and related animal models, mainly vertebrates and particularly mammals. It can be argued that invertebrates and many other taxa are important parts of all ecosystems, and, in many instances, have been shown to be also vulnerable to endocrine disruption. Thus, this work is aimed to show some observations on important marine invertebrate taxa, from an ecological point of view. The most important example of endocrine disruption in marine wild populations is the imposex response of marine gastropods, known for more than 40 years, and worldwide used to evaluate marine antifouling pollution. Among the mollusks, other important natural resources are bivalve species, used as human food sources and cephalopods, free-living, highly specialized mollusks, and also human food sources. Effects derived from endocrine disruptors in these species indicate that consumption could bring these compounds to human populations in an almost direct way, sometimes without any form of cooking or preparation. While discussing these questions, this work is also aimed to stimulate research on endocrine disruption among the invertebrate taxa that inhabited our oceans, and on which these effects are poorly known today.

Keywords: endocrine disruption, marine invertebrates, ecological risk assessment, reproduction, environmental pollution

INTRODUCTION

In the beginning of the twenty first century, the International Program on Chemical Safety (IPCS, a joint program with WHO—World Health Organization and UNEP—United Nations Environment Program and the International Labor Organization) published a document entitled *Global Assessment of the State-Of-The-Science of Endocrine Disruptors* (2). This work reunited the then available scientific information on endocrine disruption (ED). The results were indicative, not conclusive: it showed that some effects observed in wildlife could be attributed to chemical compounds that can act as endocrine disruptor chemicals (EDCs), but the causal links are weak and effects related to highly polluted areas in most cases. Furthermore, the results indicated only weak evidence of endocrine-related effects in human populations. Among the studied compounds, most are POPs such as polychlorinated biphenyls (PCBs), dioxins and dichlorodiphenyltrichloroethane (DDT). The final remark was the need for broad, collaborative and international research efforts.

Against this background and putting forward a great sum of results from new research UNEP and WHO published a new document: *State of the Science of Endocrine Disrupting Chemicals—2012* (1). This document included three sections: the first explains the basic concepts and facts on endocrine disruption; the second discusses in detail the effects of endocrine disruptors in humans and wildlife in 12 chapters, *based in the fact that endocrine systems are very similar among vertebrate species and that endocrine effects manifest themselves independently of species*. This is an important remark for the further sections. The third and final section discusses exposure of humans and wildlife to EDCs and to potential EDCs. The key concerns derived from this impressive study are briefly showed below, as the original document is available at the WHO site (http://www.who.int/ceh/publications/endocrine/en/).

- Human and wildlife are dependent on the ability to reproduce and develop normally, what is not possible without a healthy endocrine system.
- Three evidence lines indicate concern on endocrine disruption: (i) high incidence and increasing trends of endocrine-related disorders in humans; (ii) the observation of endocrine disruption related effects in wildlife populations; (iii) identification of EDCs related to disease outcomes in laboratory studies.
- About 800 compounds are known or suspect to be able to affect: (i) hormone receptors, (ii) hormone synthesis, or, (iii) hormone conversion. Only a small fraction was thoroughly investigated. *The vast majority of chemicals in commercial use have not been tested at all.*
- Humans and wildlife are exposed to EDCs worldwide, and to more compounds than those that are POPs. However, there have been a failure in addressing the environmental causes to the increase of EDCs effects.
- The speed of disease incidence increases rules out genetic factors only as an explanation, indicating in the other hand environmental and non-genetic factors, as nutrition, exposition, and so on.
- There are critical exposure windows in the organism's development, such as fetal development or puberty, in which they are more susceptible to EDCs.
- Wildlife populations of different taxa have been affected by EDCs. In some instances, these EDCs were recognized as POPs, and *bans on these compounds have led to population's recovery* (a key remark for ecological risk evaluation).
- Internationally agreed and validated protocols to the identification of EDCs still may detect only a part of the known spectrum of ED effects. *This increases the likelihood of overlooking harmful effects in humans and wildlife.* Thus, *disease risk* (and ecological risk) *related to EDCs may be significantly underestimated.*

Even considering that some of these findings have been contested (3, 4), in this broad scenario the new document and the extensive scientific evidence it provided showed clearly that ED effects could be a risk to human and wildlife health, and that much effort is still required to a better understanding of these effects and to provide the measures required for avoiding this growing treat. While this study is a basic reference for those working in this field of research, this study was focused in human health and vertebrate models. Some instances of EDCs effects in invertebrate populations were indicated, and, in this case, with a focus in interference mechanisms and populations responses. The aim of this work is to advance a step further in the direction of the ecological risk evaluation state and requirements for the marine environments, from an ecotoxicological point of view. While being important for environmental health, these aspects are out of the scope of the original work.

ENDOCRINE DISRUPTION IN MARINE INVERTEBRATES: GENERAL ASPECTS OF THIS QUESTION

Invertebrates represent more than 95% of the known species in the animal kingdom, and large groups of these species are of ecological relevance in marine ecosystems (5–7). By 1999, compounds such as the common herbicides atrazine, simazine and Diuron, metals and organometallic compounds such as mercury, cadmium, or organotins, insecticides such as Toxaphene, DDT, or Endrin, alkylphenols such as nonylphenol or PCBs such as Aroclor 1242 or natural or synthetic vertebrate steroids such as diethylstilbestrol or testosterone were implicated in causing endocrine disruption in invertebrates (8). Evidence mounted ever since, and this kind of problem is being reported for several important groups of marine invertebrates, such as amphipods (9, 10), copepods, crabs, and hermit crabs (11, 12), barnacles (13), abalones (14), echinoderms (5), and polychaetes (8). In some species, intersexuality may include a simultaneous activity of both sexes gonads, in a true hermaphroditic condition (15) or could be induced by pollutants (14). Among decapoda and branchiopoda, intersexuality is fairly common, at typical background incidences of <1%, and many common pollutants have been shown to be capable to interfere with the hormonal responses (7, 11). While it is widely known that endocrine disruptors may play a key role in the conditions of marine

Abbreviations: CONAMA, National Environmental Council of Brazil; DDT, Dichlorodiphenyltrichloroethane; DOC, Dissolved Organic Carbon; ED, Endocrine Disruption; EDC, Endocrine Disrupting Compound(s); EQS, Environmental Quality Standard; IPCS, International Program on Chemical Safety; HPG, hypothalamic-pituitary-gonadal; Oct-GnRH, Octopus Gonadotrophin-Releasing Hormone; PAH, Polycyclic Aromatic Hydrocarbon(s); PCB, Polychlorinated biphenyls; POP, Persistent Organic Pollutant(s); POC, Particulate Organic Carbon; RPLI, Relative Penis Length Index; RPSI, Relative Penis Size Index; TBT, Tributyltin; TPT, Triphenyltin; UNEP, United Nations Environment Program; VDSI, Vas Deferens Sequence Index; WHO, World Health Organization.

invertebrate communities, it was often very difficult to make extrapolations from the results of studies did at cellular and sub-cellular levels to the individual and population levels for each tested species (10). A small compilation of some studies done in the last years with marine invertebrates can show the wide range of endocrine disrupting compounds and the variety of associated responses (**Table 1**, below). It should be noted that most of these studies do not focused in combined effects, a critical point in environmental monitoring.

Even as marked changes in marine invertebrate populations in some instances where demonstrated to occur, mainly molluscan populations, whole ecosystem, multitaxonomic environmental monitoring is seldom possible due to technical and funding questions. Only in some limited instances specific populations' distributions data are available, and mostly related to monitoring species, or those of great economic value (28). In many instances of toxicity assessment, single invertebrate species are being used to perform toxicity tests to evaluate potential responses of organisms of many different phyla, as pointed out by Depledge and Billinghurst (8). However, 20 years later this approach is still being used in many, if not most, instances.

In regard of population dynamics, some very important gaps in the available knowledge about environmental effects of pollutants are still present, turning the integration of ecologic and ecotoxicologic information even more difficult. Aspects such as habitat loss due to growing human pressure (29), the lack of specific knowledge of invertebrate endocrine systems, that are very different from vertebrate ones (6, 13), the assimilation pathways of pollutants such as water exposition, dietary exposition, feeding habits (8, 29) and also the very important questions of species responses at different development phases of the reproductive cycle and to mixtures of pollutants which may show similar/dissimilar effects (30). When the great variability of natural processes in marine communities is taken in account, it is not difficult to understand why seldom population's declines in marine invertebrates' communities have been shown to be derived from external forcing such as pollutant pressure. In the particular case of endocrine disruptors, the relative potency of each compound for the studied species is badly known, what makes the evaluation of combined toxicities a still more uncertain affair (6, 29).

As a concluding remark for this introducing section, I would argue that in the case of invertebrates the most impacting effects of pollutants, including endocrine disruptors, are those that could be strongly related to the occurrence of known pollutants affecting and, in some instances, eradicating or seriously compromising natural populations, and thus, affecting the marine ecosystems from an ecological point of view, or, also, compromising biological productivity. The most striking study cases are those related to molluscan species, and these will be the focus of the next sections.

Population decline, local extinctions or reduced reproductive capacity have been demonstrated to be directly related to endocrine disruption in three different conditions: the worldwide development of imposex in marine gastropod species (31), the occurrence of intersexuality in the abalone in Japan, which also led to some documented population reduction caused by reproductive failure (14) and the case of the Basin d'Arcachon, where bivalve commercial production collapsed during the peak of organotins application as biocides in marine antifouling paints and subsequently recovered as this application was restricted, France being the first country to exert this control (32, 33). As marine bivalves and cephalopods are also part of human diet in coastal areas (34), they are further discussed.

ENDOCRINE DISRUPTION: DETECTION AND EVALUATION OF EFFECTS IN MARINE GASTROPOD POPULATIONS IN A LOW ORGANOTINS EXPOSITION SCENARIO

In respect to ED in wildlife marine invertebrate populations, the most characteristic phenomena in organotins polluted areas is a syndrome that is called "imposex" in female gastropods. This syndrome consists in the imposition of male sexual characters, such as penis and/or vas deferens in female individuals. Smith (35), introduced this term after reports of a "penis like" growth of tissue behind the right tentacle of female gastropods, in the location of the male penis. Further research indicated the antifouling biocide tributyltin (TBT), then in intensive application in any kind of vessel as the main cause, and intensive boat and shipping activities areas as the most affected ones (36–39). By 1991, this problem had been reported in 132 gastropod species, this number rising to 192 by 2005 (40). The last extensive report raised again this figure to 268 species by 2009 (41). In the other hand, these last authors indicated some 42 gastropod species that does not develop masculinization when exposed to this compound. Species differential sensitivity, phylogeny—mesogastropods are remarkably less sensitive than neogastropods—and feeding habits are possible causes for these observations. There are many theories to explain the occurrence of this kind of DE syndrome, but the complete mechanism has not yet been totally explained (6, 41, 42).

However, as reports mounted in the literature, the problem of TBT antifoulings pollution was perceived to be global, as first indicated by Ellis and Pattisina (31). Many techniques were developed for imposex evaluation when field and laboratorial studies showed that the relative development of masculine characters on the females was dose-dependent for TBT and in some species also to TPT (triphenyltin, an alternative for TBT as biocide in the paints formulation). Development of these techniques resulted in the application of imposex development indexes, other than the simpler evaluation of the percentage of affected females in each given sampled population. These indexes were based on two approaches: those that compared the penis development in males and affected females, and those that followed the development of the vas deferens in affected females. In the first case, these indexes are the Relative Penis Length Index (RPLI) or the Relative Penis Size Index (RPSI) [(43), for a full description of measurements and application]. In the second case, the index is the Vas Deferens Sequence Index or VDSI [please refer to (40, 43–45) for particular applications of this approach].

TABLE 1 | Some examples of endocrine disrupting compounds and their range of effects in marine invertebrate species.

Compounds	Tested species	Effects	References
TBT, DBT	*Mya arenaria*	Lower progesterone levels, sexual maturation delay, "F"	(16)
TBT	*Mya arenaria*	Skewed sex ratio, vitellin reduction, oestradiol-17β production in gonad reduced "F"	(17)
TBT	*Ruditapes decussata*	Increase in testosterone, oestradiol decrease "F"	(18)
TBT	*Haliotis madaka*	Intersexuality, ovary spermatogenesis, "F" **populations reduction**	(14)
North Sea Oil (NSO)	*Mytilus edulis*	Ovarian follicle development, normal spermatogenesis	(19)
NSO + PAH + Alkylphenols	*Mytilus edulis*	Male gonadal melanomacrophage centers, degeneration ovary follicles	(19)
Bisphenol A	*Mytilus edulis*	Spawning induction for both sexes, ovocyte atresia	(20)
2,2′,4,4′-tetrabromodiphenyl ether	*Mytilus edulis*	Ovocyte atresia, male spawning induction	(20)
Diallyl phthalate	*Mytilus edulis*	Follicle and ovocyte reduction, male spawning induction	(20)
PAHs, TBT	*Mytilus galloprovincialis*	Intersexuality, oocite atresia "F"	(21)
Benzo(a)pyrene	*Portunus trituberculatus*	Reduced ovarian growth, testosterone, progesterone and 17βestradiol secretion reduction	(22)
Benzo(a)pyrene	*Chlamys farreri*	Reduced testosterone and 17βestradiol production, progesterone disruption in ovary, ovarian impairment, development delay	(23)
Bisphenol A, 17βestradiol	*Mytilus galloprovincialis*	Gene transcription	(24)
Testosterone	*Brachionus calyciflorus*	Increased swimming, fertilization rate and recognition ability in males	(25)
Progesterone, flutamide (non-steroidal anti-androgen)	*Brachionus calyciflorus*	Inhibited swimming speed, suppression of fertilization and reduced recognition ability in males	(25)
Dibutyl phthalate	*Galeolaria caespitosa*	Sperm dysfunction, impaired embryogenesis	(26)
Propylparaben	*Tigriopus japonicus*	Sex ratio alteration toward females	(27)

Most were laboratory studies, while those including field studies are indicated by the letter "F." Bold letters, population reduction observed.

These techniques provided the researchers with means to evaluate the relative intensity of the pollution and the extension of the affected areas with a very simple and cost effective monitoring tool.

Obviously, the ideal case is to have parallel chemical analysis for this monitoring, being these analyses of water (44), of sediments (46), or of the animals tissues (47). In the most ideal case, the intensity of imposex in gastropod populations or the organotin body burden of the animals could have provided a proxy of mean TBT water concentrations (44), but the environmental variability is such that these approaches were never thoroughly developed. Another combined monitoring approach, using imposex in gastropods populations to guide sediments sampling to the more critical areas is of easier application. Persistence of organotin pollution in conditions such as fine-grained, organic-rich, mostly anoxic coastal sediments (48, 49) has made TBT and other organotins legacy pollutants, being considered as POPs by WHO-UNEP (1). As a matter of fact, this is probably the most important reason that would explain why imposex is still being reported in European waters (50–53), even when clear instances of improvement are being reported (54). The same occurs in other areas were organotins uses were banned, such as Korea, for instance (55, 56). In the other hand, unregulated use of these compounds have been already demonstrated in some areas, for instance, Latin America (57–59) or North Africa (60–62).

From an ecotoxicological point of view, the work of Stroben et al. (44), being multispecific, clearly demonstrated that species sensitivity could be different even in the same genus, and thus, indicated that antifouling pollution could affect marine communities as a selective pressure. In **Figure 1**, below, some results of this study are presented and discussed.

As we can see from the original data, the species *Nucella lapillus* and *Ocenebra erinacea* are much more sensible, presenting a much more developed vas deferens than *Trivia* species or *Hinia* species at a given TBT concentration. Thus, exposed to similar conditions, the pollution effects on individuals and populations will differ greatly among the different species present at each site. Surely, not all species sampled occurred at all places at the same time. In any case, at the UK environmental target concentration of 2 ng(Sn). L^{-1} (vertical line 1), for instance, the four most sensitive species will present imposex, while both less sensitive *Hinia* species will not. All tested species that present imposex in this concentration range will have females presenting a small penis and/or a partially developed vas deferens, but no sterile individuals in the populations that reach these VDSI values (please refer to the original work for the details of each species VDSI development evaluation). However, at the 10 ng(Sn). L^{-1} concentration level, vertical line 2, that was then fairly common in coastal waters, the more sensitive species VDSI values would be above stage 4, indicating that populations began to show sterile females and thus were in danger by recruitment reduction. Local extinction of the most sensitive species was observed all around the world, sometimes eradicating part of the previous species population's distributions. For instance, some two thirds of the *Stramonita brasiliensis* populations area in Guanabara Bay, a highly polluted harbor area in Brazil, were lost between the sixties and the nineties (46). About half of this area was recovered by this species by 2012 [(45); see the details in **Figure 2** below for the area extension].

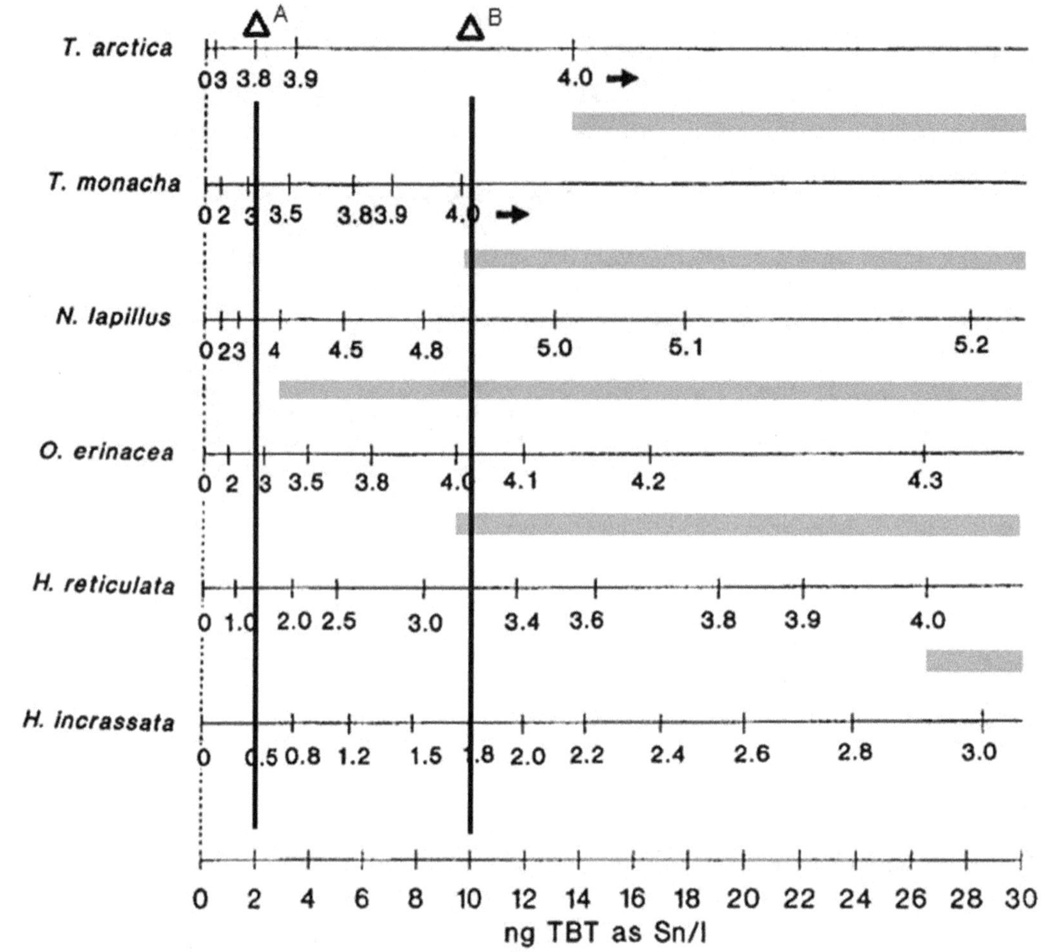

FIGURE 1 | Imposex development is different marine gastropod species at increasing water TBT concentrations. Imposex intensity: values of VDSI index measured for each species; TBT water concentrations in ng(Sn). L^{-1}. Ecological risk indicated by light gray bars indicating population damage by lack of recruitment due to female sterility. Vertical concentration lines: A: TBT EQS of the UK; B: Brazilian limit for sea waters, Class 1, CONAMA Resolution 357. Modified from Stroben et al. (44) by the author.

The recovery of affected populations after the controls on TBT application as biocide and further banning has being considered as a sure indication of pollution reduction (54). If only marine gastropods were affected by TBT, this would have been serious enough, but lack of knowledge of the response of other marine species to this compound makes the hypothesis of ecosystem recovery somewhat less consistent (63). Even in the case of gastropods, recent research indicated that resistance to TBT effects could control the distribution of two species with different organotin sensitivity of *Leucozonia* genus, at least in a heavily polluted, big harbor area (64).

Other important recent observations on imposex development are related to aphallic imposex expression, thus separating the two classic ways of imposex intensity evaluation (by females' penis lengths or by vas deferens development). Aphally in marine gastropods was first showed to occur in *Nucella lapillus* males, in a specific location in England, Dumpton Gap. This syndrome was reported as a genetic problem that caused male specimens to have undeveloped sexual characters, malformations or even to lack their penises. In the other hand, the syndrome caused a reduction in imposex development in the females, thus permitting an isolated population to survive in a heavily polluted coast. This particular condition was called "Dumpton syndrome" because it was discovered at Dumpton Gap (65, 66). By the late nineties, this syndrome has been described in Brittany (67, 68) and in the northwest coast of Spain (69). These last authors proposed a modified VDSI evaluation scheme, as sterile females *Nucella lapillus* were observed for the first time lacking penises. This observation made clear that penis development in imposex females may be independent of vas deferens development. Because of this observation, the authors pointed that in DS conditions, or, for instance, *at lower ambient organotins concentrations*, the VDSI so modified would be a better indicator of TBT pollution that indexes such as the RPLI or RPSI that would be meaningless for aphallic females. More recently, and under different experimental conditions,

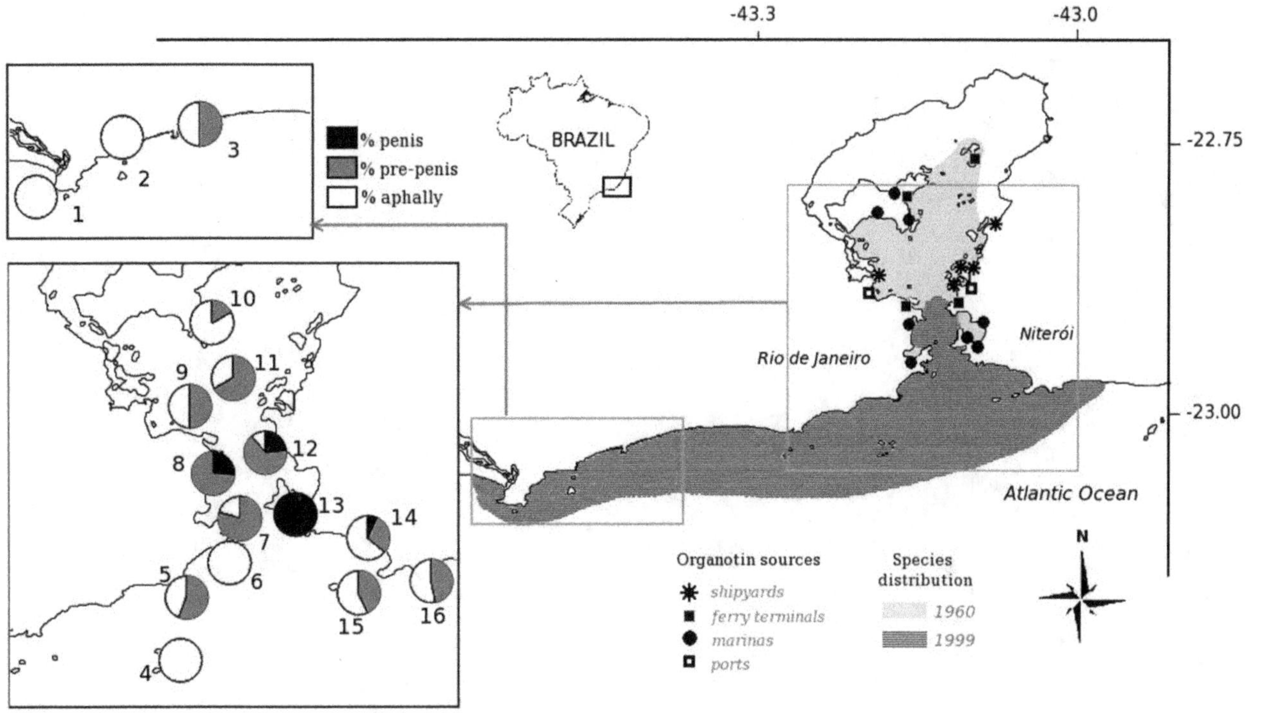

FIGURE 2 | Evolution of the marine gastropod *Stramonita brasiliensis* populations at Guanabara Bay, Brazil, between 1960 and 2013. Organotin sources and expression of imposex development are also shown. Modified from Toste et al. (45).

it was demonstrated that TPT (triphenyltin), a tri-substituted organotin used as biocide as substitute for TBT when this compound began to be controlled, mainly in Japan (70, 71) could induce aphallic imposex development in the same species (72). While these studies were related to *N. lapillus*, aphally is recorded in other gastropod species.

In the previously quoted work by Stroben et al. (44), the species *N. lapillus*, *Trivia arctica*, *T. monacha*, and *Hinia reticulata* were showed to present complete vas deferens development from near the base of the right tentacle, where the penis is located in the males, to the vulva opening, without penis development. In *Cantharus cecillei*, this same general development pattern was observed to occur, while presenting some specific differences [see (40), for the complete observations]. In these species, however, no observation was made about *male* aphally, what would indicate that these ways of imposex development were not related to DS. In another series of works with *Stramonita brasiliensis* in the Brazilian coast, female aphally was frequently observed (73, 74). The proportional incidence of female aphallic imposex development was showed to be related to the distance from the organotins sources at Guanabara Bay, along a sensible distance from the main sources area (to some 60 km distance of the organotins sources centroid, Spearman test $R = 0.6959$, $p < 0.05$), with no male aphally being observed (45). Thus, it became clear that at least for *S. brasiliensis* vas deferens development is independent of that of the penis and penis development occurred only closer to the organotin sources inside Guanabara Bay, and thus, at higher environmental concentrations.

What is more important, it was observed that imposex females could even be sterilized without the development of a penis, a very important observation for environmental monitoring using imposex response that was first demonstrated by Barreiro et al. (69) in *N. lapillus*. Based in these observations, a new imposex development scheme for VDSI in *Stramonita brasiliensis* was proposed, with low and high exposition routes, that is shown in **Figure 3**, modified from Toste et al. (45), below. These observations could be important for other imposex monitoring studies, as aphally in imposex females have been reported in some gastropod species, such as *Hexaplex trunculus*, Lahbib et al. (75); *Stramonita rustica*, Artifon et al. (76); *Thais brevidentata, Thais bisserialis, Thais kiosquiformis, Thais melones, Plicopurpura pansa, Plicopurpura columellaris*, Grimón et al. (77). These observations with other species confirmed that VDSI could be the only adequate approach for imposex intensity evaluation. With the global reduction of TBT pollution, worldwide demonstrated by dozens of published works of measured organotins concentrations worldwide in environmental matrices, the classic imposex evaluation approach seems to need a revision. The VDSI application as shown by Toste et al. (45), may even help discriminating higher from lower exposition conditions for the studied gastropod populations, what could be useful in evaluating the relative importance of the remaining organotins sources, or of their illegal use. This

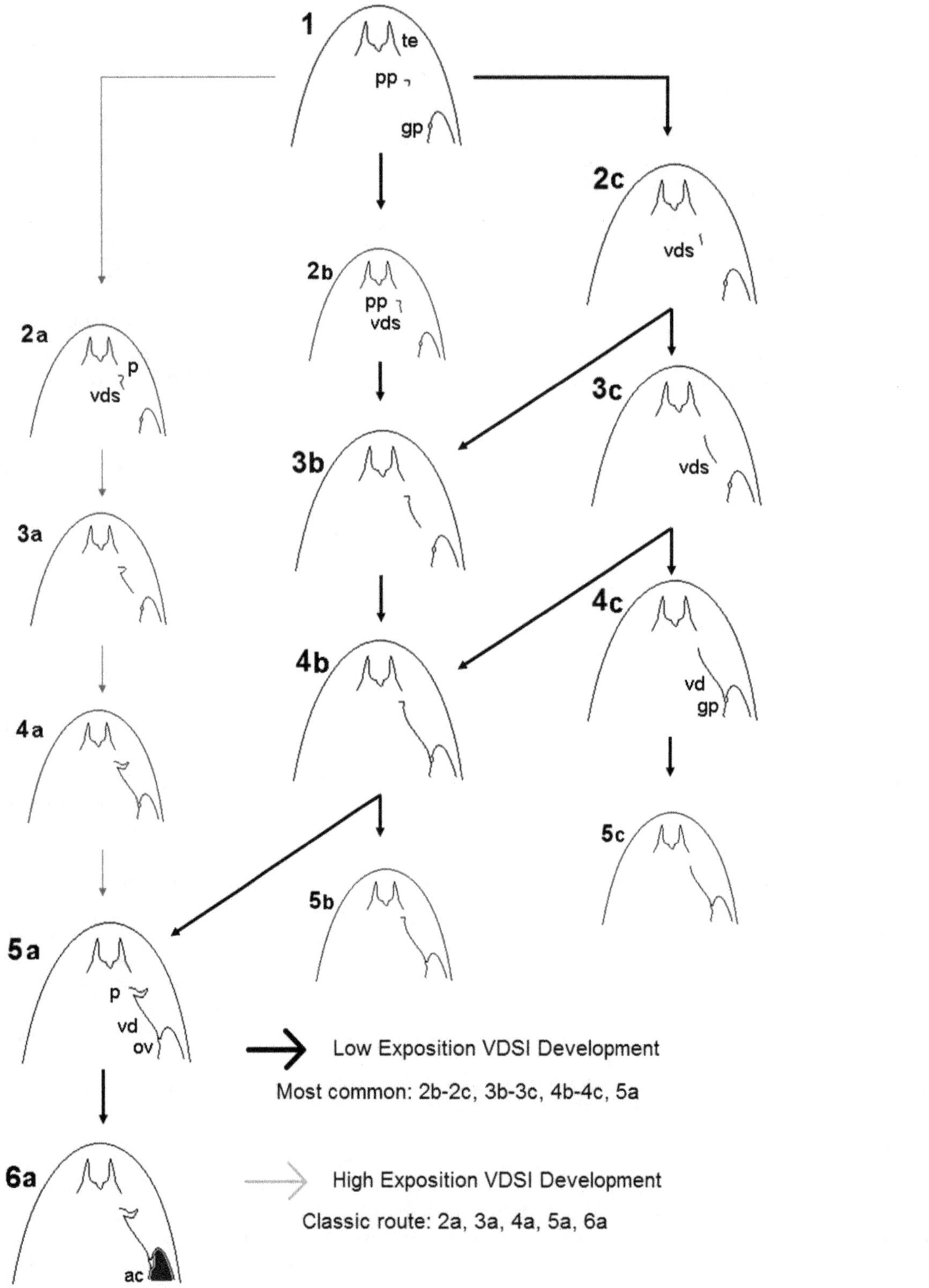

FIGURE 3 | Imposex development scheme for *Stramonita brasiliana (Stramonita haemastoma as originally published)* with high and low exposition routes, according to Toste et al. (45). Captions: te, tentacle; pp, penis primordium; gp, genital papilla; vds, vas deferens; ov, obstructed vulva; ac, aborted capsules. The inclination of the routes at the same stages is related to relative organotins exposition: the nearer to stage 1, lower expositions were indicated by distance for organotins sources in the field. Dark arrows indicate the more commonly observed routes in Southeastern Brazil.

approach, however, still requires the sacrifice of the studied animals, what would not be required by the use of a non-destructive approach such as the one developed by Fernandez et al. (73).

The widespread occurrence of imposex female aphally renders penis lengths indexes meaningless (for instance, total female aphally was recorded for 9 out of 19 stations for imposex monitoring in *Nucella lapillus* in 2014, causing values for RPLI in this species along the Portuguese coast to drop to almost zero, thus rendering its application unable to further indicate decreasing tendencies afterward but for one sampling station along the Portuguese coast [(53), **Table 1**]. The same observation was reported in *Hexaplex trunculus*, showing a temporal reduction pattern of phallic imposex development as observed in *Stramonita brasiliensis* in Brazil, by Lahbib et al. (78) in Tunisia. The use of vas deferens development only, without taking in account the penis development, for VDSI application was even indicated for *Nucella lapillus* by (79). In the other way, some recent studies done in more heavily polluted areas that still remain in Latin America, such as Peru (59, 80) and Chile (81), for instance, showed that penis-based indexes are still useful and could still provide relevant information for some time to come in the remaining hot spots areas. Anyway, the aphallic imposex development observed for *S. brasiliensis* could lead to female sterility, as previously pointed out, when the females presented only pre-penises or very small penises (45), thus making the VDSI the most relevant imposex development index to be applied in this new, mostly low exposure scenario.

There is still another complicating factor in the field imposex analysis: the quite relevant question of interference in the imposex response of the animals. This interference may arise by two different mechanisms: one is the complexation of organotins when high loads of organic matter are present in the waters at the same time. It was long known that organic matter has as very strong affinity to organotins (82) and that in anoxic sediments, degradation of organotins is very slow (83, 84). In any case, this same high affinity will be present in waters rich in POC (particulate organic carbon) and DOC (dissolved organic carbon). These organic compounds thus may act as a kind of "buffer," reducing the bioavailability of organotins to the biota, and, consequently, the imposex expression of gastropod populations. Frequently associated to organic rich waters in the coastal zone are direct sewage discharges, important artificial sources of POC and DOC. At the same time, these sewage discharges are also important sources of xenoestrogens to the same coastal areas. It has been demonstrated by bioassays with *Nucella lapillus* using sewage treatment plant effluents rich in xenoestrogens such as octylphenol, nonylphenol, and bisphenol A that exposition to these effluents could activate the estrogen receptor of this species (85) and at the same time were capable of reducing the imposex expression of TBT-treated females (86). The most affected response is, not unexpectedly, the RPLI, as we saw the growing relative importance of the aphallic vas deferens development routes before.

This interference mechanism was observed in the field for the first time at a small touristic city, called Paraty, which is located at the end of a small inlet in the southeastern coast of Rio de Janeiro state, Brazil. Coincidently, in this area, the organotin sources and organic matter sources are located very close to each other, in the inner inlet, and this particularity made possible to understand the different water residence times of each compound. Monitoring studies of imposex development in populations of *S. brasiliensis* were made in 2006 and 2011, and while a relative amelioration was observed in the inner inlet stations, the outer stations showed a relative aggravation of the imposex condition. The most likely reasons for this strange observation are that while organotins were present in the whole area, and recent input was showed to occur at the 2011 sampling by sediment analysis, the number of small boats, that are the only sources in the area, remained approximately constant while local human population has grown. Thus, organic matter and xenoestrogens inputs, aggravated by total lack of sewage treatment, also have certainly risen. Then, the "buffer" effect was enough to suppress part of the imposex development of the animals in the inner inlet. The populations recovered, while showing 100% imposex low expression incidence (only two penis bearing females recorded in the study). In the other hand, degradation of the organic matter and dispersion reduced the "buffer" effect in the outer inlet, and thus the remaining organotins are still able to produce a response in the animals. While somewhat speculative, the key to understand this process was the difference in water residence times of organotins, that are highly toxic to marine organisms, and of the sewage derived organic matter, that is highly nutritive, and thus, quickly degraded by aerobic bacteria. While not all these parameters were measured in occasion, the very color and particulate matter content of the waters from the inner inlet when compared to those of the outer inlet showed clearly where the problem was. A schematic conceptual description of this interference mechanism is shown in **Figures 4A,B**, below. For the original data and details, please refer to Borges et al. (87).

Putting all these information and ideas together, what seems clear is that in a new scenario of lower organotins inputs, in many instances derived from contaminated sediments, including in Europe (48, 88–90), the imposex response of marine gastropod populations should be evaluated with care. Under conditions of interference with this response, imposex development could be reduced in some areas, mostly in urbanized areas with parallel sewage discharge pollution. In these conditions, while the animals may show a low imposex response, the animals' body burden of organotins could still be high, even higher than in more pristine conditions. Some recent results seems to indicate this possibility with animals presenting high organotins body burden with showing low imposex responses (59, 91). Some aspects of the populations used for biomonitoring have influence on the results, such as genetics, temperature influence on metabolism or even the seasonality of the reproductive cycle, a basic aspect often not considered (92). In any case, the key to understand the animal's response would be the possibility of interference by other parameters in the water, which is dependent of each study area particularities. The conclusion that organotin pollution has been ameliorated may be doubtful in some situations. As biological monitoring is frequently used without bioassays or body burden analysis, the result of these studies must be evaluated with care. If interference is suspected,

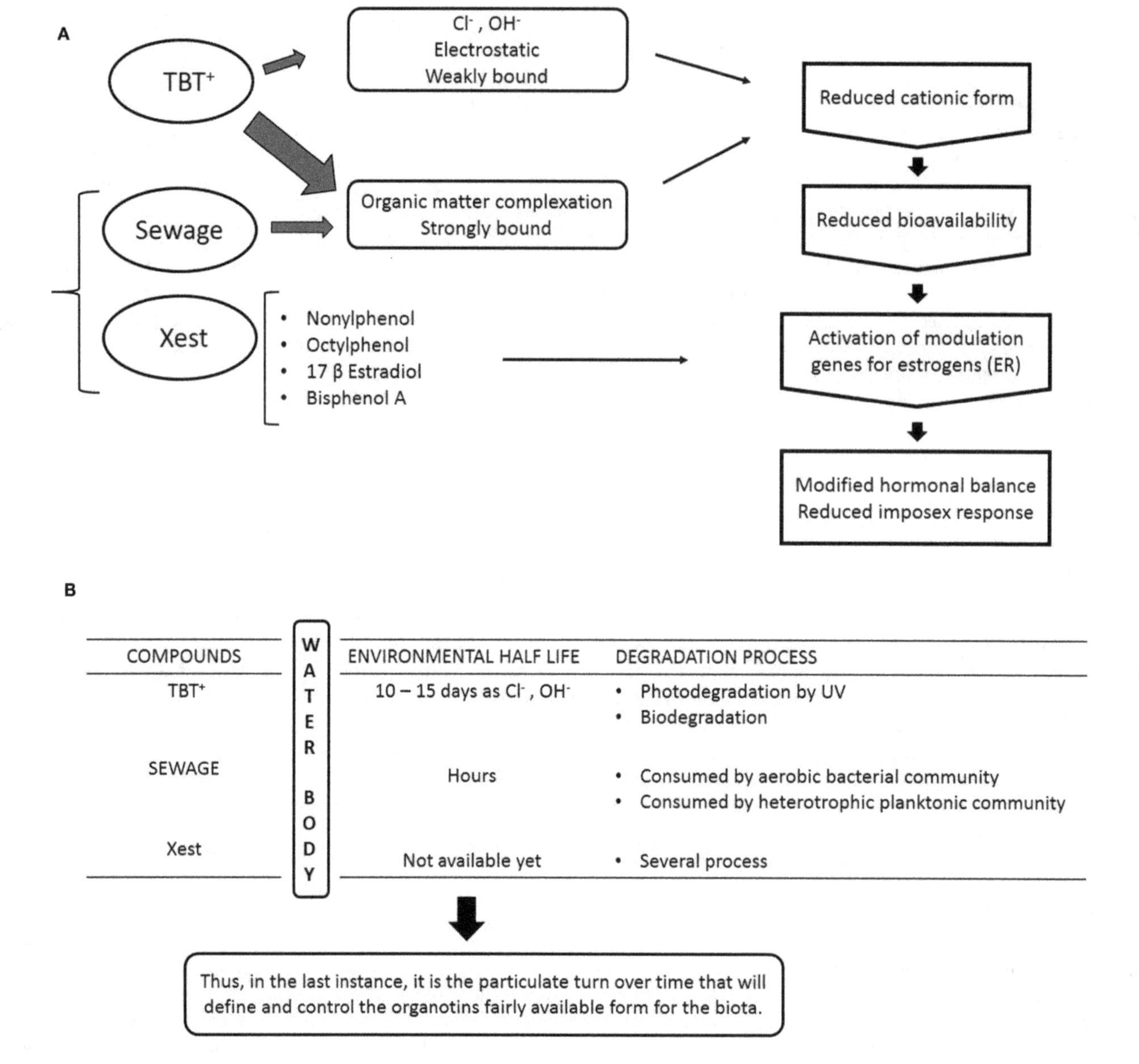

FIGURE 4 | (A) Schematic scheme for an interference mechanism in the imposex response of marine gastropod mollusk to organotin compounds. While cationic organotins are the most available form to biota, both particulate and dissolved organic matter from sewage can complex organotins, while sewage is also a source of xenoestrogens that may act as antagonists to imposex development. **(B)** Main environmental aspects of the interference mechanism proposed. Due to the multiple variables involved, only the general lines are indicated.

confirmatory chemical analysis is indicated, and occurrence of organotin pollution should be suspected. *In this case, the very occurrence of imposex in marine snails is a clue that biologically active organotin compounds are present in local waters.* It is important to remember that organotins could present a human health risk for some coastal populations, as previously reported (34, 76, 81, 93, 94). Imposex development is still the faster and cheaper biological monitoring method to evaluate the occurrence of remaining hotspots of organotin pollution, or to verify its illegal use.

ENDOCRINE DISRUPTION IN MARINE BIVALVE MOLLUSKS: GROWING IN IMPORTANCE AS BIOMONITORING ORGANISMS IN A NEAR FUTURE

Among all animal taxa, bivalve mollusks are probably the most important for monitoring the extension and intensity of marine pollution. Numerous programs of marine monitoring employed bivalve mollusks, among which the Mussel Watch was the most important. Being sessile, resistant, easily collected, these are adequate organisms for monitoring studies. The fact that bivalves are also important components of many human populations diet in coastal areas, and the object of growing mariculture investments make these species important vectors of transference of pollutants introduced in these coastal areas to human populations. Marine bivalves have also been shown to present reproductive anomalies related to endocrine disruptors. When the bivalve *Ruditapes decussatus* was transplanted to TBT polluted areas, a rising on testosterone levels with estradiol reduction was observed (18). This same observation was made on *Mya arenaria* populations (16). This last species had shown male-biased populations in another study, by Gagné et al. (17), the first instance in which hormonal alterations were reflected at population level. The occurrence of intersexuality has been showed to occur in marine bivalves (21). On the subject of endocrine disruption, the most common studies were focused in the occurrence of vitellogenin proteins in males, for instance, of *Tapes philippinarum* (95–97) or *Mytilus edulis* (19, 20, 98). This occurrence is related to availability of xenobiotics such as nonylphenol, bisphenol A, ethinylestradiol, or PAHs, common in urban sewage (99–103). In spite of many instances of endocrine disruption being observed within populations of marine bivalves, the extinction of populations was not commonly observed. From this point of view, the most studied case of extensive populational damage was the Arcachon Bay, France, and the commercial farming of *Crassostrea gigas*, the Pacific oyster.

The Basin D'Arcachon is a closed roughly triangular tidal water body with some 156 km^2 area, in which some 10,000 to 15,000 tons of commercial oysters were produced each year. From 1975 to 1982, oyster production was severely reduced, due to absence of spatfall and anomalous growth, with shell calcification anomalies (32). While these problems were reported at the same time in other areas with this same species in England and also along the Spanish Mediterranean coast, the most important and studied area was Arcachon (104). In a very interesting review, Ruiz et al. (33), indicated that from initial water concentrations of TBT of <1 ng(Sn)L^{-1} by 1960, the increased use of this compound led these concentrations to rise above 100 ng(Sn)L^{-1} by 1981–1982, when controls on application were applied by the French government. After these measures, water concentrations of TBT decreased to about 10 ng(Sn)L^{-1} by 1987, reaching again about 1 ng(Sn)L^{-1} by 1993. These same authors have also shown that besides the oyster production collapse, other important ecological changes occurred in the same area. Simultaneously, it was observed a great reduction of the local populations of the gastropod *Ocenebra erinacea*, in which the first symptoms of imposex development were reported by 1973, earlier than the oyster production collapse. With the reduction of organotin pollution, gastropod populations recovered later. Also "green tides" of *Enteromorpha* spp. were reported to occur by 1982. While clearly indicating the gaps in the original data, the authors indicated that TBT effects on other invertebrate grazers may explain this anomalous observation, a first evidence of multispecific TBT ecological disturbance. Our research group has also noted excessive algal growth and apparent reduction of herbivorous species in some organotin polluted coastal areas in Brazil. This subject is now under a closer scrutiny, as our previous studies were designed for imposex evaluation only.

It should be pointed out, also, that dioecious bivalves did not have the internal fecundation of marine gastropods that made gastropods such useful species for environmental monitoring of endocrine disruption. Reproductive conditions evaluation in marine bivalves often requires histological analysis, what precludes a quick, fast, effective monitoring methodology such as imposex evaluation. With the phasing out of TBT, and the intensive use of new antifoulings that may act as xenoestrogens or estrogen agonists, such as Irgarol 1051, the "naval version" of atrazine [see (73) for a deeper discussion], imposex will be used only in the monitoring of the remaining hotspots of legacy organotin polluted areas. The relative importance of marine bivalves as indicators of marine endocrine disruption will probably rise in a near future, including in the evaluation of health risks for coastal human populations.

POSSIBLE NEW TARGETS FOR ED COMPOUNDS: MARINE CEPHALOPOD MOLLUSKS

Cephalopods are free-living predator mollusks with high mobility and very effective sensorial capabilities, almost completely opposed to the typical oyster species in respect of adequation for environmental monitoring studies. They are in some instances important and appreciated food items, and have been included in human risk analysis for coastal areas (34). From an endocrine disruption point of view, cephalopods have a more complex nervous system than the other mollusks. While in bivalves and gastropods neurohormones secreted by nervous ganglia and gonads are responsible for sexual maturation, showing first and second order control systems, cephalopods show a third order neuroendocrine control system that is comparable to the vertebrate HPG ax [see (105)]. In this sophisticated control system, the Octopus Gonadotrophin-Releasing Hormone (Oct-GnRH) has been shown to act as modulator in functions such as feeding, memory or sensorial, as well as in steroidogenesis in *Octopus vulgaris* (106). In the other hand, it has been shown that estradiol regulates Oct-GnRH and several functions of the nervous systems in the same species (107). As cephalopods are being considered excellent candidates for mariculture in Europe (105), a cycle may be closing on them: as xenoestrogens have been shown to be present in many instances in coastal areas and can affect these animals, their use in mariculture will turn them sessile for all environmental aspects such as bioaccumulation and pollutants transference for humans. Clearly more research is required on this subject.

ENDOCRINE DISRUPTION AND ECOLOGICAL RISK ASSESSMENT

The global aspects of endocrine disruption may be inferred by the ubiquity of detection of proven or suspect endocrine disrupting compounds, even while the biological effects in invertebrate populations are not clearly shown yet. Simple and inexpensive monitoring tools as imposex induction was for organotins monitoring are still lacking, and tools as vitellogenin induction in males are not specific. Certainly a weight of evidence approach will be required at each location based on previous knowledge of possible ED compounds sources and loads. However, in the same way that imposex have been shown to occur worldwide, and to have caused many gastropod species local extinctions, there is no plausible reason today to suppose that the ubiquity of ED compounds is not producing population damage on many invertebrate species, damage that cannot be observed with current methods and approaches. It was recently demonstrated that male infertility could be induced by several environmental contaminants (108), and that even low incidence of female intersexuality in crustacean populations may have drastic effects at population level (10, 109).

Ecological risk assessment is one of the most difficult tasks today, because it requires a deep knowledge of at last three important fields that should be employed at the same time. These are: (i) the pollutant chemical properties and behavior in aquatic environments, that will define its speciation and reactivity; (ii) the physical components of dispersion and mixing that will also influence the compound's water residence time, which is the basic aspect to indicate the exposition of aquatic communities to pollutants: and (iii) the response of each individual species to the pollutant. This is the basic scenario for single pollutants exposition. Much of the current risk evaluation works relay on these three basic kinds of information. First, the available chemical data for each compound are not always complete or reliable. Second, the mean concentrations reported for the studied compounds in the literature were seldom based on modeled concentrations in any particular area, let alone thoroughly calibrated dispersion models (110–112). Third, the available database of biological effects of the ED tested compounds is very far from being complete.

While presenting today's best available technology, would these approaches be sufficient to understand the selective pressures posed by the actual sum of anthropogenic compounds present in coastal areas? I believe these are not. Experience has shown that as more studies developed, and as the legislations advance, still the biological communities change and productivity and biodiversity decreases, and the assessment of these changes depends on expensive ecological studies that are not usually made with the appropriate extension and frequency. To improve this situation, it would be important to advance along three separate lines of action at the same time:

Axis (i) the lack of knowledge on DE effects on invertebrates of many compounds in current use tool should be a priority in research. The importance of this point was shown in the particular study case of marine antifouling paints by interference these effects can induce in the evaluation of the most used biomonitoring approach.

Axis (ii) the problem of the "cocktail effect," not only by the way of sheer toxicity—what means acute or extensive effects -, but by the cumulative action of pollutants on the hormonal regulation mechanisms, should be another. This line is consistent with the results on human and vertebrate health discussed by WHO-UNEP (1).

Axis iii) the final considerations on the difficulty of tracing specific compounds effects on marine communities without knowing the "cocktail" composition, based on antifoulings examples previously discussed (112). This means a necessity for stronger simultaneous determination methods for multiple target compounds, and a relative potency scale for ED compounds in multiple marine taxa.

Certainly, there are other factors on these ecological risk evaluations, such as human population growth, that is greater in the coastal areas; climatic changes; the changing uses of littoral areas; overexploitation of marine resources (113). But we should always try to control the introduction in the environment of hazardous and potentially hazardous chemicals, including known and possible endocrine disruptors.

FINAL REMARKS

I guess in the near future it would be required to focus on the necessity of integrated studies, and on some measures required to make these studies easier to integrate. To reach this goal, we will need a relative potency scale for EDCs in marine species, an integrated database of EDCs with padronized doses and responses easily accessible to researchers and a combined chemical-ecotoxicological-ecological modeling and monitoring approach as the desired end-point. A growing number of works is appearing studying pollutants interactions to different taxa, and these efforts should be supported, because as pointed elsewhere, the interactions are not predicable. To finish this discussion, I would like to point out that specific bioindicators for ED in fieldwork in these new times would be much more probably the exception than the rule.

AUTHOR'S NOTE

My idea is that through the case of marine gastropod and bivalve mollusks to raise interest in research on the ecotoxicological and ecological effects of endocrine disruptors. Among marine invertebrates, endocrine disruption could be widespread, as I tried to show with the particular cases discussed. In the same way that the effects of endocrine disruptors are still poorly known in human and vertebrate populations, invertebrates could also be at risk, as several instances of populations extinctions and recuperation have been demonstrated. So, while by the point of view of human health research is much needed in this field, in the case of ecological damage and ecosystems functions much research is still required too. Perhaps even a specific topic may be raised on this subject.

AUTHOR CONTRIBUTIONS

The author confirms being the sole contributor of this work and has approved it for publication.

REFERENCES

1. WHO-UNEP. *State of the Science of Endocrine Disrupting Chemicals - 2012.* Geneva (2012).
2. IPCS. *Global Assessment of the State-Of-The-Science of Endocrine Disruptors.* Geneva (2002).
3. Nohynek GJ, Borgert CJ, Dietrich D, Rozman KK. Endocrine disruption: fact or urban legend? *Toxicol Lett.* (2013) 223:295–305. doi: 10.1016/j.toxlet.2013.10.022
4. Wise A, O'Brien K, Woodruff T. Are oral contraceptives a significant contributor to the estrogenicity on drinking water? *Environ Sci Technol.* (2011) 45:51–60. doi: 10.1021/es1014482
5. Janer G, Sternberg RM, LeBlanc GA, Porte C. Testosterone conjugating activities in invertebrates: are they targets for endocrine disruptors? *Aquat Toxicol.* (2005) 71:273–82. doi: 10.1016/j.aquatox.2004.11.024
6. Porte C, Janer G, Locusso LC, Oitiz-Zarragoitia M, Cajaraville MP, Fossi MC, et al. Endocrine disruptors in marine organisms. *App Persp Comp Biochem Physiol C.* (2006) 143:303–15. doi: 10.1016/j.cbpc.2006.03.004
7. Rodríguez EM, Medesani DA, Fingerman M. Endocrine disruption in crustaceans due to pollutants: a review. *Comp Biochem Physiol A.* (2007) 146:661–71. doi: 10.1016/j.cbpa.2006.04.030
8. Depledge MH, Billinghurst Z. Ecological significance of endocrine disruption in marine invertebrates. *Mar Poll Bull.* (1999) 39:32–8. doi: 10.1016/S0025-326X(99)00115-0
9. Ford AT, Fernandes TF, Rider SA, Read PA, Robinson CD, Davies IM. Endocrine disruption in a marine amphipod? Field observations of intersexuality and de-masculinization. *Mar Env Res.* (2004) 58:169–73. doi: 10.1016/j.marenvres.2004.03.013
10. Ford AT, Sambles C, Kille P. Intersexuality in crustaceans: genetic, individual and population level effects. *Mar Env Res.* (2008) 66:146–8. doi: 10.1016/j.marenvres.2008.02.067
11. Le Blanc G. Crustacean endocrine toxicology: a review. *Ecotoxicology.* (2007) 16:61–81. doi: 10.1007/s10646-006-0115-z
12. Kronenberger K, Brandis D, Türkay M, Storch V. Functional morphology of the reproductive system of *Galathea intermedia* (Decapoda:Anomura). *J Morph.* (2004) 262:500–15. doi: 10.1002/jmor.10259
13. Billinghurst Z, Clare AS, Fileman T, McEvoy J, Readman J, Depledge MH. Inhibition of barnacle settlement by the environmental oestrogen 4-nonylphenol and the natural oestrogen 17βoestradiol. *Mar Poll Bull.* (1998) 36:833–9. doi: 10.1016/S0025-326X(98)00074-5
14. Horiguchi T, Kojima M, Takiguchi N, Kaya M, Shiraishi H, Morita M. Continuing observation of disturbed reproductive cycle and ovarian spermatogenesis in the giant abalone Haliotis madaka from an organotin contamined site of Japan. *Mar Poll Bull.* (2005) 51:817–22. doi: 10.1016/j.marpolbul.2005.06.045
15. Sant'anna BS, Turra A, Zara FJ. Simultaneous activity of male and female gonads in intersex hermit crabs. *Aquat Biol.* (2010) 10:201–9. doi: 10.3354/ab00283
16. Siah A, Pellerin J, Amiard JC, Pelletier E, Viglino L. Delayed gametogenesis and progesterone levels in soft-shell clams (*Mya arenaria*) in relation to *in situ* contamination to organotins and heavy metals in the St. Lawrence river, Canada. *Comp Biochem Phisiol C.* (2003) 135:145–56. doi: 10.1016/S1532-0456(03)00085-1
17. Gagné F, Blaise CC, Pellerin J, Pelletier E, Douville M, Gauthier-Clerc S, et al. Sex alteration in soft-shell clams (*Mya Arenaria*) in an intertidal zone of the Saint Lawrence river (Quebec, Canada). *Comp Biochem Physiol C.* (2003) 134:189–98. doi: 10.1016/S1532-0456(02)00248-X
18. Morcillo Y, Porte C. Evidence of endocrine disruption in clams – *Ruditapes decussata* –transplanted to a tributyltin-polluted environment. *Environ Poll.* (2000) 107:47–52. doi: 10.1016/S0269-7491(99)00133-5
19. Aarab N, Minier C, Lemaire S, Unruh E, Hansen PD, Larsen BK. Biochemical and histological responses in mussel (*Mytilus edulis*) exposed to North Sea oil and to a mixture of North Sea oil and alkylphenols. *Mar Environ Res.* (2004) 58:437–41. doi: 10.1016/j.marenvres.2004.03.121
20. Aarab N, Lemaire S, Unruh E, Hansen PD, Larsen BK, Andersen OK. Preliminary study of responses in mussel (*Mytilus edulis*) exposed to bisphenol a, diallyl phthalate and tetrabromodiphenyl ether. *Aquat toxicol.* (2006) 78:86–92. doi: 10.1016/j.aquatox.2006.02.021
21. Ortiz-Zarragoitia M, Cajaraville MP. Intersex and oocyte atresia in a mussel population from the biosphere's reserve of Urdaibai (Bay of Biscay). *Ecol Environ Saf.* (2010) 73:693–701. doi: 10.1016/j.ecoenv.2010.04.002
22. Wen J, Pan L. Short-term exposure to benzo[a]pyrene disrupts reproductive endocrine status in the swimming crab *Portunus trituberculatus. Comp Biochem Physiol C.* (2015) 174–5:13–20. doi: 10.1016/j.cbpc.2015.06.001
23. Tian S, Pan L, Sun X. An investigation on endocrine disrupting effects and toxic mechanisms modulated by benzo[a]pyrene in female scallop *Chlamiys farreri. Aquat Toxicol.* (2013) 144:162–71. doi: 10.1016/j.aquatox.2013.09.031
24. Balbi T, Franzelitti S, Fabbri R, Montagna M, Fabbri E, Canesi L. Impact of bisphenol A (BPA) on early embryo development in the marine mussel *Mytilus galloprovincialis*: effects on genus transcription. *Environ Poll.* (2016) 218:996–1004. doi: 10.1016/j.envpol.2016.08.050
25. Jin S, Shao Li, Song X, Xiao J, Ouyang K, Zhang K, et al. Fertilization and male fertility in the rotifer *Brachiorus calyciflorus* in the presence of three environmental endocrines. *Chemsphere.* (2016) 220:146–54. doi: 10.1016/j.chemosphere.2018.12.097
26. Lu Y, Lin M, Aitken RJ. Exposure of spermatozoa to dibutyl phthalate induces abnormal embryonic development in a marine invertebrate *Galeolaria caespitosa* (Polychaeta:Serpulidae). *Aquat Toxicol.* (2017) 191:189–200. doi: 10.1016/j.aquatox.2017.08.008
27. Kang H, Kim M, Hwang U, Jeong C, Lee J. Effects of methylparaben, ethylparaben and propylparaben on life parameters and sex ratio in the marine copepod *Trigriopus japonicus. Chemosphere.* (2019) 226:388–94. doi: 10.1016/j.chemosphere.2019.03.151
28. Bowen RE, Depledge MH. Rapid assessment of marine pollution (RAMP). *Mar Poll Bull.* (2006) 53:631–9. doi: 10.1016/j.marpolbul.2006.09.002
29. Sumpter JP. Xenoendocrine disrupters - environmental impacts. *Toxicol Let.* (1998) 102–3:337–42. doi: 10.1016/S0378-4274(98)00328-2
30. Sárria MP, Santos MM, Reis-Henriques MA, Vieira NM, Monteiro NM. The umprebictable effects of mixtures of androgenic and estrogenic chemicals on fish early life. *Envirom Intern.* (2011) 37:418–24. doi: 10.1016/j.envint.2010.11.004
31. Ellis DV, Pattisina LA. Widespread neogastropod imposex: a biological indicator of global TBT contamination? *Mar Poll Bull.* (1990) 21:248–53. doi: 10.1016/0025-326X(90)90344-8
32. Alzieu C. Environmental impact of TBT: the French experience. *Sci Tot Env.* (2000) 258:99–102. doi: 10.1016/S0048-9697(00)00510-6
33. Ruiz JM, Bachelet G, Caumette P, Donard OFX. Three decades of tributyltin in the coastal environment with emphasis on Arcachon Bay, France. *Env Poll.* (1996) 93:195–203. doi: 10.1016/0269-7491(96)00029-2
34. Lee CC, Hsu YC, Kao YT, Chen HL. Health risk assessment of the intake of butyltin and phenyltin compounds from fish and sea food in Taiwanese population. *Chemosphere.* (2016) 164:568–75. doi: 10.1016/j.chemosphere.2016.08.141
35. Smith BS. Sexuality in the American mud snail, *Nassarius obsoletus* Say. *Proc Malacol Soc.* (1971) 39:377–8. doi: 10.1093/oxfordjournals.mollus.a065117
36. Smith BS. The estuarine mud snail, *Nassarius obsoletus*: abnormalities in the reproductive system. *J Moll St.* (1980) 46:247–56.
37. Smith BS. Reproductive anomalies in stenoglossan snails related to pollution from marinas. *J Appl Toxicol.* (1981) 1:15–21. doi: 10.1002/jat.2550010105
38. Smith BS. Male characteristics on female mud snails caused by antifouling bottom paints. *J Appl Toxicol.* (1981) 1:22–5. doi: 10.1002/jat.2550010106
39. Smith BS. Tributyltin compounds induce male characteristics on female mud snails *Nassarius obsoletus = Ilyanassa obsoleta. J Appl Toxicol.* (1981) 1:141–4. doi: 10.1002/jat.2550010302
40. Shi HH, Huang CJ, Zhu SX, Yu XJ, Xie WY. Generalized system of imposex and reproductive failure in female gastropods of coastal Waters of mainland China. *Mar Ecol Prog Ser.* (2005) 304:179–89. doi: 10.3354/meps304179
41. Titley O'Neal CP, Munkittrick KR, Macdonald BA. The effects of organotin in female gastropods. *J Environ Monit.* (2011) 13:2360–88. doi: 10.1039/c1em10011d
42. Stange D, Sieratowics A, Oehlmann J. Imposex development in *Nucella lapillus* – Evidence for the involvement of retinoid X receptor and androgen signaling pathways *in vivo. Aquat Toxicol.* (2012) 106–7:20–4. doi: 10.1016/j.aquatox.2011.10.010
43. Gibbs PE, Bryan GW. Biomonitoring of tributyltin (TBT) pollution using the imposex response of neogastropod molluscs. In: Kramer KJM, editor.

Biomonitoring of Coastal Waters and Estuaries. Boca Raton: CRC Press, Inc. (1994). p. 205–26.

44. Stroben E, Schulte-Oehlmann U, Fioroni P, Oehlmann J. A comparative method for easy assesment of coastal TBT pollution by the degree of imposex in prosobranch species. *Haliotis.* (1995) 24:1-12.
45. Toste R, Pessoa IA, Dore M, Parahyba M, Fernandez MA. Is aphallic vas deferens development in females related to the distance from organotin sources? A study with *Stramonita haemastoma. Ecotoxicol Environ Saf.* (2013) 91:162–70. doi: 10.1016/j.ecoenv.2013.01.026
46. Fernandez MA, Wagener ALR, Limaverde AM, Scofield AL, Pinheiro FM, Rodrigues EF. Imposex and surface sediment speciation: a combined approach to evaluate organotin contamination in Guanabara Bay, Rio de Janeiro, Brazil. *Mar Environ Res.* (2005) 59:435–52. doi: 10.1016/j.marenvres.2004.07.001
47. Leung KMY, Kwong RPY, Ng WC, Horigushi T, Qiu JW, Yang R, et al. Ecological risk assessment of endocrine disrupting organotin compounds using marine neogastropods in Hong Kong. *Chemosphere.* (2006) 65:922–38. doi: 10.1016/j.chemosphere.2006.03.048
48. Ruiz JM, Albaina N, Carro B, Barreiro R. A combined whelk watch suggests repeated TBT desorption pulses. *Sci Tot Environ.* (2015) 502:167–71. doi: 10.1016/j.scitotenv.2014.09.019
49. Santos DM, Turra A, de Marchi MRR, Montone RC. Distribution of butyltin compounds in Brazil's southern and southeastern estuarine ecosystems: assessment of spatial scales and compartiments. *Environ Sci Poll Res.* (2016) 23:16152–63. doi: 10.1007/s11356-016-6720-3
50. Guomundsdóttir LÓ, Ho KKY, Lam JCW, Svavarsson J, Leung KMY. Long-term temporal trends (1992–2008) of imposex status associated with organotin contamination in the dogwhelk *Nucella lapillus* along the Icelandic coast. *Mar Poll Bull.* (2011) 63:500–7. doi: 10.1016/j.marpolbul.2011.02.012
51. Langston WJ, Pope ND, Davey M, Langston KM, O'Hara SCM, Gibbs PE, et al. Recovery from TBT pollution in English Channel environments: a problem solved? *Mar Pol Bull.* (2015) 95:551–64. doi: 10.1016/j.marpolbul.2014.12.011
52. Ruiz JM, Carro B, Albaima N, Couceiro L, Míguez A, Quitela M, et al. Bi-species imposex monitoring in Galicia (NW Spain) shows contrasting achievement of the OSPAR Ecological Quality Objective for TBT. *Mar Poll Bull.* (2017) 114:715–23. doi: 10.1016/j.marpolbul.2016.10.058
53. Laranjeiro F, Sánchez-Marin P, Oliveira IB, Galante-Oliveira I, Barroso C. Fifteen years of imposex and tributyltin pollution monitoring along the Portuguese coast. *Environ Poll.* (2018) 232:411-2. doi: 10.1016/j.envpol.2017.09.056
54. Morton B. Recovery from imposex by a population of the dogwhelk, *Nucella lapillus* (Gastropoda: Caenogastropoda), on the southeastern coast of England since May, 2004: a 52-month study. *Mar Poll Bull.* (2009) 58:1530–8. doi: 10.1016/j.marpolbul.2009.05.012
55. Kim NS, Hong SH, Yim UH, Shin K-H, Shim WJ. Temporal changes in TBT pollution in water, sediment and oyster from Jinhae Bay after the total ban in South Korea. *Mar Poll Bull.* (2014) 86:547–54. doi: 10.1016/j.marpolbul.2014.06.035
56. Lam NH, Jeong H, Kang S, Kim D, Ju M, Horigushi T, et al. Organotins and new antifoulings biocides in water and sediments from three Korean Special Management Sea Areas following tem years of tributyltin regulation: contamination profiles and risk assessment. *Mar Poll Bull.* (2017) 121:302–12. doi: 10.1016/j.marpolbul.2017.06.026
57. Paz Villarraga CA, Castro IB, Miloslavich P, Fillmann G. Venezuellan caribbean sea under the threat of TBT. *Chemosphere.* (2015) 119:704–10. doi: 10.1016/j.chemosphere.2014.07.068
58. Batista RM, Castro IB, Fillmann G. Imposex and butyltin contamination still evidente in Chile after TBT global. *Sci Tot Env.* (2016) 566–7:446–53. doi: 10.1016/j.scitotenv.2016.05.039
59. Castro IB, Iannacone J, Santos S, Fillmann G. TBT is still a concern in Peru. *Chemospere.* (2018) 205:253–9. doi: 10.1016/j.chemosphere.2018.04.097
60. El Ayari T, Bierne N, El Menif NT. Imposex incidence in *Stramonita haemastoma* (Gastropoda: Muricidae) from the Mediterranean and Atlantic coast after Tributyltin global ban. *J Sea Res.* (2018) 134:10–5. doi: 10.1016/j.seares.2017.12.004
61. Lahbib Y, Ablidi,S., Pennec M, Flower R, El Menif NT. Imposex and butultins concentrations in snails from the lagoon of Bizerta (Northern Tunisia). *Mar Biol Res.* (2011) 6:600–7. doi: 10.1080/174510009034 37075
62. Anastasiou TI, Chatzinikolau E, Mandalakis M, Arvanitidis C. Imposex and organotin compounds in ports of the Mediterranean and Atlantic: is the story over? *Sci Tot Environ.* (2016) 569–70:1315–29. doi: 10.1016/j.scitotenv.2016.06.209
63. Matthiessen P. The impact of organotin pollution on aquatic invertebrate communities – are molluscs the only group whose populations have been affected? *Env Sci Heal.* (2019) 11:13–20. doi: 10.1016/j.coesh.2019.06.003
64. Costa MB, Zamprogno GAC, Pedruzzi FC, Morais L, Tognella M, Godoi AF, et al. Differential organotin sensitivity in two *Leucozonia* species from a ship traffic area in southeastern Brazil. *Mar Biol Res.* (2014) 10:712–24. doi: 10.1080/17451000.2013.850512
65. Gibbs PE. A male genital defect in the dog-whelk, *Nucella lapillus* (neogastropoda), favouring survival in a TBT-polluted area. *J Mar Biol Assoc UK.* (1993) 73:667–78. doi: 10.1017/S0025315400033208
66. Gibbs PE. Male genital defect (Dumpton Syndrome) in the dog-whelk Nucella lapillus (Neogastropoda): Mendelian inheritance inferred, based in laboratory breeding experiments. *J Mar Biol Assoc UK.* (2005) 85:143–50. doi: 10.1017/S0025315405010969h
67. Huet M, Paulet YM, Glémarec M. Tributyltin (TBT) pollution in the coastal waters of west Brittany as indicated by imposex in *Nucella lapillus. Mar Environ Res.* (1996) 41:157–67. doi: 10.1016/0141-1136(95)00152-2
68. Huet M, Le Goïc N, Gibbs PE. Appearance of a genetically-based pollution resistance in a marine gastropod, *Nucella Lapillus,* in south-west Brittany: a new case of Dumpton Syndrome. *J Mar Biol Assoc UK.* (2008) 88:1475–9. doi: 10.1017/S0025315408002038
69. Barreiro R, Quintela M, Ruiz JM. Aphally and imposex in *Nucella lapillus* from Galicia (NW Spain): incidence, geographical distribution and consequences for the biomonitoring of TBT contamination. *Mar Ecol Prog Ser.* (1999) 185:229–38. doi: 10.3354/meps185229
70. Horiguchi T, Shiraishi H, Shimizu M, Morita M. Imposex and organotin compounds in *Thais clavigera e T. bronni* in Japan. *J Mar Biol Assoc UK.* (1994) 74:651–69. doi: 10.1017/S002531540004772X
71. Horiguchi T, Shiraishi H, Shimizu M, Morita M. Effects of triphenyltin chloride and five other organotin compounds on the development of imposex in the rock shell, *Thais clavigera. Env Poll.* (1997) 95:85–91. doi: 10.1016/S0269-7491(96)00093-0
72. Laranjeiro F, Sánchez-Marin P, Barros A, Galante-Oliveira S, Moscoso-Pérez C, Fernández-González V, et al. Triphenyltin induces imposex in *Nucella lapillus* through an aphallic route. *Aquat Toxicol.* (2016) 175:127–31. doi: 10.1016/j.aquatox.2016.03.005
73. Fernandez MA, Pinheiro FM, Quadros JP, Camillo E Jr. An easy, non-destructive, probalistic method to evaluate the imposex response of neogastropod populations. *Mar Environ Res.* (2007) 63:41–54. doi: 10.1016/j.marenvres.2006.06.002
74. Quadros JP, De., Camillo E Jr, Pinheiro FM, Fernandez MAS. Imposex as an indicator of organotin pollution at Rio de Janeiro South coast: Sepetiba and Ilha Grande Bays. *Thalas.* (2009) 25:19–30. Available online at: https://www.semanticscholar.org/paper/IMPOSEX-AS-AN-INDICATOR-OF-ORGANOTIN-POLLUTION-AT-Quadros-Camillo/7a68875c4dcf98c361dd17fa618d30bbea34350b
75. Lahbib Y, Boumaïza M, Trigui El Menif N. Imposex expression in *Hexaplex trunculus* from the North Tunis Lake transplated to Bizerta Channel (Tunisia). *Ecol Ind.* (2008) 8:239–45. doi: 10.1016/j.ecolind.2007.02.003
76. Artifon V, Castro IB, Fillmann G. Spatiotemporal appraisal of TBT contamination and imposex along a tropical bay (Todos os Santos Bay, Brazil). *Environ Sci Poll Res.* (2016) 23:16047–55. doi: 10.1007/s11356-016-6745-7
77. Grimón ROR, Osorio MFA, Freitas DM, Castro IB. Tributyltin impacts in Galapagos Islands and Ecuadorian shore: marine protected áreas under treat. *Mar Pol.* (2016) 69:24–31. doi: 10.1016/j.marpol.2016.03.017
78. Lahbib Y, Ablidi S, Trigui El Menif N. First assessment of the effectiveness of the internation convention on the control of harmful antifouling systems on ships in Tunisia using using imposex in *Hexaplex trunculus* as biomarker. *Mar Poll Bull.* (2018) 128:17–23. doi: 10.1016/j.marpolbul.2018.01.012
79. Sánchez-Marín P, Oliveira IB, Souza ACA, Takahashi S, Tanabe S, Galante-Oliveira S. Evaluation of female aphally in imposex-affected populations of

Nucella lapillus at the southernmost distributional limit of the species in Europe. *J Moll Stud.* (2016) 82:144–53. doi: 10.1093/mollus/eyv043

80. Castro IB, Fillmann G. High tributyltin and imposex levels in the commercial muricid *Thais chocolata* from two Peruvian harbour areas. *Env Tox Chem.* (2012) 31–5:955–60. doi: 10.1002/etc.1794
81. Mattos Y, Stotz WB, Romero MS, Bravo M, Fillmann G, Castro IB. Butyltin contamination in Northern Chilean coast: is there a potential risk for consumers? *Sci Tot Environ.* (2017) 595:209–17. doi: 10.1016/j.scitotenv.2017.03.264
82. Langston WJ, Pope ND. determinants of TBT adsorption and desorption in estuarine sediments. *Mar Poll Bull.* (1995) 31:32–43. doi: 10.1016/0025-326X(95)91269-M
83. Dowson PH, Bubb JM, Willians TP, Lester JN. Degradation of tributyltin in freshwater and estuarine marina sediments. *Wat Sci Tech.* (1993) 28:133–7. doi: 10.2166/wst.1993.0611
84. Dowson DH, Bubb JM, Lester JN. A study of the partitioning and sorptive behavior of butyltins in the aquatic environment. *Appl Organomet Chem.* (1996) 7:623–33. doi: 10.1002/aoc.590070805
85. Castro LF, Melo C, Guillot R, Mendes I, Queirós S, Lima D, et al. The estrogen receptor of the gastropod Nucella lapillus: modulation following exposure to an estrogenic effluent? *Aquat Toxicol.* (2007) 84:465–8. doi: 10.1016/j.aquatox.2007.07.008
86. Santos MM, Reis-Henriques MA, Guillot R, Lima D, Franco-Duarte R, Mendes I, et al. Anti-androgenic effects of sewage treatment plant effluents in the prosobranch gastropod Nucella lapillus. *Comp Biochem Physiol C.* (2008) 148:87–93. doi: 10.1016/j.cbpc.2008.03.012
87. Borges CLL, Fernandez MA, Castro IB, Fillmann G. Organotin pollution from pleasure craft at Paraty, a tourist area of southeastern Brazil: amelioration or interference? *Braz J Ocean.* (2013) 61:177–86. doi: 10.1590/S1679-87592013000300002
88. Egardt J, Nilsson P, Dahllöf I. Sediment indicates the continued use of banned antifouling compounds. *Mar Poll Bull.* (2017) 125:282–8. doi: 10.1016/j.marpolbul.2017.08.035
89. Choi M, Moon H-B, Yu J, Cho H, Choi H-G. Temporal trends (2004–2009) of imposex in rock shells *Thais clavigera* collected along the Korean coast associated with tributyltin regulation in 2003 and 2008. *Arch Environ Contam Toxicol.* (2013) 64:448–55. doi: 10.1007/s00244-012-9839-3
90. Briant N, Bancon-Montigny C, Freydier R, Delpoux S, Elbaz-Poulichet F. Behavior of butyltin compounds in the sediment pore Waters of a contamined marina (Port Camargue, South of France). *Chemosphere.* (2016) 150:123–9. doi: 10.1016/j.chemosphere.2016.02.022
91. Rossato M, Castro IB, Paganini CL, Colares EP, Fillmann G, Pinho GLL. Sex steroid imbalances in the muricid Stramonita haemastoma from TBT contamined sites. *Environ Sci Poll Res.* (2016) 23:7861–8. doi: 10.1007/s11356-015-5942-0
92. Rossato M, Costa MB, Castro IB, Pinho GLL. Size, season and origino f gastropods matter in imposex assessments. *Ecotox Environ Saf.* (2018) 159:324–31. doi: 10.1016/j.ecoenv.2018.05.013
93. Chien LC, Hung TC, Chaoang KY. Daily intake of TBT, Cu, Zn, Cd and As for fishermen in Taiwan. *Sci Tot Environ.* (2002) 285:117–85. doi: 10.1016/S0048-9697(01)00916-0
94. Fernandez MA, Limaverde AM, Scofield A, Wagener A De LR. Preliminary evaluation of human health risks derived from ingestion of organotin contamined seafood in Brazil. *Braz J Ocean.* (2005) 53:75–7. doi: 10.1590/S1679-87592005000100008
95. Matozzo V, Marin MG. Can 4-nonylphenol induce vitellogenin-like proteins in the clam Tapes philippinarum? *Environ Res.* (2005) 97:43–9. doi: 10.1016/j.envres.2004.03.002
96. Matozzo V, Marin MG. First evidence of altered vitellogenin-like protein levels in clam Tapes philippinarum and in cockle Cerastoderma glaucum from the Lagoon of Venice. *Mar Poll Bull.* (2007) 55:494–504. doi: 10.1016/j.marpolbul.2007.09.010
97. Matozzo V, Marin MG. Can 17-β estradiol induce vitellogenin-like proteins in the clam Tapes philippinarum? *Environ Toxicol Pharm.* (2008) 26:38–44. doi: 10.1016/j.etap.2008.01.001
98. Puinean AM, Labadie P, Hill EM, Osada M, Kishida M, Nakao R. Laboratory exposure to 17β-estradiol fails to induce vitellogenin and estrogen receptor gene expression in the marine invertebrate *Mytilus edulis. Aquat Toxicol.* (2006) 79:376–83. doi: 10.1016/j.aquatox.2006.07.006
99. Chambers PA, Allard M, Walker SL, Marsalek J, Lawrence J. Impacts of municipal wastewater effluents on Canadian waters: a review. *Wat Qual Res J Canada.* (1997) 32:659–713. doi: 10.2166/wqrj.1997.038
100. Kummerer K. Drugs in the environment: emission of drugs, diagnostic aids and desinfectants into wastewater by hospitals in relation to other sources – review. *Chemosphere.* (2001) 45:957–69. doi: 10.1016/S0045-6535(01)00144-8
101. Weigel S, Kuhlmann J, Huhnerfuss H. Drugs and personal care products as ubiquitous pollutants: occurrence and distribution of clofibric acid, caffeine and DEET in the North Sea. *Sci Total Environ.* (2002) 295:131–41. doi: 10.1016/S0048-9697(02)00064-5
102. Andreozzi R, Raffaele M, Nicklas P. Pharmaceuticals in effluents and their solar photodegradation in aquatic environment. *Chemosphere.* (2003) 50:1319–30. doi: 10.1016/S0045-6535(02)00769-5
103. Gagné F, Blaise G, Hellou J. Endocrine disruption and health effects of caged mussels, *Elliptio complanata,* placed downstream from a primary treated municipal effluent plume for one year. *Comp Biochem Physiol C.* (2004) 138:33–44. doi: 10.1016/j.cca.2004.04.006
104. Alzieu CL, SanJuan J, Deltreil P, Borel M. Tin ontamination in Arcachon Bay: effects in oyster shell anomalies. *Mar Poll Bull.* (1986) 17:494–98. doi: 10.1016/0025-326X(86)90636-3
105. Di Cosmo A, Polese G. Neuroendocrine-Immune systems response to environmental stressors in the cephalopod *Octopus vulgaris. Front Physiol.* (2016) 7:434. doi: 10.3389/fphys.2016.00434
106. Minakata H, Shigeno S, Kano N, Haraguchi S, Osugi T, Tsutsui K. Octopus gonadotrophin-realesing hormone: a multifunctional peptide in the endocrine and nervous system of ths cephalopod. *J Neuroendocrinol.* (2009) 21:322–6. doi: 10.1111/j.1365-2826.2009.01852.x
107. De Lisa E, and Paolucci M, Di Cosmo A. Conservative nature of oestradiol signalling pathways in the brain lobes of Octopus vulgaris involved in reproduction, learning and motor coordination. *J Neuroendocrinol.* (2011) 24:275–84. doi: 10.1111/j.1365-2826.2011.02240.x
108. Lewis C, Ford AT. Infertility in male aquatic invertebrates: a review. *Aquat Toxicol.* (2012) 120–1:79–89. doi: 10.1016/j.aquatox.2012.05.002
109. Ford AT, Martins I, Fernandes TF. Population level effects of intersexuality in the marine environment. *Sci Tot Env.* (2007) 374:102–11. doi: 10.1016/j.scitotenv.2006.12.046
110. Horiguchi F, Yamamoto J, Nakata K. Model study of environmental concentrations of TBT in Tokio bay: development of a Windows version prototype. *Environ Modell Soft.* (2006) 21:229–33. doi: 10.1016/j.envsoft.2004.04.016
111. Pinheiro FM, Fernandez MA, Fragoso MR, Quadros JP, Camillo E Jr, et al. Assessing the impacts of organotins compounds at Ilha Grande Bay (Rio de Janeiro, Brazil): imposex and a multiple-source dispersion model. *J Coast Res SI.* (2006) 39:1383–8. Available online at: https://www.academia.edu/1149443/Assessing_the_Impacts_of_Organotin_Compounds_in_Ilha_Grande_Bay_Rio_de_Janeiro_Brazil_Imposex_and_a_Multiple-Source_Dispersion_Model
112. Fernandez MA, Pinheiro FM. New approaches for monitoring the marine environment: the case of antifouling paints. *Int J Environ Health.* (2007) 1:427. doi: 10.1504/IJENVH.2007.017875
113. UNEP. In: Nellermann C, Hain S, Alder J, editors. *Dead Water – Merging of Climate Change With Pollution, Over-Harvest and Infestations in the World's Fishing Grounds.* United Nations Environmental Programme, GRID-Arendal, Norway (2008).

6

Molecular cloning and characterization of the allatotropin precursor and receptor in the desert locust, *Schistocerca gregaria*

Els Lismont[1], *Rut Vleugels*[1], *Elisabeth Marchal*[1,2], *Liesbeth Badisco*[1], *Pieter Van Wielendaele*[1], *Cynthia Lenaerts*[1], *Sven Zels*[1], *Stephen S. Tobe*[2], *Jozef Vanden Broeck*[1] *and Heleen Verlinden*[1]*

[1] Molecular Developmental Physiology and Signal Transduction, KU Leuven, Leuven, Belgium, [2] Department of Cell and Systems Biology, University of Toronto, Toronto, ON, Canada

Edited by:
Eric W. Roubos,
Radboud University Nijmegen,
Netherlands

Reviewed by:
Young-Joon Kim,
Gwangju Institute of Science and Technology,
South Korea
Jan Adrianus Veenstra,
Universite de Bordeaux,
France

***Correspondence:**
Heleen Verlinden,
Molecular Developmental Physiology and Signal Transduction,
KU Leuven,
Naamsestraat 59, PO Box 02465,
B-3000 Leuven, Belgium
heleen.verlinden@bio.kuleuven.be

Allatotropins (ATs) are pleiotropic neuropeptides initially isolated from the tobacco hornworm, *Manduca sexta*. In 2008, the first receptor for AT-like peptides (ATR) was characterized in *Bombyx mori*. Since then, ATRs have also been characterized in *M. sexta*, *Tribolium castaneum*, *Aedes aegypti* and *Bombus terrestris*. These receptors show sequence similarity to vertebrate orexin (ORX) receptors. When generating an EST-database of the desert locust (*Schistocerca gregaria*) central nervous system, we found cDNA sequences encoding the *Schgr*-AT precursor and a fragment of its putative receptor. This receptor cDNA has now been completed and functionally expressed in mammalian cell lines. Activation of this receptor, designated as *Schgr*-ATR, by *Schgr*-AT caused an increase in intracellular calcium ions, as well as cyclic AMP (cAMP), with an EC_{50} value in the nanomolar range. In addition, the transcript distribution of both the *Schgr*-AT precursor and *Schgr*-ATR was investigated by means of quantitative real-time PCR. Moreover, we found more evidence for the myotropic and allatostimulatory actions of *Schgr*-AT in the desert locust. These data are discussed and situated in a broader context by comparison with literature data on AT and ATR in insects.

Keywords: GPCR, insect, juvenile hormone, neuropeptide, orexin, peptide, motility

Introduction

Allatotropin (AT) was originally identified as an amidated tridecapeptide isolated from the nervous system of the lepidopteran *Manduca sexta*. It was named after its first known biological function, namely the ability to stimulate juvenile hormone (JH) biosynthesis in the *corpora allata* (CA) *in vitro* (Kataoka et al., 1989). Most ATs have a conserved C-terminal pentapeptide that consists of a TARGFa motif although the hymenopteran AT has an exceptional TAYGFa C-terminal (Veenstra et al., 2012). There are also AT-like peptides (ATLs) that contain more variation in their C-terminal motif but they can elicit allatotropic activity as well (Lee et al., 2002). ATs have been isolated from numerous arthropod species, identified from the sequences of cloned genes, or deduced *in silico* from nucleotide sequence databases (Elekonich and Horodyski, 2003; Weaver and Audsley, 2009; Egekwu et al., 2014). Despite its widespread appearance in numerous insects, neither the AT precursor gene nor the AT receptor gene have been identified in *Drosophila melanogaster* or in any other members of this genus (Hewes and Taghert, 2001; Vanden Broeck, 2001). Related peptides have been reported in other phyla beyond Arthropoda. These were isolated in mollusks (Harada et al., 1993; Li et al., 1993; Veenstra, 2010), flatworms (Adami et al., 2011) and annelids (Ukena et al., 1995; Veenstra, 2011), and recent phylogenetic analysis also showed the presence of this peptidergic system in other protostomes, but not in nematodes, and in some deuterostomes (Mirabeau and Joly, 2013).

AT has pleiotropic functions in a variety of insect species. It stimulates visceral muscle activity (Paemen et al., 1991; Duve et al., 1999, 2000), heart activity (Veenstra et al., 1994), ventral diaphragm oscillation (Koladich et al., 2002), plays a role in the photic entrainment of the circadian clock (Petri et al., 2002), controls the release of digestive enzymes in the midgut (Lwalaba et al., 2010), inhibits active ion transport in the midgut (Lee et al., 1998) and stimulates the secretion of saliva and the contractions of the muscles surrounding the salivary glands (Masood and Orchard, 2014). In *Culex pipiens*, ovarian development was arrested when nondiapausing females were injected with AT dsRNA immediately after adult eclosion, mimicking the diapausing phenotype (Kang et al., 2014). Furthermore, in *T. castaneum*, disrupted adult development and fecundity was observed after injections of AT dsRNA in young pupae (Abdel-latief and Hoffmann, 2014).

It has been suggested that the ancestral role for this peptide family is related to its myotropic role, while the stimulation of JH biosynthesis evolved secondarily in some insect groups (Elekonich and Horodyski, 2003). The myotropic activity of AT on the gut was also suggested to be important for feeding, since gut contractions are necessary to allow food motility and the flow of digestive enzymes (Oeh et al., 2001; Audsley and Weaver, 2009; Nagata et al., 2012).

ATs exert effects on their cellular targets by binding to receptors with high affinity binding sites that are members of the family of rhodopsin-like G protein-coupled receptors (GPCRs). The AT receptors (ATRs) are orthologous to vertebrate orexin/hypocretin receptors. To date, five ATRs have been characterized; namely the neuropeptide 16 receptor in *Bombyx mori* (Yamanaka et al., 2008), the receptors of *M. sexta* (Horodyski et al., 2011), *Tribolium castaneum* (Vuerinckx et al., 2011), *Aedes aegypti* (Nouzova et al., 2012) and *Bombus terrestris* (Verlinden et al., 2013). The first three were dose-dependently activated by *Manse*-AT. The *T. castaneum* receptor was also activated by *Schgr*-AT (which is identical to *Lom*-AG-MT1, the AT from *Locusta migratoria*) and by an endogenous AT-like peptide (*Trica*-ATL) predicted from the *Tribolium* genome (Vuerinckx et al., 2011). The ATR receptor of *B. terrestris* also responded to *Manse-AT*, *Schgr*-AT, and *Trica*-ATL, but much higher concentrations were needed for generating these pharmacological effects (Verlinden et al., 2013). Activation of these AT(L) receptors resulted in an elevation of intracellular calcium and cAMP concentrations (Horodyski et al., 2011; Vuerinckx et al., 2011; Verlinden et al., 2013).

ATR-like receptor genes can also be found in the genomes of the mosquitoes *Anopheles gambiae* and *Culex quinquefasciatus*, the pea aphid *Acyrthosiphon pisum*, the kissing bug *Rhodnius prolixus*, the monarch butterfly *Danaus plexippus*, the jewel wasp *Nasonia vitripennis*, the honey bee *Apis mellifera*, the alfalfa leafcutter bee *Megachile rotundata*; the ant species *Harpegnathos saltator*, *Acromyrmex echinatior* and *Solenopsis invicta* and various other insect species (Caers et al., 2012 and unpublished BLAST analysis).

In *Locusta migratoria* a member of the AT family was first identified as the accessory gland myotropin 1, since it was isolated from the male accessory glands and shown to stimulate contractility of the locust oviduct (Paemen et al., 1991, 1992). In *S. gregaria*, AT was found in the brain (protocerebrum, antennal lobes, and tritocerebrum), the circumoesophageal connectives, the suboesophageal ganglion (SOG), the stomatogastric nervous system and all thoracic and abdominal ganglia. No mass peak corresponding to AT was found in the locust *corpora cardiaca* (CC) or retrocerebral complex (Homberg et al., 2004; Clynen and Schoofs, 2009).

We now complement the data obtained in the above mentioned lepidopteran, coleopteran, dipteran and hymenopteran species with a quantitative analysis of the AT precursor and receptor transcripts in different tissues of a representative of the hemimetabolous insects, *S. gregaria*. In addition, we show more evidence for the allatostimulatory and myoactive roles of *Schgr*-AT in the desert locust.

Materials and Methods

Rearing of Animals

Gregarious desert locusts were reared under crowded conditions with controlled temperature ($30 \pm 1°C$), light (14 h photoperiod) and ambient relative humidity (40–60%). The locusts were kept at high density (>200 locusts/cage) in special wooden cages and fed daily with fresh cabbage leaves supplemented with dry oat flakes. Mature females deposited their eggs in pots filled with a slightly moistened sterile sand mixture (7 parts sand, 3 parts peat, and 1 part water). After oviposition, these pots were collected once a week and set apart in empty cages, resulting in pools of hatched first instar hoppers, which differed by no more than 7 days in age. Depending on the experimental conditions, the locusts were further synchronized at the time of ecdysis (Badisco et al., 2011a; Marchal et al., 2011).

The breeding of solitarious desert locusts was performed under isolated conditions according to the method described by Hoste et al. (2002). Newly hatched hoppers were separated at the day of eclosion and were placed in individual containers. Temperature, light-dark photoperiods and food supply were similar for isolated-reared and crowded-reared locusts. All solitarious animals came from stocks that were reared under isolated conditions for at least three generations. To characterize the phase status of crowded-reared and isolated-reared locusts, morphometric measurements of femur length (F), caput width (C), and elytra (E) were performed (Dirsch, 1953). The F/C ratio increased, whereas the E/F ratio decreased in successive isolated-reared generations, indicating that individuals shifted toward the solitarious phase. The color and behavioral characteristics of crowded- and isolated-reared locusts were very typical for the gregarious and solitarious phase, respectively.

Tissue Collection

The locust tissues were dissected under a binocular microscope and immediately snap frozen in liquid nitrogen. In a first experiment, we collected three pools of each tissue (brain, optic lobes, *corpora cardiaca*, *corpora allata*, prothoracic gland, SOG, salivary gland, prothoracic ganglion, mesothoracic ganglion, metathoracic ganglion, gonads, fatbody, flight muscle, foregut, midgut, hindgut, Malpighian tubules, and male accessory gland) of 10 day old gregarious and solitarious males and females. The three pools consist of respectively 40, 10, and 10 animals. In a second tissue collection the abdominal ganglia were dissected from 10 day old gregarious animals. The first three (1–3) abdominal ganglia are fused to the metathoracic ganglion and the last four (8–11) are fused to each other and form the terminal abdominal ganglion (Burrows, 1996). Abdominal ganglia 4-5 and 6-7 were dissected together. The three pools males and females each consist of 10 animals. Until further processing, we stored all the tissue samples at −80°C to prevent degradation.

RNA Extraction and cDNA Synthesis

The dissected pooled tissues (<100 mg) were collected in "MagNa Lyser green beads" 2.0 ml tubes (Roche). Semi-automated homogenization of these samples was performed in a MagNA Lyser® Instrument (Roche, Mannheim, Germany) according to the manufacturer's instructions. Total RNA was extracted from the tissue homogenate utilizing an "RNeasy® Lipid Tissue Mini Kit" (Qiagen, Germantown, MD) in combination with a DNase treatment (RNase-free DNase set, Qiagen) to eliminate potential genomic DNA contamination.

After verification of the RNA quantity and quality with the Nanodrop (Thermo Fisher Scientific Inc.), we transcribed the resulting total RNA using the SuperScript® III Reverse Transcriptase (Invitrogen™ Life Technologies, Carlsbad, CA) utilizing random hexamers and oligodT's as described in the protocol. Afterwards, the resulting cDNA was diluted tenfold.

Molecular Cloning

The *Schgr*-AT precursor and a partial fragment of the putative *Schgr*-ATR were found by scanning the EST database of *S. gregaria* (Badisco et al., 2011b). The sequence of the *Schgr*-AT precursor was confirmed by sequencing the plasmid that was used to produce the cDNA library. Additional sequence information of *Schgr-ATR* was obtained by 3′ and/or 5′ rapid amplification of cDNA-ends (RACE) using the "5′/3′ RACE Kit, 2nd Generation" (Roche) in combination with *Schgr*-ATR gene specific primers (see Supplementary Table 1).

cDNA covering the entire *Schgr*-ATR was amplified using a three step procedure. In the first step gene specific cDNA was made using the "Transcriptor High Fidelity cDNA Synthesis Kit" (Roche) and the gene specific primer 5′-TGATAAACA TCACTCTGTAT-3′. Next, two PCR rounds were performed using the "Pwo DNA Polymerase" (Roche). The following cycle program was used twice: 94°C for 180 s followed by 30 cycles of 94°C for 45 s, 61°C for 60 s, 72°C for 120 s. The program ended at 4°C after a final elongation at 72°C for 10 min. In the first PCR round, the forward primer: 5′-TCTGCCCACAGTACA TCCAA-3′ and the reverse primer: 5′-CACTCCACTAGCGAC CACAA-3′ were used and in the second PCR round the forward primer: 5′-CACCATGACAGAGAACGAAAC-3′ and the reverse primer: 5′-GTTGCGGGTAAGGAGGTGT-3′ were used. After the first PCR round a PCR clean-up was performed using the "GenElute™ PCR Clean-Up Kit" (Sigma-Aldrich®).

The resulting PCR products were purified from a 1% agarose gel with the "GenElute™ Gel extraction Kit" (Sigma-Aldrich®). The *Schgr*-AT precursor was cloned in a "pCR™4-TOPO" vector (Invitrogen™) and the *Schgr*-ATR was cloned into a "pcDNA™3.1/V5-His TOPO®" vector (Invitrogen™) following the manufacturer's instructions. The vector was transformed into One Shot® TOP10 chemical competent *E. coli* cells (Invitrogen) and grown on LB agar plates (35 g/l; Sigma-Aldrich®) with ampicillin (10 mg/ml; Invitrogen™). Colonies with an insert were collected and grown in LB medium (Sigma-Aldrich®) with ampicillin (10 mg/ml). The plasmid was purified using the "GenElute™ Plasmid Miniprep Kit" (Sigma-Aldrich®). DNA Sequences were determined using the ABI PRISM 3130 Genetic Analyzer (Applied Biosystems®) following the protocol outlined in the "BigDye® Terminator v1.1 Cycle Sequencing Kit" (Applied Biosystems®).

Phylogenetic and Structural Analysis

We compared the *Schgr*-ATR sequence with other insect ATR(-like) sequences. We aligned the following sequences with MUltiple Sequence Comparison by Log- Expectation (MUSCLE; Edgar, 2004): *S. gregaria* ATR (GenBank acc. no. **JN543509**), *M. sexta* ATR (GenBank acc. no. **ADX66344**), and *T. castaneum* ATR (GenBank acc. no. **XP_973738**). In addition, a phylogenetic tree was constructed with the neighbor-joining method, using the amino acid sequences [starting from transmembranic region (TM) 1 and ending with the TM7] from the *Schgr*-ATR, ATR-like receptors of insect organisms [the ones mentioned above, *B. terrestris* ATR (GenBank acc. no. **XP_003402490**), the *A. mellifera* ATR (GenBank acc. no. **XP_001120335**), *M. rotundata* ATR (GenBank acc. no. **XP_003708421**), *N. vitripennis* ATR (GenBank acc. no. **XP_008217710**), *R. prolixus* ATR (GenBank acc. no. **AHE41431**), *A. aegypti* ATR (GenBank acc. no. **AEN03789**), *B. mori* neuropeptide A5 and A16 receptor (GenBank acc. no. **NP_001127740** and **NP_001127714**), and *D. plexippus* ATR (GenBank acc. no. **EHJ74388**)] and the FMRFamide receptor of *D. melanogaster* (GenBank acc. no. **AAF47700**), to root the tree (MEGA software vs. 6; Tamura et al., 2013; 1000-fold bootstrap resampling).

Cell Culture and Transfections

Pharmacological analyses were performed in Chinese hamster ovary (CHO) WTA11 cells stably co-expressing the bioluminescent protein apoaequorin (Brough and Shah, 2009) and the promiscuous $G_{\alpha16}$ subunit, which couples most agonist-induced GPCRs to the phospholipase C and calcium pathway, irrespective of their natural signaling cascade (Offermans and Simon, 1995; Milligan et al., 1996 cell lines were obtained from the Free University of Brussels and Euroscreen, Belgium). In subsequent experiments, CHO-PAM28 cells stably expressing apoaequorin, but not the promiscuous $G_{\alpha16}$, and human embryonic kidney

(HEK) 293 cells (Invitrogen™) were used to measure the *Schgr*-ATR downstream signaling properties via calcium and cAMP, respectively.

CHO-WTA11 cells, CHO-PAM28 cells and HEK293 cells were cultured in monolayers in Dulbecco's Modified Eagles Medium nutrient mixture F12-Ham (DMEM/F12) (Sigma-Aldrich®) supplemented with 100 U/ml penicillin and 100 μg/ml streptomycin (Sigma-Aldrich®) to prevent bacterial contamination of gram-positive and gram-negative bacteria, respectively. The medium was also supplemented with 10% fetal bovine serum (Sigma-Aldrich®). For CHO-WTA11 cells, 250 mg/ml zeocin (Invitrogen™) was added to the medium, whereas for CHO-PAM28 cells, 5 μg/ml puromycin (Sigma-Aldrich®) was added to the medium. Puromycin and zeocin were initially used to select for cells stably expressing apoaequorin (CHO-PAM28) (Torfs et al., 2002), or both apoaequorin and $G_{\alpha 16}$ (CHO-WTA11) (Blanpain et al., 1999) and are thus still used as additional antibiotics in the appropriate screens. All cells were maintained in an incubator at 37°C with a constant supply of 5% CO_2.

Transfections with pcDNA™3.1-*Schgr*ATR or empty pcDNA™3.1 vector were carried out in T75 flasks at 60–80% confluency. Transfection medium for CHO cells was prepared using the Lipofectamine LTX Kit (Invitrogen™) with 2.5 ml DMEM/F12, 12.5 μl PlusTM Reagent and 5 μg vector construct (pcDNA™3.1-*Schgr*ATR or empty pcDNA™3.1 vector) in 5 ml polystyrene round-bottom tubes. After a 5 min incubation period at room temperature, 30 μl LTX was added to the medium. After a further incubation period of 30 min at room temperature, the medium was removed from the cells and the DNA/LTX mix was added dropwise to the cells followed by 3 ml of fresh complete medium. The transfection medium used for HEK293 cells was similar to that used for CHO cells except that in addition to 4 μg of pcDNA™3.1-*Schgr*ATR expression construct (or empty pcDNA3.1 vector plasmid), cells were co-transfected with 2 μg of reporter CRE(6×)-Luc plasmid. This reporter plasmid contains six tandem repeats of a cAMP Responsive Element (CRE) in front of a minimum collate promoter and the ORF of luciferase (this reporter plasmid was also used in various other studies: for example Hearn et al., 2002; Johnson et al., 2004). Following transfection, cells were incubated overnight (37°C, 5% CO_2), then 10 ml of cell medium was added followed by a second overnight incubation (37°C, 5% CO_2). Ligand-induced changes in either, intracellular calcium or cAMP were then monitored in the cells as described below.

Calcium Reporter Assay in CHO Cells

CHO cells (CHO-WTA11 or CHO-PAM28) transfected with receptor expression construct (or empty vector) were detached with PBS, complemented with 0.2% EDTA (pH 8.0), and rinsed off the flask with DMEM/F12 without phenolred (Gibco®). The number of viable and nonviable cells was determined using a NucleoCounter® NC-100™ (Chemometic). The cells were pelleted for 4 min at 800 rpm and resuspended to a density of 5×10^6 cells/ ml in sterile filtered bovine serum albumin (BSA) medium (DMEM/F12 with L-glutamine and 15 mM Hepes, without phenolred, supplemented with 0.1% BSA) and loaded with 5 μM Coelenterazine_h (Invitrogen™). Next, the cells were incubated for 4 h in the dark, at room temperature, while gently shaken to reconstitute the holo-enzyme aequorin. After a tenfold dilution 30 min prior to the screening, 50 μl cell solution was injected in the wells (~25000 cells/well) and exposed to *Schgr*-AT (GL Biochem, Shanghai, China) reconstituted in several dilutions in BSA medium distributed in the 96-well plate. In every row, BSA medium without potential ligands was placed in one well to serve as the blank for that row. The calcium response was recorded for 30 s on a multimode microplate reader Mithras LB 940 at a wavelength of 469 nm (Berthold Technologies). After 30 s, 0.1% Triton X-100 was added and the signal was measured for another 10 s. Triton X-100 is a non-ionic surfactant that will break the cell membranes so the total cellular calcium content can be measured. The total calcium signal (ligand + Triton X-100) is representative for the amount of cells present in the well. The response of each blank (small signal caused by cells ruptured by the injection in the wells) was subtracted from the luminescence obtained for wells within the same row. Calculations were made using the output file from the Microwin software (Berthold Technologies) in Excel (Microsoft). Further analysis was done in Excel and GraphPad Prism 5. An illustration of this assay is shown in Supplementary Figure S1.

Cyclic AMP (cAMP) Reporter Assay in HEK293 Cells

To monitor changes in intracellular cAMP levels, HEK293 cells co-transfected with receptor construct (or empty vector) and reporter gene plasmid ($CRE_{6\times}$-luciferase) were detached with PBS, complemented with 0.2% EDTA (pH 8.0), and rinsed off the flask with DMEM/F12 without phenolred (Gibco®). The number of viable and nonviable cells was determined using the NucleoCounter® NC-100™. The cells were pelleted for 4 min at 800 rpm and finally resuspended to a density of 1×10^6 cells/ml in DMEM/F12 without phenolred, but containing 200 μM 3-isobutyl-1-methylxanthine (IBMX, Sigma–Aldrich®; 20 μl of 0.1 M IBMX in DMSO in 10 ml DMEM/F12) to prevent cAMP breakdown. Into each well of a white 96-well plate 50 μl of cell suspension (~50000 cells/well) was added to either 50 μl of DMEM/F-12 (with IBMX, but without phenolred) or DMEM/F-12 [with IBMX, without phenolred and containing 10 μM NKH-477 (a forskolin analog; used to enhance cAMP levels in the cells)] containing various concentrations of the allatotropin peptide (GL Biochem, Shanghai, China). In each row of the plate at least one well with only phenol red-free DMEM/F-12 with IBMX was measured. This well is used to calculate the blank level. The cells were then incubated (37°C, 5% CO_2) for 3–4 h. Hereafter 100 μl of steadylite plus™ substrate (PerkinElmer) was added to each well using a multichannel pipette and the plate was incubated for 15 min in the dark. Finally, light emission resulting from the luciferase enzymatic activity was recorded at 0 s and 5 s on a multimode microplate reader Mithras LB 940 at a wavelength of 469 nm. The signal of the two measurements (0 and 5 s) was almost identical; an average of these two was used for further analysis. Results were analyzed by using Excel and Graphpad Prism 5 Software. An illustration of this assay is shown in Supplementary Figure S2.

qRT-PCR Study of Transcript Levels

Accurate normalization of the raw data was obtained by using the optimal combination of endogenous control genes. The best combination of reference genes was determined using GeNorm (Vandesompele et al., 2002) as described by Van Hiel et al. (2009) and Verlinden et al. (2010). The PCR reactions were performed in a 20 µl reaction volume following the manufacturer's instructions for the Fast SYBR® Green Master Mix (2×) (Applied Biosystems®). The final concentration of the primers was 500 nM. Primers for the endogenous controls, as well as for the *Schgr*-ATR and *Schgr*-AT target genes, were designed by means of the Primer Express® Software v2.0 (Applied Biosystems®). For primer sequences, see **Table 1**.

To identify efficient primersets for the qRT-PCR, relative standard curves for the endogenous controls and the *Schgr*-ATR and *Schgr*-AT transcripts were generated with serial (10×) dilutions of a brain cDNA sample. Reactions were run in duplicate on a StepOne™ Plus System (ABI Prism, Applied Biosystems®) using the following thermal cycling profile: 95°C for 10 min, followed by 40 steps of 95°C for 3 s and 60°C for 30 s. After 40 cycles, samples were run for the dissociation protocol (i.e., melting curve analysis). Analysis of the dissociation curves of the different amplification products revealed a single melting peak. In addition, we analyzed the PCR products via agarose gel electrophoresis, showing the presence of a single band of the expected size for each transcript. Furthermore, sequencing of the PCR products ultimately confirmed the identity of the amplified DNA with their respective target sequences.

To study the transcript levels, we normalized, for each sample, the relative amount of transcript to the endogenous controls (Actin and GADPH) and calculated transcript levels relative to a calibrator sample (in this case, a mix of all measured tissues of males and females, gregarious and solitarious). The tissue, phase and sex distribution experiments were repeated three times with independent biological pools of adult *S. gregaria* tissues (40, 10, and 10 animals per pool). We detected no amplification of the fluorescent signal in any negative control sample, proving that the extraction procedure, including the DNase treatment, effectively removed genomic DNA from all the RNA samples and that there was no contamination. Statistical analysis was performed by means of SPSS (v17.0, SPSS Inc., Chicago, Illinois), using the Mann-Whitney U test for comparing two independent groups. A level of $P < 0.05$ was considered significant.

In a second qRT-PCR we studied the transcript levels in the abdominal ganglia in males and females of gregarious animals. The first three abdominal ganglia are fused to the metathoracic ganglion hence the same samples as in the first transcript study were used. For each sample the relative transcript amounts were normalized to the housekeeping genes coding for Actin and GADPH. The brain sample of the females (a sample from the first tissue distribution) was used as the calibrator sample.

TABLE 1 | Oligonucleotide primers for qRT-PCR used in this study.

	Forward primer	Reverse primer
Actin	5′-AATTACCATTGGTA ACGAGCGATT-3′	5′-TGCTTCCATAC CCAGGAATGA-3′
GAPDH	5′-GTCTGATGAC AACAGTGCAT-3′	5′-GTCCATCACGCC ACAACTTTC-3′
Schgr-AT	5′-ATGCAGAACA ACCCGGAACT-3′	5′-CTGGTTAGCGT CCACGAACTT-3′
Schgr-ATR	5′-CGTCAACCCAGT CATCTACAACTT-3′	5′-TAGGCGCAC GTCCAGAACA-3′

Abbreviations used: GAPDH, Glyceraldehyde-3-phosphate dehydrogenase; Schgr, Schistocerca gregaria.

Schgr-AT Bioassay

Schgr-AT was tested on an isolated gut preparation, as described by Schoofs et al. (1990). The midgut from a sexually mature male was ligated at both ends with strings by which the gut was suspended between the arm of a transducer and the bottom of a plastic chamber containing 2.5 ml *S. gregaria* saline (1L: 8.766 g NaCl; 0.188 g $CaCl_2$; 0.746 g KCl; 0.407 g $MgCl_2$; 0.336 g $NaHCO_3$; 30.807 g sucrose; 1.892 g trehalose; pH 7.2) at room temperature (Supplementary Figure S3). The transducer monitored the contractions of the gut, which were visualized on a connected recorder (LKB 2210 recorder). When a constant rhythm of contractions was reached, 25 µl of 10 mM M *Schgr*-AT (GL Biochem, Shanghai, China) dissolved in saline (to reach a final concentration of one micromolar) or the same volume of saline without peptide was added to the chamber. In between two measurements the chamber was rinsed three times with saline; after this the constant contraction rhythm was restored.

In Vitro Measurement of JH Biosynthesis—Radiochemical Assay (RCA)

Rates of JH release and the JH content were measured by the *in vitro* radiochemical assay (RCA) originally described by Tobe and Pratt (Pratt and Tobe, 1974; Tobe and Pratt, 1974) and further discussed by Feyereisen and Tobe (1981) and Yagi and Tobe (2001). The RCA measures the rate of incorporation of the methyl group from [Methyl-14C] methionine (50 µM, 2.11 GBq/mmol, New England Nuclear Co.) into JH in isolated CA. CA were dissected out of the head of vitellogenic adult females, since it is known that their CA produce a high amount of JH (Tobe and Pratt, 1975). The dissected CA were directly transferred to conical glass vials holding 50 µl of radioactive TC199 medium [3 µCi/ml medium; lacking L-methionine, glucose, acetate and calcium (Gibco®, with Hank's sals, HEPES 25 mM)]. The individual CA were shaken at 30°C during the first incubated period of 3 h. Next, CA were transferred to fresh radioactive TC199 medium supplemented with 30 µM farnesoic acid (FA) to stimulate JH synthesis. 1 µM *Schgr*-AT was added to the experimental CA. 8 control CA and 9 *Schgr*-AT treated CA were tested. Incubation medium was extracted using 300 µl of iso-octane. The samples were vortexed and centrifuged for 10 min at 2000 rpm. The top 200 µl of the iso-octane layer was removed and put into scintillation vials containing 3 ml of scintillant (ICN) and measured in a liquid scintillation counter (Beckman, LS-6500).

The effect of *Schgr*-AT on the JH production of the CA was calculated by dividing the difference of the JH production during the second incubation and the JH production during the first incubation by the JH production during the second incubation. Significance was determined with a student's *t*-test in GraphPad Prism 5.

Results

Cloning and Sequence Analysis

As described in the *S. gregaria* EST paper (Badisco et al., 2011b), a partial fragment of an orexin 2 receptor-like/ ATR-like receptor and the *Schgr*-AT precursor are represented in the EST database. These sequences were confirmed by PCR, cloning, and sequencing. We further completed the sequence of the *Schgr*-ATR by rapid amplification of cDNA ends (RACE). The *Schgr*-ATR amino acid sequence is shown in **Figure 1**. The receptor belongs to the rhodopsin-like GPCRs and contains seven transmembrane domains [analyzed with a hidden Markov model for predicting transmembrane regions (Sonnhammer et al., 1998; Krogh et al., 2001)]. The sequence of the precursor *Schgr*-AT is displayed in **Figure 2**. The sequence contains a signal peptide predicted by SignalP 4.1 (Petersen et al., 2011) and two recognition motifs for proteolytic processing of the preproallatotropin. The G-residue at the C-terminal may be a substrate for peptidyl amidating monooxygenase (PAM) resulting in an amidated neuropeptide (Rouillé et al., 1995; Veenstra, 2000; Veenstra et al., 2012). The obtained nucleotide sequence of the *Schgr*-ATR fragment and the sequence of *Schgr*-AT have been submitted to the European Bioinformatics Institute (EBI) database (*Schgr-ATR*: GenBank accession no. **JN543509**; *Schgr-AT*: GenBank accession no. **KP233881**).

Analysis of Phylogenetic Relationships

Amino acid sequence comparisons between the *Schgr*-ATR and other insect ATR-like receptors show high overall amino acid similarity (identical and conservatively substituted residues; **Figure 1**). The amino acid sequences (TM1-7) of the ATR-like receptors and the FMRFamide receptor from *D. melanogaster*,

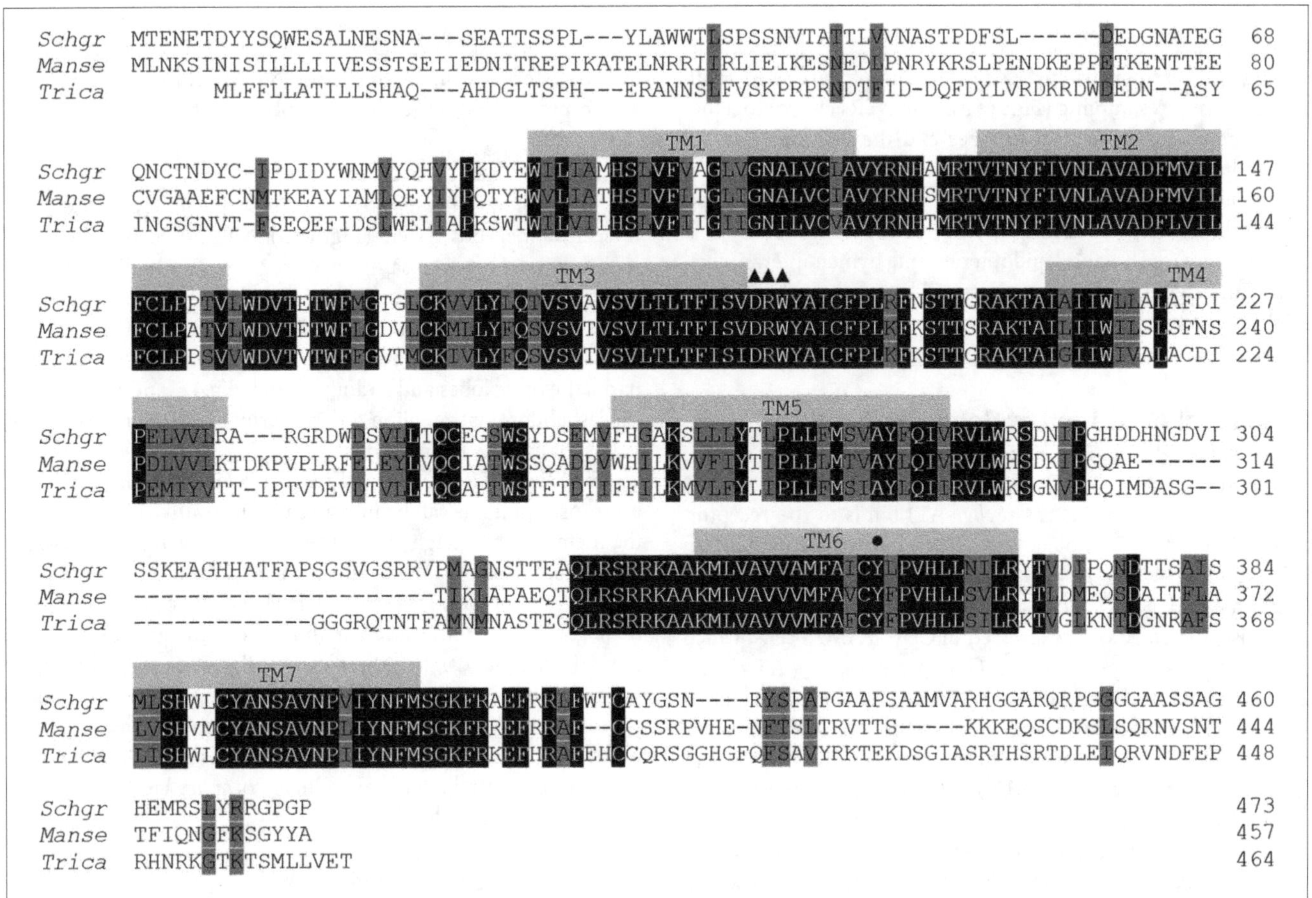

FIGURE 1 | Amino acid sequence of the *Schgr*-ATR (GenBank acc. no. JN543509) and homologous receptors from *Manduca sexta* (GenBank acc. no. ADX66344) and *Tribolium castaneum* (GenBank acc. no. XP_973738). The amino acid position is indicated at the right. Identical residues between the aligned sequences are highlighted in black, and conservatively substituted residues in gray. Dashes indicate gaps that were introduced to maximize homologies. Putative transmembrane regions (TM1-TM7) are indicated by gray bars. The position of the W (here changed to Y) (•) that is usually conserved in many rhodopsin-like GPCRs and the DRW motif (▲▲▲) are labeled.

ATG	CGC	TGC	GCC	GCC	GCC	GCC	CTG	TGC	CTG	CTG	GTC	GCC	CTC	GCC
M	R	C	A	A	A	A	L	C	L	L	V	A	L	A
GCC	CTC	TGC	GCC	GCC	GCC	GCC	GCC	GCC	CCC	GCG	GCT	CAC	TAC	GGC
A	L	C	A	A	A	A	A	A	P	A	A	H	Y	G
CGC	GGC	TCC	CGC	CCC	CGC	ACG	ATA	CGG	GGC	TTC	AAG	AAC	GTG	GCA
R	G	S	R	P	R	T	I	R	G	F	K	N	V	A
CTC	TCC	ACC	GCG	CGG	GGC	TTC	GGC	AAG	CGA	GAC	GGC	AAC	CAG	CTG
L	S	T	A	R	G	F	G	K	R	D	G	N	Q	L
GAG	GCC	GCG	CTC	GCT	GAC	CGC	GAC	ACC	ACC	CTC	CCG	GAC	AGC	TTC
E	A	A	L	A	D	R	D	T	T	L	P	D	S	F
CCT	GTG	GAA	TGG	TTC	GCC	GCC	GAG	ATG	CAG	AAC	AAC	CCG	GAA	CTG
P	V	E	W	F	A	A	E	M	Q	N	N	P	E	L
GCT	CGC	ATG	ATC	GTC	AGC	AAG	TTC	GTG	GAC	GCT	AAC	CAG	GAT	GGA
A	R	M	I	V	S	K	F	V	D	A	N	Q	D	G
GAA	CTG	ACG	GCA	GAG	GAA	CTC	CTC	AGG	CCC	ACT	TAC	TGA		
E	L	T	A	E	E	L	L	R	P	T	Y	STOP		

FIGURE 2 | Precursor sequence of *Schgr*-AT. The sequence of AT is highlighted in green. The predicted signal peptide sequence is shown in orange and the recognition sites for proteolytic processing of the proneuropeptide are shown in blue. The G-residue predicted to be transformed into the C-terminal amide is shown in yellow.

to root the tree, were aligned with MUSCLE. A neighbor-joining tree was constructed using MEGA software with 1000-fold bootstrap resampling (**Figure 3**). The ATRs cluster together as compared to the root of the tree and the lepidopteran and hymenopteran ATRs cluster within their insect class. The overall insect phylogeny is however not respected in the tree. Bootstrap values already indicate that the power of some nodes is less as compared to the lepidopteran and hymenopteran cluster. Future characterization projects will hopefully result in more ATR sequences from diverse phylogenetic classes and will hopefully increase the overall power of phylogenetic studies.

Functional Activation of *Schgr*-ATR with AT

The *Schgr*-ATR was expressed in CHO-WTA11 cells, which express the promiscuous $G_{\alpha 16}$ protein that can induce a calcium rise if an agonist (in this case *Schgr*-AT) binds to the receptor. *Schgr*-AT elicits a sigmoidal dose-dependent response with an EC_{50} value of 4.43×10^{-9} M (**Figure 4A**; $\log EC_{50} = -8.354 \pm 0.025$, mean ± SEM). To test if the receptor can induce a calcium rise, the receptor is expressed in CHO-PAM28 cells, which do not express the promiscuous $G_{\alpha 16}$ protein. *Schgr*-AT clearly induced an intracellular calcium response with an EC_{50} value of 5.57×10^{-9} M (**Figure 4B**; $\log EC_{50} = -8.254 \pm 0.067$, mean ± SEM). HEK293 cells were used to test whether the receptor can also signal through cAMP. NKH-477 (a forskolin-analog), which activates adenylyl cyclase, will be responsible for an increase of intracellular cAMP levels. If the receptor couples negatively to adenylyl cyclase, a reduction of intracellular cAMP levels would be expected following administration of *Schgr*-AT. This was not observed when *Schgr*-ATR was expressed in the HEK293 cells (results not shown). However, in the absence of NKH-477, a specific increase of luciferase reporter activity was observed with an EC_{50} value of 8.10×10^{-8} M (**Figure 4C**; $\log EC_{50} = -7.09 \pm 0.123$, mean ± SEM). CHO-WTA11, CHO-PAM28 and HEK293 cells transfected with an empty pcDNA 3.1 vector did not show any response to *Schgr*-AT (results not shown).

Transcript Level Studies

The expression of the *Schgr-AT* precursor is largely restricted to the central nervous system (**Figure 5**). No significant differences were observed between samples of gregarious and solitarious animals, hence they are represented together. Females in general show higher *Schgr-AT* precursor transcript levels as compared to males. The effect is significant ($p < 0.05$) in the central brain parts, the optic lobes and abdominal ganglia 4-5 and 6-7. Only in the last abdominal ganglion the transcript levels are higher in the males than in the females ($p < 0.05$).

The *Schgr-ATR* is also mainly expressed in the CNS. The highest transcript levels can be measured in the brain, the optic lobes, the metathoracic ganglion and the abdominal ganglia (**Figure 5**). The receptor also shows relatively high transcript levels in the Malpighian tubules, intestine, male accessory glands, mesothoracic ganglion, prothoracic ganglion, fat body, gonads, CA and the salivary glands. No significant differences were observed between sexes, or phases. Nor did we observe significant differences between the transcript levels in larval and adult CA (results not shown). The *Schgr*-ATR transcript levels are 200–1000- fold lower in the central nervous system as compared to the *Schgr*-AT precursor transcript levels.

Gut Motility Bio-Assay

Schgr-AT was added to the midgut preparation *in vitro* when a constant contraction rhythm was observed. This led to an immediate tetanus (**Figure 6A** left). After rinsing, the tetanus disappeared and normal contraction rhythm was restored (results not shown). No change in contraction strength or rhythm of the

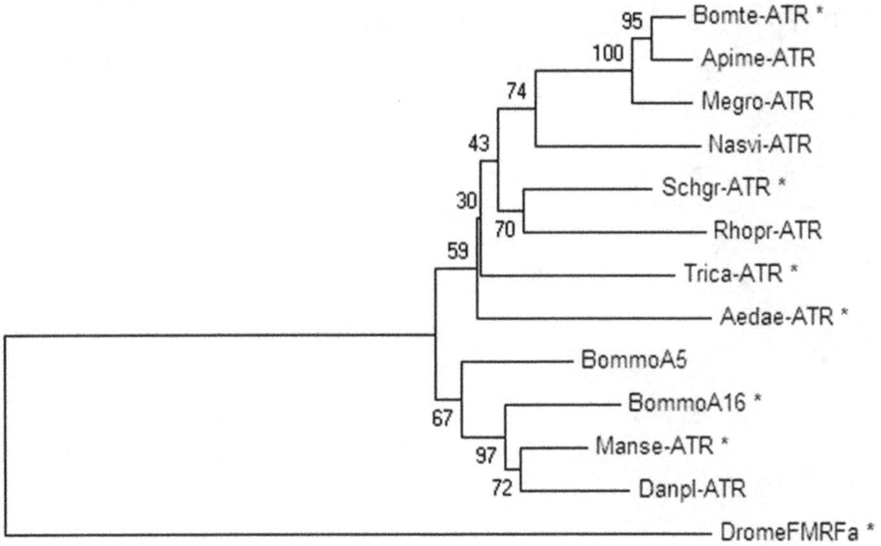

FIGURE 3 | Neighbor-joining tree of insect ATR-like receptors in dendrogram display with representative branch length. Phylogenetic and molecular evolutionary analyses were conducted by using MEGA version 6. The FMRFamide-receptor of *D. melanogaster* (GenBank acc. no. **AAF47700**) was used as an outgroup to root the tree. Proteins marked with an asterisk were functionally characterized. Bootstrap-support values are based on 1000 replicates and are indicated on the nodes. The other GenBank accession numbers are: *S. gregaria* ATR (**JN543509**), *M. sexta* ATR (**ADX66344**), *T. castaneum* ATR (**XP_973738**), *B. terrestris* ATR (**XP_003402490**), *A. mellifera* ATR (**XP_001120335**), *M. rotundata* ATR (**XP_003708421**), *N. vitripennis* ATR (**XP_008217710**), *R. prolixus* ATR (**AHE41431**), *A. aegypti* ATR (**AEN03789**), *B. mori* neuropeptide A5 and A16 receptor (**NP_001127740** and **NP_001127714**), and *D. plexippus* ATR (**EHJ74388**).

midgut was observed when we added saline without the peptide (results not shown). The entire procedure was repeated and again only change in contraction of the midgut could be observed when adding *Schgr*-AT (**Figure 6B** right).

In Vitro Measurement of JH Biosynthesis—Radiochemical Assay (RCA)

In the control CA the JH production was slightly lower during the second incubation period when compared to the first incubation. This is likely the result of the natural decrease in JH biosynthesis by senescence of the CA cells or a decrease in JH precursor pools as in the *in vitro* nature of the experiment. However, if the CA were treated with AT during the second incubation period, the JH production increased significantly ($p < 0.05$; **Figure 7**).

Discussion

Molecular Cloning and Phylogeny

In the present study, we have characterized *Schgr*-ATR, an AT receptor of the desert locust, *S. gregaria*. The obtained sequence has considerable similarity with orthologous receptors from other insects (**Figure 1**) (Horodyski et al., 2011; Vuerinckx et al., 2011; Nouzova et al., 2012; Verlinden et al., 2013). The sequence contains a DRW (instead of the typical DRY) motif in the second intracellular loop, as it is the case for other AT receptors. AT and its receptor seem to be present in both hemimetabolous and holometabolous insect species (**Figure 3**), although exceptions exist. *Drosophila* appears to lack both the ligand (Hewes and Taghert, 2001; Vanden Broeck, 2001) and its receptor. It was first thought that the hymenopteran insects, *A. mellifera* (Hummon et al., 2006) and *N. vitripennis* (Hauser et al., 2010) also lacked an AT-like peptide. However, after a more thorough search, a hymenopteran *AT* gene was found (Veenstra et al., 2012) and, meanwhile, an AT receptor was characterized in the hymenopteran species *B. terrestris* (Verlinden et al., 2013).

The ATRs show large sequence similarity to the mammalian orexin (ORX) receptors. Although the ORX and AT peptides do not display any obvious sequence similarity and ORX does not activate the invertebrate receptors (Vuerinckx et al., 2011), Mirabeau and Joly found evidence for a common origin of the AT and ORX precursor genes (Mirabeau and Joly, 2013).

Functional Receptor Characterization

We demonstrated that *Schgr*-AT activates the *Schgr*-ATR *in vitro* and causes an increase in both intracellular calcium ion and cAMP levels with an EC_{50} value in the nanomolar range (**Figure 4**). The higher standard deviation measured in the HEK293 cells compared to the CHO cells can be explained by the absence of a normalization step for the total amount of cells per well, which was used in the calcium reporter assays. The measurement of the bioluminescence in the cAMP reporter assay is dependent on a CRE and thus dependent on the phosphorylation of CREB (cAMP Responsive Element Binding protein). Therefore, it has been speculated that a change in bioluminescence may also be caused by calcium, since CREB can also be phosphorylated by calcium/calmodulin-dependent protein kinase (Johannessen et al., 2004). However, an earlier study of another neuropeptide receptor (*Schgr*-sNPFR) that makes use

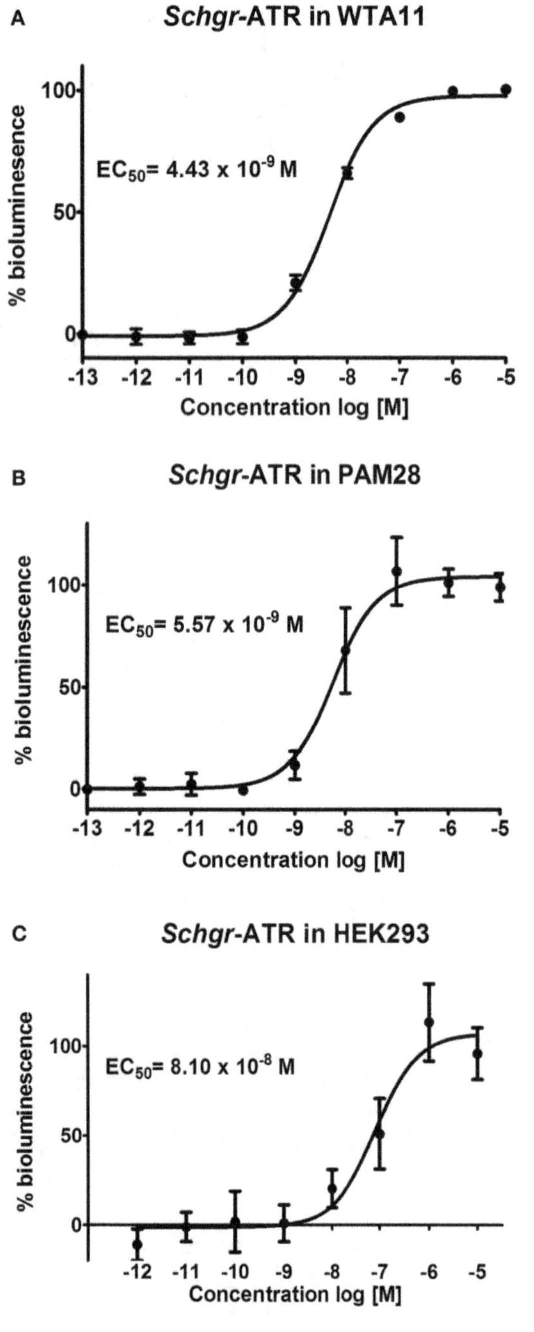

FIGURE 4 | Dose-response curve for bioluminescence responses induced in (A) CHO-WTA11-*Schgr*-ATR cells, (B) CHO-PAM28-*Schgr*-ATR cells, (C) HEK293- *Schgr* -ATR cells. In all cell lines, the bioluminescence was measured in two independent transfections in triplicate and data are given in percentage (±S.D.) of the maximal response. The zero response level corresponds to treatment with BSA buffer only.

of the same assays, showed increased intracellular calcium levels (CHO cell screen), but no increase in bioluminescence in the HEK293 cell screen, which would be expected if the calcium was responsible for the increase in bioluminescence in this screen (Dillen et al., 2013). In addition, the reporter plasmid was also used in various other studies (for example Hearn et al., 2002; Johnson et al., 2004). These facts suggest that an increase in bioluminescence in this assay is caused directly by an increase in intracellular cAMP levels and not (indirectly) by the increase in intracellular calcium levels.

Our pharmacological data correspond well with previous pharmacological characterizations of ATRs in other insects. Upon activation by their endogenous AT, the AT(L)Rs of *M. sexta*, *T. castaneum* and *B. terrestris* also stimulate intracellular calcium and cAMP levels, although lower EC_{50} values were measured (Horodyski et al., 2011; Vuerinckx et al., 2011; Verlinden et al., 2013). The fact that the EC_{50} value of the receptor expressed in HEK293 cells is higher than the EC_{50} value of the receptor expressed in CHO-PAM28 cells might indicate that the calcium response of *Schgr*-ATR is more sensitive than the cAMP response, although the difference may (in part) be explained by the use of different assays.

Tissue Distribution and Functions of Allatotropin

Schgr-AT precursor expression seems to be largely restricted to the central nervous system (**Figure 5**). This is as expected, since neuropeptides are usually produced in the nervous system and transported toward their target tissues (Caers et al., 2012). Our qRT-PCR data correspond very well with previous immunological and mass spectrometry data obtained in *L. migratoria* (Paemen et al., 1992) and *S. gregaria* (Homberg et al., 2004; Clynen and Schoofs, 2009) confirming the presence of this neuropeptide in extensive areas of the locust brain, including all neuropils in the optic lobe, the antennal lobes, and most areas in the protocerebrum. The first "AT-related" peptide in locusts was originally purified from male accessory glands of *L. migratoria* (*Lom*-AG-MT1) (Paemen et al., 1991) and is identical to *Schgr*-AT. The AT present in the male accessory glands (which show very low relative expression levels) is presumably originating from the (last) abdominal ganglia. Moreover, in other insect species specific neuroendocrine cells in the abdominal ganglia appear to be the most abundant source of AT (Veenstra et al., 1994, 2012; Veenstra and Costes, 1999; Rudwall et al., 2000; Neupert et al., 2009).

The *Schgr*-AT precursor shows 100–1000 fold higher transcript levels in the central nervous system as compared to the *Schgr*-ATR. This can be explained by the fact that neuropeptides are released in large quantities into the periphery, where they will bind to their receptors, to execute their functions. Moreover, the half-life of a peptide is expected to be shorter than the turnover rate of receptors.

The high abundance of ATR in the central nervous systems suggests a critical role in sensory processing, learning and memory and motor control (Elekonich and Horodyski, 2003). In *Leucophaea maderae*, injections of AT near the accessory medulla, which is identified as the location of the circadian clock in this cockroach and part of the optic lobes, resulted in changes in circadian locomotor activity (Petri et al., 2002). Also in *S. gregaria* high expression levels of ATR were measured in the optic lobes.

The ATR expression in the CA is probably related to the stimulatory role of AT on the biosynthesis and release of JH. Already,

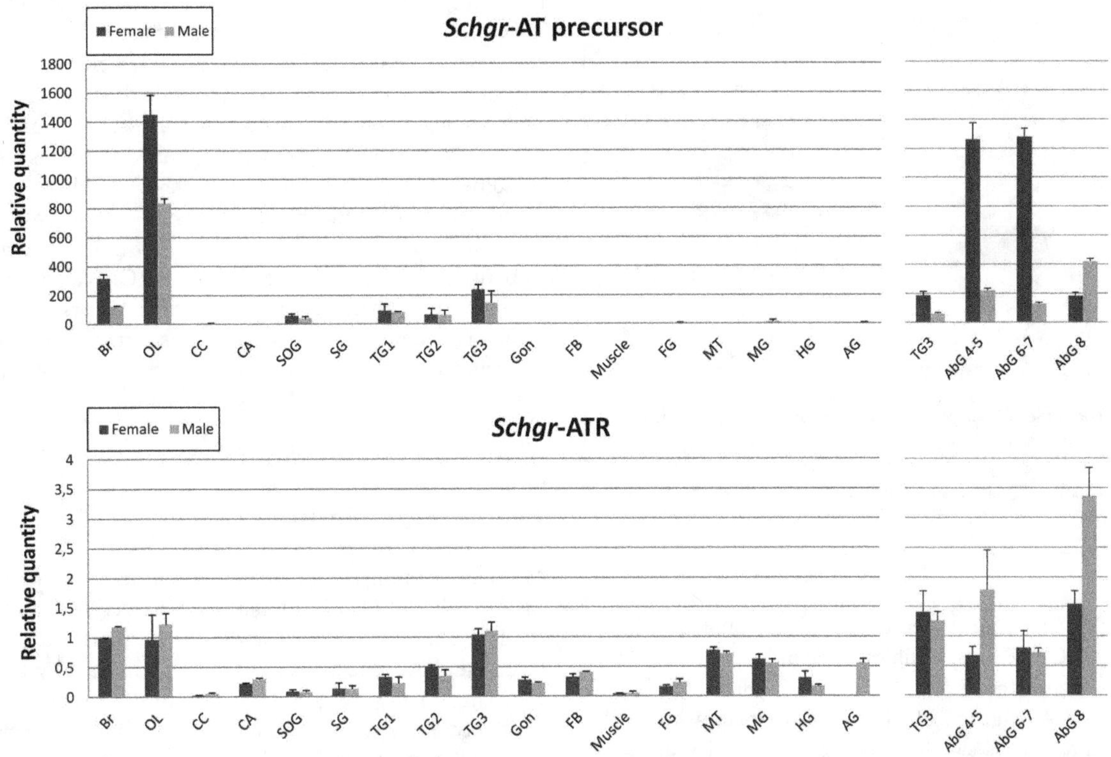

FIGURE 5 | Graphic representation of the transcript levels of the precursor of *Schgr*-AT and the *Schgr*-ATR measured in sexually mature *S. gregaria* in two experiments. The data represent mean values ± S.E.M. of three independent tissue samples run in duplicate, normalized relative to Actin and GAPDH transcript levels. Abbreviations used: Br, brain; OL, optic lobes; CC, *corpora cardiaca*; CA, *corpora allata*; PG, prothoracic gland; SOG, suboesophageal ganglion; SG, salivary gland; TG1, prothoracic ganglion; TG2, mesothoracic ganglion; TG3, metathoracic ganglion; Gon, gonads; FB, fat body; Muscle, flight muscle; FG, foregut; MT, Malpighian tubules; MG, midgut; HG, hindgut; AG, male accessory glands, AbG, abdominal ganglia. The first three abdominal ganglia (1–3) are fused to the metathoracic ganglion (TG3). On the left the results of the first qRT-PCR study are depicted. The data of the gregarious and solitarious animals are represented together. On the right the results of the second qRT-PCR study are depicted.

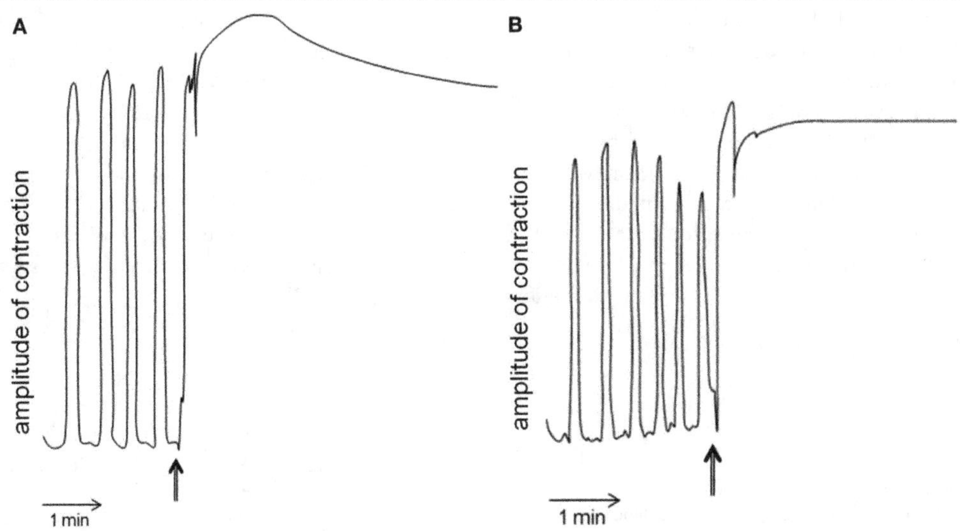

FIGURE 6 | Myotropic activity of *Schgr*-AT on the midgut of *Schistocerca gregaria*. Arrows indicate the administration of *Schgr*-AT. **(A)** and **(B)** represent two independent measurements on the same midgut.

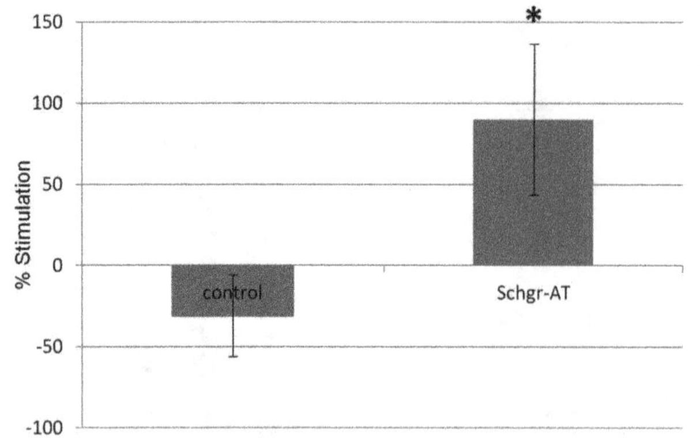

FIGURE 7 | The effect of *Schgr*-AT on the rate of JH biosynthesis in the CA as measured in an *in vitro* radio-chemical assay (RCA). The bars represent averages ± S.E.M. of 8 control and 9 *Schgr*-AT treated, individual CA dissected from vitellogenic adult females. Significant differences ($p < 0.05$) are indicated by an asterisk (*).

Tobe et al. (1977) demonstrated that an allatostimulatory factor released by the CA was responsible for the production of JH. We now also confirmed that *Sch*gr-AT indeed stimulates the JH production in the CA (**Figure 7**). This may also explain why the AT precursor expression is significantly higher in 10 day old adult females as compared to males (**Figure 5**), since JH (regulated by AT) was demonstrated to be important in females of this age for vitellogenin production and oocyte growth (Pratt and Tobe, 1974; Sevala et al., 1995; Glinka and Wyatt, 1996; Wyatt et al., 1996). The difference was especially pronounced in the abdominal ganglia, hence they could be responsible for activation of the CA.

The high expression levels of *Schgr*-ATR in the Malpighian tubules were also observed in *M. sexta* and suggest that AT may have a role in osmoregulation (Horodyski et al., 2011). The expression of the *Schgr*-ATR in the salivary glands can be related to a role in the stimulation of saliva secretion as was recently discovered in *R. prolixus* (Masood and Orchard, 2014). High transcript levels of *Schgr*-ATR were measured in the digestive system as well. This can be explained by the fact that AT affects the intestinal motility, as was shown with the bio-assay (**Figure 6**). Another link that can be made with the digestive system, is the impact of the nutritional status on the transcript levels of the AT precursor. In larvae of *M. sexta* and the armyworm *Mythimna separate* it was shown that starvation led to higher transcript levels of AT (Lee and Horodyski, 2002, 2006; Zhang et al., 2008). In larvae, starvation causes an additional molt, indicating that JH levels are elevated. This gives the larvae the opportunity to acquire additional nutrients once they become available in order to successfully complete development to a robust reproductive adult. In contrast, starvation of some insects during the adult stage inhibited oocyte maturation as a consequence of decreasing JH biosynthesis (Tobe and Chapman, 1979; Zhang et al., 2008). The overall regulation of JH titer is complex, since the CA can be influenced by multiple stimulatory and inhibitory factors, and since JH catabolism and binding to JH transport proteins also plays a major role in the control of JH titer (Lee and Horodyski, 2006).

Author Contributions

Molecular cloning and EST database analyses were performed by LB, PV, HV and EL. Functional tests with AT were performed by PV, HV, CL, RV and SZ. The radio chemical assay was performed by EM and ST. The dissections were performed by EM, LB and HV. The pharmacological characterization was performed by EL. Guidance of the study, writing and correction of the manuscript were performed by HV, EL and JV.

Acknowledgments

The authors would like to thank the anonymous reviewers for their constructive comments. We would like to thank Roger Jonckers and Evelien Herinckx for maintaining the locusts, Marijke Christiaens for help with the figures and Joost Van Duppen for technical support. We would like to thank Marc Parmentier (Free University of Brussels, Belgium) and Michel Detheux (Euroscreen S.A., Belgium) for providing CHO-WTA11 and CHO-PAM28 cells. We gratefully acknowledge the Interuniversity Attraction Poles (IAP) programs (Belgian Science Policy Grant (P7/40)), the Research Foundation of Flanders (FWO) and the KU Leuven Research Foundation (GOA/11/02) for financial support. HV was supported by the FWO (the research fund of the Flemish region), RV, CL and SZ were supported by a PhD fellowship of the IWT.

References

Abdel-latief, M., and Hoffmann, K. H. (2014). Functional activity of allatotropin and allatostatin in the pupal stage of a holometablous insect, *Tribolium castaneum* (Coleoptera, Tenebrionidae). *Peptides* 53, 172–184. doi: 10.1016/j.peptides.2013.10.007

Adami, M. L., Damborenea, C., and Ronderos, J. R. (2011). Expression of a neuropeptide similar to allatotropin in free living turbellaria (platyhelminthes). *Tissue Cell.* 43, 377–383. doi: 10.1016/j.tice.2011.07.005

Audsley, N., and Weaver, R. J. (2009). Neuropeptides associated with the regulation of feeding in insects. *Gen. Comp. Endocrinol.* 162, 93–104. doi: 10.1016/j.ygcen.2008.08.003

Badisco, L., Huybrechts, J., Simonet, G., Verlinden, H., Marchal, E., Huybrechts, R., et al. (2011b). Transcriptome analysis of the desert locust central nervous system: production and annotation of a *Schistocerca gregaria* EST database. *PLoS ONE* 6:e17274. doi: 10.1371/journal.pone.0017274

Badisco, L., Marchal, E., Van Wielendaele, P., Verlinden, H., Vleugels, R., and Vanden Broeck, J. (2011a). RNA interference of insulin-related peptide and neuroparsins affects vitellogenesis in the desert locust *Schistocerca gregaria*. *Peptides* 32, 573–580. doi: 10.1016/j.peptides.2010.11.008

Blanpain, C., Lee, B., Vakili, J., Doranz, B. J., Govaerts, C., Miqeotte, I., et al. (1999). Extracellular cysteines of CCR5 are required for chemokine binding, but dispensable for HIV-1 coreceptor activity. *J. Biol. Chem.* 274, 18902–18908. doi: 10.1074/jbc.274.27.18902

Brough, S. J., and Shah, P. (2009). Use of aequorin for G protein-coupled receptors hit identification and compound profiling. *Methods Mol. Biol.* 552, 181–198. doi: 10.1007/978-1-60327-317-6_13

Burrows, M. (1996). *The Neurobiology of an Insect Brain*. New York, NY: Oxford University Press. doi: 10.1093/acprof:oso/9780198523444.001.0001

Caers, J., Verlinden, H., Zels, S., Vandersmissen, H. P., Vuerinckx, K., and Schoofs, L. (2012). More than two decades of research on insect neuropeptide GPCRs: an overview. *Front. Endocrinol.* 3:151. doi: 10.3389/fendo.2012.00151

Clynen, E., and Schoofs, L. (2009). Peptidomic survey of the locust neuroendocrine system. *Insect Biochem. Mol. Biol.* 39, 491–507. doi: 10.1016/j.ibmb.2009.06.001

Dillen, S., Zels, S., Verlinden, H., Spit, J., Van Wielendaele, P., and Vanden Broeck, J. (2013). Functional characterization of the short neuropeptide F receptor in the desert locust, *Schistocerca gregaria*. *PLoS ONE* 8:e53604. doi: 10.1371/journal.pone.0053604

Dirsch, V. M. (1953). Morphological studies on phases of the desert locust (*Schistocerca gregaria* Forskal). *Anti Locust Bul.* 16, 1–34.

Duve, H., Audsley, N., Weaver, R. J., and Thorpe, A. (2000). Triple co-localization of two types of allatostatin and an allatotropin in the frontal ganglion of the lepidopteran *Lacanobia oleracea* (Noctuidae): innervation and action on the foregut. *Cell Tissue Res.* 300, 153–163. doi: 10.1007/s004410050056

Duve, H., East, P. D., and Thorpe, A. (1999). Regulation of lepidopteran foregut movement by allatostatins and allatotropin from the frontal ganglion. *J. Comp. Neurol.* 413, 405–416.

Edgar, R. C. (2004). MUSCLE: multiple sequence alignment with high accuracy and high throughput. *Nucleic Acids Res.* 32, 1792–1797. doi: 10.1093/nar/gkh340

Egekwu, N., Sonenshine, D. E., Bissinger, B. W., and Roe, R. M. (2014). Transcriptome of the female synganglion of the black-legged tick *Ixodes scapularis* (Acari: Ixodidae) with comparison between Illumina and 454 systems. *PLoS ONE* 9:e102667. doi: 10.1371/journal.pone.0102667

Elekonich, M. M., and Horodyski, F. M. (2003). Insect allatotropins belong to a family of structurally-related myoactive peptides present in several invertebrate phyla. *Peptides* 24, 1623–1632. doi: 10.1016/j.peptides.2003.08.011

Feyereisen, R., and Tobe, S. S. (1981). A rapid partition assay for routine analysis of *corpora allata* release by insect *corpora allata*. *Anal. Biochem.* 111, 372–375. doi: 10.1016/0003-2697(81)90575-3

Glinka, A. V., and Wyatt, G. R. (1996). Juvenile hormone activation of gene transcription in locust fat body. *Insect Biochem. Mol. Biol.* 26, 13–18. doi: 10.1016/0965-1748(95)00045-3

Harada, A., Yoshida, M., Minakata, H., Nomoto, K., Muneoka, Y., and Kobayashi, M. (1993). Structure and function of the molluscan myoactive tetradecapeptides. *Zool. Sci.* 10, 257–265.

Hauser, F., Neupert, S., Williamson, M., Predel, R., Tanaka, Y., and Grimmelikhuijzen, C. J. P. (2010). Genomics and peptidomics of neuropeptides and protein hormones present in the parasitic wasp *Nasonia vitripennis*. *J. Proteome Res.* 9, 5296–5310. doi: 10.1021/pr100570j

Hearn, M. G., Ren, Y., McBride, E. W., Reveillaud, I., Beinborn, M., and Kopin, A. S. (2002). A *Drosophila* dopamine 2-like receptor: molecular characterization and identification of multiple alternatively spliced variants. *Proc. Natl. Acad. Sci. U.S.A.* 99, 14554–14559. doi: 10.1073/pnas.202498299

Hewes, R. S., and Taghert, P. H. (2001). Neuropeptides and neuropeptide receptors in the *Drosophila melanogaster* genome. *Genome Res.* 11, 1126–1142. doi: 10.1101/gr.169901

Homberg, U., Brandl, C., Clynen, E., Schoofs, L., and Veenstra, J. A. (2004). Mas-allatotropin/Lom-AG-myotropin I immunostaining in the brain of the locust, *Schistocerca gregaria*. *Cell Tissue Res.* 318, 439–457. doi: 10.1007/s00441-004-0913-7

Horodyski, F., Verlinden, H., Filkin, N., Vandersmissen, H. P., Fleury, C., Reynolds, S. E., et al. (2011). Isolation and functional characterization of an allatotropin receptor from *Manduca sexta*. *Insect Biochem. Mol. Biol.* 41, 804–814. doi: 10.1016/j.ibmb.2011.06.002

Hoste, B., Luyten, L., Claeys, I., Clynen, E., Rahman, M. M., De Loof, A., et al. (2002). An improved breeding method for solitarious locusts. *Entomol. Exp. Appl.* 104, 281–288. doi: 10.1046/j.1570-7458.2002.01014.x

Huang, J., Marchal, E., Hult, E. F., Zels, S., Vanden Broeck, J., and Tobe, S. S. (2014). Mode of action of allatostatins in the regulation of juvenile hormone biosynthesis in the cockroach, *Diploptera punctata*. *Insect Biochem. Mol. Biol.* 54, 61–68. doi: 10.1016/j.ibmb.2014.09.001

Hummon, A. B., Richmond, T. A., Verleyen, P., Baggerman, G., Huybrechts, J., Ewing, M. A., et al. (2006). From the genome to the proteome: uncovering peptides in the *Apis* brain. *Science* 314, 647–649. doi: 10.1126/science.1124128

Johannessen, M., Delghandi, M. P., and Moens, U. (2004). What turns CREB on? *Cell. Signal.* 6, 1211–1227. doi: 10.1016/j.cellsig.2004.05.001

Johnson, E. C., Bohn, L. M., and Taghert, P. H. (2004). *Drosophila* CG8422 encodes a functional diuretic hormone receptor. *J. Exp. Biol.* 207, 743–748. doi: 10.1242/jeb.00818

Kang, D. S., Denlinger, D. L., and Sim, C. (2014). Suppression of allatotropin simulates reproductive diapause in the mosquito Culex pipiens. *J. Insect Physiol.* 64, 48–53. doi: 10.1016/j.jinsphys.2014.03.005

Kataoka, H., Toschi, A., Li, J. P., Carney, R. L., Schooley, D. A., and Kramer, S. J. (1989). Identification of an allatotropin from adult *Manduca sexta*. *Science* 243, 1481–1483. doi: 10.1126/science.243.4897.1481

Knight, P. J., Pfeifer, T. A., and Grigliatti, T. A. (2003). Functional assay for G-protein-coupled receptors using stably transformed insect tissue culture cell lines. *Anal. Biochem.* 320, 88–103. doi: 10.1016/S0003-2697(03)00354-3

Koladich, P. M., Cusson, M., Bendena, W. G., Tobe, S. S., and McNeil, J. N. (2002). Cardioacceleratory effects of *Manduca sexta* allatotropin in the true armyworm moth *Pseudaletia unipuncta*. *Peptides* 23, 645–651. doi: 10.1016/S0196-9781(01)00658-1

Krogh, A., Larsson, B., von Heijne, G., and Sonnhammer, E. L. (2001). Predicting transmembrane protein topology with a hidden Markov model: application to complete genomes. *J. Mol. Biol.* 305, 567–580. doi: 10.1006/jmbi.2000.4315

Lee, K. Y., Chamberlin, M. E., and Horodyski, F. M. (2002). Biological activity of *Manduca sexta* allatotropin-like peptides, predicted products of tissue-specific and developmentally regulated alternatively spliced mRNAs. *Peptides* 23, 1933–1941. doi: 10.1016/S0196-9781(02)00181-X

Lee, K. Y., and Horodyski, F. M. (2002). Restriction of nutrient intake results in the increase of a specific *Manduca sexta* allatotropin (*Manse*-AT) mRNA in the larval nerve cord. *Peptides* 23, 653–661. doi: 10.1016/S0196-9781(01)00659-3

Lee, K. Y., and Horodyski, F. M. (2006). Effects of starvation and mating on *corpora allata* activity and allatotropin (*Manse*-AT) gene expression in *Manduca sexta*. *Peptides* 27, 567–574. doi: 10.1016/j.peptides.2005.08.024

Lee, K. Y., Horodyski, F. M., and Chamberlin, M. E. (1998). Inhibition of midgut ion transport by allatotropin (*Mas*-At) and *Manduca* FRLFamides in the tobacco hornworm *Manduca sexta*. *J. Exp. Biol.* 201, 3067–3074.

Li, K. W., Holling, T., de With, N. D., and Geraerts, W. P. M. (1993). Purification and characterization of a novel tetradecapeptide that modulates oesophagus motility in *Lymnaea stagnalis*. *Biochem. Biophys. Res. Commun.* 197, 1056–1061. doi: 10.1006/bbrc.1993.2585

Lwalaba, D., Hoffmann, K. H., and Woodring, J. (2010). Control of the release of digestive enzyme in the larvae of the fall armworm, *Spodoptera frugiperda*. *Arch. Insect Biochem. Physiol.* 73, 14–29. doi: 10.1002/arch.20332

Marchal, E., Badisco, L., Verlinden, H., Vandersmissen, T.,Van Soest, S., Van Wielendaele, P., et al. (2011). Role of the Halloween genes, Spook and Phantom in ecdysteroidogenesis in the desert locust, *Schistocerca gregaria*. *J. Insect Physiol.* 41, 815–822. doi: 10.1016/j.jinsphys.2011.05.009

Masood, M., and Orchard, I. (2014). Molecular characterization and possible biological roles of allatotropin in *Rhodnius prolixus*. *Peptides* 53, 159–171. doi: 10.1016/j.peptides.2013.10.017

Milligan, G., Marshall, F., and Rees, S. (1996). G16 as a universal G protein adapter: implications for agonist screening strategies. *Trends Pharmacol. Sci.* 17, 235–237. doi: 10.1016/0165-6147(96)10026-2

Mirabeau, O., and Joly, J. S. (2013). Molecular evolution of peptidergic signaling systems in bilaterians. *Proc. Natl. Acad. Sci. U.S.A.* 110, E2028–E2037. doi: 10.1073/pnas.1219956110

Nagata, S., Matsumoto, S., Mizoguchi, A., and Nagasawa, H. (2012). Identification of cDNAs encoding allatotropin and allatotropin-like peptides from the silkworm, *Bombyx mori*. *Peptides* 34, 98–105. doi: 10.1016/j.peptides.2012.01.002

Neupert, S., Schattschneider, S., and Predel, R. (2009). Allatotropin-related peptide in cockroaches: identification via mass spectrometric analysis of single identified neurons. *Peptides* 30, 489–494. doi: 10.1016/j.peptides.2008.10.023

Nouzova, M., Brockhoff, A., Mayoral, J. G., Goodwin, M., Meyerhof, W., and Noriega, F. G. (2012). Functional characterization of an allatotropin receptor expressed in the *corpora allata* of mosquitoes. *Peptides* 34, 201–208. doi: 10.1016/j.peptides.2011.07.025

Oeh, U., Dyker, H., Lösel, P., and Hoffmann, K. H. (2001). *In vivo* effects of *Manduca sexta* allatotropin and allatostatin on development and reproduction in the fall armyworm, *Spodoptera frugiperda* (Lepidoptera, Noctuidae). *Invertebr. Repr. Dev.* 39, 239–247. doi: 10.1080/07924259.2001.9652488

Offermans, S., and Simon, M. I. (1995). Gα15 and Gα16 couple a wide variety of receptors to phospholipase C. *J. Biol. Chem.* 25, 15175–15180. doi: 10.1074/jbc.270.25.15175

Paemen, L., Schoofs, L., and De Loof, A. (1992). Localization of *Lom*-AG-myotropin I-like substances in the male reproductive and nervous tissue of the locust, *Locusta migratoria*. *Cell Tissue Res.* 268, 91–97. doi: 10.1007/BF00338057

Paemen, L., Tips, A., Schoofs, L., Proost, P., Van Damme, J., and De Loof, A. (1991). *Lom*-AG-myotropin: a novel myotropic peptide from the male accessory glands of *Locusta migratoria*. *Peptides* 12, 7–10. doi: 10.1016/0196-9781(91)90158-L

Petersen, T. N., Brunak, S., von Heijne, G., and Nielsen, H. (2011). SignalP 4.0: discriminating signal peptides from transmembrane regions. *Nat. Methods* 8, 785–786. doi: 10.1038/nmeth.1701

Petri, B., Homberg, U., Loesel, R., and Stengl, M. (2002). Evidence for a role of GABA and Mass-allatotropin in photic entrainment of the circadian clock of the cockroach *Leucophaea maderae*. *J. Exp. Biol.* 205, 1459–1469.

Pratt, G. E., and Tobe, S. S. (1974). Juvenile hormones radiobiosynthesised by *corpora allata* of adult female locusts *in vitro*. *Life Sci.* 14, 575–586. doi: 10.1016/0024-3205(74)90372-5

Rouillé, Y., Duguay, S. J., Lund, K., Furuta, M., Gong, Q., Lipkind, G., et al. (1995). Proteolytic processing mechanisms in the biosynthesis of neuroendocrine peptides: the subtilisin-like proprotein convertases. *Front. Neuroendocrinol.* 16, 322–361. doi: 10.1006/frne.1995.1012

Rudwall, A. J., Sliwowska, J., and Nässel, D. R. (2000). Allatotropin-like neuropeptide in the cockroach abdominal nervous system: myotropic actions, sexually dimorphic distribution and colocalization with serotonin. *J. Comp. Neurol.* 428, 159–173. doi: 10.1002/1096-9861(20001204)428:1<159::AID-CNE11>3.0.CO;2-Y

Schoofs, L., Holman, M. G., Hayes, T. K., Nachman, R. J., Vandesande, F., and De Loof, A. (1990). Isolation, identification and synthesis of locustamyotropin II, an additional neuropeptide of *Locusta migratoria*: member of the cephalomyotropic peptide family. *Insect Biochem.* 20, 479–484. doi: 10.1016/0020-1790(90)90029-T

Sevala, V. L., Davey, K. G., and Prestwich, G. D. (1995). Photoaffinity labeling and characterization of a juvenile hormone binding protein in the membranes of follicle cells of *Locusta migratoria*. *Insect Biochem. Mol. Biol.* 25, 267–273. doi: 10.1016/0965-1748(94)00065-P

Sonnhammer, E. L., von Heijne, G., and Krogh, A. (1998). A hidden Markov model for predicting transmembrane helices in protein sequences. *Proc. Int. Conf. Intell. Syst. Mol. Biol.* 6, 175–182.

Tamura, K., Stecher, G., Peterson, D., Filipski, A., and Kumar, S. (2013). MEGA6: molecular evolutionary genetics analysis version 6.0. *Mol. Biol. Evol.* 30, 2725–2729. doi: 10.1093/molbev/mst197

Tobe, S. S., and Chapman, C. S. (1979). The effects of starvation and subsequent feeding on juvenile hormone synthesis and oocyte growth in *Schistocerca gregaria*. *J. Insect Physiol.* 25, 701–708. doi: 10.1016/0022-1910(79)90122-7

Tobe, S. S., Chapman, C. S., and Pratt, G. E. (1977). Decay in juvenile hormone biosynthesis by insect *corpus allatum* after nerve transection. *Nature* 268, 728–730. doi: 10.1038/268728a0

Tobe, S. S., and Pratt, G. E. (1974). The influence of substrate concentrations on the rate of insect juvenile hormone biosynthesis by corpora allata of the desert locust *in vitro*. *Biochem. J.* 144, 107–113.

Tobe, S. S., and Pratt, G. E. (1975). *Corpus allatum in vitro* during ovarian maturation in the desert locust, *Schistocerca gregaria*. *J. exp. Biol.* 62, 611–627.

Torfs, H., Detheux, M., Oonk, H. B., Akerman, K. E., Poels, J., Van Loy, T., et al. (2002). Analysis of C-terminally substituted tachykinin-like peptide agonists by means of aequorin-based luminescent assays for human and insect neurokinin receptors. *Biochem. Pharmacol.* 63, 1675–1682. doi: 10.1016/S0006-2952(02)00914-0

Ukena, K., Oumi, T., Matsushima, O., Ikeda, T., Fujita, T., Minakata, H., et al. (1995). A novel gut tetradecapeptide isolated from the earthworm, *Eisenia foetida*. *Peptides* 16, 995–999. doi: 10.1016/0196-9781(95)00071-Q

Vanden Broeck, J. (2001). Neuropeptides and their precursors in the fruitfly, *Drosophila melanogaster*. *Peptides* 22, 241–254. doi: 10.1016/S0196-9781(00)00376-4

Vandesompele, J., De Preter, K., Pattyn, F., Poppe, B., Van Roy, N., De Paepe, A., et al. (2002). Accurate normalization of real-time quantitative RT-PCR data by geometric averaging of multiple internal control genes. *Genome Biol.* 3:research0034. doi: 10.1186/gb-2002-3-7-research0034

Van Hiel, M. B., Van Wielendaele, P., Temmerman, L., Van Soest, S., Vuerinckx, K., Huybrechts, R., et al. (2009). Identification and validation of housekeeping genes in brains of the desert locust *Schistocerca gregaria* under different developmental conditions. *BMC Mol. Biol.* 10:56. doi: 10.1186/1471-2199-10-56

Veenstra, J. A. (2000). Mono- and dibasic proteolytic cleavage sites in insect neuroendocrine peptide precursors. *Arch. Insect Biochem. Physiol.* 43, 49–63. doi: 10.1002/(SICI)1520-6327(200002)43:2<49::AID-ARCH1>3.0.CO;2-M

Veenstra, J. A. (2010). Neurohormones and neuropeptides encoded by the genome of *Lottia gigantea*, with reference to other mollusks and insects. *Gen. Comp. Endocrinol.* 167, 86–103. doi: 10.1016/j.ygcen.2010.02.010

Veenstra, J. A. (2011). Neuropeptide evolution: neurohormones and neuropeptides predicted from the genomes of *Capitella teleta* and *Helobdella robusta*. *Gen. Comp. Endocrinol.* 171, 160–175. doi: 10.1016/j.ygcen.2011.01.005

Veenstra, J. A., and Costes, L. (1999). Isolation and identification of a peptide and its cDNA from the mosquito Aedes aegypti related to *Manduca sexta* allatotropin. *Peptides* 20, 1145–1151. doi: 10.1016/S0196-9781(99)00117-5

Veenstra, J. A., Lehman, H. K., and Davis, N. T. (1994). Allatotropin is a cardioacceleratory peptide in *Manduca sexta*. *J. Exp. Biol.* 188, 347–354.

Veenstra, J. A., Rodriguez, L., and Weaver, R. J. (2012). Allatotropin, leucokinin and AKH in honey bees and other Hymenoptera. *Peptides* 35, 122–130. doi: 10.1016/j.peptides.2012.02.019

Verlinden, H., Lismont, E., Bil, M., Urlacher, E., Mercer, A., Vanden Broeck, J., et al. (2013). Characterisation of the allatotropin receptor in *Bombus terrestris* (Hymenoptera, Apidae). *Gen. Comp. Endocrinol.* 193, 193–200. doi: 10.1016/j.ygcen.2013.08.006

Verlinden, H., Vleugels, R., Marchal, E., Badisco, L., Tobback, J., Pflüger, H.-J., et al. (2010). The cloning, phylogenetic relationship and distribution pattern of two new putative GPCR-type octopamine receptors in the desert locust (*Schistocerca gregaria*). *J. Insect Physiol.* 56, 868–875. doi: 10.1016/j.jinsphys.2010.03.003

Verlinden, H., Vleugels, R., Verdonck, R., Urlacher, E., Vanden Broeck, J., and Mercer, A. (2015). Pharmacological and signalling properties of a D2-like dopamine receptor (Dop3) in *Tribolium castaneum*. *Insect Biochem. Mol. Biol.* 56, 9–20. doi: 10.1016/j.ibmb.2014.11.002

Vleugels, R., Lenaerts, C., Vanden Broeck, J., and Verlinden, H. (2014). Signalling properties and pharmacology of a 5-HT7 -type serotonin receptor from *Tribolium castaneum*. *Insect. Mol. Biol.* 23, 230–243. doi: 10.1111/imb.12076

Vuerinckx, K., Verlinden, H., Lindemans, M., Vanden Broeck, J., and Huybrechts, R. (2011). Characterization of an allatotropin-like peptide receptor in the red flour beetle, *Tribolium castaneum*. *Insect Biochem. Mol. Biol.* 41, 815–822. doi: 10.1016/j.ibmb.2011.06.003

Weaver, R. J., and Audsley, N. (2009). Neuropeptide regulators of juvenile hormone synthesis: structures, functions, distribution, and unanswered questions. *Ann. N.Y. Acad. Sci.* 1163, 316–329. doi: 10.1111/j.1749-6632.2009.04459.x

Wyatt, G. R., Braun, R. P., and Zhang, J. (1996). Priming effect in gene activation by juvenile hormone in locust fat body. *Arch. Insect Biochem. Physiol.* 32, 633–640.

Yagi, K. J., and Tobe, S. S. (2001). The radiochemical assay for juvenile hormone biosynthesis in insects: problems and solutions. *J. Insect. Physiol.* 47, 1227–1234. doi: 10.1016/S0022-1910(01)00124-X

Yamanaka, N., Yamamoto, S., Zitnan, D., Watanabe, K., Kawada, T., Satake, H., et al. (2008). Neuropeptide receptor transcriptome reveals unidentified neuroendocrine pathways. *PLoS ONE* 3:e3048. doi: 10.1371/journal.pone.0003048

Zels, S., Verlinden, H., Dillen, S., Vleugels, R., Nachman, R. J., and Vanden Broeck, J. (2014). Signaling properties and pharmacological analysis of two sulfakinin receptors from the red flour beetle, *Tribolium castaneum*. *PLoS ONE* 9:e94502. doi: 10.1371/journal.pone.0094502

Zhang, L., Luo, L., and Jiang, X. (2008). Starvation influences allatotropin gene expression and juvenile hormone titer in the female adult oriental armyworm, *Mythimna separata*. *Arch. Insect Biochem. Physiol.* 68, 63–70. doi: 10.1002/arch.20255

7

Endocrinology of the aging prostate: Current concepts

Rossella Cannarella, Rosita A. Condorelli, Federica Barbagallo, Sandro La Vignera and Aldo E. Calogero*

Department of Clinical and Experimental Medicine, University of Catania, Catania, Italy

Edited by:
Marc R. Blackman, Washington DC VA Medical Center, United States

Reviewed by:
Carla Pelusi, University of Bologna, Italy
Antonello Lorenzini, University of Bologna, Italy

***Correspondence:**
Sandro La Vignera
sandrolavignera@unict.it

Benign prostate hyperplasia (BPH), one of the most common diseases in older men, adversely affects quality-of-life due to the presence of low urinary tract symptoms (LUTS). Numerous data support the presence of an association between BPH-related LUTS (BPH-LUTS) and metabolic syndrome (MetS). Whether hormonal changes occurring in MetS play a role in the pathogenesis of BPH-LUTS is a debated issue. Therefore, this article aimed to systematically review the impact of hormonal changes that occur during aging on the prostate, including the role of sex hormones, insulin-like growth factor 1, thyroid hormones, and insulin. The possible explanatory mechanisms of the association between BPH-LUTS and MetS are also discussed. In particular, the presence of a male polycystic ovarian syndrome (PCOS)-equivalent may represent a possible hypothesis to support this link. Male PCOS-equivalent has been defined as an endocrine syndrome with a metabolic background, which predisposes to the development of type II diabetes mellitus, cardiovascular diseases, prostate cancer, BPH and prostatitis in old age. Its early identification would help prevent the onset of these long-term complications.

Keywords: low urinary tract symptoms, metabolic syndrome, aging, insulin, male PCOS-equivalent, benign prostate hyperplasia

INTRODUCTION

Prostate diseases, usually diagnosed in the elderly, mainly include benign prostatic hyperplasia (BPH) and prostate cancer (PCa). BPH is defined as an increased prostate volume, largely due to the cellular proliferation occurring in the transition zone, namely the portion of the prostatic tissue that surrounds the urethra. BPH is an age-dependent disease which can obstruct the prostatic urethra. Its prevalence varies between 5% and 10% in men aged 40, but reaches 80% in men aged 70–80 (1). PCa represents the second cause of mortality for oncologic diseases in Western countries (2). Although ethnicity also influences the epidemiology of PCa (3), increasing age is a widely-accepted risk factor for the development of this malignant tumor. Accordingly, it is more frequently diagnosed in aging men, whereas it is quite uncommon before the age of 45 (4).

Hormonal changes occurring in aging may play a role in the pathogenesis of prostate diseases. These include changes of sexual hormones, insulin-like growth factor 1 (IGF1), thyroid hormones, cortisol and insulin. Importantly, hyperinsulinemia seems to impact on prostate tissue and is associated with prostate inflammation and hyperplasia. However, the mechanisms of this association are not well-recognized yet. This review aims to provide comprehensive and updated insights into the endocrinology of the aging prostate, including possible pathogenic mechanisms linking prostate to endocrinological and metabolic health.

SEX HORMONES AND PROSTATE IN AGING

Prostate diseases and androgen decline represent some of the most common conditions in the aging male. Several large cross-sectional studies have shown an approximate 1%–2% annual decline in testosterone (T) levels in men during aging (5, 6). In middle-age men, the combination of low T and hypogonadism-related symptoms is known as "late-onset hypogonadism (LOH)." LOH has an estimated prevalence of 2.1% (7), but it reaches 15% when only biochemical criteria are used for its diagnosis (8). However, the presence of various diseases plays a crucial role in the decrease of T production during aging. These include obesity, type 2 diabetes mellitus and metabolic syndrome (MetS), which can also lead to an estrogen increase (9). Considering the high prevalence of these diseases in elderly men, it is important to understand the role of sex hormones, and, therefore, of their age-related change, in the development and the treatment for prostate disorders.

Androgens

Androgens and Prostate Physiology

Androgens are essential for the development and the growth of the male genital system, including the prostate. The effects of androgens on the prostate are mainly mediated by the androgen receptor (AR), which is expressed in both prostatic stromal and epithelial cells (10). T, produced by Leydig cells of the testes, is the main circulating androgen in men and it is converted to its more potent metabolite, the 5α-dihydro-testosterone (DHT) by 5α-reductase whose type 2 is the isoform mostly expressed in the prostate tissue (11). Other androgens include adrenally-derived dehydroepiandrosterone (DHEA), androstenedione and 5α-androstenedione, which can be converted to sex steroids with higher potency and act on the prostate.

During development, androgens stimulate differentiation and proliferation of both the epithelial and the stromal compartments of the gland (12). Prostate differentiation and growth start at the 10–12th week of gestation (13). The increase of T that occurs shortly after birth and then, in the period known as "mini-puberty," has a crucial role in prostate development (13). After mini-puberty, T levels and prostate volume decrease and prostate growth is quiescent until puberty (14). During puberty, a second phase of prostate growth starts and the prostate size increases from about 10 g at early puberty to almost 20 g around the age of twenty (15). In middle age, a third phase of prostate proliferation begins and continues up to the elderly (15). However, this third phase is different from the first two phases of prostate growth. First, the proliferation involves only one of the three anatomical areas of the prostate, the transitional zone surrounding the urethra, while the entire gland grows during the first two phases. Second, an age-related decline in serum T levels begins in middle age. Therefore, although androgens are responsible for prostate growth in the first two phases, the role of androgens is the object of great debate for middle-aged and elderly men (10). Indeed, a clear association between higher circulating T levels and benign prostatic hyperplasia (BPH) has never been demonstrated (16).

Androgens and Prostate Diseases

Androgens and Benign Prostate Hyperplasia

LUTS and BPH have long been considered a relative contraindication to testosterone replacement therapy (TRT). However, recent studies have contradicted the classic idea that androgens inevitably stimulate prostate growth (17). According to the saturation model, the prostate is sensitive to changes in androgen levels when they occur in a severe low range, but this sensitivity is lost for T levels corresponding to mild hypogonadism or eugonadal. Indeed, prostate ARs become saturated at relatively low T levels and thus, the gland becomes unresponsive to further increases in T levels (18). Experimental and clinical studies suggest that the saturation point for human prostate tissue probably occurs in the very low range of T levels, but a precise cutoff value has not been established; it could vary among men (17). According to this model, the association between T and prostate-specific antigen (PSA) is represented by a sigmoid curve. T levels of 8 nmol/L corresponds to the plateau value below which small changes in T levels cause greater variations in PSA (19). As reported in recent reviews (12, 17), studies evaluating the link between TRT and BPH/LUTS have mostly shown that TRT does not have any effect on BPH symptoms [measured by the International Prostate Symptom Score (IPSS)] and occasionally the IPSS score may decrease (20–22). A recent meta-analysis did not show a worsening of LUTS severity in hypogonadal patients treated with T vs. placebo (23). The safety of TRT in patients with severe LUTS remains to be established and the presence of LUTS of moderate-intensity (IPSS ≤19) is not a contraindication to TRT (23).

However, although current evidence suggests that higher T levels are not involved in BPH development, T seems to have a role in this pathogenic process by stimulating inflammation within prostate tissue. Inflammation has a crucial role in the pathogenesis of BPH and low, rather than high, T may stimulate prostate inflammation (12). Nevertheless, an anti-inflammatory effect of T in the prostate has also been described. In an experimental study using human prostatic stromal cell cultures, the treatment *in-vitro* with different pro-inflammatory stimuli, such as tumor necrosis factor α (TNF-α) or lipopolysaccharide (LPS), or co-culturing with activated CD4β lymphocytes, significantly enhanced the secretion of several cytokines and growth factors (24). The pre-treatment of BPH stromal cells with DHT inhibited the secretion of several inflammatory/growth factors and the proliferation of activated CD4β lymphocytes in a dose-dependent manner (24). The same authors developed a rabbit model of MetS, by feeding New Zealand male rabbits with a high-fat diet (HFD) for

12 weeks (25). Rabbits with MetS developed glucose intolerance, dyslipidemia, hypertension, increased visceral fat accumulation, hypogonadotropic hypogonadism, hyperestrogenism, and prostate inflammation. TRT has been shown to protect rabbits from prostatic hypoxia, fibrosis, and inflammation induced by the high-fat diet that appears to play a role in the development and even progression of BPH/LUTS (25). Interestingly, they found that MetS severity was associated with an increase of *AR* and *estrogen receptor* α (*ERα*), but not of *estrogen receptor β* (ER*β*) gene expression within the prostate (10). This suggests that the prostate could become more sensitive to sex hormone changes that occur during MetS. Indeed, TRT not only corrects the low T levels and the rise of estrogen levels which are typical of MetS, but it also normalizes the majority of MetS-induced prostate alterations (25).

Accordingly, in human BPH stromal cells, AR activation by DHT inhibited TNFα, LPS, or CD4 (+) T cell-induced secretion of inflammatory/growth factors, including interleukin (IL)-6, IL-8, and basic fibroblast growth factor (bFGF), by blocking the nuclear translocation of the nuclear factor kappa-B (NF- κB) (24). Moreover, HFD prostates had increased phosphodiesterase type 5 (PDE5) expression. This was associated with a higher expression of *cyclooxygenase 2* (*COX2*) and *TNFα* among inflammatory genes and of *TGFβ*, *Rho-associated coiled-coil-containing protein kinase 2* (*ROCK2*) and *α spinal muscular atrophy* (*αSMA*) among those genes specifically involved in fibrosis and myofibroblast activation. Interestingly, HFD-induced *PDE5* overexpression was counteracted by T treatment (26). Therefore, recent evidence suggests that the treatment of hypogonadism, which is frequently associated with MetS, not only does not seem to be dangerous for prostate health, but could even prevent the inflammatory process of this gland (12).

Even in inflammation of the prostate caused by *Escherichia coli*, the most frequent bacterial infection due to the reflux of infected urine into the prostate ducts (ascending urethral infection), T seems to play a protective role. Ho and colleagues have shown that T not only inhibits the invasion and colonization of the uropathogenic *Escherichia coli* (UPEC), but has also reduced the levels of pro-inflammatory cytokines (IL-1β, IL-6, and IL- 8) induced by UPEC in a dose-dependent manner. In particular, T plays an anti-inflammatory role in LPS-induced prostate cell inflammation by down-regulating *Janus kinases, signal transducer and activator of transcription proteins* (JAK/STAT1) signaling pathway (JAK/STAT1) (27).

Androgens and Prostate Cancer

The concern that T promotes the development of PCa has been the object of great debate since the discovery of PCa dependency on androgen in the 1940s thanks to the pioneering studies of Huggins and Hodges, who found that castration resulted in regression of metastatic PCa (28). However, according to the saturation model, androgen-dependency of prostate growth is evident only in hypogonadism (18). Thus, the relationship between T and the risk of PCa remains poorly understood. Several studies have shown an increased risk of PCa in men with hypogonadism (29). This hypothesis was firstly reported in 1996 by Morgentaler and colleagues, who found a higher prevalence of biopsy-detectable PCa in men with low total or free testosterone levels (30) and it was supported by subsequent studies (31–34). In contrast, studies assessing the relationship between high endogenous T levels and the development of PCa are less clear (29). However, there is evidence that previous T levels may influence Gleason scores, clinical outcomes and recurrence (29).

More controversial remains the safety of TRT in patients with a history of PCa after treatment. T could cause the growth of subclinical cancers that are frequently hidden in the prostate of older men (35). Aside, metastases of PCa are hormone-dependent, therefore T should not be administered to these patients (35). However, some clinicians have suggested considering TRT for patients with a history of organ-confined PCa if they have undergone radical prostatectomy, have undetectable PSA for at least two years and low-grade PCa (Gleason score <7). The possible risks and benefits of TRT should be discussed with the patient and TRT should be followed up with appropriate monitoring by experienced physicians (36).

Also, although adrenal androgens have weak androgenic effects, 11-oxy-androgens of adrenal origin can be metabolized in peripheral tissues to potent androgens which might have a role in the development of PCa. Moreover, emerging evidence suggests the role of microbiome components in the development of PCa that are only beginning to be understood. Recent studies have shown that gut bacteria are capable of metabolizing C21 glucocorticoids to 11-oxygenated C19 androgens *via* an enzyme known as steroid-17,20-desmolase (*desAB*) encoded by the *desAB* gene. A cortisol-inducible operon (*desABCD*) was previously identified in *Clostridium scindens* ATCC 35704 encoding enzyme involved in anaerobic side-chain cleavage. This operon also encodes a transketolase (desAB) which have steroid-17,20-desmolase activity (37). Interestingly, the compounds cleaved by steroid-17,20-desmolase, 11-ketoandrostenedione (11 KT), and 1,4-androstadiene-3,11,17- trione (AT) were found to stimulate proliferation of PCa cells (LNCaP), to a greater extent than dihydrotestosterone. Further researches are needed to fully understand the mechanism through which these compounds stimulate cell proliferation and the potential clinical role in the development and treatment of prostate cancer (38).

Estrogens and Prostate

Prostate is commonly considered a target of androgens, but also estrogens can play an important role in prostate growth and differentiation. In fact, both ERα and ERβ are expressed in the prostate. ERα is mainly located in the stromal cells and its activation regulates the growth of both stromal and epithelial prostatic cells *via* paracrine mediators like stromal bFGF, epidermal growth factor (EGF), and IGF1 (39, 40). In contrast, ERβ is located in epithelial cells and their activation modulates the estrogenic signals in the prostate (41).

17ß-Estradiol (E_2) is considered the most potent estrogen in men and it mainly originates from aromatization of T in fat and muscle, whereas about 20% is secreted by Leydig cells (42).

In aging men, paralleling the decrease of T levels, the ratio of estrogens to androgens shows an important increase (43). There are several endogenous and exogenous estrogens which may play an important role in prostate. Endogenous estrogens include estrone (E_1), which is considered to have minimal influence within the prostate, and estriol (E_3), the main estrogen of pregnancy, which is present in minimal concentrations in men. However, E_2 can be a potent inducer of prostatic proliferation (44). Local steroids with ER agonist activity include also 5α-androstane-3β, 17β-diol (3βAdiol), and 7α-hydroxy-DHEA (7HD). The effects of these sex steroids are not fully understood but they seem to influence prostate hyperplasia (44). Exogenous estrogens include therapeutic drugs, phytoestrogens, and endocrine disruptors. ERs have a high affinity for environmental estrogens such as bisphenol A (BPA), phthalates, pesticides, etc. In rodent studies, developmental BPA, DES, or E_2 exposure affects prostate epigenome and thus causes increased prostate susceptibility to dysplasia and hormonal carcinogenesis with aging (45).

Estrogen hormone action in the prostate depends not only on the types of estrogens but most of all, from the type of ER. Specifically, ERα activation is associated with prostate hyperplasia, inflammation, and dysplasia (46). However, the main stimulation of inflammation in BPH by estrogens seem to be mediated by the membrane ER G protein-coupled receptor 30 (GPR30) or G protein-coupled ER (GPER), which are also expressed in prostate stromal cells (47). On the contrary, ERβ inhibits proliferation and its knockout results in prostate hyperplasia (48). The prostatic hyperplasia observed in ERβ knockout mice is attributed to the unopposed action to ERα, suggesting that the ratio ERα/ERβ is an important factor in estrogen-induced proliferation (44).

Estrogens and Benign Prostate Hyperplasia

Recent studies suggest that not only low T levels, but also an increase of estrogens may favor BPH/LUTS progression (10). Marmorston and colleagues first reported that the E_2/T ratio in 24-h urinary collections was elevated in men with BPH compared to normal controls (49). Other epidemiologic studies have found an association between BPH and higher serum estrogen levels or estrogen/androgen ratio (50, 51). As previously reported, prostate inflammation could be amplified and maintained by metabolic alteration occurring in conditions such as MetS. Vignozzi and colleagues showed that HFD rabbits had higher E_2 to T ratio and lower urinary tract fibrosis, which improved with TRT (25). Recent evidence has also shown that leptin, a hormone produced by adipocytes, induces proliferative effects in prostate cells. This effect may be partially mediated by the direct effect of leptin on estrogen metabolism, as leptin induces aromatase expression (52).

Therefore, ERα, as a key mediator, is also a potential therapeutic target in BPH. The block of conversion of androgens to estrogens by aromatase inhibitors seems to prevent prostate hyperplasia (12). Similar to aromatase inhibitors, selective estrogen receptor modulators (SERMs) have shown anti-proliferative effects on prostate tissue (53).

Estrogens and Prostate Cancer

Evidence suggests that ERα mediates the harmful effects of estrogen not only promoting BPH/LUTS, but also prostate carcinogenesis. In the early 1980s, Noble showed the estrogen-dependence of PCa in a rat model (54). In aromatase knockout (KO) mice, high T levels only lead to prostate hypertrophy and hyperplasia, whereas high E_2 and low T levels induced also premalignant lesions (55). Indeed, prostatic intraepithelial neoplasia does not occur in ERαKO mice and SERMs that bind and inhibit ERα prevent PCa progression in mice and men (56–58). Epidemiological studies have confirmed the role of estrogens on PCa (59). African-American men, who have high serum E_2 levels, present an increased risk of developing PCa (60). Indeed, ERα expression is significantly associated with high Gleason score and poor survival in PCa patients (61), whereas the expression of ERβ seems decreased or lost in PCa samples (62). Therefore, preclinical and clinical results suggest that ERβ agonists may be useful in PCa therapy, especially in the early stage (59).

Since the discovery of estrogen dependence of PCa, numerous clinical trials were conducted and molecular and functional effects of antiestrogen treatment in PCa have been conducted. Androgen deprivation therapy (ADT) is the first line of treatment for PCa. Nonetheless, ADT frequently induces resistance and PCa can progress toward an androgen-independent form, known as castration-resistant PCa, characterized by worse prognosis. For this reason, alternative approaches to androgen ablation have been investigated to prevent the progression of PCa. Currently, molecular networks of estrogenic signaling *via* ERα, ERβ, and GPR30 in PCa have not been fully understood but new compounds, whose efficacy has been successfully tested in preclinical and clinical models of PC, opened the way for novel therapeutic strategies for treating prostatic diseases (41, 59).

In conclusion, the above-mentioned evidence suggests a role for age-related changes in sex hormones; in particular, hypogonadism and the increase in estrogen levels related to obesity play a pivotal role in the pathogenesis of age-related prostatic diseases.

INSULIN-LIKE GROWTH FACTOR 1 AND PROSTATE

Several studies indicate that IGF1 declines with age (63). Interestingly, IGF1 seems to have an important role in the pathogenesis of metabolic syndrome. Indeed, several studies, both *in-vitro* and *in-vivo* have shown the association between low levels of IGF1 and altered lipid metabolism, cardiovascular disease and diabetes (64). Nevertheless, increased levels of IGF1 have also been reported in patients with diabetes mellitus (65).

A large body of evidence shows that the growth hormone (GH)- IGF1 endocrine axis has a pivotal role in the growth and development of prostate in normal physiology as in pathological conditions (66–69). IGF1 is secreted mainly by the liver under

GH stimulation, but it is also expressed locally within the stromal and epithelial cells of the prostate, where it can act in autocrine/paracrine manner (70). The binding of IGF1 to the IGF1 receptor (IGF1R) or the insulin receptor (IR) in the prostate gland, activates the phosphoinositide 3-kinase (PI3K)/protein kinase B (AKT) pathway and RAF/MAPK pathway, which promote cell survival and proliferation (70).

Some studies have shown a greater prevalence of prostate enlargement and BPH in patients with acromegaly (67, 69). Kumar and colleagues documented structural changes in acromegalic patients by prostatic biopsy (71). They found that patients with acromegaly have higher IPSS, an increased rate of prostate enlargement on rectal exploration and ultrasound, higher PSA levels and obstructive pattern on uroflowmetry, and structural prostate changes, regardless of their age, disease activity, or gonadal status (71). These results suggest that the hyper-activation of the GH/IGF1 axis plays an important role in the pathogenesis of BPH in patients with acromegaly. This is further supported by the decrease of prostate volume in patients with inactive disease (for more than 24 months) (71).

Also, there is ample evidence that IGF1 and the signal transduction network that it regulates have important roles in the development of tumors (72). Epidemiological studies have reported that high circulating levels of IGF1 are associated with an increased risk of PCa, particularly advanced disease (70, 73). Experimental studies have shown that the binding of IGF1 to both the IGF1R and IR promotes mitogen signaling events, increases cell proliferation and inhibits apoptosis (72). Both IGF1R and IR are overexpressed in PCa tissue (74). Moreover, the expression of the components of the GH, insulin, and IGF1 axes can be finely modulated in the prostate by environmental factors such as the diet. As previously described, it was well documented that obesity promotes structural changes in the prostate (12). Prostate of obese mice presents altered mRNA expression levels of GH receptor (GHR) and glucose transporter 4 (GLUT4) and an up-regulation in IGF-binding protein 3 (Igfbp3) expression, which might have pathophysiological implications (75). Emerging evidence suggests a direct regulation of IGF/insulin signaling to the *transmembrane serine protease 2* (*TMPRSS2*)/*V-ETS avian erythroblastosis E26 oncogene homolog* (*ERG*) gene fusion, one of the main somatic events in PCa (76). It has been hypothesized that ERG-positive tumors may be more sensitive to IGF/insulin signaling, which could promote PCa progression (70). Furthermore, another possible mechanism is the activation of AR. IGF1 signaling stimulates ARs by attenuating forkhead box-containing protein O subfamily (Foxol) inhibition (77). Recent researches have highlighted the involvement of not only IGF1 signaling but also of GH itself. GH is responsible for the activation of transcription 5 (STAT5) protein which is involved in the development of several tumors including PCa (78). GHRH antagonists have been shown to decrease directly prostate volume without involving the androgen pathway (79).

Neoplastic, cardiovascular and respiratory disorders are common causes of mortality and morbidity in patients with acromegaly. Nonetheless the higher prevalence of "prostate structural changes" and a possibly increased risk of PCa in patients with acromegaly, no guidelines recommend screening for prostatic disorders. Therefore, a prostatic evaluation may be useful in the work-up of all male patients with acromegaly (71). Actual evidence supports the possible involvement of GH/IGF1 in the pathogenesis of BPH and PCa also in the general population and therapeutic agents targeting the IGF1R may be beneficial in the treatment of prostate diseases.

Finally, the increase of IGF1 seems to play a role in the pathogenesis of BPH and PCa, since it stimulates prostate cell proliferation. Notably, this hormone usually declines with age, although metabolic abnormalities and acromegaly leads to IGF1 increase. Therefore, IGF1 levels should be assessed in patients with prostatic diseases, when diabetes (or other metabolic alterations) or acromegalic features concomitantly occur.

THYROID HORMONES AND PROSTATE

Thyroid hormones (THs) are involved in cellular growth, metabolism and differentiation. Their effects are mainly mediated by triiodothyronine (T3) that, by binding the nuclear TH receptors (TRs), activates TH response elements (TREs) in the promoter of TH target genes. However, non-classical or non-genomic effects of TH have also been described (80).

The prevalence of thyroid dysfunction increases in the elderly. Recent data from observational studies suggest that serum thyroid-stimulating hormone (TSH) levels increase in older people. The US National Health and Nutritional Examination Survey (NHANES) III study showed that serum TSH concentrations, as well as serum thyroid peroxidase (TPOAb) and thyroglobulin (TgAb) antibodies, increased with age in both men and women (81). Hyperthyroidism is less common than hypothyroidism in the elderly and mainly caused by autonomously functioning thyroid nodules (82).

TRs are strongly expressed in the human prostate (83) and several studies have investigated the role of THs in the development of prostate diseases. Epidemiological studies have found that men with BPH or PCa have significantly increased serum T3 levels compared with euthyroid men (84, 85). Accordingly, Eldhose and colleagues found significantly increased levels of free T3 (FT3) and free thyroxine (FT4) and decreased levels of TSH in patients with BPH compared with controls. They also found that FT3 correlated positively and TSH negatively with prostate volume (86). It has also been shown that patients with hypothyroidism have a decreased risk of developing PCa compared to euthyroid men (87). A recent meta-analysis has shown that hyperthyroidism was associated with higher risks of PCa (pooled risk ratio: 1.35, 95%CI: 1.05-1.74) compared with euthyroidism (88). Experimental studies have shown that THs increase PCa cell proliferation *in-vitro* (89). Specifically, Hsieh and Juang found that T3 can enhance LNCaP cell proliferation and that this effect is cell-specific. LNCaP cells are androgen-sensitive and well-differentiated cells, derived from metastatic lymph nodes of a PCa patient (90). Other studies also indicated that T3 has an important role in the regulation of growth and differentiation of LNCaP cells and PSA expression (91–93). Specifically, a direct effect of T3 on PSA expression was described. Zhu and Young identified a functional TRE in the PSA promoter region, suggesting that T3 regulates PSA expression at the transcription level (93). Also, it has been described that T3 upregulates the proliferation of LNCaP cells through downregulation of the *B-cell translocation gene 2* (*BTG2*), a gene involved in cell-cycle regulation, through the TRE pathway (94). Experimental studies have also shown that THs promote carcinogenesis by inducing angiogenesis (95). Non-classical mechanisms of THs may be also responsible for the effects on the prostate. The binding of TH to plasma membrane receptor integrin avb3 might activate various pro-carcinogenic pathways, including protein inhibitor 3 kinases (PI-3 K) and mitogen activated-protein kinases 1/2 (MAPK 1/2), thereby increasing cell proliferation and angiogenesis (80).

In conclusion, although a relationship between TH and prostate seems clear, the exact mechanisms by which they act need to be further investigated and targeting TH actions might become an alternative adjuvant therapy against PCa proliferation. Due to the age-related rise in TSH levels and the negative correlation between serum TSH levels and prostate volume (81), the role of this hormone in the pathogenesis of prostate diseases in the aging male seems unlikely.

ROLE OF INSULIN IN PROSTATE DISEASES

Insulin, Metabolic Syndrome, and Benign Prostate Hyperplasia

BPH is considered an age-dependent disease, whose etiology is currently poorly understood. Several studies address to insulin-resistance and hyperinsulinemia, which are components of MetS, a role in the pathogenesis of BPH and LUTS. Accordingly, hyperinsulinemia has been shown to enhance prostatic epithelial cell proliferation *in-vitro* (96) and, conversely, hypoinsulinemia decreases prostate volume (97). In line with these findings, patients with serum insulin levels >13 mU/l have a greater prostate volume and annual BPH growth rate compared with those with insulin levels <7 mU/l (98).

Data from the second Nord-Trondelag Health Study, carried out in 21,694 patients, revealed a significantly higher risk for LUTS in patients with diabetes mellitus than in non-diabetic men (99). Also, the risk for developing LUTS has been esteemed twice in patients with diabetes compared with non-diabetic men (100). Accordingly, insulin-resistance is an independent predictor of severe LUTS development (101). This may be attributed to the autonomic nervous system hyperactivity, mainly involving the α-adrenergic pathway, which is closely associated with hyperinsulinemia and is involved in the pathogenesis of LUTS (102).

A recent retrospective study carried out in about 900 patients reported that, after correction for age, insulin levels and insulin-resistance are significantly associated with prostate volume. Interestingly, MetS predicted BPH/LUTS clinical progression (103), thus pointing to the additional role of MetS, other than insulin, in BPH/LUTS. A systematic review with meta-analysis performed on 8,476 participants, including 5,554 (30.1%) with and 12,922 (69.9%) without MetS showed a significantly higher prostate volume in patients compared to controls (104).

The National Cholesterol Education Program adult treatment panel III (2005 revision) defines MetS as the presence of three or more criteria among the following: i) abdominal obesity (waist circumference >102 cm), ii) hypertriglyceridemia (>150 mg/dl) or medications, iii) low high-density lipoprotein (HDL) cholesterol (<40 mg/dl) or medications, iv) hypertension (>130/85 mmHg) or medication, v) high fasting glucose (>110 mg/dl) or medication (105). The evidence supports an association between BPH and each of the MetS components (102).

In greater detail, a BMI >35 Kg/m^2 has been associated with a 3.5-fold higher risk of developing an increased prostate volume (>40 ml) (106) and with a 1.2-fold higher risk of developing LUTS compared to those with a BMI <25 kg/m^2 (107). Data obtained in 21,694 patients have confirmed these findings by showing that BMI is a predictor for LUTS development (99). Other reports also support such conclusions (100, 108).

Notably, dyslipidemia is also associated with BPH. Patients with lower HDL cholesterol show increased prostate volume and a higher annual BPH growth rate compared with higher HDL cholesterol values (109). Also, patients with BPH have higher total and low-density lipoprotein (LDL) cholesterol than those without BPH (110) and an association between LDL cholesterol and BPH has been already shown (111). Also, among patients with diabetes, those with the highest LDL cholesterol levels have a 4-fold higher risk of developing BPH (111). These findings suggest that dyslipidemia strongly associates with BPH in the presence of other signs of MetS.

Results from 2,372 patients enrolled in the Third National Health and Nutrition Examination Survey (NHANES III) provide a role for the association between hypertension and LUTS-BPH. Particularly, those with a positive anamnesis for hypertension have increased odds for LUTS compared to those with no hypertension (112). These findings have been largely confirmed also elsewhere (100). Moreover, patients with hypertension showed larger prostate volume and a higher annual BPH growth rate compared with controls (109).

In addition to mechanisms closely associated to hyperinsulinemia, the impairment of nitric oxide (NO) and NO synthase (NOS) activity, the Rho kinase system, the pro-inflammatory status and the abnormality of sexual hormones seems also to be involved in BPH/LUTS pathogenesis in patients with MetS (102, 113). However, the hypothesis of the existence of a male polycystic ovary syndrome (PCOS) equivalent may represent an additional pathogenic mechanism deserving of consideration (please see *Male PCOS Equivalent Exists: A New Syndrome*)?.

Insulin and Prostate Cancer

Several lines of experimental evidence have pointed to the role of insulin in the enhancement of prostate carcinogenesis, particularly in advanced PCa. More in detail, androgens are known to induce epithelial differentiation in prostate cells (114). Androgen deprivation therapy (ADT), usually prescribed in patients with advanced PCa, leads to cellular de-differentiation and transdifferentiation (114–116). Under such conditions, hyperinsulinemia, a common side effect of ADT, enhances PCa cell plasticity, thus increasing tumor migration and invasiveness, by upregulating the Forkhead Box Protein C2 (FOXC2) transcription factor (117). Furthermore, PCa cell lines have an increased ratio of pyruvate dehydrogenase flux to citrate synthase flux following exposure to insulin, which correlates with an insulin dose-dependent increase in cell division (118). This experimental evidence suggests that ADT-induced hyperinsulinemia may likely impact on cancer progression and metastasis.

In line with these *in-vitro* findings, hyperinsulinemia has been associated with a greater PCa mortality (119–122) and treatment failure (122). A retrospective study evaluating the effects of MetS on the time to develop tumor progression in patients with PCa and ADT reported a significantly shorter time to PSA progression (16 vs. 36 months) and a trend toward a shorter overall survival (36.5 vs. 46.7 months) when MetS is present compared with those who do not have it (122). Some Authors have even proposed to define PCa as a component of MetS, since hyperisulinemia prospectively is a risk factor for PCa deaths (119). A long-term survival analysis performed on 2,546 patients who developed PCa, found that patients with weight excess and high C-peptide levels have a four-fold higher risk of mortality compared with those with a BMI <25 kg/m^2 and low C-peptide levels, independently of other clinical predictors (120).

Supporting these data, the IR is expressed in PCa cells and, interestingly, its expression increases with the Gleason score (74, 123) and ADT (124).

Despite such findings, whether treatment with metformin or other insulin-sensitizing drugs may play a role in PCa therapy is still a matter of debate. An *in-vitro* study reported that GSK1838705A, a potent insulin-like growth factor-1 receptor (IGF1R)/IR inhibitor, is capable of decreasing docetaxel-resistant PCa cell viability and migration, as well as *in-vivo* tumor growth. Therefore, a role for this drug for the treatment of advanced resistant PCa has been postulated (125). Also, by blocking IGF1R, metformin has been reported to significantly inhibit PCa cell proliferation, migration and invasiveness, suggesting a role in PCa treatment (126). Furthermore, tyrphostin NT157, which inhibits the insulin receptor substrates 1 and 2 (IRS1 and IRS2), was shown to decrease proliferation and increase apoptosis of PCa cell lines (127).

On these premises, a population-based study carried out in a cohort of 1,001 patients with PCa and 942 controls showed a lower PCa prevalence in patients using metformin compared with non-users. Also, it showed an inverse relationship between PCa risk and metformin length of treatment, intensity of use and cumulative dosage (128). Similarly, a population-based study on 24,723 case-control pairs found a lower PCa risk in men using antidiabetic medication (129). Other evidence supports a beneficial effect of metformin in lowering PCa incidence and overall survival (130–132).

In conclusion, despite the evidence on the possible role of antidiabetic drugs as adjuvant therapy in patients with PCa, particularly in those on ADT, is growing, there is still insufficient data from randomized trials to suggest their use in the clinical practice (133).

MALE PCOS EQUIVALENT EXISTS: A NEW SYNDROME?

PCOS is a very common endocrine disorder in women of reproductive age, with a prevalence of 6-15% (134). A genetic background and environmental factors are involved in its etiology. Despite PCOS diagnostic criteria mainly include hyperandrogenism, oligo-ovulation, or anovulation and polycystic ovaries (135), the role of metabolic dysfunction in the pathogenesis of this syndrome is widely accepted. Indeed, up to 75% of patients with PCOS are insulin-resistant and some are hyperinsulinemic (135). Accordingly, the presence of polycystic ovaries, which gave the name to the syndrome, is only one of the many downstream clinical manifestations of PCOS and it is not the pivotal pathogenic factor leading to the development of this syndrome (136, 137).

Since a genetic background has been observed in PCOS, this hereditary predisposition can be potentially inherited by the male sibling of the affected patients. Interestingly, the brothers and the

TABLE 1 | Biochemical and clinical parameters in male relatives of women with polycystic ovarian syndrome, in young and elderly men with early androgenetic alopecia (146).

Parameter	Male relatives of women with PCOS	Men with early-onset androgenetic alopecia	Clinical findings in elderly men with AGA
Serum free testosterone levels	–	↑	–
Serum SHBG levels	–	↓	–
Free testosterone index	–	↑	–
Serum LH levels	–	↑	–
Serum FSH levels	–	↓	–
LH/FSH ratio	–	↑	–
LH and FSH response to GnRH analog	↑	–	–
Serum AMH levels	↑	–	–
Serum DHEAS levels	↑	↑	–
Serum 17α hydroxy-progesterone	–	↑	–
Serum adiponectin levels	↑	–	–
Serum glucose levels	–	↑	–
Serum insulin levels	↑	↑	↑
Risk for insulin-resistance	↑	↑	–
Serum cholesterol levels	↑	↑	–
Risk for metabolic syndrome	–	↑	↑
Risk for type II diabetes mellitus	–	–	↑
Risk for endothelial dysfunction	↑	–	–
Blood pressure	↑	↑	↑
Serum aldosterone levels	–	–	↑
Serum fibrinogen levels	–	–	↑
Risk for atheromatous plaques	–	–	↑
Risk for ischemic heart disease	–	–	↑
Risk for benign prostate hyperplasia	–	–	↑
Risk for prostate cancer	–	–	↑

↑, increased; ↓, decreased; -, non-reported.

AGA, androgenetic alopecia; AMH, anti-Müllerian hormone; DHEAS, dehydroepiandrosterone sulfate; FSH, follicle-stimulating hormone; GnRH, gonadotropin-realizing hormone; LH, luteinizing hormone; SHBG, sex hormone binding globulin.

relatives of women with PCOS have a high prevalence of hormonal and metabolic abnormalities (138–140). They also show a greater prevalence of early-onset androgenetic alopecia (AGA) (141), which has been suggested as a clinical sign of the male PCOS equivalent (142–144). The occurrence of hormonal and metabolic abnormalities in men with early-onset AGA (younger than 35 years) has been reported (145, 146) (**Table 1**). A meta-analytic study performed in 1009 unrelated men found increased luteotropic hormone (LH) and dehydroepiandrosterone (DHEAS), decreased sex hormone-binding globulin (SHBG), a downward trend for FSH and an upward trend for the LH/FSH ratio in patients with early-onset AGA compared with controls. This hormonal pattern somewhat resembles that found in female PCOS. The same meta-analysis showed a significant increase in insulin levels and HOMA index, total and LDL cholesterol and triglycerides in patients vs. controls, already before the age of 35 (147).

Large cohort studies in older men with early-onset AGA have clearly shown a higher prevalence of type II diabetes mellitus (148) and a greater risk for cardiovascular disease (CVD) (149). Thus, AGA has been suggested as an independent predictor of mortality for diabetes mellitus and CVD (150). Curiously, these men have also a higher prevalence of prostate diseases, such as BPH (151–155), PCa (156), and prostatitis (157), which are known to be influenced by the metabolic status. In this view, prostate diseases may be seen as long-term complications of the male PCOS equivalent syndrome (**Table 2**) (146). This concept supports the association between metabolic abnormalities and prostate diseases in the elderly. The acknowledgment and timely diagnosis of this syndrome may be of great utility to early identify and treat metabolic disorders in men, preventing the long-term complications, including diabetes, CVD and prostate diseases.

TABLE 2 | Age-related features of the male polycystic ovarian syndrome (PCOS) equivalent.

Age	
<35 years	Clinical signs of hyperandrogenism (early-onset AGA, acne or hypertrichosis) PCOS-like hormonal pattern (e.g., increased DHEAS, 17α-OH-progesterone, FAI, LH/FSH, decreased FSH) Metabolic abnormalities (insulin-resistance, low SHBG levels, hyperglycemia, hyperinsulinemia), and/or a trend towards higher BMI values A familiar history positive for PCOS
Elderly men	Diabetes mellitus, cardiovascular diseases, benign prostatic hyperplasia, prostatitis, prostate cancer

CONCLUSION

In conclusion, the receptors for sex hormones, IGF1, THs and insulin expressed in the prostate cells indicate the close relationship between the prostate and hormones (**Figure 1**). Also, serum levels of these hormones vary with aging and are influenced by several comorbidities such as gonadal dysfunction, thyroid disease, obesity, MetS, insulin-resistance and diabetes mellitus. In particular, the evidence attributes a role in the pathogenesis of prostate inflammation, BPH and PCa to the age-related change in T levels as well as the increase in obesity-

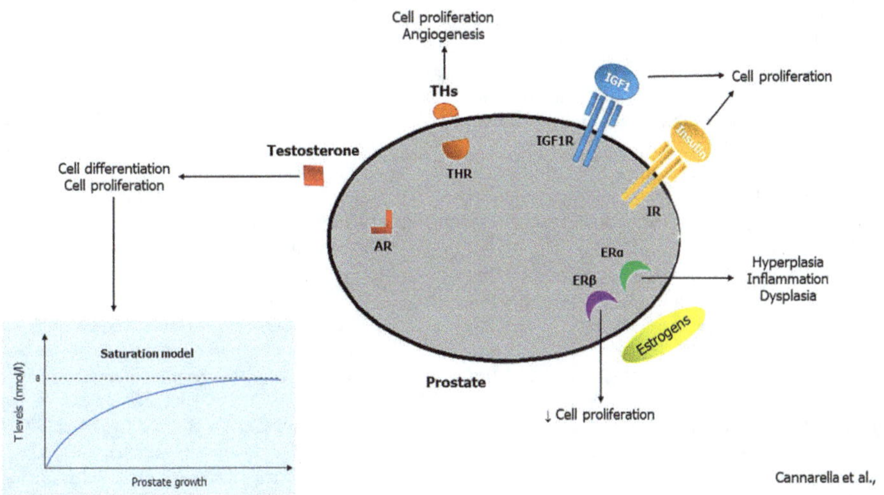

FIGURE 1 | Hormonal effects in the prostatic tissue. By binding to the androgen receptor (AR), testosterone (T) stimulates cell differentiation in prenatal life. According to the saturation model, it induces cell proliferation when its serum levels are in the hypogonadal range (<8 nmol/l). Thyroid hormones (THs) enhance prostate cell proliferation and angiogenesis, triggering the TH receptor (THR). Insulin-like growth factor 1 (IGF1) and insulin induce cell proliferation by interacting with their receptors (IGF1R and IR, respectively). Finally, estrogens can trigger the estrogen receptor α (ERα) that stimulates cell hyperplasia, inflammation, and dysplasia, or the estrogen receptor β (ERβ) that hinders cell proliferation.

related estrogen levels. Furthermore, the increase in IGF1, which occurs in diabetic or acromegalic patients, leads to the proliferation of prostate cells. In contrast, the age-related decline in serum TSH levels is unlikely to be involved in the pathogenesis of prostate disease. Finally, metabolic abnormalities can lead to insulin (but also to IGF1 and E_2)-mediated prostate inflammation and hyperplasia. This justifies the importance of endocrine counseling in patients with prostate diseases, which primarily allows the identification of endocrine or metabolic comorbidities responsible for an increased cardiovascular risk. Further research is needed to confirm the existence of a male-PCOS equivalent.

AUTHOR CONTRIBUTIONS

RC conceived the study and contributed to writing the draft of the paper. RAC contributed to write the draft of the paper and critically revised the final version of the paper. FB searched the studies and contributed to write the draft of the paper. SL contributed to writing the final version of the paper and critically revised it. AC was the project administrator. He contributed to writing the final version of the paper and critically revised it. All authors contributed to the article and approved the submitted version.

REFERENCES

1. Vuichoud C, Loughlin KR. Benign prostatic hyperplasia: epidemiology, economics and evaluation. *Can J Urol* (2015) 22(1):1–6.
2. Siegel RL, Miller KD, Jemal A. Cancer statistics, 2016. *CA Cancer J Clin* (2016) 66:7–30. doi: 10.3322/caac.21332
3. De Santis CE, Siegel RL, Sauer AG, Miller KD, Fedewa SA, Alcaraz KI, et al. Cancer statistics for African Americans, 2016: Progress and opportunities in reducing racial disparities. *CA Cancer J Clin* (2016) 66(4):290–308. doi: 10.3322/caac.21340
4. Daniyal M, Siddiqui ZA, Akram M, Asif HM, Sultana S, Khan A. Epidemiology, etiology, diagnosis and treatment of prostate cancer. *Asian Pac J Cancer Prev* (2014) 15(22):9575–8. doi: 10.7314/APJCP.2014.15.22.9575
5. Feldman HA, Longcope C, Derby CA, Johannes CB, Araujo AB, Coviello, et al. Age trends in the level of serum testosterone and other hormones in middle-aged men: longitudinal results from the Massachusetts male aging study. *J Clin Endocrinol Metab* (2002) 87(2):589–98. doi: 10.1210/jcem.87.2.8201
6. O'Donnell AB, Araujo AB, McKinlay JB. The health of normally aging men: The Massachusetts Male Aging Study (1987–2004). *Exp Gerontol* (2004) 39:975–84. doi: 10.1016/j.exger.2004.03.023
7. Tajar A, Huhtaniemi IT, O'Neill TW, Finn JD, Pye SR, Lee DM, et al. Characteristics of androgen deficiency in late-onset hypogonadism: results from the European Male Aging Study (EMAS). *J Clin Endocrinol Metab* (2012) 97(5):1508–16. doi: 10.1210/jc.2011-2513
8. Buvat J, Maggi M, Guay A, Torres LO. Testosterone deficiency in men: systematic review and standard operating procedures for diagnosis and treatment. *J Sex Med* (2013) 10(1):245–84. doi: 10.1111/j.1743-6109.2012.02783.x
9. Huhtaniemi I. Late-onset hypogonadism: Current concepts and controversies of pathogenesis, diagnosis and treatment. *Asian J Androl* (2014) 16:192–202. doi: 10.4103/1008-682X.122336
10. Corona G, Vignozzi L, Rastrelli G, Lotti F, Cipriani S, Maggi M. Benign prostatic hyperplasia: a new metabolic disease of the aging male and its correlation with sexual dysfunctions. *Int J Endocrinol* (2014) 2014:329456. doi: 10.1155/2014/329456
11. Bartsch G, Rittmaster RS, Klocker H. Dihydrotestosterone and the concept of 5alpha-reductase inhibition in human benign prostatic hyperplasia. *Eur Urol* (2000) 37(4):367–80. doi: 10.1159/000020181
12. Rastrelli G, Vignozzi L, Corona G, Maggi M. Testosterone and Benign Prostatic Hyperplasia. *Sex Med Rev* (2019) 7(2):259–71. doi: 10.1016/j.sxmr.2018.10.006
13. Kellokumpu-Lehtinen P, Santti R, Pelliniemi LJ. Correlation of early cytodifferentiation of the human fetal prostate and Leydig cells. *Anat Rec* (1980) 196:263–73. doi: 10.1002/ar.1091960302
14. Cunha GR, Alarid ET, Turner T, Donjacour AA, Boutin EL, Foster BA. Normal and abnormal development of the male urogenital tract. Role of androgens, mesenchymal-epithelial interactions, and growth factors. *J Androl* (1992) 13(6):465–75.
15. Schauer IG, Rowley DR. The functional role of reactive stroma in benign prostatic hyperplasia. *Differentiation* (2011) 82:200–10. doi: 10.1016/j.diff.2011.05.007
16. Liu CC, Huang SP, Li WM, Wang CJ, Chou YH, Li CC, et al. Relationship between serum testosterone and measures of benign prostatic hyperplasia in aging men. *Urology* (2007) 70(4):677–80. doi: 10.1016/j.urology.2007.05.025
17. Miranda EP, Torres LO. Late-onset hypogonadism: Prostate safety. *Andrology* (2020) 8(6):1606–13. doi: 10.1111/andr.12772 (in press).
18. Morgentaler A, Traish AM. Shifting the paradigm of testosterone and prostate cancer: the saturation model and the limits of androgen-dependent growth. *Eur Urol* (2009) 55(2):310–20. doi: 10.1016/j.eururo.2008.09.024
19. Rastrelli G, Corona G, Vignozzi L, Maseroli E, Silverii A, Monami M, et al. Serum PSA as a predictor of testosterone deficiency. *J Sex Med* (2013) 10 (10):2518–28. doi: 10.1111/jsm.12266
20. Karazindiyanoğlu S, Cayan S. The effect of testosterone therapy on lower urinary tract symptoms/bladder and sexual functions in men with symptomatic late-onset hypogonadism. *Aging Male* (2008) 11(3):146–9. doi: 10.1080/13685530802290438
21. Haider A, Gooren LJ, Padungtod P, Saad F. Concurrent improvement of the metabolic syndrome and lower urinary tract symptoms upon normalisation of plasma testosterone levels in hypogonadal elderly men. *Andrologia* (2009) 41(1):7–13. doi: 10.1111/j.1439-0272.2008.00880.x
22. Shigehara K, Sugimoto K, Konaka H, Iijima M, Fukushima M, Maeda Y, et al. Androgen replacement therapy contributes to improving lower urinary tract symptoms in patients with hypogonadism and benign prostate hypertrophy: a randomised controlled study. *Aging Male* (2011) 14(1):53–8. doi: 10.3109/13685538.2010.518178
23. Kohn TP, Mata DA, Ramasamy R, Lipshultz LI. Effects of Testosterone Replacement Therapy on Lower Urinary Tract Symptoms: A Systematic Review and Meta-analysis. *Eur Urol* (2016) 69(6):1083–90. doi: 10.1016/j.eururo.2016.01.043
24. Vignozzi L, Cellai I, Santi R, Lombardelli L, Morelli A, Comeglio P, et al. Antiinflammatory effect of androgen receptor activation in human benign prostatic hyperplasia cells. *J Endocrinol* (2012) 214(1):31–43. doi: 10.1530/JOE-12-0142
25. Vignozzi L, Morelli A, Sarchielli E, Comeglio P, Filippi S, Cellai I, et al. Testosterone protects from metabolic syndrome-associated prostate inflammation: an experimental study in rabbit. *J Endocrinol* (2012) 212 (1):71–84. doi: 10.1530/JOE-11-0289
26. Morelli A, Comeglio P, Filippi S, Sarchielli E, Vignozzi L, Maneschi E, et al. Mechanism of action of phosphodiesterase type 5 inhibition in metabolic syndrome-associated prostate alterations: an experimental study in the rabbit. *Prostate* (2013) 73(4):428–41. doi: 10.1002/pros.22584
27. Ho CH, Fan CK, Yu HJ, Wu CC, Chen KC, Liu SP, et al. Testosterone suppresses uropathogenic Escherichia coli invasion and colonization within prostate cells and inhibits inflammatory responses through JAK/STAT-1 signaling pathway. *PloS One* (2017) 12(6):e0180244. [published correction appears in PLoS One. 12 (12), e0190317]. doi: 10.1371/journal.pone.0180244
28. Huggins C, Hodges CV. Studies on prostatic cancer. I. The effect of castration, of estrogen and androgen injection on serum phosphatases in metastatic carcinoma of the prostate. *CA Cancer J Clin* (1972) 22(4):232–40. doi: 10.3322/canjclin.22.4.232

29. Rodriguez KM, Pastuszak AW, Khera M. The Role of Testosterone Therapy in the Setting of Prostate Cancer. *Curr Urol Rep* (2018) 19(8):67. doi: 10.1007/s11934-018-0812-1
30. Morgentaler A, Bruning CO, DeWolf WC. Occult prostate cancer in men with low serum testosterone levels. *JAMA* (1996) 276(23):1904–6. doi: 10.1001/jama.276.23.1904
31. Shin BS, Hwang EC, Im CM, Kim SO, Jung SI, Kang TW, et al. Is a decreased serum testosterone level a risk factor for prostate cancer? A cohort study of Korean men. *Korean J Urol* (2010) 51(12):819–23. doi: 10.4111/kju.2010.51.12.819
32. García-Cruz E, Piqueras M, Huguet J, Peri L, Izquierdo L, Musquera M, et al. Low testosterone levels are related to poor prognosis factors in men with prostate cancer prior to treatment. *BJU Int* (2012) 110(11):541–6. doi: 10.1111/j.1464-410X.2012.11232.x
33. Mearini L, Zucchi A, Nunzi E, Villirillo T, Bini V, Porena M. Low serum testosterone levels are predictive of prostate cancer. *World J Urol* (2013) 31 (2):247–52. doi: 10.1007/s00345-011-0793-x
34. Bayar G, Şirin H, Aydın M, Özağarı A, Tanrıverdi O, Kadıhasanoğlu M, et al. Low free and bioavailable testosterone levels may predict pathologically-proven high-risk prostate cancer: a prospective, clinical trial. *Turk J Urol* (2017) 43(3):289–96. doi: 10.5152/tud.2017.35467
35. Bhasin S, Brito JP, Cunningham GR, Hayes FJ, Hodis HN, Matsumoto AM, et al. Testosterone Therapy in Men With Hypogonadism: An Endocrine Society Clinical Practice Guideline. *J Clin Endocrinol Metab* (2018) 103 (5):1715–44. doi: 10.1210/jc.2018-00229
36. Heidenreich A, Bastian PJ, Bellmunt J, Bolla M, Joniau S, van der Kwast T, et al. EAU guidelines on prostate cancer. part 1: screening, diagnosis, and local treatment with curative intent-update 2013. *Eur Urol* (2014) 65(1):124–37. doi: 10.1016/j.eururo.2013.09.046
37. Ridlon JM, Ikegawa S, Alves JM, Zhou B, Kobayashi A, Iida T, et al. Clostridium scindens: a human gut microbe with a high potential to convert glucocorticoids into androgens. *J Lipid Res* (2013) 54(9):2437–49. doi: 10.1194/jlr.M038869
38. Ly LK, Rowles JL, Paul HM, Alves JMP, Yemm C, Wolf PM, et al. Bacterial steroid-17,20-desmolase is a taxonomically rare enzymatic pathway that converts prednisone to 1,4-androstanediene-3,11,17-trione, a metabolite that causes proliferation of prostate cancer cells. *J Steroid Biochem Mol Biol* (2019) 199:105567. doi: 10.1016/j.jsbmb.2019.105567
39. Bacher M, Rausch U, Goebel HW, Polzar B, Mannherz HG, Aumüller G. Stromal and epithelial cells from rat ventral prostate during androgen deprivation and estrogen treatment–regulation of transcription. *Exp Clin Endocrinol* (1993) 101(2):78–86. doi: 10.1055/s-0029-1211211
40. Gupta C. The role of estrogen receptor, androgen receptor and growth factors in diethylstilbestrol-induced programming of prostate differentiation. *Urol Res* (2000) 28(4):223–9. doi: 10.1007/s002400000107
41. Lau KM, To KF. Importance of Estrogenic Signaling and Its Mediated Receptors in Prostate Cancer. *Int J Mol Sci* (2016) 17(9):E1434. doi: 10.3390/ijms17091434
42. Vermeulen A, Kaufman JM, Goemaere S, van Pottelberg I. Estradiol in elderly men. *Aging Male* (2002) 5:98–102. doi: 10.1080/713604678
43. Belanger A, Candas B, Dupont A, Cusan L, Diamond P, Gomez JL, et al. Changes in serum concentrations of conjugated and unconjugated steroids in 40- to 80-year-old men. *J Clin Endocrinol Metab* (1994) 79:1086–90. doi: 10.1210/jcem.79.4.7962278
44. Nicholson TM, Ricke WA. Androgens and estrogens in benign prostatic hyperplasia: past, present and future. *Differentiation* (2011) 82(4-5):184–99. doi: 10.1016/j.diff.2011.04.006
45. Ho SM, Tang WY, Belmonte de Frausto J, Prins GS. Developmental exposure to estradiol and bisphenol A increases susceptibility to prostate carcinogenesis and epigenetically regulates phosphodiesterase type 4 variant 4. *Cancer Res* (2006) 66(11):5624–32. doi: 10.1158/0008-5472.CAN-06-0516
46. Ellem SJ, Risbridger GP. The dual, opposing roles of estrogen in the prostate. *Ann N Y Acad Sci* (2009) 1155:174–86. doi: 10.1111/j.1749-6632.2009.04360.x
47. Comeglio P, Morelli A, Cellai I, Vignozzi L, Sarchielli E, Filippi S, et al. Opposite effects of tamoxifen on metabolic syndrome-induced bladder and prostate alterations: a role for GPR30/GPER? *Prostate* (2014) 74(1):10–28. doi: 10.1002/pros.22723
48. Krege JH, Hodgin JB, Couse JF, Enmark E, Warner M, Mahler JF, et al. Generation and reproductive phenotypes of mice lacking estrogen receptor beta. *Proc Natl Acad Sci U S A* (1998) 95(26):15677–82. doi: 10.1073/pnas.95.26.15677
49. Marmorston J, Lombardo LJ, Myers SM, Gierson H, Stern E, Hopkins CE. Urinary excretion of estrone, estradiol and estriol by patients with prostatic cancer and benign prostate hypertrophy. *J Urol* (1965) 93(2):287–95. doi: 10.1016/S0022-5347(17)63760-1
50. Roberts RO, Jacobson DJ, Rhodes T, Klee GG, Leiber MM, Jacobsen SJ. Serum sex hormones and measures of benign prostatic hyperplasia. *Prostate* (2004) 61(2):124–31. doi: 10.1002/pros.20080
51. Hammarsten J, Damber JE, Karlsson M, Knutson T, Ljunggren O, Ohlsson C, et al. Insulin and free oestradiol are independent risk factors for benign prostatic hyperplasia. *Prostate Cancer Prostatic Dis* (2009) 12(2):160–5. doi: 10.1038/pcan.2008.50
52. Habib CN, Al-Abd AM, Tolba MF, Khalifa AE, Khedr A, Mosli HA, et al. Leptin influences estrogen metabolism and accelerates prostate cell proliferation. *Life Sci* (2015) 121:10–5. doi: 10.1016/j.lfs.2014.11.007
53. Nomura H, Kawashima H, Masaki S, Hosono TY, Matsumura K, Tamada S, et al. Effect of selective estrogen receptor modulators on cell proliferation and estrogen receptor activities in normal human prostate stromal and epithelial cells. *Prostate Cancer Prostatic Dis* (2009) 12:375–81. doi: 10.1038/pcan.2009.20
54. Noble RL. Production of NB rat carcinoma of the dorsal prostate and response of estrogen-dependent transplants to sex hormones and tamoxifen. *Cancer Res* (1980) 40:3547–50.
55. Ellem SJ, Risbridger GP. Aromatase and regulating the estrogen: androgen ratio in the prostate gland. *J Steroid Biochem Mol Biol* (2010) 118:246–51. doi: 10.1016/j.jsbmb.2009.10.015
56. Raghow S, Hooshdaran MZ, Katiyar S, Steiner MS. Toremifene prevents prostate cancer in the transgenic adenocarcinoma of mouse prostate model. *Cancer Res* (2002) 62:1370–6.
57. Price D, Stein B, Sieber P, Tutrone R, Bailen J, Goluboff E, et al. Toremifene for the prevention of prostate cancer in men with high grade prostatic intraepithelial neoplasia: results of a double-blind, placebo-controlled, phase IIB clinical trial. *J Urol* (2006) 176:965–70. doi: 10.1016/j.juro.2006.04.011
58. Ricke WA, McPherson SJ, Bianco JJ, Cunha GR, Wang Y, Risbridger GP. Prostatic hormonal carcinogenesis is mediated by in situ estrogen production and estrogen receptor alpha signaling. *FASEB J* (2008) 22:1512–20. doi: 10.1096/fj.07-9526com
59. Di Zazzo E, Galasso G, Giovannelli P, Di Donato M, Castoria G. Estrogens and Their Receptors in Prostate Cancer: Therapeutic Implications. *Front Oncol* (2018) 8:2:2. doi: 10.3389/fonc.2018.00002
60. Ross RK, Bernstein L, Lobo RA, Shimizu H, Stanczyk FZ, Pike MC, et al. 5-alpha-reductase activity and risk of prostate cancer among Japanese and US white and black males. *Lancet* (1992) 339:887–9. doi: 10.1016/0140-6736(92)90927-U
61. Takizawa I, Lawrence MG, Balanathan P, Rebello R, Pearson HB, Garg E, et al. Estrogen receptor alpha drives proliferation in PTEN-deficient prostate carcinoma by stimulating survival signaling, MYC expression and altering glucose sensitivity. *Oncotarget* (2015) 6:604–16. doi: 10.18632/oncotarget.2820
62. Bardin A, Boulle N, Lazennec G, Vignon F, Pujol P. Loss of ERbeta expression as a common step in estrogen-dependent tumor progression. *Endocr Relat Cancer* (2004) 11:537–51. doi: 10.1677/erc.1.00800
63. Sonntag WE, Lynch CD, Cefalu WT, Ingram RL, Bennett SA, Thornton PL, et al. Pleiotropic effects of growth hormone and insulin-like growth factor (IGF)-1 on biological aging: inferences from moderate caloric-restricted animals. *J Gerontol A Biol Sci Med Sci* (1999) 54(12):521–38. doi: 10.1093/gerona/54.12.B521
64. Aguirre GA, De Ita JR, de la Garza RG, Castilla-Cortazar I. Insulin-like growth factor-1 deficiency and metabolic syndrome. *J Transl Med* (2016) 14:3. doi: 10.1186/s12967-015-0762-z
65. Neam Ţu MC, Avramescu ET, Marcu IR, Turcu-Ştiolică A, Boldeanu MV, NeamŢu OM, et al. The correlation between insulin-like growth factor with glycemic control, glomerular filtration rate, blood pressure, hematological

changes or body mass index in patients with type 2 diabetes mellitus. *Rom J Morphol Embryol* (2017) 58(3):857–61.

66. Mantzoros CS, Tzonou A, Signorello LB, Stampfer M, Trichopoulos D, Adami HO. Insulin-like growth factor 1 in relation to prostate cancer and benign prostatic hyperplasia. *Br J Cancer* (1997) 76(9):1115–8. doi: 10.1038/bjc.1997.520
67. Colao A, Marzullo P, Spiezia S, Ferone D, Giaccio A, Cerbone G, et al. Effect of growth hormone (GH) and insulin-like growth factor I on prostate diseases: an ultrasonographic and endocrine study in acromegaly, GH deficiency, and healthy subjects. *J Clin Endocrinol Metab* (1999) 84 (6):1986–91. doi: 10.1210/jcem.84.6.5776
68. Corrêa LL, Lima GA, Paiva HB, Silva CM, Cavallieri SA, Miranda LC, et al. Prostate cancer and acromegaly. *Arq Bras Endocrinol Metabol* (2009) 53 (8):963–8. doi: 10.1590/S0004-27302009000800009
69. Corrêa LL, Balarini Lima GA, Cavallieri SA, Miranda LC, Gadelha MR. Prostatic disorders in acromegalic patients experience of a Brazilian center. *Int Braz J Urol* (2013) 39(3):393–401. doi: 10.1590/S1677-5538.IBJU.2013.03.13
70. Ahearn TU, Peisch S, Pettersson A, Ebot EM, Zhou CK, Graff RE, et al. Expression of IGF/insulin receptor in prostate cancer tissue and progression to lethal disease. *Carcinogenesis* (2018) 39(12):1431–7. doi: 10.1093/carcin/bgy112
71. Kumar S, Yadav RN, Gupta P, Gaspar BL, Kakkar N, Verma A, et al. Prostatic hyperplasia in acromegaly, a myth or reality: a case-control study. *Eur J Endocrinol* (2015) 172(2):97–106. doi: 10.1530/EJE-14-0698
72. Pollak M. Insulin and insulin-like growth factor signalling in neoplasia. *Nat Rev Cancer* (2008) 8(12):915–28. doi: 10.1038/nrc2536
73. Price AJ, Allen NE, Appleby PN, Crowe FL, Travis RC, Tipper SJ, et al. Insulin-like growth factor-I concentration and risk of prostate cancer: results from the European Prospective Investigation into Cancer and Nutrition. *Cancer Epidemiol Biomarkers Prev* (2012) 21(9):1531–41. doi: 10.1158/1055-9965.EPI-12-0481-T
74. Cox ME, Gleave ME, Zakikhani M, Bell RH, Piura E, Vickers E, et al. Insulin receptor expression by human prostate cancers. *Prostate* (2009) 69:33–40. doi: 10.1002/pros.20852
75. L-López F, Sarmento-Cabral A, Herrero-Aguayo V, Gahete MD, Castaño JP, Luque RM. Obesity and metabolic dysfunction severely influence prostate cell function: role of insulin and IGF1. *J Cell Mol Med* (2017) 21(9):1893–904. doi: 10.1111/jcmm.13109
76. Tomlins SA, Bjartell A, Chinnaiyan AM, Jenster G, Nam RK, Rubin MA, et al. ETS gene fusions in prostate cancer: from discovery to daily clinical practice. *Eur Urol* (2009) 56(2):275–86. doi: 10.1016/j.eururo.2009.04.036
77. Yanase T, Fan W. Modification of androgen receptor function by IGF-1 signaling implications in the mechanism of refractory prostate carcinoma. *Vitam Horm* (2009) 80:649–66. doi: 10.1016/S0083-6729(08)00623-7
78. Levy DE, Gilliland DG. Divergent roles of STAT1 and STAT5 in malignancy as revealed by gene disruptions in mice. *Oncogene* (2000) 19(21):2505–10. doi: 10.1038/sj.onc.1203480
79. Rick FG, Schally AV, Block NL, Nadji M, Szepeshazi K, Zarandi M, et al. Antagonists of growth hormone-releasing hormone (GHRH) reduce prostate size in experimental benign prostatic hyperplasia. *Proc Natl Acad Sci U S A* (2011) 108(9):3755–60. doi: 10.1073/pnas.1018086108
80. Moeller LC, Broecker-Preuss M. Transcriptional regulation by nonclassical action of thyroid hormone. *Thyroid Res* (2011) 4(1):6. doi: 10.1186/1756-6614-4-S1-S6
81. Hollowell JG, Staehling NW, Flanders WD, Hannon WH, Gunter EW, Spencer CA, et al. Serum TSH, T(4), and thyroid antibodies in the United States population (1988 to 1994): National Health and Nutrition Examination Survey (NHANES III). *J Clin Endocrinol Metab* (2002) 87 (2):489–99. doi: 10.1210/jcem.87.2.8182
82. Laurberg P, Pedersen KM, Vestergaard H, Sigurdsson G. High incidence of multinodular toxic goitre in the elderly population in a low iodine intake area vs. high incidence of Graves' disease in the young in a high iodine intake area: Comparative surveys of thyrotoxicosis epidemiology in East-Jutland Denmark and Iceland. *J Intern Med* (1991) 229:415–20. doi: 10.1111/j.1365-2796.1991.tb00368.x
83. Sakurai A, Nakai A, DeGroot LJ. Expression of three forms of thyroid hormone receptor in human tissues. *Mol Endocrinol* (1989) 3(2):392–9. doi: 10.1210/mend-3-2-392
84. Lehrer S, Diamond EJ, Bajwa AM, Kornreich R, Stagger S, Stone NN, et al. Association between serum triiodothyronine (t3) level and risk of disease recurrence in men with localized prostate cancer. *Prostate Cancer Prostatic Dis* (2001) 4(4):232–4. doi: 10.1038/sj.pcan.4500542
85. Lehrer S, Diamond EJ, Stone NN, Droller MJ, Stock RG. Serum triiodothyronine is increased in men with prostate cancer and benign prostatic hyperplasia. *J Urol* (2002) 168(6):2431–3. doi: 10.1016/S0022-5347(05)64161-4
86. Eldhose A, Nandeesha H, Dorairajan LN, Sreenivasulu K, Arul Vijaya Vani S. Thyroid and parathyroid hormones in benign prostatic hyperplasia. *Br J Biomed Sci* (2016) 73(2):94–6. doi: 10.1080/09674845.2016.1173333
87. Mondul AM, Weinstein SJ, Bosworth T, Remaley AT, Virtamo J, Albanes D. Circulating thyroxine, thyroid-stimulating hormone, and hypothyroid status and the risk of prostate cancer. *PloS One* (2012) 7(10):e47730. doi: 10.1371/journal.pone.0047730
88. Tran TV, Kitahara CM, de Vathaire F, Boutron-Ruault MC, Journy N. Thyroid dysfunction and cancer incidence: a systematic review and meta-analysis. *Endocr Relat Cancer* (2020) 27(4):245–59. doi: 10.1530/ERC-19-0417 pii: ERC-19-0417.R2.
89. Hsieh ML, Juang HH. Cell growth effects of triiodothyronine and expression of thyroid hormone receptor in prostate carcinoma cells. *J Androl* (2005) 26 (3):422–8. doi: 10.2164/jandrol.04162
90. Horoszewicz JS, Leong SS, Kawinski E, Karr JP, Rosenthal H, Chu TM, et al. LNCaP model of human prostatic carcinoma. *Cancer Res* (1983) 43(4):1809–18.
91. Hedlund TE, Miller GJ. A serum-free defined medium capable of supporting growth of four established human prostatic carcinoma cell lines. *Prostate* (1994) 24(5):221–8. doi: 10.1002/pros.2990240502
92. Zhang S, Hsieh ML, Zhu W, Klee GG, Tindall DJ, Young CY. Interactive effects of triiodothyronine and androgens on prostate cell growth and gene expression. *Endocrinology* (1999) 140(4):1665–71. doi: 10.1210/endo.140.4.6666
93. Zhu W, Young CY. Androgen-Dependent transcriptional regulation of the prostate-specific antigen gene by thyroid hormone 3,5,3′-L-triiodothyronine. *J Androl* (2001) 22(1):136–41.
94. Tsui KH, Hsieh WC, Lin MH, Chang PL, Juang HH. Triiodothyronine modulates cell proliferation of human prostatic carcinoma cells by downregulation of the B-cell translocation gene 2. *Prostate* (2008) 68 (6):610–9. doi: 10.1002/pros.20725
95. Pinto M, Soares P, Ribatti D. Thyroid hormone as a regulator of tumor-induced angiogenesis. *Cancer Lett* (2011) 301(2):119–26. doi: 10.1016/j.canlet.2010.11.011
96. Vikram A, Jena GB, Ramarao P. Increased cell proliferation and contractility of prostate in insulin-resistant rats: linking hyperinsulinemia with benign prostate hyperplasia. *Prostate* (2010) 70:79–89. doi: 10.1002/pros.21041
97. Vikram A, Tripathi DN, Ramarao P, Jena GB. Intervention of D-glucose ameliorates the toxicity of streptozotocin in accessory sex organs of rat. *Toxicol Appl Pharmacol* (2008) 226:84–93. doi: 10.1016/j.taap.2007.09.006
98. Hammarsten J, Högstedt B. Hyperinsulinaemia as a risk factor for developing benign prostatic hyperplasia. *Eur Urol* (2001) 39:151–8. doi: 10.1159/000052430
99. Seim A, Hoyo C, Ostbye T, Vatten L. The prevalence and correlates of urinary tract symptoms in Norwegian men: the HUNT study. *BJU Int* (2005) 96:88–92. doi: 10.1111/j.1464-410X.2005.05573.x
100. Joseph MA, Harlow SD, Wei JT, Sarma AV, Dunn RL, Taylor JM, et al. Risk factors for lower urinary tract symptoms in a population-based sample of African-American men. *Am J Epidemiol* (2003) 157:906–14. doi: 10.1093/aje/kwg051
101. Russo GI, Cimino S, Fragalà E, Privitera S, La Vignera S, Condorelli R, et al. Insulin resistance is an independent predictor of severe lower urinary tract symptoms and erectile dysfunction: results from a cross-sectional study. *J Sex Med* (2014) 11(8):2074–82. doi: 10.1111/jsm.12587
102. Abdollah F, Briganti A, Suardi N, Castiglione F, Gallina A, Capitanio U, et al. Metabolic syndrome and benign prostatic hyperplasia: evidence of a potential relationship, hypothesized etiology, and prevention. *Korean J Urol* (2011) 52(8):507–16. doi: 10.4111/kju.2011.52.8.507
103. Xia BW, Zhao SC, Chen ZP, Chen C, Liu TS, Yang F, et al. The underlying mechanism of metabolic syndrome on benign prostatic hyperplasia and prostate volume. *Prostate* (2020) 80(6):481–90. doi: 10.1002/pros.23962

104. Russo GI, Castelli T, Urzì D, Privitera S, Fragalà E, La Vignera S, et al. Connections between lower urinary tract symptoms related to benign prostatic enlargement and metabolic syndrome with its components: a systematic review and meta-analysis. *Aging Male* (2015) 18(4):207–16. doi: 10.3109/13685538.2015.1062980
105. Huang PL. A comprehensive definition for metabolic syndrome. *Dis Model Mech* (2009) 2:231–7. doi: 10.1242/dmm.001180
106. Parsons JK, Carter HB, Partin AW, Windham BG, Metter EJ, Ferrucci L, et al. Metabolic factors associated with benign prostatic hyperplasia. *J Clin Endocrinol Metab* (2006) 91:2562–8. doi: 10.1210/jc.2005-2799
107. Kristal AR, Arnold KB, Schenk JM, Neuhouser ML, Weiss N, Goodman P, et al. Race/ethnicity, obesity, health-related behaviors and the risk of symptomatic benign prostatic hyperplasia: results from the prostate cancer prevention trial. *J Urol* (2007) 177:1395–400. doi: 10.1016/j.juro.2006.11.065
108. Laven BA, Orsini N, Andersson SO, Johansson JE, Gerber GS, Wolk A. Birth weight, abdominal obesity and the risk of lower urinary tract symptoms in a population-based study of Swedish men. *J Urol* (2008) 179:1891–5. doi: 10.1016/j.juro.2008.01.029
109. Hammarsten J, Högstedt B, Holthuis N, Mellström D. Components of the metabolic syndrome-risk factors for the development of benign prostatic hyperplasia. *Prostate Cancer Prostatic Dis* (1998) 1:157–62. doi: 10.1038/sj.pcan.4500221
110. Nandeesha H, Koner BC, Dorairajan LN, Sen SK. Hyperinsulinemia and dyslipidemia in non-diabetic benign prostatic hyperplasia. *Clin Chim Acta* (2006) 370:89–93. doi: 10.1016/j.cca.2006.01.019
111. Parsons JK, Bergstrom J, Barrett-Connor E. Lipids, lipoproteins and the risk of benign prostatic hyperplasia in community-dwelling men. *BJU Int* (2008) 101:313–8. doi: 10.1111/j.1464-410X.2007.07332.x
112. Rohrmann S, Smit E, Giovannucci E, Platz EA. Association between markers of the metabolic syndrome and lower urinary tract symptoms in the Third National Health and Nutrition Examination Survey (NHANES III). *Int J Obes (Lond)* (2005) 29:310–6. doi: 10.1038/sj.ijo.0802881
113. Russo GI, Cimino S, Castelli T, Favilla V, Gacci M, Carini M, et al. Benign Prostatic Hyperplasia, Metabolic Syndrome and Non-Alcoholic Fatty Liver Disease: Is Metaflammation the Link? *Prostate* (2016) 76(16):1528–35. doi: 10.1002/pros.23237
114. Nouri M, Ratther E, Stylianou N, Nelson CC, Hollier BG, Williams ED. Androgen-targeted therapy-induced epithelial-mesenchymal plasticity and neuroendocrine transdifferentiation in prostate cancer: an opportunity for intervention. *Front Oncol* (2014) 4:370:370. doi: 10.3389/fonc.2014.00370
115. Li P, Yang R, Gao WQ. Contributions of epithelial-mesenchymal transition and cancer stem cells to the development of castration resistance of prostate cancer. *Mol Cancer* (2014) 13:55. doi: 10.1186/1476-4598-13-55
116. Bishop JL, Davies A, Ketola K, Zoubeidi A. Regulation of tumor cell plasticity by the androgen receptor in prostate cancer. *Endocr Relat Cancer* (2015) 22:165–82. doi: 10.1530/ERC-15-0137
117. Chaki SP, Barhoumi R, Rivera GM. Nck adapter proteins promote podosome biogenesis facilitating extracellular matrix degradation and cancer invasion. *Cancer Med* (2019) 8(17):7385–98. doi: 10.1002/cam4.2640
118. Rabin-Court A, Rodrigues MR, Zhang XM, Perry RJ. Obesity-associated, but not obesity-independent, tumors respond to insulin by increasing mitochondrial glucose oxidation. *PloS One* (2019) 14(6):e0218126. doi: 10.1371/journal.pone.0218126
119. Hammarsten J, Hogstedt B. Hyperinsulinaemia: a prospective risk factor for lethal clinical prostate cancer. *Eur J Cancer* (2005) 41:2887–95. doi: 10.1016/j.ejca.2005.09.003
120. Ma J, Li H, Giovannucci E, Mucci L, Qiu W, Nguyen PL, et al. Prediagnostic body-mass index, plasma C-peptide concentration, and prostate cancer-specific mortality in men with prostate cancer: a long-term survival analysis. *Lancet Oncol* (2008) 9:1039–47. doi: 10.1016/S1470-2045(08)70235-3
121. Faris JE, Smith MR. Metabolic sequelae associated with androgen deprivation therapy for prostate cancer. *Curr Opin Endocrinol Diabetes Obes* (2010) 17:240–6. doi: 10.1097/MED.0b013e3283391fd1
122. Flanagan J, Gray PK, Hahn N, Hayes J, Myers LJ, Carney-Doebbeling C, et al. Presence of the metabolic syndrome is associated with shorter time to castration-resistant prostate cancer. *Ann Oncol* (2011) 22:801–7. doi: 10.1093/annonc/mdq443
123. Heni M, Hennenlotter J, Scharpf M, Lutz SZ, Schwentner C, Todenhofer T, et al. Insulin receptor isoforms A and B as well as insulin receptor substrates1 and–2 are differentially expressed in prostate cancer. *PloS One* (2012) 7: e50953. doi: 10.1371/journal.pone.0050953
124. Lubik AA, Gunter JH, Hollier BG, Fazli L, Ettinger S, Stylianou N, et al. Insulin-like growth factor-2 increases de novo steroidogenesis in prostate cancer cells. *Endocr Relat Cancer* (2013) 20:173–86. doi: 10.1530/ERC-12-0250
125. Zhou F, Chen X, Fan S, Tai S, Jiang C, Zhang Y, et al. GSK1838705A, an insulin-like growth factor-1 receptor/insulin receptor inhibitor, induces apoptosis and reduces viability of docetaxel-resistant prostate cancer cells both in vitro and in vivo. *Onco Targets Ther* (2015) 8:753–60. doi: 10.2147/OTT.S79105
126. Kato H, Sekine Y, Furuya Y, Miyazawa Y, Koike H, Suzuki K. Metformin inhibits the proliferation of human prostate cancer PC-3 cells via the downregulation of insulin-like growth factor 1 receptor. *Biochem Biophys Res Commun* (2015) 461(1):115–21. doi: 10.1016/j.bbrc.2015.03.178
127. Ibuki N, Ghaffari M, Reuveni H, Pandey M, Fazli L, Azuma H, et al. The tyrphostin NT157 suppresses insulin receptor substrates and augments therapeutic response of prostate cancer. *Mol Cancer Ther* (2014) 13 (12):2827–39. doi: 10.1158/1535-7163.MCT-13-0842
128. Wright JL, Stanford JL. Metformin use and prostate cancer in Caucasian men: results from a population-based case-control study. *Cancer Causes Control* (2009) 20(9):1617–22. doi: 10.1007/s10552-009-9407-y
129. Murtola TJ, Tammela TL, Lahtela J, Auvinen A. Antidiabetic medication and prostate cancer risk: a population-based case-control study. *Am J Epidemiol* (2008) 168(8):925–31. doi: 10.1093/aje/kwn190
130. He XX, Tu SM, Lee MH, Yeung SJ. Thiazolidinediones and metformin associated with improved survival of diabetic prostate cancer patients. *Ann Oncol* (2011) 22(12):2640–5. doi: 10.1093/annonc/mdr020
131. Ruiter R, Visser LE, van Herk-Sukel MP, Coebergh JW, Haak HR, Geelhoed-Duijvestijn PH, et al. Lower risk of cancer in patients on metformin in comparison with those on sulfonylurea derivatives: results from a large population-based follow-up study. *Diabetes Care* (2012) 35(1):119–24. doi: 10.2337/dc11-0857
132. Margel D, Urbach DR, Lipscombe LL, Bell CM, Kulkarni G, Austin PC, et al. Metformin use and all-cause and prostate cancer-specific mortality among men with diabetes. *J Clin Oncol* (2013) 31(25):3069–75. doi: 10.1200/JCO.2012.46.7043
133. Whitburn J, Edwards CM, Sooriakumaran P. Metformin and Prostate Cancer: a New Role for an Old Drug. *Curr Urol Rep* (2017) 18(6):46. doi: 10.1007/s11934-017-0693-8
134. Yu HF, Chen HS, Rao DP, Gong J. Association between polycystic ovary syndrome and the risk of pregnancy complications: A PRISMA-compliant systematic review and meta-analysis. *Medicine (Baltimore)* (2016) 95(51): e4863. doi: 10.1097/MD.0000000000004863
135. Goodman NF, Cobin RH, Futterweit W, Glueck JS, Legro RS, Carmina E, et al. American association of clinical endocrinologists, American college of endocrinology, and androgen excess and PCOS society disease state clinical review: guide to the best practices in the evaluation and treatment of polycystic ovary syndrome. *Endocr Pract* (2015) 21(12):1415–26. doi: 10.4158/EP15748.DSCPT2
136. Benítez R, Sir-Petermann T, Palomino A, Angel B, Maliqueo M, Pérez F, et al. Prevalence of metabolic disorders among family members of patients with polycystic ovary syndrome. *Rev Med Chil* (2001) 129(7):707–12. doi: 10.4067/S0034-98872001000700001
137. Yilmaz M, Bukan N, Ersoy R, Karakoç A, Yetkin I, Ayvaz G, et al. Glucose intolerance, insulin resistance and cardiovascular risk factors in first degree relatives of women with polycystic ovary syndrome. *Hum Reprod* (2005) 20 (9):2414–20. doi: 10.1093/humrep/dei070
138. Legro RS, Driscoll D, Strauss JF, Fox J, Dunaif A. Evidence for a genetic basis for hyperandrogenemia in polycystic ovary syndrome. *Proc Natl Acad Sci USA* (1998) 95(25):14956–60. doi: 10.1073/pnas.95.25.14956
139. Legro RS, Kunselman AR, Demers L, Wang SC, Bentley-Lewis R, Dunaif A. Elevated dehydroepiandrosterone sulfate levels as the reproductive phenotype in the brothers of women with polycystic ovary syndrome. *J Clin Endocrinol Metab* (2002) 87:2134–8. doi: 10.1210/jcem.87.5.8387

140. Lenarcik A, Bidzińska-Speichert B, Tworowska-Bardzińska U, Krępuła K. Hormonal abnormalities in first-degree relatives of women with polycystic ovary syndrome (PCOS). *Endokrynol Pol* (2011) 62(2):129–33.
141. Lunde O, Magnus P, Sandvik L, Høglo S. Familial clustering in the Polycystic Ovarian syndrome. *Gynecol Obstet Invest* (1989) 28:23–30. doi: 10.1159/000293493
142. Carey AH, Chan KL, Short F, White D, Williamson R, Franks S. Evidence for a single gene effect causing polycystic ovaries and male pattern baldness. *Clin Endocrinol* (1993) 38:653–8. doi: 10.1111/j.1365-2265.1993.tb02150.x
143. Govind A, Obhrai MS, Clayton RN. Polycystic ovaries are inherited as an autosomal dominant trait: analysis of 29 polycystic ovary syndrome and 10 control families. *J Clin Endocrinol Metab* (1999) 84:38–53. doi: 10.1210/jcem.84.1.5382
144. Legro RS. Is there a male phenotype in polycystic ovary syndrome families? *J Pediatr Endocrinol Metab* (2000) 13:1307–9.
145. Cannarella R, Condorelli RA, Dall'Oglio F, La Vignera S, Mongioì LM, Micali G, et al. Increased DHEAS and Decreased Total Testosterone Serum Levels in a Subset of Men with Early-Onset Androgenetic Alopecia: Does a Male PCOS-Equivalent Exist? *Int J Endocrinol* (2020) 2020:1942126. doi: 10.1155/2020/1942126
146. Cannarella R, Condorelli RA, Mongioì LM, La Vignera S, Calogero AE. Does a male polycystic ovarian syndrome equivalent exist? *J Endocrinol Invest* (2018) 41(1):49–57. doi: 10.1007/s40618-017-0728-5
147. Cannarella R, La Vignera S, Condorelli RA, Calogero AE. Glycolipid and hormonal profiles in young men with early-onset androgenetic alopecia: A meta-analysis. *Sci Rep* (2017) 7(1):7801. doi: 10.1038/s41598-017-08528-3
148. Lotufo PA, Chae CU, Ajani UA, Hennekens CH, Manson JE. Male pattern baldness and coronary heart disease: the Physicians' Health Study. *Arch Intern Med* (2000) 160(2):165–71. doi: 10.1001/archinte.160.2.165
149. Lesko SM, Rosenberg L, Shapiro S. A case-control study of baldness in relation to myocardial infarction in men. *JAMA* (1993) 269(8):998–1003. doi: 10.1001/jama.269.8.998
150. Su LH, Chen LS, Lin SC, Chen HH. Association of androgenetic alopecia with mortality from diabetes mellitus and heart disease. *JAMA Dermatol* (2013) 149:601–6. doi: 10.1001/jamadermatol.2013.130
151. Oh BR, Kim SJ, Moon JD, Kim HN, Kwon DD, Won YH, et al. Association of benign prostatic hyperplasia with male pattern baldness. *Urology* (1998) 51 (5):744–8. doi: 10.1016/S0090-4295(98)00108-3
152. Chen W, Yang CC, Chen GY, Wu MC, Sheu HM, Tzai TS. Patients with a large prostate show a higher prevalence of androgenetic alopecia. *Arch Dermatol Res* (2004) 296(6):245–9. doi: 10.1007/s00403-004-0514-z
153. Kaplan SA. Patients with a large prostate show a higher prevalence of androgenetic alopecia. *J Urol* (2005) 174(5):1905. doi: 10.1016/S0022-5347 (01)68832-3
154. Kaplan SA. Re: Androgenetic alopecia as an early marker of benign prostatic hyperplasia. *J Urol* (2012) 188(5):1846–7. doi: 10.1016/j.juro.2012.07.079
155. Arias-Santiago S, Arrabal-Polo MA, Buendía-Eisman A, Arrabal-Martín M, Gutiérrez-Salmerón MT, Girón-Prieto MS, et al. Androgenetic alopecia as an early marker of benign prostatic hyperplasia. *J Am Acad Dermatol* (2012) 66:401–8. doi: 10.1016/j.jaad.2010.12.023
156. Amoretti A, Laydner H, Bergfeld W. Androgenetic alopecia and risk of prostate cancer: a systematic review and meta-analysis. *J Am Acad Dermatol* (2013) 68(6):937–43. doi: 10.1016/j.jaad.2012.11.034
157. Kucerova R, Bienova M, Kral M, Bouchal J, Trtkova KS, Burdova A, et al. Androgenetic alopecia and polymorphism of the androgen receptor gene (SNP rs6152) in patients with benign prostate hyperplasia or prostate cancer. *J Eur Acad Dermatol Venereol* (2015) 29(1):91–6. doi: 10.1111/jdv.12468

8

A multi-oscillatory circadian system times female reproduction

Valérie Simonneaux[1] and Thibault Bahougne[1,2]*

Institut des Neurosciences Cellulaires et Intégratives, CNRS (UPR 3212), Strasbourg, France, [2] Service d'Endocrinologie et Diabète, Hôpital Civil, Hôpitaux Universitaires de Strasbourg, Strasbourg, France

Edited by:
Hubert Vaudry, University of Rouen, France

Reviewed by:
Yoshitaka Oka, University of Tokyo, Japan
Vance Trudeau, University of Ottawa, Canada

***Correspondence:**
Valérie Simonneaux, Institut des Neurosciences Cellulaires et Intégratives, CNRS (UPR 3212), 5 rue Blaise Pascal, Strasbourg 67084, France
simonneaux@inci-cnrs.unistra.fr

Rhythms in female reproduction are critical to insure that timing of ovulation coincides with oocyte maturation and optimal sexual arousal. This fine tuning of female reproduction involves both the estradiol feedback as an indicator of oocyte maturation, and the master circadian clock of the suprachiasmatic nuclei (SCN) as an indicator of the time of the day. Herein, we are providing an overview of the state of knowledge regarding the differential inhibitory and stimulatory effects of estradiol at different stages of the reproductive axis, and the mechanisms through which the two main neurotransmitters of the SCN, arginine vasopressin, and vasoactive intestinal peptide, convey daily time cues to the reproductive axis. In addition, we will report the most recent findings on the putative functions of peripheral clocks located throughout the reproductive axis [kisspeptin (Kp) neurons, gonadotropin-releasing hormone neurons, gonadotropic cells, the ovary, and the uterus]. This review will point to the critical position of the Kp neurons of the anteroventral periventricular nucleus, which integrate both the stimulatory estradiol signal, and the daily arginine vasopressinergic signal, while displaying a circadian clock. Finally, given the critical role of the light/dark cycle in the synchronization of female reproduction, we will discuss the impact of circadian disruptions observed during shift-work conditions on female reproductive performance and fertility in both animal model and humans.

Keywords: female reproduction, circadian clock, suprachiasmatic nuclei, kisspeptin, GnRH, LH, estradiol, shift-work

Introduction

Ovulation in female mammals is a complex process, which is exquisitely regulated by a number of environmental (time of day, time of year, food resources, and stress level) and internal (development stage, hormonal milieu, and metabolic rate) factors. Indeed, female reproduction is a long-term, demanding process and therefore, it is important that a limiting critical status is reached to ensure successful reproductive outcome. In adult females where all these criteria are attained, there are still two important cues that time ovulation: the circulating level of gonadal hormones, specifically estradiol, which is an indicator of oocyte maturation, and the time of day arising from biological clocks. This dual regulation ensures that the timing of ovulation coincides with the period of maximal activity and sexual motivation. Most mechanistic studies aimed at understanding this subtle timing of ovulation have been performed in laboratory rodents, but ovulation in humans is also gated by similar hormonal and circadian inputs. Hence, this review will not only focus on the mechanisms regulating the timing of reproduction in female rodents, but will also discuss human female fertility, including the desynchronization associated with modern life styles (shift work, jet lag, and sleep alteration).

Female Reproduction is Rhythmic

Reproductive activity in female mammals displays a regular cycle (menstrual cycles in women, estrous cycles in rodents) driven by a complex interaction of the circadian system, hypothalamic neuropeptides, gonadotropins [luteinizing hormone (LH) and follicle-stimulating hormone (FSH), both secreted by the pituitary gonadotroph cells], and sex steroid hormones produced by the ovaries. The final output of this regulatory process is to combine the production of a mature oocyte (ovulation) with a receptive reproductive tract, which will ensure the embryo's development.

During the first part of the reproductive cycle (follicular phase in women; metestrus–diestrus in rodents), gonadotrophs produce more FSH than LH. This relative FSH preponderance contributes to the recruitment and development of ovarian follicles. FSH promotes follicular growth leading to a progressive increase of the sex steroid hormone, estradiol, and increases LH receptor expression in granulosa cells (1). During this early phase, LH pulses occur with a high frequency (period of 1–2 h in women, 20 min in rodents) and uniform amplitude, and the pulse frequency tends to increase toward the end of the phase. The second part of the reproductive cycle (luteal phase in women; proestrus–estrus in rodents) begins with a marked and transient secretion of LH (**Figures 1A,D**). The LH surge has three functions: (1) induction of ovulation of mature follicles, (2) resumption of oocyte meiosis, and (3) arrest of granulosa cell proliferation and luteum induction. After the LH surge, ovulation generally follows a few hours later in rodents, and 24–48 h in women. The preovulatory LH surge takes place approximately every 4–5 days in rodents and every 28 days in women and its occurrence depends on high circulating estradiol levels (2, 3). Additionally, the LH surge requires a daily signal since it arises at a very specific time of day, usually at the end of the resting period, thus in the late afternoon in nocturnal rodents and the end of the night/early morning in the diurnal rodent Arvicanthis (4) and in humans (5–7). Indeed, in 80% of women, the LH surge occurs around 8 a.m. At the end of the reproductive cycle, LH pulse frequency decreases significantly down to a pulse interval of 2–6 h with variable amplitude (8).

The secretion of both LH and FSH is under the control of a hypothalamic neurohormone, gonadotropin-releasing hormone (GnRH), which is synthesized in neurons scattered throughout the preoptic area (POA) and the organum vasculosum laminae terminalis. These neurons project to the median eminence where they release GnRH in the portal circulation in a pulsatile manner. GnRH activates specific receptors located on pituitary gonadotrophs inducing the synthesis and release of LH and FSH. GnRH is essential for reproduction as mutations in the gene coding for GnRH (10) and GnRH receptor (11) are proposed to be responsible for idiopathic hypogonadotropic hypogonadism (IHH), characterized by delayed puberty and infertility (11). The pulsatility of GnRH release is critical to induce proper gonadotropin secretion, and there is a tight correlation between GnRH and LH pulsatilities. Pulsatile administration of exogenous GnRH (one pulse per hour) is capable of restoring the preovulatory surge, ovulation, and normal menstrual cycles in patients suffering from Kallmann syndrome (12, 13). In contrast, continuous GnRH administration induces a reversible blockage of the pituitary gonadotroph cells' secretion (14).

Various (neuro)transmitters had been proposed to regulate GnRH neuronal activity until the neuropeptide kisspeptin (Kp) was discovered as a potent activator of GnRH release. In 1996, the *Kiss1* gene was discovered and reported to encode a peptide called metastin, because of its anti-metastatic property on malignant melanoma cells (15). However, the receptor of this peptide, GPR54, was later found to play a critical role in reproductive physiology when two groups reported that mutation of the *GPR54* receptor results in IHH in humans, with an identical phenotype observed in mice with a targeted deletion in this receptor (16, 17). The *Kiss1* gene was shown to encode a family of Kps from an initial 145 amino acid propeptide, Kp-145, which is cleaved into peptides of different sizes from Kp-54 (previously named metastin) to Kp-10. The discovery of Kp's role in reproductive function has been a milestone in the field of reproductive biology, and numerous studies now indicate that Kps are critical regulators of sexual differentiation and maturation as well as of normal adult reproductive functioning across mammalian species, including humans (18). Kp neurons are localized within two hypothalamic areas, in the arcuate nucleus (ARN) and the rostral periventricular nucleus of the third ventricle, also called anteroventral periventricular nucleus (AVPV), or the preotic area (according to species). They send projections mainly to the GnRH neuron cell bodies (AVPV Kp neurons) and nerve terminals [ARN Kp neurons (19–22)] (**Figure 1A**). The AVPV presents a marked sexual dimorphism, with more Kp neurons in females as compared to males (20, 23). The AVPV Kp neurons are the main drivers of the preovulatory GnRH/LH surge (24). In contrast, the ARN Kp neurons are not sexually dimorphic (20, 23). The Kp receptor, Kiss1R (formerly GPR54), is highly expressed in GnRH neurons but also in other brain areas (25, 26) and in most endocrine tissues like the pituitary gland, ovary, and placenta (27). Kp has a very potent stimulatory action on GnRH release and, therefore, gonadotropin secretion in all mammalian species investigated so far (18, 19, 28, 29). Central injection of doses as low as 0.1–1 pmol Kp10 is indeed sufficient to evoke robust LH secretion in rats and monkeys (28, 30). Kp injections must be short and at least 2 h apart to induce the LH peak since the repeated administration of Kp induces Kiss1R desensitization (31, 32). Notably, Kp release in the stalk-median eminence is pulsatile (33), and pulsatile Kp drives LH secretion in juvenile monkeys (34). A recent study reported that pulsatile administration of Kp was able to evoke dramatic synchronous activation of *GnRH* gene transcription with robust stimulation of GnRH secretion in murine-cultured hypothalamic explants (35). The preeminent phenotypes of impaired reproduction (abnormal sexual maturation, small uterus, ovaries without mature follicles, no estrous cycles) often arise from mutations in *Kiss1* (36, 37) and *Kiss1R* (16, 38, 39), which suggest that the Kiss1/Kiss1R complex is essential for the central regulation of the gonadotropic axis.

Other classical neurotransmitters and neuropeptides have been reported to regulate GnRH neuron activity albeit not to the same extent as Kp. GABA and glutamate fibers are found close to GnRH perikarya in the POA and axons in the median eminence. Both neurotransmitters have been shown to play a role in the regulation of GnRH release. Glutamate stimulates *Gnrh* gene

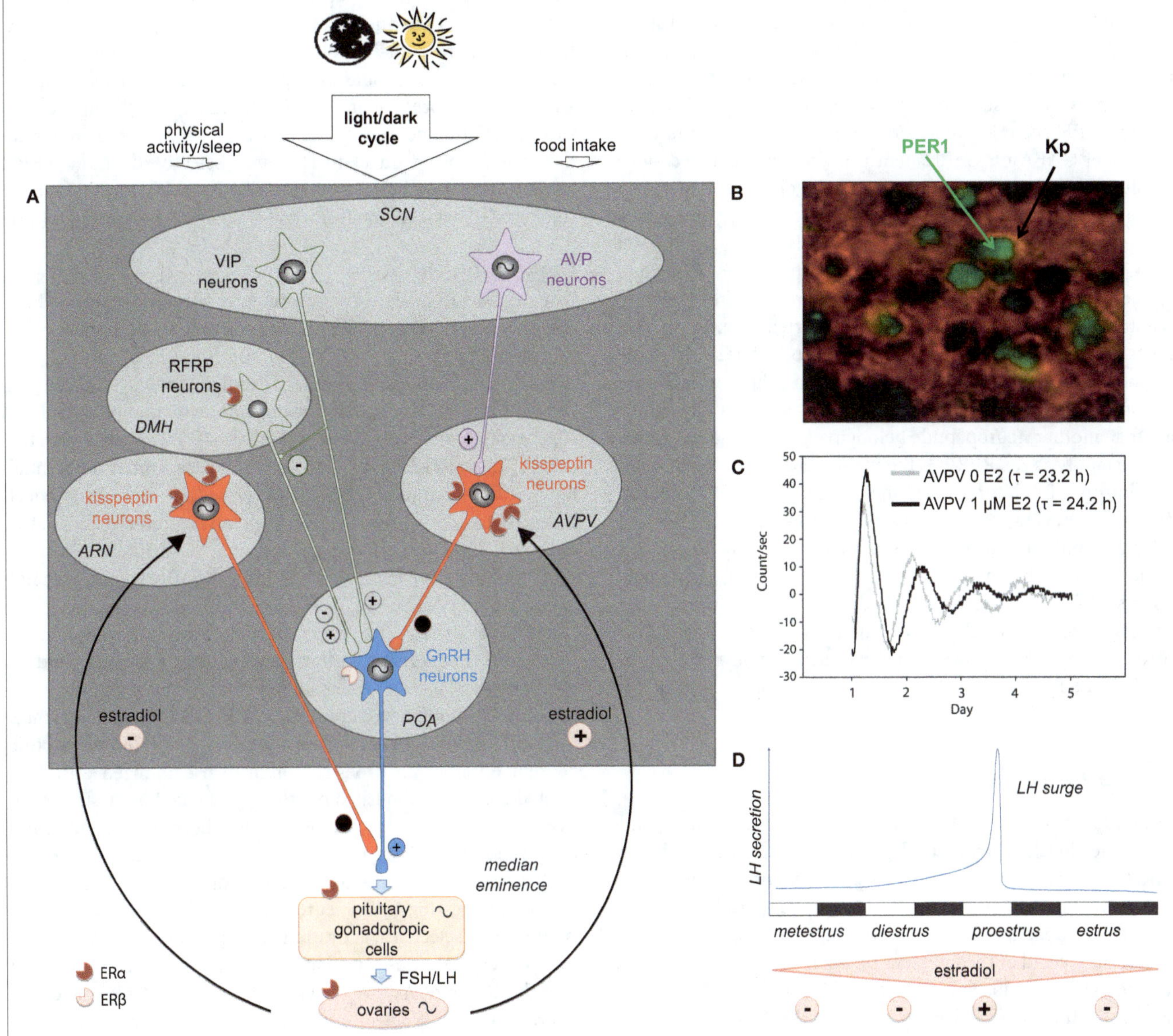

FIGURE 1 | The multi-oscillatory network of the female hypothalamic–pituitary gonadal axis in rodents. (A) Schematic representation of the neuroendocrine pathway timing female reproduction: the master circadian clock located in the hypothalamic suprachiasmatic nucleus (SCN) is synchronized to the daily cycle mostly via the light/dark cycle and to a less extend by other time cues (food intake and sleep/wake activity); two SCN peptidergic transmitters forward the daily information to the reproductive axis: arginine vasopressin (AVP) is the most essential daily transmitter projecting to the kisspeptin (Kp) neurons of the anteroventral periventricular nuclei (AVPV), which in turn strongly activate the GnRH neurons located in the preoptic area (POA); vasoactive intestinal peptide (VIP) directly modulates GnRH neuron activity and possibly indirectly via neurons of the dorsomedial hypothalamus (DMH), which express RF-related peptide (RFRP); GnRH released in the portal blood system activates the synthesis and release of the gonadotropins luteinizing hormone (LH) and folliculo-stimulating hormone (FSH), which in turn regulate oocyte maturation, estradiol synthesis, and finally ovulation triggered by the LH surge; throughout the estrous cycle, estradiol feeds back onto different levels of the reproductive axis principally via the nuclear estrogen receptor α (ERα) and to a less extend via ERβ. Kp neurons are the main estradiol targets with an inhibitory effect of low estradiol on Kp neurons of the arcuate nucleus (ARN) and a stimulatory action of high estradiol on AVPV Kp neurons. In addition to the master SCN clock, peripheral clocks are located in the AVPV Kp neurons, GnRH neurons, pituitary gonadotrophs, and the different cell types of the ovary. **(B)** Representative pictures showing PER1 immunoreactivity (green) in Kp immunoreactive neurons (red) in the AVPV of female mice sampled at zeitgeber time 20 (8 h after lights off on a 12 h light/12 h dark schedule) on the day of proestrus [adapted from Ref. (9)]. **(C)** Representative bioluminescence traces from isolated AVPV explants of PER2:LUCIFERASE female mice, in absence (0 E2, light gray line) or in presence of estradiol (1 µM E2, black line) in the culture medium; τ indicates the period of the circadian AVPV oscillations in both conditions [adapted from Ref. (9)]. **(D)** Schematic representation of the mouse estrus cycle including the four stages: metestrus, diestrus, proestrus (the stage at which the LH concentration raises as an LH surge), and estrus; during the first part of the reproductive cycle, low circulating level of estradiol displays a negative feedback, whereas at proestrus, high estradiol levels exert a positive feedback, causing a synchronized activation of GnRH neurons leading to the preovulatory surge of LH; notably, the LH surge occurs at the end of the resting period, which is late day in nocturnal species.

expression and GnRH release during the LH surge, whereas a glutamate antagonist blocks *Gnrh* gene expression and the LH surge when administered in the morning (40–42). Administration of an AMPA agonist enhances the *in vivo* LH secretion in OVX rats only with estradiol substitution, whereas glutamate stimulates *in vitro* GnRH secretion in a estradiol-independent matter (43). The role of GABA on GnRH neuronal activity is debated since inhibitory and stimulatory effects have been observed depending on the protocols used, the presence of sex steroid treatment, the timing in the estrus cycle and the hypothalamic region studied (44, 45). Fibers containing the orexigenic neuropeptide Y contact a majority of GnRH neurons, which express neuropeptide Y receptors. This neuropeptide has been reported to exert variable effects depending on the metabolic and reproductive status of the animal, but most of the studies describe an inhibitory effect of neuropeptide Y on GnRH neurons (46–48). Recent studies indicate that another neuropeptide belonging to the same RF-amide peptide family as Kp, RFRP-3 (the mammalian homolog of avian gonadotropin-inhibitory hormone), regulates GnRH neuron activity [for review, see Ref. (49–51)]. Unlike Kp, RFRP-3 can activate or inhibit the reproductive axis according to gender, species, and environmental conditions (26, 51–53). In female rodents RFRP neuronal activity is decreased at the time of the LH surge, possibly to relieve the inhibitory effect of RFRP-3 on GnRH neurons (54). However, mice bearing a null mutation of GPR147, the RFRP-3 receptor, present only a mild reproductive phenotype (55).

Estrogenic Regulation

Estradiol produced by the ovaries exerts both positive and negative feedback upstream of the reproductive axis, modulating GnRH neuron activity and anterior pituitary gonadotroph cells. During the first part of the reproductive cycle, estradiol induces a negative feedback, whereas when estradiol concentration is the highest (at the end of the follicular phase in humans or proestrus in rodents) the feedback becomes positive, causing a synchronized activation of GnRH neurons leading to GnRH release in the hypophyseal portal blood and finally the preovulatory LH surge (56) (**Figures 1A,D**). The effect of estradiol is mediated via two types of nuclear estrogen receptors (ERs), which induce long lasting genomic action, ERα and ERβ (57, 58), but it can also have a rapid action via membrane bound estradiol receptors, including the GPR30 (59, 60).

GnRH Neurons

Gonadotropin-releasing hormone neurons contain few, if any, ERα (61–63), but do express ERβ (64–66) and GPR30 (67). Estradiol application to cultured primate GnRH neurons induces a rapid increase in action potential firing frequency (68) and intracellular calcium oscillations (69). Similar effects have been reported in the mouse GnRH neurons (70). This rapid effect of estradiol is proposed to be mediated via GPR30 in primates (67) and ERβ in mice (70, 71). Using an *in vitro* GnRH neuronal model, the GT1-7 cells, it was reported that *Kiss1R* expression is estradiol dependant, with a Kp-induced GnRH increase only in cells treated with estradiol (72, 73). A primary effect of estradiol on GnRH neurons has been hypothesized to upregulate expression of channel transcripts (TRPC4 channels and HCN1 channels) that orchestrate the downstream signaling of Kiss1R in GnRH neurons (74, 75). Therefore, estradiol could be a potent regulator of ion channel and receptor expression in GnRH cells, hence controlling the sensitivity of GnRH neurons to Kp. However, a recent study reported that mutant mice with a GnRH neuron-selective deletion of ERβ exhibit normal cycles and negative feedback, leaving the critical role for ERβ in GnRH neuron activity still an open question (76).

Kisspeptin Neurons

In contrast to GnRH, Kp neurons have a high density of ERα and are, therefore, considered as the intermediate node for the estradiol feedback on GnRH neurons (19, 20, 32, 61, 77–79) (**Figure 1A**). Interestingly, the estradiol feedback in rodents depends on the Kp neuron localization as estradiol stimulates *Kiss1* expression in the AVPV and inhibits *Kiss1* expression in the ARN (77, 80–82). In non-rodent mammals, a similar differential regulation by estradiol is also observed with a stimulatory effect in the rostral periventricular/POA and an inhibitory effect in the ARN (83, 84). The mechanism underlying these differences in the regulation of *Kiss1* expression by ERα in both structures is not yet fully understood. AVPV *Kiss1* activation requires an estrogen response element (ERE)-dependent pathway, whereas inhibition of *Kiss1* expression in the ARN involves ERE-independent mechanisms (80, 85). Recent studies have reported that estradiol additionally modulates daily activity of AVPV Kp neurons. Hence, the daily variation in c-Fos activation, *Kiss1* mRNA and peptide content observed in proestrus or in ovariectomized estradiol-treated rodents is abolished or strongly reduced in diestrus or in ovariectomized animals (9, 86–88). Furthermore, estradiol has been reported to increase the number of arginine vasopressin (AVP) synaptic contacts onto Kp neurons (89), regulate AVP_{1a} receptor expression by Kp neurons (88) and be permissive for the AVP-induced electrical activation of Kp neurons (90). Altogether these observations indicate that high circulating levels of estradiol gate the action of AVP onto AVPV Kp neurons (see Role of the Suprachiasmatic Nuclei for the role of AVPV on Kp neurons).

Circadian System

Estradiol is also suggested to influence daily functions since shifts are observed during the pubertal period, pregnancy, menopause, and throughout the reproductive cycle (91–93). In rodents, ERα and ERβ are expressed in the retina, the retino-hypothalamic tract, the geniculohypothalamic tract and raphe nuclei-derived serotonergic inputs, all major inputs to the suprachiasmatic nuclei (SCN), which contain the master circadian clock (94). In mice, the second half of the proestrus night is often, but not consistently, characterized by increased motor activity compared to the remaining nights of the estrous cycle (95, 96). Furthermore, ovariectomy reduces total motor activity, and estradiol reverses this effect, while also shortening the length of the free running period and advancing the onset of wheel running activity (96). Estradiol may act directly on SCN clock gene oscillation since estradiol treatment in ovariectomized rats decreased *Cry2* mRNA levels (97) and estradiol application to SCN slices increased the spontaneous firing frequency and depolarized cell membranes of the SCN neurons (98). However, other studies reported that estradiol treatment of SCN explants from PER2:LUCIFERASE mice has no effect on the period and amplitude of the circadian oscillations (9, 99). Alternatively, estradiol may alter rhythms in running activity via indirect effects on the medial POA or striatum (100, 101).

Pituitary

Pituitary gonadotrophs express ERα, and estradiol has been proposed to exert a direct negative feedback effect on gonadotropin secretion (102–104). Chronic treatment with estradiol induces negative feedback effects on gonadotrophin secretion after GnRH supraphysiologic stimulation in ewes (105) or humans (106). Interestingly, a recent study reported that mice with a selective deletion of ERα in pituitary gonadotroph cells had elevated serum LH and estradiol values, and displayed irregular estrous cycles punctuated by prolonged periods of disorganized cycling, pointing to ERα participation in the estradiol negative feedback at the pituitary level (107). It is worth mentioning that this phenotype was much less severe than the one observed after a total ERα deletion. Although the role of Kiss/Kiss1R at the pituitary is still the subject of debate, it is interesting to note that the activation of pituitary ERα up-regulates *Kiss1* expression, whereas chronic exposure to estradiol down regulates *Kiss1R* expression on pituitary gonadotrophs (108).

Uterus

The uterus expresses high levels of ERα, and is an important site for the estrogenic control of reproductive physiology (109, 110). Estradiol, together with progesterone, regulates uterine growth and differentiation, which in turn control embryo-endometrial interactions during early pregnancy (110). Furthermore, estradiol treatment also shortens the period of the circadian clock in the uterus (99).

Daily and Circadian Regulations

Role of the Suprachiasmatic Nuclei

The Hypothalamic Suprachiasmatic Nuclei Host the Master Biological Clock

Most biological functions, including female reproduction, are synchronized to the daily variation of environmental factors. Among these factors, the recurring light/dark cycle is the most predictable environmental cue used by mammals to adjust their behavior and physiology appropriately. The mechanisms by which light and dark synchronize biological functions involve the master biological clock located in the hypothalamic SCN and a retino-hypothalamic tract, which forwards the non-visual light to the SCN.

The demonstration that a biological clock located in the basal hypothalamus was driving circadian rhythms came from experiments showing that SCN lesions in rodents abolished circadian rhythms in locomotor activity, which were restored following exogenous SCN implants (111, 112). The circadian activity of SCN neurons relies on a complex molecular system cycling endogenously with a period of about 1 day (*circa dies*). This molecular clockwork is composed of transcription–translation loops, which are now well described (113, 114). Dimers of the CLOCK and BMAL1 proteins bind to a specific E-box promoter to induce the transcription of four clock genes *Per1*, *Per2*, *Cry1*, and *Cry2*, which after translation produce proteins which form dimers to repress their own transcription by competing with the CLOCK/BMAL1 binding. Following degradation of the inhibitory proteins, the transcription–translation loop starts over for another circadian cycle. When SCN explants or dissociated cells are kept *in vitro*, the endogenous circadian oscillations continue for weeks or months, providing that the culture medium gets enough nutrients and oxygen for the cell metabolism. A very interesting animal model used to demonstrate these sustained endogenous oscillations is the PER2:LUCIFERASE mice, where the expression of the *luciferase* gene is driven by the *Per2* promoter (115, 116). When explants or dissociated cells of PER2:LUCIFERASE mouse SCN are placed in a culture medium containing luciferine, the rhythmic expression of PER2 drives a rhythmic expression of luciferase, which by oxidizing luciferin causes the emission of a bioluminescent signal with a circadian period.

In order to achieve its role in adjusting biological functions with the astronomical daily cycles, the SCN circadian activity has to be synchronized with the time of day and transmit this timing information to the rest of the body. Light has long been known to be the main synchronizer of the SCN circadian clock, but interestingly it uses a specific non-visual pathway, which includes melanopsin-containing intrinsically photosensitive retinal ganglion cells projecting directly to the SCN (117, 118). Upon light activation, these ganglion cell terminals release glutamate and pituitary activating cAMP peptide, which change the phase (synchronizes) of the circadian clock. The synchronizing property of light depends on the time of application during the day, and the characteristics of the phase responses depend on species. The astronomical light/dark alternation synchronizes the circadian clock in order to attain a daily rhythm of a precise 24-h period. The CLOCK/BMAL1 dimers not only activate canonical clock gene expression, but other clock-controlled genes whose promoters display E-boxes and therefore undergo rhythmic expression. This mechanism was first demonstrated for the gene encoding AVP, an important output of the SCN clock (119). Levels of SCN AVP mRNA are markedly higher during the day than at night, but in *Clock* KO mice the SCN AVP rhythm is strongly dampened (120).

SCN Lesion or Clock Gene Mutations Alter the Reproductive Cycle

Various experiments aiming at impairing clock function were performed to delineate whether functional SCN neurons are required for the daily timing of the LH surge, mostly in female rodents. Early experiments of SCN lesions (121) or SCN-POA neuronal connection cut (122) resulted in an impaired LH surge and estrous cyclicity in female rats. Furthermore, female mice carrying mutations of *Clock* or *Bmal1* displayed disrupted estrous cycles (123–127). $Clock^{-/-}$ mutant mice, for example, have extended and disrupted estrous cycles under both a light/dark cycle and during continuous darkness. In humans, it was reported that women with single-nucleotide polymorphisms in the ARNTL (*Bmal1*) have more miscarriages and less pregnancies than those without (128). Although these experiments have pointed to a crucial role of the SCN in the proper timing of estrous cyclicity, reproductive impairment following clock gene mutations could as well result from peripheral clock desynchronization (see Other Clocks in the Reproductive System). Interestingly, the reproductive phenotypes of young Clock-, Bmal1-, or Per1/Per2-mutated mice resemble that of middle-aged (over 10-month old) wild-type mice, with increased length and decreased frequency of estrous cycles (129, 130). These observations indicate that alterations in central or peripheral clocks may lead to advanced reproductive senescence (130).

The preovulatory LH surge is initiated by a SCN-derived stimulatory signal, at a time closely preceding general activity onset. However, this signal is effective at stimulating GnRH neurons to produce the LH surge only when estradiol concentrations have reached a critical threshold. Prior to the day of proestrus, the developing ovarian follicles secrete insufficient estradiol to fulfill this criteria and therefore, the SCN signal does not trigger the LH surge (56). The occurrence of the daily stimulatory SCN signal can be unmasked by implanting female rodents with estradiol capsules that result in proestrus concentrations of this hormone; in this case, a LH surge occurs every day (3, 56, 131).

SCN Neuropeptides Involved in the Timing of the GnRH/LH Surge

Transplant of fetal SCN tissue into bilaterally SCN-lesioned hamsters restores locomotor, but not endocrine rhythms in the absence of neural outgrowth, suggesting that intact neural connections are required for endocrine rhythmicity, whereas behavioral rhythms can be supported by a diffusible signal (132). Neuroanatomical studies have pointed to two putative SCN neural outputs signaling daily information to the reproductive axis, AVP and vasoactive intestinal peptide (VIP). Early experiments have identified SCN-originating, VIP-containing fibers contacting GnRH neurons (133, 134), which express the VIP receptor VPAC2 (135). However, more recent studies indicate that the SCN signals the time of day to GnRH neurons indirectly via AVP fibers projecting to the Kp neurons of the AVPV (78, 89).

Anterograde tracing studies show that a number of AVP-containing axons originating in the SCN make appositions to Kp neurons, whereas very few or no VIP terminals were found apposed to Kp neurons (87, 89). Furthermore, AVP is released with a peak coinciding with the onset of the LH surge (136) and AVPV Kp neurons express V1a receptors (87). Interestingly, the AVP input to Kp neurons is sensitive to estradiol since estradiol treatment significantly increases the number of AVP terminal appositions on individual Kp neurons (89) and circadian expression of V1a mRNA is abolished in ovariectomized animals (88). Furthermore, AVP signaling onto Kp neurons is critically dependent on circulating estradiol as AVP no longer activates Kp neurons in ovariectomized mice, an effect that is fully restored by estradiol treatment (90). Altogether, these results are consistent with the hypothesis that Kp neurons located in the rodent AVPV receive daily information from the SCN via an AVPergic monosynaptic pathway, a signal which is modulated (gated) by circulating estradiol (**Figure 1A**).

In line with these neuroanatomical observations, earlier physiological experiments pointed to a functional role of AVP in the GnRH/LH surge timing, even though the importance of Kp neurons was not yet known. Inhibition of AVP signaling with a V1a antagonist resulted in a reduction in the estradiol-induced LH surge (137), while intracerebroventricular infusion of AVP in SCN-lesioned, ovarectomized, and estradiol-treated rats was able to induce an LH surge (138). Furthermore, in co-cultures of POA and SCN, the GnRH surge was coordinated with the rhythm in AVP, but not VIP, and administration of AVP, not VIP, to preoptic explants in the presence of estradiol significantly increased GnRH release, providing further evidence for an important role of AVP in the LH surge generation (139). Finally, a recent study reported that intracerebroventricular administration of AVP in female Syrian hamsters activates Kp neurons similarly in the early or late part of the day, while in the same animals GnRH neurons are activated only late in the day (87). This observation was further confirmed by *in vitro* electrophysiological recordings of Kp-GFP neurons showing that AVP increases the firing rate of most Kp neurons during proestrus, independently of the time of day (90). Altogether these findings indicate that AVP activates Kp neurons every day, and the daytime gating of the GnRH/LH surge does not take place through SCN AVP–AVPV Kp signaling but rather downstream at the AVPV Kp–POA GnRH signaling.

A significant role of the SCN-derived VIP output in female reproduction should not be excluded (**Figure 1A**). Indeed, VIP afferents on GnRH neurons are sexually dimorphic, with female rats exhibiting higher VIPergic innervation than males (134). Furthermore, central administration of VIP antiserum reduces the LH surge (140), while central infusion of VIP is able to rescue the LH surge in middle-aged female rats (141). Finally, blocking the $VPAC_2$ receptor attenuates GnRH neuronal cell firing during the afternoon surge in female, estradiol-treated mice (142). A recent study reported that the SCN-derived VIP neurons project to RFRP-3 neurons and central administration of VIP markedly suppresses RFRP-3 cellular activity in the evening, but not the morning, therefore indicating a specific role of VIP on neurons expressing RFRP-3, a neuropeptide thought to participate in the circadian-timed removal of estradiol negative feedback (143).

Other Clocks in the Reproductive System

It has long been thought that the SCN-driven outputs are the sole source forwarding circadian signals to the female reproductive system. However, a growing body of evidence now suggests that structures and organs that are part of the gonadotropic axis might also play an intrinsic role in the timing of female reproduction.

In mammals, the timing system is now described as a multioscillator hierarchy of coordinated and synchronized cell and tissue clocks (144). The use of *Per1-luc* transgenic rats (145) and Per2:LUCIFERASE transgenic mice (115), where the *Per1* or *Per2* promoter drives expression of the *luciferase* gene, was decisive for the demonstration that non-SCN central structures and peripheral organs can sustain endogenous circadian oscillations. Thus, central structures (e.g., olfactory bulb, ARN, and retrochiasmatic area) and peripheral organs (e.g., liver, lung, heart, and kidney) are able to display endogenous-sustained circadian rhythmicity. The phase and the period of these "peripheral" clocks are tissue characteristic and different from those of the "central" clock of the SCN. The strength of their endogenous oscillations is often lesser than that of the SCN since according to tissues (and transgenic mice) the oscillations last from 2 to 20 cycles on average, whereas those of SCN can last several months. The oscillations generated by the peripheral clocks are independent of the SCN activity (they persist in SCN-lesioned animals) but their rhythms appear synchronized by the master clock, which is sometimes referred to as the conductor of the organism's multi-oscillatory network. In the context of such a complex circadian network, recent evidence now suggests that the hypothalamo-pituitary gonadal axis is also a functional multi-oscillatory axis. Indeed, reproductive tissues from hypothalamic Kp and GnRH neurons down to the ovaries and the uterus display endogenous circadian oscillations of clock genes, as explained below. However, the functional role of these reproductive clocks with regards to the timing of reproduction (ovulation, implantation, and parturition) has yet to be determined.

Kisspeptin Neurons

Daily and circadian activities of Kp neurons in the AVPV area have been investigated in female rodents because of their strategic position between the integration of SCN-derived AVP input on one hand (87, 89) and the triggering of the preovulatory GnRH/LH surge on the other (19). Additionally, the modulatory effect of circulating estradiol on the daily activity of Kp neurons has also been investigated because of the potent effect of estradiol on Kp synthesis (77). Under high circulating estradiol levels, either in proestrus or in ovariectomized + estradiol-supplemented rodents, Kp neuronal activity (as seen by c-FOS activation) and Kiss1 mRNA are significantly increased about 3 h before lights off, thus 2 h before the LH surge (9, 86–88). Furthermore, we recently reported that Kp immunoreactivity is markedly but transiently decreased at the same time (9). In contrast, in low circulating estradiol conditions, in diestrus or ovariectomized animals, the daily variation in neuronal activity, Kiss1 mRNA and Kp immunoreactivty is abolished or strongly dampened (9, 86, 88). The daily activation of Kp neurons is triggered by the SCN AVP input since central injection of AVP induces c-FOS in Kp neurons and increases Kiss1 mRNA (87). Although AVP is released from the SCN neurons in the afternoon (146), AVP can activate Kp neurons in the morning or in the afternoon, indicating that the daily control of the LH surge is not gated by the AVPV Kp neurons (87). A recent study recording Kp neuron electrical activity confirmed that Kp neuron responsiveness to AVP depends on the concentrations of estradiol (90). Altogether these data indicate that under high circulating estradiol (when oocytes are mature enough to be released), Kp neurons can be activated by the SCN-derived AVP to increase Kp synthesis and release in order to induce GnRH neuronal activation and the downstream LH surge. In addition to the AVP activation of Kp neurons, we recently reported that these neurons host an intrinsic circadian clock, named Kiss-Clock (9). A preliminary study reported that the clock genes *Per1* and *Bmal1* are expressed in the rat AVPV, but their cellular localization was not established (88). We further demonstrated that virtually all AVPV Kp neurons express the PER1 protein (**Figure 1B**) with a daily rhythm both in proestrus and diestrus, but with a phase delay of about 3 h in diestrus as compared to proestrus (9). Furthermore, we reported that isolated Kp-expressing AVPV explants from PER2:LUCIFERASE mice display endogenous circadian oscillations with a period of 23.2 h (thus 1 h shorter than the SCN circadian period of the same mice), confirming the presence of an intrinsic circadian oscillator in AVPV Kp neurons (9) (**Figure 1C**). Remarkably, the period of this circadian clock is increased by 1 h in the presence of estradiol in the culture medium (**Figure 1C**), which is in line with the observed phase difference in PER1 expression according to the estrous stage. In contrast, the period of the SCN clock is not altered by environmental estradiol either *in vivo* or *in vitro* (9). The role of this Kiss-Clock has yet to be established. However, according to previous studies one might hypothesize that it could time sensitivity to estradiol since *ERα* gene expression can be regulated by the BMAL1/CLOCK dimer (147), or it could also impact *Kiss1* gene expression since a circadian transcriptional factor, albumin D-site binding protein (Dbp), was reported to trigger *Kiss1* transcription via the D-box (148).

GnRH Neurons

Because of their pulsatile activity and critical role in timing the LH surge, GnRH neurons were the first in the reproductive system to be reported to express clock genes and display circadian activity. Indeed, all core clock genes (*Clock*, *Bmal1*, *Per1/2*, and *Cry1/2*) are expressed and cycle with a circadian period in both GT1-7 GnRH neuronal cell lines and GnRH neurons (149–152). Disruption of the circadian clock by transient expression of Clock Δ 19 in GT1-7 cells decreases the GnRH pulse frequency, while overexpression of *Cry1* in the same cells increases GnRH pulse amplitude (149). The GnRH clock could also regulate the timing of the neuronal sensitivity to upstream inputs. Indeed, the ability of VIP to activate GnRH neurons depends on the time of day and the estradiol environment (153), and the sensitivity of GT1-7 cells to release GnRH upon Kp or VIP treatment is time dependent (151). This time-dependent sensitivity may explain why central infusion of Kp fails to advance the onset of the LH surge in either naturally cycling or ovariectomized estradiol-supplemented female rodents (154, 155). Finally, the stimulatory and synchronizing effects of Kp on GnRH release are reduced in preoptic explants of *Bmal1* KO mice (35). Therefore, the circadian clock in GnRH neurons may provide a time-keeping mechanism to appropriately release GnRH under Kp, and possibly VIP, stimulation.

Pituitary Gland and Gonadotroph Cells

The pituitary, as a whole, was among the first peripheral oscillators found to display strong sustained circadian oscillations with a circadian period of about 23.8 h in *Per1*- or PER2-luciferase transgenic rodents (115, 145). It was further established that all clock genes expressed a daily rhythm in the whole pituitary but with a different profile according to the estrus stage (127, 156). The pituitary gland is made of different cell types, which could host several circadian oscillators with different phases. Expression of all cognate clock genes was identified in the alphaT3-1 gonadotroph cell line (147) and GnRH activation was reported to selectively increase *mPer1* expression in gonadotroph cells (157).

Furthermore, the gene coding for the GnRH receptor contains non-canonical E-box promoter elements and *Bmal1* knockdown in a gonadotrope cell line reduces GnRH receptor mRNA (147). These studies raised the hypothesis that an intrinsic clock in gonadotrophs could directly regulate GnRH signaling and LH surge timing. To test this hypothesis, a specific BMAL1 KO disruption was performed in the gonadotrophs (127). The mutated mice still displayed a preovulatory LH surge and estrous cyclicity (although with a significant increase in cycle length variance) and the average time of puberty and fertility performance was not altered. Taken together, these data suggest that the intrinsic clock in gonadotroph cells is dispensable for LH surge regulation but contributes to estrous cycle robustness (127).

Ovaries

The ovarian circadian clock is very well documented in many mammalian and non-mammalian species and its function has been thoroughly investigated both *in vivo* and *in vitro* (158–161). Each cell type of the ovary, including theca cells, granulosa cells, and oocytes have a circadian clock (162). Further analyses reported that clock gene rhythms are only observed in mature granulosa and luteal cells, indicating that these rhythms are activated at a specific stage of follicle development, possibly under the control of FSH acting as a synchronizer of follicular cell activities (163). Ovarian physiology is strongly regulated by gonadotropins, and current studies indicate that LH stimulates various clock genes in the ovaries (159, 164). Furthermore, the endogenous rhythm of Per-driven oscillations in isolated ovaries is significantly shifted by LH and FSH indicating that the ovarian circadian clock is entrained by hormonal signals from the pituitary (160). Recently, a study reported that mice with a conditional KO of *Bmal1* in steroidogenic cells show severe deficits in implantation success and compromised progesterone secretion (165). A previous study demonstrated a circadian rhythm in ovarian sensitivity to LH with a greater ovarian response at night as compared to day, indicating that the ovarian circadian clock may set its responsiveness to the LH surge (161). Finally, various ovarian genes, including those encoding for the LH receptor and enzymes involved in steroid hormone biosynthesis, display circadian rhythms in granulosa cells and these rhythms are altered following the silencing of *Bmal1* expression (163). Altogether, these findings indicate that the clock in the ovary may be involved in the timing of ovulation, steroid hormone synthesis, and follicular growth and differentiation.

Uterus and Oviduct

Global knockout of the *Bmal1* or *Clock* gene disrupts implantation, increases fetal reabsorption during pregnancy, and leads to a high rate of full-term pregnancy failures (124, 166). Early in 2002, clock genes were found to be expressed in the uterus and oviduct of mice (167). Furthermore, the oviduct was reported to display a daily rhythm of several clock genes and clock-controlled gene (168). In the uterus, the presence of sustained endogenous clock oscillations was demonstrated in tissue explants of PER2:LUCIFERASE mice (99). These uterine oscillations were sustained even during pregnancy suggesting that embryos may be submitted to the maternal clock *in utero* (169). Interestingly, the period of the uterine clock oscillations changes according to the estrous stage and it is decreased when the tissue is incubated with estradiol (99). Additionally, a targeted deletion of *Bmal1* in the myometrium indicates a role for myometrial *Bmal1* in maintaining normal timing of parturition (170). Although additional studies are required to determine the physiological role of the uterine and oviduct clocks, the data obtained so far suggest that the developing embryo may be subjected to rhythmic changes in the oviduct during transit to the uterus and in the uterus during pregnancy.

Shift-Work Consequences on Reproductive Cycles and Fertility

Shift Work

The modern 24-h-functioning society requires that an increasing number of employees work outside of the natural active period, in shifted conditions. According to the International Labor Organization (ILO; 1990), working in shifts is "a method of organization of working time in which workers succeed one another at the workplace so that the establishment can operate longer than the hours of work of individual workers" at different daily and night hours. Under a fixed-shift system, working time can be organized in two or three shifts: the early, late, and/or nightshifts. Under a rotating-shift system, workers might be assigned to work shifts that vary regularly over time.

Over the last 20 years in United States, almost 27% of men and 16% of women experienced shift work (171). In 2012, 15% of French workers, including 9.3% women, were working under shift work either occasionally (8%) or permanently (7.4%). An increasing number of analyses report that alteration in working schedule is often associated with an increased risk of developing cardiovascular/metabolic/gastrointestinal disorders, some types of cancer, and mental disorders including depression and anxiety (172–174). Hence, in 2007, shift work was reclassified from a possible to a probable human carcinogen (class 2A) by the International Agency for Research on Cancer. A French law passed on December 20, 2014 listed shift work as a risk factor increasing professional arduousness.

Given the importance of the circadian systems in the regulation of female reproduction, and given the fetal exposure to the maternal daily rhythms in temperature, substrates, and hormones, female shift workers may display reproductive alterations, such as an increased risk of irregular menstrual cycles, endometriosis, miscarriage, low birth weight, or pre-term delivery (175–177). Such disturbances may result from altered SCN clock synchronization with rest-activity and feed-fast cycles and/or internal desynchronization amongst peripheral clocks, especially those of the reproductive axis. Indeed, a recent study reported that peripheral clock genes in lymphocytes of shift workers are strongly altered as compared to day workers (178). Additionally, recent animal studies have shown that the functioning of fetal clocks depends on maternal hormones (179) and possibly feeding and activity, then maternal circadian disruption during pregnancy may lead to fetal SCN and peripheral clocks desynchronization.

In addition to the effect of circadian dysregulation, it should be kept in mind that shift work-related alterations in other daily functions, particularly food intake and sleep, may indirectly impact female reproduction. Thus, obesity, which is often associated with shift work, has a strong impact on reproductive performance (180) and sleep disturbance in prepubertal girls can alter estradiol-dependent pubertal development (181).

Modeling Shift Work in Rodents

Shift work is a very complex situation and therefore, it is difficult to design animal model conditions that mimic human shift work. A recent review listed four relevant models that use altered timing of food intake, activity, sleep or light exposure, or a combination of several (182).

Very few *in vivo* animal studies have investigated the alteration of fertility or the LH surge after a shift in the light/dark cycle or a photoperiod change (6, 56, 183). In one study, female Syrian hamsters were submitted to a 3-h phase advance or delay (183). When the phase advance was applied between 1 and 3 days before estrous, the LH surge was not fully resynchronized to the new schedule, even after 3 days. However, when hamsters were submitted to a 3-h phase delay, the LH surge was synchronized to the dark onset more rapidly. Similarly, in ovariectomized transgenic GnRH-GFP mice, a dark phase advance led to an advance in the LH surge (56). When the photoperiod length was modified in female hamsters, the timing of the LH surge was shifted in a similar manner to the nocturnal onset of locomotor activity (6).

In mice, exposure to either phase advances or delays at the beginning and throughout pregnancy leads to a significant decrease in pregnancy success (184). Interestingly, an *in vitro* study analyzed the effect of a 6-h phase advance on endogenous circadian oscillation of the SCN and various peripheral clocks and found that the ovarian clock was not fully resynchronized 6 days after the phase shift (185).

Although these few studies indicate that shifts in light/dark cycle alter the timing of the preovulatory LH surge and the synchrony amongst reproductive clocks, it is obvious that new animal studies have to be developed in order to understand the mechanisms underlying the various effect of shift work on reproduction and fertility in females.

Reproductive Consequence in Women Under Shift Work

A number of studies have investigated the relationship between fertility and shift work or night work in women working in pharmaceutical industries, hospitals, slaughter houses, and canneries (175, 178, 186–200). Although human studies are limited in their use for understanding causality and underlying mechanisms of health consequences of shift work, most of the above studies have reported a negative impact of shift work on fertility. However, there is a large heterogeneity among these analyses especially regarding the fertility criteria examined: body temperature curve, menstrual disorders, time to get pregnant, etc. Furthermore, it is important to stress that clinical or biological criteria can be misinterpreted since irregular cycles, as an indicator of the reproductive axis sensibility to shift work, may have no correlation with subfertility and pregnancy capacity (197).

Using body temperature curves to follow menstrual cycles, shift work was found to be associated with higher rates of short cycles and inadequate luteal phases (188). Furthermore, a higher prevalence of menstrual disorders is often found in female shift workers as compared to the non-shift workers. For example, in the most relevant studies including the largest populations, irregular cycles are reported in 12–20% of shift workers and 7–10% in non-shift workers (175, 192). In a large Danish population (17,531 daytime workers and 3,907 shift workers), it was reported that fixed evening and fixed night female workers took longer to get pregnant with adjusted odds ratio around 0.80, compared to daytime workers, but there was no unequivocal evidence of a causal association between shift work and subfecundity since this reduction may be mediated by pregnancy planning bias or differential options for sexual contacts (187). Only a few studies have examined reproductive hormones with various conclusions. It has been reported that FSH and LH levels are not different between shift and day workers (190, 192), but a single measurement of LH without a gynecologic examination and cycle characterization is difficult to interpret. The levels of 17-β-estradiol were found to be significantly increased (178, 201) in female shift workers possibly due to a prolonged follicular phase (186). Some studies have reported no significant relationship between shift work and subfertility or dysmenorrhea (196–200). However, among these studies, one has only a few women included with a surprising 35% of control women displaying irregular cycles (196). Another study reported no significant subfertility in shift-working women 1 year after birth control termination but yet, these women displayed a delay to get pregnant twice as long compared to the day-working group (199).

The pineal hormone melatonin, whose nocturnal production is profoundly affected by shifts in light/dark conditions, has been proposed to display potential anti-estrogenic effects (202, 203). Urinary melatonin excretion tends to be lower with a delayed peak of production during shift work (190, 193, 201, 204). The combination of inhibition on melatonin secretion with estradiol mistiming has been proposed to be involved in the hormone-related cancers observed in night shift workers (204, 205).

The conflicting results regarding the negative effect of shift work on female reproduction probably reflect large differences in the shift-work schedules, duration, and age of exposure, with a high number of confounding factors (like stress, fatigue, obesity, etc.) as well as methodological limitations (206, 207). Despite these considerations, cycling disorders should be considered as a sensitivity or intolerance to shift work. Shift work during pregnancy has adverse effects including increased risk of miscarriage (208), although this is somewhat controversial (209). Yet, most authors recommend avoiding shift work during pregnancy.

Conclusion

Daily and estrogenic regulations of female reproduction allow the timing of ovulation to coincide with optimal reproductive tract functioning (oocyte maturation and receptive reproductive tract), maximal arousal (general activity and sexual motivation), and the best environmental conditions (food resources and stress level). These general coordinations confer maximum adaptive advantage to insure the success of this high energy-demanding reproductive function. Although the central role of the master SCN clock in the daily regulation of the LH surge has been well documented, the recent evidence that other peripheral clocks are located all along the gonadotropic axis, from Kp and GnRH neurons to the ovaries and uterus, raises the question of their role in the timing of reproduction. The latest findings indicate that these local clocks may optimize circadian cell sensitivity to upstream signals and set appropriate timing of the downstream reproductive responses. Notably, application of phase shifts leads to different rates of clock resynchronization between the SCN and reproductive organs, suggesting internal desynchronization of the reproductive axis, as seen in other functional axes. In our current society, where a significant number of female workers are working night or evening shifts, the delicate timing of organization in the reproductive network can easily be disrupted. While numerous studies have reported negative consequences of shift work on metabolic and cardiovascular functions as well as cancer occurrence, there are surprisingly few epidemiologic studies in humans and mechanistic studies in animal models reporting the incidence of shift work on female fertility. Future studies in the field should, therefore, investigate the impact of daily rhythm alterations, as observed under shift-work conditions, jet lag, or sleep disturbance, on reproductive cycle and fertility both in animal models and humans.

Author Contributions

VS and TB contributed equally to the writing of this review.

Acknowledgments

Authors are very grateful to Caroline Ancel and Matthew Beymer for their scientific advice and English correction. TB is supported by the Fondation pour la Recherche Médicale for his PhD research stay (FDM20140630371).

References

1. Hillier SG. Current concepts of the roles of follicle stimulating hormone and luteinizing hormone in folliculogenesis. *Hum Reprod* (1994) **9**:188–91.
2. Norman RL, Blake CA, Sawyer CH. Estrogen-dependent 24-hour periodicity in pituitary LH release in the female hamster. *Endocrinology* (1973) **93**:965–70. doi:10.1210/endo-93-4-965
3. Legan SJ, Karsch FJ. A daily signal for the LH surge in the rat. *Endocrinology* (1975) **96**:57–62. doi:10.1210/endo-96-1-57
4. McElhinny TL, Sisk CL, Holekamp KE, Smale L. A morning surge in plasma luteinizing hormone coincides with elevated Fos expression in gonadotropin-releasing hormone-immunoreactive neurons in the diurnal rodent, *Arvicanthis niloticus*. *Biol Reprod* (1999) **61**:1115–22. doi:10.1095/biolreprod61.4.1115
5. Bronson FH, Vom Saal FS. Control of the preovulatory release of luteinizing hormone by steroids in the mouse. *Endocrinology* (1979) **104**:1247–55. doi:10.1210/endo-104-5-1247
6. Moline ML, Albers HE, Todd RB, Moore-Ede MC. Light-dark entrainment of proestrous LH surges and circadian locomotor activity in female hamsters. *Horm Behav* (1981) **15**:451–8. doi:10.1016/0018-506X(81)90009-X
7. Kerdelhué B, Brown S, Lenoir V, Queenan JT, Jones GS, Scholler R, et al. Timing of initiation of the preovulatory luteinizing hormone surge and its relationship with the circadian cortisol rhythm in the human. *Neuroendocrinology* (2002) **75**:158–63. doi:10.1159/000048233
8. Melmed S, Kaiser Ursula B. Gonadotropin hormones. In: *The Pituitary*. 3rd edn (2010). p. 205–60.
9. Chassard D, Bur I, Poirel V-J, Mendoza J, Simonneaux V. Evidence for a putative circadian Kiss-Clock in the hypothalamic AVPV in female mice. *Endocrinology* (2015) **156**:2999–3011. doi:10.1210/en.2014-1769
10. Bouligand J, Ghervan C, Tello JA, Brailly-Tabard S, Salenave S, Chanson P, et al. Isolated familial hypogonadotropic hypogonadism and a GNRH1 mutation. *N Engl J Med* (2009) **360**:2742–8. doi:10.1056/NEJMoa0900136
11. Chevrier L, Guimiot F, de Roux N. GnRH receptor mutations in isolated gonadotropic deficiency. *Mol Cell Endocrinol* (2011) **346**:21–8. doi:10.1016/j.mce.2011.04.018
12. Crowley WF, McArthur JW. Simulation of the normal menstrual cycle in Kallman's syndrome by pulsatile administration of luteinizing hormone-releasing hormone (LHRH). *J Clin Endocrinol Metab* (1980) **51**:173–5. doi:10.1210/jcem-51-1-173
13. Chryssikopoulos A, Gregoriou O, Papadias C, Loghis C. Gonadotropin ovulation induction and pregnancies in women with Kallmann's syndrome. *Gynecol Endocrinol* (1998) **12**:103–8. doi:10.3109/09513599809024958
14. Knobil E, Plant TM, Wildt L, Belchetz PE, Marshall G. Control of the rhesus monkey menstrual cycle: permissive role of hypothalamic gonadotropin-releasing hormone. *Science* (1980) **207**:1371–3. doi:10.1126/science.6766566
15. Lee JH, Miele ME, Hicks DJ, Phillips KK, Trent JM, Weissman BE, et al. KiSS-1, a novel human malignant melanoma metastasis-suppressor gene. *J Natl Cancer Inst* (1996) **88**:1731–7. doi:10.1093/jnci/88.23.1731
16. De Roux N, Genin E, Carel J-C, Matsuda F, Chaussain J-L, Milgrom E. Hypogonadotropic hypogonadism due to loss of function of the KiSS1-derived peptide receptor GPR54. *Proc Natl Acad Sci U S A* (2003) **100**:10972–6. doi:10.1073/pnas.1834399100
17. Seminara SB, Messager S, Chatzidaki EE, Thresher RR, Acierno JS, Shagoury JK, et al. The GPR54 gene as a regulator of puberty. *N Engl J Med* (2003) **349**:1614–27. doi:10.1056/NEJMoa035322
18. Pinilla L, Aguilar E, Dieguez C, Millar RP, Tena-Sempere M. Kisspeptins and reproduction: physiological roles and regulatory mechanisms. *Physiol Rev* (2012) **92**:1235–316. doi:10.1152/physrev.00037.2010
19. Gottsch ML, Cunningham MJ, Smith JT, Popa SM, Acohido BV, Crowley WF, et al. A role for kisspeptins in the regulation of gonadotropin secretion in the mouse. *Endocrinology* (2004) **145**:4073–7. doi:10.1210/en.2004-0431
20. Clarkson J, Herbison AE. Postnatal development of kisspeptin neurons in mouse hypothalamus; sexual dimorphism and projections to gonadotropin-releasing hormone neurons. *Endocrinology* (2006) **147**:5817–25. doi:10.1210/en.2006-0787
21. Clarkson J, d'Anglemont de Tassigny X, Colledge WH, Caraty A, Herbison AE. Distribution of kisspeptin neurones in the adult female mouse brain. *J Neuroendocrinol* (2009) **21**:673–82. doi:10.1111/j.1365-2826.2009.01892.x
22. Hoong Yip S, Boehm U, Herbison AE, Campbell RE. Conditional viral tract-tracing delineates the projections of the distinct kisspeptin neuron populations to gonadotropin-releasing hormone (GnRH) neurons in the mouse. *Endocrinology* (2015) **156**:2582–94. doi:10.1210/en.2015-1131
23. Kauffman AS, Gottsch ML, Roa J, Byquist AC, Crown A, Clifton DK, et al. Sexual differentiation of Kiss1 gene expression in the brain of the rat. *Endocrinology* (2007) **148**:1774–83. doi:10.1210/en.2006-1540
24. Smith JT, Popa SM, Clifton DK, Hoffman GE, Steiner RA. Kiss1 neurons in the forebrain as central processors for generating the preovulatory luteinizing hormone surge. *J Neurosci* (2006) **26**:6687–94. doi:10.1523/JNEUROSCI.1618-06.2006
25. Herbison AE, de Tassigny Xd, Doran J, Colledge WH. Distribution and postnatal development of Gpr54 gene expression in mouse brain and gonadotropin-releasing hormone neurons. *Endocrinology* (2010) **151**:312–21. doi:10.1210/en.2009-0552
26. Simonneaux V, Ancel C, Poirel VJ, Gauer F. Kisspeptins and RFRP-3 act in concert to synchronize rodent reproduction with seasons. *Front Neurosci* (2013) **7**:22. doi:10.3389/fnins.2013.00022

27. Kotani M, Detheux M, Vandenbogaerde A, Communi D, Vanderwinden JM, Le Poul E, et al. The metastasis suppressor gene KiSS-1 encodes kisspeptins, the natural ligands of the orphan G protein-coupled receptor GPR54. *J Biol Chem* (2001) **276**:34631–6. doi:10.1074/jbc.M104847200
28. Navarro VM, Castellano JM, Fernández-Fernández R, Tovar S, Roa J, Mayen A, et al. Characterization of the potent luteinizing hormone-releasing activity of KiSS-1 peptide, the natural ligand of GPR54. *Endocrinology* (2005) **146**:156–63. doi:10.1210/en.2004-0836
29. Dhillo WS, Chaudhri OB, Patterson M, Thompson EL, Murphy KG, Badman MK, et al. Kisspeptin-54 stimulates the hypothalamic-pituitary gonadal axis in human males. *J Clin Endocrinol Metab* (2005) **90**:6609–15. doi:10.1210/jc.2005-1468
30. Plant TM, Ramaswamy S, Dipietro MJ. Repetitive activation of hypothalamic G protein-coupled receptor 54 with intravenous pulses of kisspeptin in the juvenile monkey (Macaca mulatta) elicits a sustained train of gonadotropin-releasing hormone discharges. *Endocrinology* (2006) **147**:1007–13. doi:10.1210/en.2005-1261
31. Tovar S, Vázquez MJ, Navarro VM, Fernández-Fernández R, Castellano JM, Vigo E, et al. Effects of single or repeated intravenous administration of kisspeptin upon dynamic LH secretion in conscious male rats. *Endocrinology* (2006) **147**:2696–704. doi:10.1210/en.2005-1397
32. d'Anglemont de Tassigny X, Fagg LA, Carlton MBL, Colledge WH. Kisspeptin can stimulate gonadotropin-releasing hormone (GnRH) release by a direct action at GnRH nerve terminals. *Endocrinology* (2008) **149**:3926–32. doi:10.1210/en.2007-1487
33. Keen KL, Wegner FH, Bloom SR, Ghatei MA, Terasawa E. An increase in kisspeptin-54 release occurs with the pubertal increase in luteinizing hormone-releasing hormone-1 release in the stalk-median eminence of female rhesus monkeys in vivo. *Endocrinology* (2008) **149**:4151–7. doi:10.1210/en.2008-0231
34. Plant TM. The role of KiSS-1 in the regulation of puberty in higher primates. *Eur J Endocrinol* (2006) **155**(Suppl):S11–6. doi:10.1530/eje.1.02232
35. Choe HK, Kim H-D, Park SH, Lee H-W, Park J-Y, Seong JY, et al. Synchronous activation of gonadotropin-releasing hormone gene transcription and secretion by pulsatile kisspeptin stimulation. *Proc Natl Acad Sci U S A* (2013) **110**:5677–82. doi:10.1073/pnas.1213594110
36. Topaloglu AK, Tello JA, Kotan LD, Ozbek MN, Yilmaz MB, Erdogan S, et al. Inactivating KISS1 mutation and hypogonadotropic hypogonadism. *N Engl J Med* (2012) **366**:629–35. doi:10.1056/NEJMoa1111184
37. d'Anglemont de Tassigny X, Fagg LA, Dixon JPC, Day K, Leitch HG, Hendrick AG, et al. Hypogonadotropic hypogonadism in mice lacking a functional Kiss1 gene. *Proc Natl Acad Sci U S A* (2007) **104**:10714–9. doi:10.1073/pnas.0704114104
38. Brioude F, Bouligand J, Francou B, Fagart J, Roussel R, Viengchareun S, et al. Two families with normosmic congenital hypogonadotropic hypogonadism and biallelic mutations in KISS1R (KISS1 receptor): clinical evaluation and molecular characterization of a novel mutation. *PLoS One* (2013) **8**:e53896. doi:10.1371/journal.pone.0053896
39. Wahab F, Quinton R, Seminara SB. The kisspeptin signaling pathway and its role in human isolated GnRH deficiency. *Mol Cell Endocrinol* (2011) **346**:29–36. doi:10.1016/j.mce.2011.05.043
40. Petersen SL, Ottem EN, Carpenter CD. Direct and indirect regulation of gonadotropin-releasing hormone neurons by estradiol. *Biol Reprod* (2003) **69**:1771–8. doi:10.1095/biolreprod.103.019745
41. Donoso AO, Seltzer AM, Navarro CE, Cabrera RJ, López FJ, Negro-Vilar A. Regulation of luteinizing hormone-releasing hormone and luteinizing hormone secretion by hypothalamic amino acids. *Braz J Med Biol Res* (1994) **27**:921–32.
42. Ottem EN, Godwin JG, Petersen SL. Glutamatergic signaling through the N-methyl-D-aspartate receptor directly activates medial subpopulations of luteinizing hormone-releasing hormone (LHRH) neurons, but does not appear to mediate the effects of estradiol on LHRH gene expression. *Endocrinology* (2002) **143**:4837–45. doi:10.1210/en.2002-220707
43. Arias P, Jarry H, Leonhardt S, Moguilevsky JA, Wuttke W. Estradiol modulates the LH release response to N-methyl-D-aspartate in adult female rats: studies on hypothalamic luteinizing hormone-releasing hormone and neurotransmitter release. *Neuroendocrinology* (1993) **57**:710–5. doi:10.1159/000126429
44. Watanabe M, Fukuda A, Nabekura J. The role of GABA in the regulation of GnRH neurons. *Front Neurosci* (2014) **8**:387. doi:10.3389/fnins.2014.00387
45. Morello H, Caligaris L, Haymal B, Taleisnik S. Daily variations in the sensitivity of proestrous LH surge in the inhibitory effect of intraventricular injection of 5-HT or GABA in rats. *Can J Physiol Pharmacol* (1992) **70**:447–51. doi:10.1139/y92-057
46. Xu J, Kirigiti MA, Cowley MA, Grove KL, Smith MS. Suppression of basal spontaneous gonadotropin-releasing hormone neuronal activity during lactation: role of inhibitory effects of neuropeptide Y. *Endocrinology* (2009) **150**:333–40. doi:10.1210/en.2008-0962
47. Klenke U, Constantin S, Wray S. Neuropeptide Y directly inhibits neuronal activity in a subpopulation of gonadotropin-releasing hormone-1 neurons via Y1 receptors. *Endocrinology* (2010) **151**:2736–46. doi:10.1210/en.2009-1198
48. Kiyokawa M, Matsuzaki T, Iwasa T, Ogata R, Murakami M, Kinouchi R, et al. Neuropeptide Y mediates orexin A-mediated suppression of pulsatile gonadotropin-releasing hormone secretion in ovariectomized rats. *J Med Invest* (2011) **58**:11–8. doi:10.2152/jmi.58.11
49. Williams WP, Kriegsfeld LJ. Circadian control of neuroendocrine circuits regulating female reproductive function. *Front Endocrinol* (2012) **3**:60. doi:10.3389/fendo.2012.00060
50. Khan AR, Kauffman AS. The role of kisspeptin and RFamide-related peptide-3 neurones in the circadian-timed preovulatory luteinising hormone surge. *J Neuroendocrinol* (2012) **24**:131–43. doi:10.1111/j.1365-2826.2011.02162.x
51. Simonneaux V, Bur I, Ancel C, Ansel L, Klosen P. A kiss for daily and seasonal reproduction. *Prog Brain Res* (2012) **199**:423–37. doi:10.1016/B978-0-444-59427-3.00024-1
52. Kriegsfeld LJ, Mei DF, Bentley GE, Ubuka T, Mason AO, Inoue K, et al. Identification and characterization of a gonadotropin-inhibitory system in the brains of mammals. *Proc Natl Acad Sci U S A* (2006) **103**:2410–5. doi:10.1073/pnas.0511003103
53. Ubuka T, Inoue K, Fukuda Y, Mizuno T, Ukena K, Kriegsfeld LJ, et al. Identification, expression, and physiological functions of Siberian hamster gonadotropin-inhibitory hormone. *Endocrinology* (2012) **153**:373–85. doi:10.1210/en.2011-1110
54. Gibson EM, Humber SA, Jain S, Williams WP, Zhao S, Bentley GE, et al. Alterations in RFamide-related peptide expression are coordinated with the preovulatory luteinizing hormone surge. *Endocrinology* (2008) **149**:4958–69. doi:10.1210/en.2008-0316
55. León S, García-Galiano D, Ruiz-Pino F, Barroso A, Manfredi-Lozano M, Romero-Ruiz A, et al. Physiological roles of gonadotropin-inhibitory hormone signaling in the control of mammalian reproductive axis: studies in the NPFF1 receptor null mouse. *Endocrinology* (2014) **155**:2953–65. doi:10.1210/en.2014-1030
56. Christian CA, Mobley JL, Moenter SM. Diurnal and estradiol-dependent changes in gonadotropin-releasing hormone neuron firing activity. *Proc Natl Acad Sci U S A* (2005) **102**:15682–7. doi:10.1073/pnas.0504270102
57. White JO, Herschman MJ, Parmar G, Philipson KA, Elder MG, Habib NA, et al. Activated oestrogen receptor in human breast cancer: clinical and biochemical correlates. *Br J Surg* (1987) **74**:588–90. doi:10.1002/bjs.1800740715
58. Radovick S, Levine JE, Wolfe A. Estrogenic regulation of the GnRH neuron. *Front Endocrinol* (2012) **3**:52. doi:10.3389/fendo.2012.00052
59. Filardo EJ. Epidermal growth factor receptor (EGFR) transactivation by estrogen via the G-protein-coupled receptor, GPR30: a novel signaling pathway with potential significance for breast cancer. *J Steroid Biochem Mol Biol* (2002) **80**:231–8. doi:10.1016/S0960-0760(01)00190-X
60. Filardo EJ, Quinn JA, Bland KI, Frackelton AR. Estrogen-induced activation of Erk-1 and Erk-2 requires the G protein-coupled receptor homolog, GPR30, and occurs via trans-activation of the epidermal growth factor receptor through release of HB-EGF. *Mol Endocrinol* (2000) **14**:1649–60. doi:10.1210/mend.14.10.0532
61. Herbison AE, Theodosis DT. Localization of oestrogen receptors in preoptic neurons containing neurotensin but not tyrosine hydroxylase, cholecystokinin or luteinizing hormone-releasing hormone in the male and female rat. *Neuroscience* (1992) **50**:283–98. doi:10.1016/0306-4522(92)90423-Y
62. Dorling AA, Todman MG, Korach KS, Herbison AE. Critical role for estrogen receptor alpha in negative feedback regulation of gonadotropin-releasing hormone mRNA expression in the female mouse. *Neuroendocrinology* (2003) **78**:204–9. doi:10.1159/000073703
63. Wintermantel TM, Campbell RE, Porteous R, Bock D, Gröne H-J, Todman MG, et al. Definition of estrogen receptor pathway critical for estrogen

positive feedback to gonadotropin-releasing hormone neurons and fertility. *Neuron* (2006) **52**:271–80. doi:10.1016/j.neuron.2006.07.023
64. Hrabovszky E, Shughrue PJ, Merchenthaler I, Hajszán T, Carpenter CD, Liposits Z, et al. Detection of estrogen receptor-beta messenger ribonucleic acid and 125I-estrogen binding sites in luteinizing hormone-releasing hormone neurons of the rat brain. *Endocrinology* (2000) **141**:3506–9. doi:10.1210/endo.141.9.7788
65. Skinner DC, Dufourny L. Oestrogen receptor beta-immunoreactive neurones in the ovine hypothalamus: distribution and colocalisation with gonadotropin-releasing hormone. *J Neuroendocrinol* (2005) **17**:29–39. doi:10.1111/j.1365-2826.2005.01271.x
66. Wolfe A, Wu S. Estrogen receptor-β in the gonadotropin-releasing hormone neuron. *Semin Reprod Med* (2012) **30**:23–31. doi:10.1055/s-0031-1299594
67. Noel SD, Keen KL, Baumann DI, Filardo EJ, Terasawa E. Involvement of G protein-coupled receptor 30 (GPR30) in rapid action of estrogen in primate LHRH neurons. *Mol Endocrinol* (2009) **23**:349–59. doi:10.1210/me.2008-0299
68. Abe H, Terasawa E. Firing pattern and rapid modulation of activity by estrogen in primate luteinizing hormone releasing hormone-1 neurons. *Endocrinology* (2005) **146**:4312–20. doi:10.1210/en.2005-0435
69. Abe H, Keen KL, Terasawa E. Rapid action of estrogens on intracellular calcium oscillations in primate luteinizing hormone-releasing hormone-1 neurons. *Endocrinology* (2008) **149**:1155–62. doi:10.1210/en.2007-0942
70. Chu Z, Andrade J, Shupnik MA, Moenter SM. Differential regulation of gonadotropin-releasing hormone neuron activity and membrane properties by acutely applied estradiol: dependence on dose and estrogen receptor subtype. *J Neurosci* (2009) **29**:5616–27. doi:10.1523/JNEUROSCI.0352-09.2009
71. Abrahám IM, Han S-K, Todman MG, Korach KS, Herbison AE. Estrogen receptor beta mediates rapid estrogen actions on gonadotropin-releasing hormone neurons in vivo. *J Neurosci* (2003) **23**:5771–7.
72. Jacobi JS, Martin C, Nava G, Jeziorski MC, Clapp C, Martínez de la Escalera G. 17-Beta-estradiol directly regulates the expression of adrenergic receptors and kisspeptin/GPR54 system in GT1-7 GnRH neurons. *Neuroendocrinology* (2007) **86**:260–9. doi:10.1159/000107770
73. Tonsfeldt KJ, Goodall CP, Latham KL, Chappell PE. Oestrogen induces rhythmic expression of the Kisspeptin-1 receptor GPR54 in hypothalamic gonadotrophin-releasing hormone-secreting GT1-7 cells. *J Neuroendocrinol* (2011) **23**:823–30. doi:10.1111/j.1365-2826.2011.02188.x
74. Bosch MA, Tonsfeldt KJ, Rønnekleiv OK. mRNA expression of ion channels in GnRH neurons: subtype-specific regulation by 17β-estradiol. *Mol Cell Endocrinol* (2013) **367**:85–97. doi:10.1016/j.mce.2012.12.021
75. Rønnekleiv OK, Zhang C, Bosch MA, Kelly MJ. Kisspeptin and gonadotropin-releasing hormone neuronal excitability: molecular mechanisms driven by 17β-estradiol. *Neuroendocrinology* (2014). doi:10.1159/000370311
76. Cheong RY, Porteous R, Chambon P, Abrahám I, Herbison AE. Effects of neuron-specific estrogen receptor (ER) α and ERβ deletion on the acute estrogen negative feedback mechanism in adult female mice. *Endocrinology* (2014) **155**:1418–27. doi:10.1210/en.2013-1943
77. Smith JT, Cunningham MJ, Rissman EF, Clifton DK, Steiner RA. Regulation of Kiss1 gene expression in the brain of the female mouse. *Endocrinology* (2005) **146**:3686–92. doi:10.1210/en.2005-0488
78. Revel FG, Saboureau M, Masson-Pévet M, Pévet P, Mikkelsen JD, Simonneaux V. Kisspeptin mediates the photoperiodic control of reproduction in hamsters. *Curr Biol* (2006) **16**:1730–5. doi:10.1016/j.cub.2006.07.025
79. Greives TJ, Mason AO, Scotti M-AL, Levine J, Ketterson ED, Kriegsfeld LJ, et al. Environmental control of kisspeptin: implications for seasonal reproduction. *Endocrinology* (2007) **148**:1158–66. doi:10.1210/en.2006-1249
80. Gottsch ML, Navarro VM, Zhao Z, Glidewell-Kenney C, Weiss J, Jameson JL, et al. Regulation of Kiss1 and dynorphin gene expression in the murine brain by classical and nonclassical estrogen receptor pathways. *J Neurosci* (2009) **29**:9390–5. doi:10.1523/JNEUROSCI.0763-09.2009
81. Ansel L, Bolborea M, Bentsen AH, Klosen P, Mikkelsen JD, Simonneaux V. Differential regulation of kiss1 expression by melatonin and gonadal hormones in male and female Syrian hamsters. *J Biol Rhythms* (2010) **25**:81–91. doi:10.1177/0748730410361918
82. Adachi S, Yamada S, Takatsu Y, Matsui H, Kinoshita M, Takase K, et al. Involvement of anteroventral periventricular metastin/kisspeptin neurons in estrogen positive feedback action on luteinizing hormone release in female rats. *J Reprod Dev* (2007) **53**:367–78. doi:10.1262/jrd.18146
83. Hoffman GE, Le WW, Franceschini I, Caraty A, Advis JP. Expression of fos and in vivo median eminence release of LHRH identifies an active role for preoptic area kisspeptin neurons in synchronized surges of LH and LHRH in the ewe. *Endocrinology* (2011) **152**:214–22. doi:10.1210/en.2010-0066
84. Tomikawa J, Homma T, Tajima S, Shibata T, Inamoto Y, Takase K, et al. Molecular characterization and estrogen regulation of hypothalamic KISS1 gene in the pig. *Biol Reprod* (2010) **82**:313–9. doi:10.1095/biolreprod.109.079863
85. Huijbregts L, de Roux N. KISS1 is down-regulated by 17beta-estradiol in MDA-MB-231 cells through a nonclassical mechanism and loss of ribonucleic acid polymerase II binding at the proximal promoter. *Endocrinology* (2010) **151**:3764–72. doi:10.1210/en.2010-0260
86. Robertson JL, Clifton DK, de la Iglesia HO, Steiner RA, Kauffman AS. Circadian regulation of Kiss1 neurons: implications for timing the preovulatory gonadotropin-releasing hormone/luteinizing hormone surge. *Endocrinology* (2009) **150**:3664–71. doi:10.1210/en.2009-0247
87. Williams WP, Jarjisian SG, Mikkelsen JD, Kriegsfeld LJ. Circadian control of kisspeptin and a gated GnRH response mediate the preovulatory luteinizing hormone surge. *Endocrinology* (2011) **152**:595–606. doi:10.1210/en.2010-0943
88. Smarr BL, Gile JJ, de la Iglesia HO. Oestrogen-independent circadian clock gene expression in the anteroventral periventricular nucleus in female rats: possible role as an integrator for circadian and ovarian signals timing the luteinising hormone surge. *J Neuroendocrinol* (2013) **25**:1273–9. doi:10.1111/jne.12104
89. Vida B, Deli L, Hrabovszky E, Kalamatianos T, Caraty A, Coen CW, et al. Evidence for suprachiasmatic vasopressin neurones innervating kisspeptin neurones in the rostral periventricular area of the mouse brain: regulation by oestrogen. *J Neuroendocrinol* (2010) **22**:1032–9. doi:10.1111/j.1365-2826.2010.02045.x
90. Piet R, Fraissenon A, Boehm U, Herbison AE. Estrogen permits vasopressin signaling in preoptic kisspeptin neurons in the female mouse. *J Neurosci* (2015) **35**:6881–92. doi:10.1523/JNEUROSCI.4587-14.2015
91. Morin LP, Fitzgerald KM, Zucker I. Estradiol shortens the period of hamster circadian rhythms. *Science* (1977) **196**:305–7. doi:10.1126/science.557840
92. Takahashi JS, Menaker M. Interaction of estradiol and progesterone: effects on circadian locomotor rhythm of female golden hamsters. *Am J Physiol* (1980) **239**:R497–504.
93. Albers HE. Gonadal hormones organize and modulate the circadian system of the rat. *Am J Physiol* (1981) **241**:R62–6.
94. Bailey M, Silver R. Sex differences in circadian timing systems: implications for disease. *Front Neuroendocrinol* (2014) **35**:111–39. doi:10.1016/j.yfrne.2013.11.003
95. Kopp C, Ressel V, Wigger E, Tobler I. Influence of estrus cycle and ageing on activity patterns in two inbred mouse strains. *Behav Brain Res* (2006) **167**:165–74. doi:10.1016/j.bbr.2005.09.001
96. Royston SE, Yasui N, Kondilis AG, Lord SV, Katzenellenbogen JA, Mahoney MM. ESR1 and ESR2 differentially regulate daily and circadian activity rhythms in female mice. *Endocrinology* (2014) **155**:2613–23. doi:10.1210/en.2014-1101
97. Nakamura TJ, Shinohara K, Funabashi T, Kimura F. Effect of estrogen on the expression of Cry1 and Cry2 mRNAs in the suprachiasmatic nucleus of female rats. *Neurosci Res* (2001) **41**:251–5. doi:10.1016/S0168-0102(01)00285-1
98. Fatehi M, Fatehi-Hassanabad Z. Effects of 17beta-estradiol on neuronal cell excitability and neurotransmission in the suprachiasmatic nucleus of rat. *Neuropsychopharmacology* (2008) **33**:1354–64. doi:10.1038/sj.npp.1301523
99. Nakamura TJ, Sellix MT, Menaker M, Block GD. Estrogen directly modulates circadian rhythms of PER2 expression in the uterus. *Am J Physiol Endocrinol Metab* (2008) **295**:E1025–31. doi:10.1152/ajpendo.90392.2008
100. Ogawa S, Chan J, Gustafsson J-A, Korach KS, Pfaff DW. Estrogen increases locomotor activity in mice through estrogen receptor alpha: specificity for the type of activity. *Endocrinology* (2003) **144**:230–9. doi:10.1210/en.2002-220519
101. Krizo JA, Mintz EM. Sex differences in behavioral circadian rhythms in laboratory rodents. *Front Endocrinol* (2014) **5**:234. doi:10.3389/fendo.2014.00234
102. Clarke IJ, Cummins JT. Direct pituitary effects of estrogen and progesterone on gonadotropin secretion in the ovariectomized ewe. *Neuroendocrinology* (1984) **39**:267–74. doi:10.1159/000123990

103. Friend KE, Chiou YK, Lopes MB, Laws ER, Hughes KM, Shupnik MA. Estrogen receptor expression in human pituitary: correlation with immunohistochemistry in normal tissue, and immunohistochemistry and morphology in macroadenomas. *J Clin Endocrinol Metab* (1994) **78**:1497–504. doi:10.1210/jcem.78.6.7515390
104. Scully KM, Gleiberman AS, Lindzey J, Lubahn DB, Korach KS, Rosenfeld MG. Role of estrogen receptor-alpha in the anterior pituitary gland. *Mol Endocrinol* (1997) **11**:674–81. doi:10.1210/mend.11.6.0019
105. Clarke IJ, Cummins JT, Crowder ME, Nett TM. Long-term negative feedback effects of oestrogen and progesterone on the pituitary gland of the long-term ovariectomized ewe. *J Endocrinol* (1989) **120**:207–14. doi:10.1677/joe.0.1200207
106. Shaw ND, Histed SN, Srouji SS, Yang J, Lee H, Hall JE. Estrogen negative feedback on gonadotropin secretion: evidence for a direct pituitary effect in women. *J Clin Endocrinol Metab* (2010) **95**:1955–61. doi:10.1210/jc.2009-2108
107. Singh SP, Wolfe A, Ng Y, DiVall SA, Buggs C, Levine JE, et al. Impaired estrogen feedback and infertility in female mice with pituitary-specific deletion of estrogen receptor alpha (ESR1). *Biol Reprod* (2009) **81**:488–96. doi:10.1095/biolreprod.108.075259
108. Richard N, Galmiche G, Corvaisier S, Caraty A, Kottler M-L. KiSS-1 and GPR54 genes are co-expressed in rat gonadotrophs and differentially regulated in vivo by oestradiol and gonadotrophin-releasing hormone. *J Neuroendocrinol* (2008) **20**:381–93. doi:10.1111/j.1365-2826.2008.01653.x
109. Wang H, Masironi B, Eriksson H, Sahlin L. A comparative study of estrogen receptors alpha and beta in the rat uterus. *Biol Reprod* (1999) **61**:955–64. doi:10.1095/biolreprod61.4.955
110. Hamilton KJ, Arao Y, Korach KS. Estrogen hormone physiology: reproductive findings from estrogen receptor mutant mice. *Reprod Biol* (2014) **14**:3–8. doi:10.1016/j.repbio.2013.12.002
111. Lehman MN, Silver R, Gladstone WR, Kahn RM, Gibson M, Bittman EL. Circadian rhythmicity restored by neural transplant. Immunocytochemical characterization of the graft and its integration with the host brain. *J Neurosci* (1987) **7**:1626–38.
112. Ralph MR, Foster RG, Davis FC, Menaker M. Transplanted suprachiasmatic nucleus determines circadian period. *Science* (1990) **247**:975–8. doi:10.1126/science.2305266
113. Lowrey PL, Takahashi JS. Genetics of circadian rhythms in Mammalian model organisms. *Adv Genet* (2011) **74**:175–230. doi:10.1016/B978-0-12-387690-4.00006-4
114. Albrecht U, Eichele G. The mammalian circadian clock. *Curr Opin Genet Dev* (2003) **13**:271–7. doi:10.1016/S0959-437X(03)00055-8
115. Yoo S-H, Yamazaki S, Lowrey PL, Shimomura K, Ko CH, Buhr ED, et al. PERIOD2:LUCIFERASE real-time reporting of circadian dynamics reveals persistent circadian oscillations in mouse peripheral tissues. *Proc Natl Acad Sci U S A* (2004) **101**:5339–46. doi:10.1073/pnas.0308709101
116. Yoo S-H, Ko CH, Lowrey PL, Buhr ED, Song E, Chang S, et al. A noncanonical E-box enhancer drives mouse Period2 circadian oscillations in vivo. *Proc Natl Acad Sci U S A* (2005) **102**:2608–13. doi:10.1073/pnas.0409763102
117. Berson DM, Dunn FA, Takao M. Phototransduction by retinal ganglion cells that set the circadian clock. *Science* (2002) **295**:1070–3. doi:10.1126/science.1067262
118. Provencio I, Rollag MD, Castrucci AM. Photoreceptive net in the mammalian retina. This mesh of cells may explain how some blind mice can still tell day from night. *Nature* (2002) **415**:493. doi:10.1038/415493a
119. Jin X, Shearman LP, Weaver DR, Zylka MJ, de Vries GJ, Reppert SM. A molecular mechanism regulating rhythmic output from the suprachiasmatic circadian clock. *Cell* (1999) **96**:57–68. doi:10.1016/S0092-8674(00)80959-9
120. Miller G. Neurobiology. Despite mutated gene, mouse circadian clock keeps on ticking. *Science* (2006) **312**:673. doi:10.1126/science.312.5774.673
121. Brown-Grant K, Raisman G. Abnormalities in reproductive function associated with the destruction of the suprachiasmatic nuclei in female rats. *Proc R Soc Lond B Biol Sci* (1977) **198**:279–96. doi:10.1098/rspb.1977.0098
122. Wiegand SJ, Terasawa E, Bridson WE, Goy RW. Effects of discrete lesions of preoptic and suprachiasmatic structures in the female rat. Alterations in the feedback regulation of gonadotropin secretion. *Neuroendocrinology* (1980) **31**:147–57. doi:10.1159/000123066
123. Van der Horst GT, Muijtjens M, Kobayashi K, Takano R, Kanno S, Takao M, et al. Mammalian Cry1 and Cry2 are essential for maintenance of circadian rhythms. *Nature* (1999) **398**:627–30. doi:10.1038/19323
124. Miller BH, Olson SL, Turek FW, Levine JE, Horton TH, Takahashi JS. Circadian clock mutation disrupts estrous cyclicity and maintenance of pregnancy. *Curr Biol* (2004) **14**:1367–73. doi:10.1016/j.cub.2004.07.055
125. Dolatshad H, Campbell EA, O'Hara L, Maywood ES, Hastings MH, Johnson MH. Developmental and reproductive performance in circadian mutant mice. *Hum Reprod* (2006) **21**:68–79. doi:10.1093/humrep/dei313
126. Ratajczak CK, Boehle KL, Muglia LJ. Impaired steroidogenesis and implantation failure in Bmal1-/- mice. *Endocrinology* (2009) **150**:1879–85. doi:10.1210/en.2008-1021
127. Chu A, Zhu L, Blum ID, Mai O, Leliavski A, Fahrenkrug J, et al. Global but not gonadotrope-specific disruption of Bmal1 abolishes the luteinizing hormone surge without affecting ovulation. *Endocrinology* (2013) **154**:2924–35. doi:10.1210/en.2013-1080
128. Kovanen L, Saarikoski ST, Aromaa A, Lönnqvist J, Partonen T. ARNTL (BMAL1) and NPAS2 gene variants contribute to fertility and seasonality. *PLoS One* (2010) **5**:e10007. doi:10.1371/journal.pone.0010007
129. Pilorz V, Steinlechner S. Low reproductive success in Per1 and Per2 mutant mouse females due to accelerated ageing? *Reproduction* (2008) **135**:559–68. doi:10.1530/REP-07-0434
130. Miller BH, Takahashi JS. Central circadian control of female reproductive function. *Front Endocrinol* (2013) **4**:195. doi:10.3389/fendo.2013.00195
131. Legan SJ, Coon GA, Karsch FJ. Role of estrogen as initiator of daily LH surges in the ovariectomized rat. *Endocrinology* (1975) **96**:50–6. doi:10.1210/endo-96-1-50
132. Silver R, LeSauter J, Tresco PA, Lehman MN. A diffusible coupling signal from the transplanted suprachiasmatic nucleus controlling circadian locomotor rhythms. *Nature* (1996) **382**:810–3. doi:10.1038/382810a0
133. Van der Beek EM, Horvath TL, Wiegant VM, Van den Hurk R, Buijs RM. Evidence for a direct neuronal pathway from the suprachiasmatic nucleus to the gonadotropin-releasing hormone system: combined tracing and light and electron microscopic immunocytochemical studies. *J Comp Neurol* (1997) **384**:569–79. doi:10.1002/(SICI)1096-9861(19970811)384:4<569::AID-CNE6>3.0.CO;2-0
134. Horvath TL, Cela V, van der Beek EM. Gender-specific apposition between vasoactive intestinal peptide-containing axons and gonadotrophin-releasing hormone-producing neurons in the rat. *Brain Res* (1998) **795**:277–81. doi:10.1016/S0006-8993(98)00208-X
135. Smith MJ, Jiennes L, Wise PM. Localization of the VIP2 receptor protein on GnRH neurons in the female rat. *Endocrinology* (2000) **141**:4317–20. doi:10.1210/endo.141.11.7876
136. Kalsbeek A, Buijs RM, Engelmann M, Wotjak CT, Landgraf R. In vivo measurement of a diurnal variation in vasopressin release in the rat suprachiasmatic nucleus. *Brain Res* (1995) **682**:75–82. doi:10.1016/0006-8993(95)00324-J
137. Funabashi T, Aiba S, Sano A, Shinohara K, Kimura F. Intracerebroventricular injection of arginine-vasopressin V1 receptor antagonist attenuates the surge of luteinizing hormone and prolactin secretion in proestrous rats. *Neurosci Lett* (1999) **260**:37–40. doi:10.1016/S0304-3940(98)00940-9
138. Palm IF, Van Der Beek EM, Wiegant VM, Buijs RM, Kalsbeek A. Vasopressin induces a luteinizing hormone surge in ovariectomized, estradiol-treated rats with lesions of the suprachiasmatic nucleus. *Neuroscience* (1999) **93**:659–66. doi:10.1016/S0306-4522(99)00106-2
139. Funabashi T, Shinohara K, Mitsushima D, Kimura F. Gonadotropin-releasing hormone exhibits circadian rhythm in phase with arginine-vasopressin in co-cultures of the female rat preoptic area and suprachiasmatic nucleus. *J Neuroendocrinol* (2000) **12**:521–8. doi:10.1046/j.1365-2826.2000.00481.x
140. Van der Beek EM, Swarts HJ, Wiegant VM. Central administration of antiserum to vasoactive intestinal peptide delays and reduces luteinizing hormone and prolactin surges in ovariectomized, estrogen-treated rats. *Neuroendocrinology* (1999) **69**:227–37. doi:10.1159/000054423
141. Sun Y, Shu J, Kyei K, Neal-Perry GS. Intracerebroventricular infusion of vasoactive intestinal Peptide rescues the luteinizing hormone surge in middle-aged female rats. *Front Endocrinol* (2012) **3**:24. doi:10.3389/fendo.2012.00024
142. Christian CA, Moenter SM. Critical roles for fast synaptic transmission in mediating estradiol negative and positive feedback in the neural control of ovulation. *Endocrinology* (2008) **149**:5500–8. doi:10.1210/en.2008-0453

143. Russo KA, La JL, Stephens SBZ, Poling MC, Padgaonkar NA, Jennings KJ, et al. Circadian control of the female reproductive axis through gated responsiveness of the RFRP-3 system to VIP signaling. *Endocrinology* (2015) **156**:2608–18. doi:10.1210/en.2014-1762
144. Menaker M, Murphy ZC, Sellix MT. Central control of peripheral circadian oscillators. *Curr Opin Neurobiol* (2013) **23**:741–6. doi:10.1016/j.conb.2013.03.003
145. Abe M, Herzog ED, Yamazaki S, Straume M, Tei H, Sakaki Y, et al. Circadian rhythms in isolated brain regions. *J Neurosci* (2002) **22**:350–6.
146. Kalsbeek A, Fliers E, Hofman MA, Swaab DF, Buijs RM. Vasopressin and the output of the hypothalamic biological clock. *J Neuroendocrinol* (2010) **22**:362–72. doi:10.1111/j.1365-2826.2010.01956.x
147. Resuehr D, Wildemann U, Sikes H, Olcese J. E-box regulation of gonadotropin-releasing hormone (GnRH) receptor expression in immortalized gonadotrope cells. *Mol Cell Endocrinol* (2007) **278**:36–43. doi:10.1016/j.mce.2007.08.008
148. Xu Z, Kaga S, Tsubomizu J, Fujisaki J, Mochiduki A, Sakai T, et al. Circadian transcriptional factor DBP regulates expression of Kiss1 in the anteroventral periventricular nucleus. *Mol Cell Endocrinol* (2011) **339**:90–7. doi:10.1016/j.mce.2011.03.020
149. Chappell PE, White RS, Mellon PL. Circadian gene expression regulates pulsatile gonadotropin-releasing hormone (GnRH) secretory patterns in the hypothalamic GnRH-secreting GT1-7 cell line. *J Neurosci* (2003) **23**:11202–13.
150. Gillespie JMA, Chan BPK, Roy D, Cai F, Belsham DD. Expression of circadian rhythm genes in gonadotropin-releasing hormone-secreting GT1-7 neurons. *Endocrinology* (2003) **144**:5285–92. doi:10.1210/en.2003-0802
151. Zhao S, Kriegsfeld LJ. Daily changes in GT1-7 cell sensitivity to GnRH secretagogues that trigger ovulation. *Neuroendocrinology* (2009) **89**:448–57. doi:10.1159/000192370
152. Hickok JR, Tischkau SA. In vivo circadian rhythms in gonadotropin-releasing hormone neurons. *Neuroendocrinology* (2010) **91**:110–20. doi:10.1159/000243163
153. Christian CA, Moenter SM. Estradiol induces diurnal shifts in GABA transmission to gonadotropin-releasing hormone neurons to provide a neural signal for ovulation. *J Neurosci* (2007) **27**:1913–21. doi:10.1523/JNEUROSCI.4738-06.2007
154. Roa J, Castellano JM, Navarro VM, Handelsman DJ, Pinilla L, Tena-Sempere M. Kisspeptins and the control of gonadotropin secretion in male and female rodents. *Peptides* (2009) **30**:57–66. doi:10.1016/j.peptides.2008.08.009
155. Neal-Perry G, Lebesgue D, Lederman M, Shu J, Zeevalk GD, Etgen AM. The excitatory peptide kisspeptin restores the luteinizing hormone surge and modulates amino acid neurotransmission in the medial preoptic area of middle-aged rats. *Endocrinology* (2009) **150**:3699–708. doi:10.1210/en.2008-1667
156. Bur IM, Cohen-Solal AM, Carmignac D, Abecassis P-Y, Chauvet N, Martin AO, et al. The circadian clock components CRY1 and CRY2 are necessary to sustain sex dimorphism in mouse liver metabolism. *J Biol Chem* (2009) **284**:9066–73. doi:10.1074/jbc.M808360200
157. Olcese J, Sikes HE, Resuehr D. Induction of PER1 mRNA expression in immortalized gonadotropes by gonadotropin-releasing hormone (GnRH): involvement of protein kinase C and MAP kinase signaling. *Chronobiol Int* (2006) **23**:143–50. doi:10.1080/07420520500521996
158. Fahrenkrug J, Georg B, Hannibal J, Hindersson P, Gräs S. Diurnal rhythmicity of the clock genes Per1 and Per2 in the rat ovary. *Endocrinology* (2006) **147**:3769–76. doi:10.1210/en.2006-0305
159. Karman BN, Tischkau SA. Circadian clock gene expression in the ovary: effects of luteinizing hormone. *Biol Reprod* (2006) **75**:624–32. doi:10.1095/biolreprod.106.050732
160. Yoshikawa T, Sellix M, Pezuk P, Menaker M. Timing of the ovarian circadian clock is regulated by gonadotropins. *Endocrinology* (2009) **150**:4338–47. doi:10.1210/en.2008-1280
161. Sellix MT. Clocks underneath: the role of peripheral clocks in the timing of female reproductive physiology. *Front Endocrinol* (2013) **4**:91. doi:10.3389/fendo.2013.00091
162. Sellix MT. Circadian clock function in the mammalian ovary. *J Biol Rhythms* (2015) **30**:7–19. doi:10.1177/0748730414554222
163. Chen H, Zhao L, Kumazawa M, Yamauchi N, Shigeyoshi Y, Hashimoto S, et al. Downregulation of core clock gene Bmal1 attenuates expression of progesterone and prostaglandin biosynthesis-related genes in rat luteinizing granulosa cells. *Am J Physiol Cell Physiol* (2013) **304**:C1131–40. doi:10.1152/ajpcell.00008.2013
164. He P-J, Hirata M, Yamauchi N, Hashimoto S, Hattori M-A. Gonadotropic regulation of circadian clockwork in rat granulosa cells. *Mol Cell Biochem* (2007) **302**:111–8. doi:10.1007/s11010-007-9432-7
165. Liu Y, Johnson BP, Shen AL, Wallisser JA, Krentz KJ, Moran SM, et al. Loss of BMAL1 in ovarian steroidogenic cells results in implantation failure in female mice. *Proc Natl Acad Sci U S A* (2014) **111**:14295–300. doi:10.1073/pnas.1209249111
166. Ratajczak CK, Herzog ED, Muglia LJ. Clock gene expression in gravid uterus and extra-embryonic tissues during late gestation in the mouse. *Reprod Fertil Dev* (2010) **22**:743–50. doi:10.1071/RD09243
167. Johnson MH, Lim A, Fernando D, Day ML. Circadian clockwork genes are expressed in the reproductive tract and conceptus of the early pregnant mouse. *Reprod Biomed Online* (2002) **4**:140–5. doi:10.1016/S1472-6483(10)61931-1
168. Kennaway DJ, Varcoe TJ, Mau VJ. Rhythmic expression of clock and clock-controlled genes in the rat oviduct. *Mol Hum Reprod* (2003) **9**:503–7. doi:10.1093/molehr/gag067
169. Akiyama S, Ohta H, Watanabe S, Moriya T, Hariu A, Nakahata N, et al. The uterus sustains stable biological clock during pregnancy. *Tohoku J Exp Med* (2010) **221**:287–98. doi:10.1620/tjem.221.287
170. Ratajczak CK, Asada M, Allen GC, McMahon DG, Muglia LM, Smith D, et al. Generation of myometrium-specific Bmal1 knockout mice for parturition analysis. *Reprod Fertil Dev* (2012) **24**:759–67. doi:10.1071/RD11164
171. Pati A, Chandrawanshi A, Reinberg A. Shift work: consequences and management. *Curr Sci* (2001) **81**:32–52.
172. Boivin DB, Tremblay GM, James FO. Working on atypical schedules. *Sleep Med* (2007) **8**:578–89. doi:10.1016/j.sleep.2007.03.015
173. Chen J-D, Lin Y-C, Hsiao S-T. Obesity and high blood pressure of 12-hour night shift female clean-room workers. *Chronobiol Int* (2010) **27**:334–44. doi:10.3109/07420520903502242
174. Matheson A, O'Brien L, Reid J-A. The impact of shiftwork on health: a literature review. *J Clin Nurs* (2014) **23**:3309–20. doi:10.1111/jocn.12524
175. Lawson CC, Whelan EA, Lividoti Hibert EN, Spiegelman D, Schernhammer ES, Rich-Edwards JW. Rotating shift work and menstrual cycle characteristics. *Epidemiology* (2011) **22**:305–12. doi:10.1097/EDE.0b013e3182130016
176. Rocheleau CM, Lawson CC, Whelan EA, Rich-Edwards JW. Shift work and adverse pregnancy outcomes: comments on a recent meta-analysis. *BJOG* (2012) **119**:378. doi:10.1111/j.1471-0528.2011.03211.x author reply 379–80,
177. Gamble KL, Resuehr D, Johnson CH. Shift work and circadian dysregulation of reproduction. *Front Endocrinol* (2013) **4**:92. doi:10.3389/fendo.2013.00092
178. Bracci M, Manzella N, Copertaro A, Staffolani S, Strafella E, Barbaresi M, et al. Rotating-shift nurses after a day off: peripheral clock gene expression, urinary melatonin, and serum 17-β-estradiol levels. *Scand J Work Environ Health* (2014) **40**:295–304. doi:10.5271/sjweh.3414
179. Torres-Farfan C, Mendez N, Abarzua-Catalan L, Vilches N, Valenzuela GJ, Seron-Ferre M. A circadian clock entrained by melatonin is ticking in the rat fetal adrenal. *Endocrinology* (2011) **152**:1891–900. doi:10.1210/en.2010-1260
180. Klenov VE, Jungheim ES. Obesity and reproductive function: a review of the evidence. *Curr Opin Obstet Gynecol* (2014) **26**:455–60. doi:10.1097/GCO.0000000000000113
181. Shaw ND, Goodwin JL, Silva GE, Hall JE, Quan SF, Malhotra A. Obstructive sleep apnea (OSA) in preadolescent girls is associated with delayed breast development compared to girls without OSA. *J Clin Sleep Med* (2013) **9**:813–8. doi:10.5664/jcsm.2928
182. Opperhuizen A-L, van Kerkhof LWM, Proper KI, Rodenburg W, Kalsbeek A. Rodent models to study the metabolic effects of shiftwork in humans. *Front Pharmacol* (2015) **6**:50. doi:10.3389/fphar.2015.00050
183. Moline ML, Albers HE. Response of circadian locomotor activity and the proestrous luteinizing hormone surge to phase shifts of the light-dark cycle in the hamster. *Physiol Behav* (1988) **43**:435–40. doi:10.1016/0031-9384(88)90116-3
184. Summa KC, Vitaterna MH, Turek FW. Environmental perturbation of the circadian clock disrupts pregnancy in the mouse. *PLoS One* (2012) **7**:e37668. doi:10.1371/journal.pone.0037668

185. Yamazaki S, Numano R, Abe M, Hida A, Takahashi R, Ueda M, et al. Resetting central and peripheral circadian oscillators in transgenic rats. *Science* (2000) **288**:682–5. doi:10.1126/science.288.5466.682
186. Lohstroh PN, Chen J, Ba J, Ryan LM, Xu X, Overstreet JW, et al. Bone resorption is affected by follicular phase length in female rotating shift workers. *Environ Health Perspect* (2003) **111**:618–22. doi:10.1289/ehp.5878
187. Zhu JL, Hjollund NH, Boggild H, Olsen J. Shift work and subfecundity: a causal link or an artefact? *Occup Environ Med* (2003) **60**:E12. doi:10.1136/oem.60.9.e12
188. Hatch MC, Figa-Talamanca I, Salerno S. Work stress and menstrual patterns among American and Italian nurses. *Scand J Work Environ Health* (1999) **25**:144–50. doi:10.5271/sjweh.417
189. Ahlborg G, Axelsson G, Bodin L. Shift work, nitrous oxide exposure and subfertility among Swedish midwives. *Int J Epidemiol* (1996) **25**:783–90. doi:10.1093/ije/25.4.783
190. Miyauchi F, Nanjo K, Otsuka K. Effects of night shift on plasma concentrations of melatonin, LH, FSH and prolactin, and menstrual irregularity. *Sangyo Igaku* (1992) **34**:545–50. doi:10.1539/joh1959.34.545
191. Messing K, Saurel-Cubizolles MJ, Bourgine M, Kaminski M. Menstrual-cycle characteristics and work conditions of workers in poultry slaughterhouses and canneries. *Scand J Work Environ Health* (1992) **18**:302–9. doi:10.5271/sjweh.1572
192. Attarchi M, Darkhi H, Khodarahmian M, Dolati M, Kashanian M, Ghaffari M, et al. Characteristics of menstrual cycle in shift workers. *Glob J Health Sci* (2013) **5**:163–72. doi:10.5539/gjhs.v5n3p163
193. Davis S, Mirick DK, Chen C, Stanczyk FZ. Night shift work and hormone levels in women. *Cancer Epidemiol Biomarkers Prev* (2012) **21**:609–18. doi:10.1158/1055-9965.EPI-11-1128
194. Wan G-H, Chung F-F. Working conditions associated with ovarian cycle in a medical center nurses: a Taiwan study. *Jpn J Nurs Sci* (2012) **9**:112–8. doi:10.1111/j.1742-7924.2011.00191.x
195. Labyak S, Lava S, Turek F, Zee P. Effects of shiftwork on sleep and menstrual function in nurses. *Health Care Women Int* (2002) **23**:703–14. doi:10.1080/07399330290107449
196. Chung F-F, Yao C-CC, Wan G-H. The associations between menstrual function and life style/working conditions among nurses in Taiwan. *J Occup Health* (2005) **47**:149–56. doi:10.1539/joh.47.149
197. Stocker LJ, Macklon NS, Cheong YC, Bewley SJ. Influence of shift work on early reproductive outcomes: a systematic review and meta-analysis. *Obstet Gynecol* (2014) **124**:99–110. doi:10.1097/AOG.0000000000000321
198. Olsen J. Cigarette smoking, tea and coffee drinking, and subfecundity. *Am J Epidemiol* (1991) **133**:734–9.
199. Spinelli A, Figà-Talamanca I, Osborn J. Time to pregnancy and occupation in a group of Italian women. *Int J Epidemiol* (1997) **26**:601–9. doi:10.1093/ije/26.3.601
200. Tuntiseranee P, Olsen J, Geater A, Kor-anantakul O. Are long working hours and shiftwork risk factors for subfecundity? A study among couples from southern Thailand. *Occup Environ Med* (1998) **55**:99–105. doi:10.1136/oem.55.2.99
201. Gómez-Acebo I, Dierssen-Sotos T, Papantoniou K, García-Unzueta MT, Santos-Benito MF, Llorca J. Association between exposure to rotating night shift versus day shift using levels of 6-sulfatoxymelatonin and cortisol and other sex hormones in women. *Chronobiol Int* (2014) **32**:128–35. doi:10.3109/07420528.2014.958494
202. Alvarez-García V, González A, Martínez-Campa C, Alonso-González C, Cos S. Melatonin modulates aromatase activity and expression in endothelial cells. *Oncol Rep* (2013) **29**:2058–64. doi:10.3892/or.2013.2314
203. Cos S, Martínez-Campa C, Mediavilla MD, Sánchez-Barceló EJ. Melatonin modulates aromatase activity in MCF-7 human breast cancer cells. *J Pineal Res* (2005) **38**:136–42. doi:10.1111/j.1600-079X.2004.00186.x
204. Papantoniou K, Pozo OJ, Espinosa A, Marcos J, Castaño-Vinyals G, Basagaña X, et al. Increased and mistimed sex hormone production in night shift workers. *Cancer Epidemiol Biomarkers Prev* (2015) **24**:854–63. doi:10.1158/1055-9965.EPI-14-1271
205. Hill SM, Belancio VP, Dauchy RT, Xiang S, Brimer S, Mao L, et al. Melatonin: an inhibitor of breast cancer. *Endocr Relat Cancer* (2015) **22**:R183–204. doi:10.1530/ERC-15-0030
206. Gold EB, Tomich E. Occupational hazards to fertility and pregnancy outcome. *Occup Med* (1994) **9**:435–69.
207. Weinberg CR, Baird DD, Wilcox AJ. Sources of bias in studies of time to pregnancy. *Stat Med* (1994) **13**:671–81. doi:10.1002/sim.4780130528
208. Axelsson G, Ahlborg G, Bodin L. Shift work, nitrous oxide exposure, and spontaneous abortion among Swedish midwives. *Occup Environ Med* (1996) **53**:374–8. doi:10.1136/oem.53.6.374
209. Bonde JP, Jørgensen KT, Bonzini M, Palmer KT. Miscarriage and occupational activity: a systematic review and meta-analysis regarding shift work, working hours, lifting, standing, and physical workload. *Scand J Work Environ Health* (2013) **39**:325–34. doi:10.5271/sjweh.3337

9

A crab is not a fish: Unique aspects of the crustacean endocrine system and considerations for endocrine toxicology

Thomas Knigge[1], Gerald A. LeBlanc[2] and Alex T. Ford[3]*

[1] Normandy University, FR CNRS 3730 SCALE, UMR-I 02 INERIS-URCA-ULH Environmental Stress and Aquatic Biomonitoring (SEBIO), Université Le Havre Normandie, Le Havre, France, [2] Department of Biological Sciences, North Carolina State University, Raleigh, NC, United States, [3] School of Biological Sciences, Institute of Marine Sciences, University of Portsmouth, Portsmouth, United Kingdom

Edited by:
Heinrich Dircksen, Stockholm University, Sweden

Reviewed by:
Taisen Iguchi, National Institute for Basic Biology, Japan
Lynn M. Riddiford, University of Washington, United States

***Correspondence:**
Thomas Knigge
thomas.knigge@univ-lehavre.fr

Crustaceans—and arthropods in general—exhibit many unique aspects to their physiology. These include the requirement to moult (ecdysis) in order to grow and reproduce, the ability to change color, and multiple strategies for sexual differentiation. Accordingly, the endocrine regulation of these processes involves hormones, receptors, and enzymes that differ from those utilized by vertebrates and other non-arthropod invertebrates. As a result, environmental chemicals known to disrupt endocrine processes in vertebrates are often not endocrine disruptors in crustaceans; while, chemicals that disrupt endocrine processes in crustaceans are often not endocrine disruptors in vertebrates. In this review, we present an overview of the evolution of the endocrine system of crustaceans, highlight endocrine endpoints known to be a target of disruption by chemicals, and identify other components of endocrine signaling that may prove to be targets of disruption. This review highlights that crustaceans need to be evaluated for endocrine disruption with consideration of their unique endocrine system and not with consideration of the endocrine system of vertebrates.

Keywords: endocrine disruption, neuroendocrine disruption, ecdysteroid signaling, color change, sexual differentiation

---

Abbreviations: AG, androgenic gland; AGH, androgenic gland hormone; CCAP, crustacean cardioactive peptide; CHH, crustacean hyperglycemic hormone; Cyp19, aromatase; EcR, ecdysone receptor; EDC, endocrine disrupting chemical; EH, eclosion hormone; ETH, ecdysis triggering hormone; FAMeT, farnesoic-O-methyl transferase; HMGCR, 3-hydroxy-3methyl-glutaryl coenzyme A reductase; IAG, insulin-like androgenic gland factor; MET, methoprene tolerant; MF, methyl farnesoate; MfR, methyl farnesoate receptor; MIH, moult inhibiting hormone; NE, norepinephrine; NMDAR, N-methyl-D-aspartate receptor; PCBs, polychlorinated biphenyls; PDH, pigment dispersing hormone; PoA, ponasterone; RPCH, red pigment concentrating hormone; RPCHR, red pigment concentrating hormone receptor; RNAi, RNA interference; RXR, retinoid-X-receptor; SRC, steroid receptor coactivator; US EPA, United States Environmental Protection Agency; XO/SG, X-organ/sinus gland; 5-HT, 5-hydroxytryptamine, serotonin; 20E, 20-hydroxyecdysone.

INTRODUCTION

Over the last two decades, both the scientific community and the lay public have become increasingly aware of the risk associated with endocrine disruption. Environmental authorities in Europe, the United States and many other countries are preoccupied with the identification of Endocrine Disrupting Chemicals (EDCs) and their effects on human health and wildlife. In 2012, a report on the state of endocrine disruption was composed under the auspices of the United Nations Environment Program (UNEP) and the World Health Organization (WHO). This report stated that in spite of numerous reports of reproductive disorders, skewed sex ratios and intersex phenomena, the understanding of endocrine disruption in invertebrates—including crustaceans—was limited (1). Since then some progress has been made, but knowledge about the effects of EDCs on the endocrine system of crustaceans remains scarce and concerns mainly pesticides designed to disrupt moulting in insects (2, 3). Among the vast array of chemical compounds listed on the Toxic Substances Control Act (TSCA) inventory (US EPA)—and many others not regulated under the TSCA—there will certainly be many other chemicals that have the potential to interfere with the crustacean endocrine system.

With about 68,000 extant species of crustaceans described—and still more to be discovered—these predominantly aquatic invertebrates form a large and very diverse arthropod taxon (4–6). As predators, scavengers, or filter feeders, they take important positions within the aquatic ecosystems at various levels of the food web. They also provide high-value fishery products and contribute with over 14 million tons—of which half are wild stock captures—to about 8% of the worldwide seafood resources (7).

This ecological and economical wealth is, however, endangered by habitat loss, climate change, pollution, overexploitation, invasive species and other anthropogenic stressors (8). In the early nineties, drastic declines of amphipods were reported in some of the Great Lakes (9, 10). Similarly, populations of the amphipod *Gammarus lacustris* significantly declined in the Selenga River delta, the main tributary to Lake Baikal (11). Although pollution, such as polychlorinated biphenyls (PCBs) or pulp mill effluents, respectively, were given consideration, the actual cause-effect relationships were complex and difficult to establish. Massive decreases in blue crab populations of Chesapeake Bay occurred in the nineties, where spawning stock abundance declined by about 80% (12). Similarly, catches of the edible crab, *Cancer pagurus*, in the English Channel were halved from 2012 to 2018 with no clear cause for this decline (13). Even if overfishing, increasing temperatures, and ocean acidification are contributing causes, reproduction impairment due to endocrine disruption could be adding to the declines, or hampering the recovery of stocks. A contribution of EDCs in these declines of marine and freshwater crustaceans is difficult to discern. Firstly, it is generally challenging to determine the quantitative contribution of individual challenges to population sustainability. Secondly, it is difficult to identify endocrine disruption without knowing how to measure it. In any case, no prominent example of endocrine disruption, comparable to imposex in prosobranch gastropods, is known for crustaceans. Examples of intersex that appear to be related to pollution have been reported for different crustacean species (14–19). But no cause-effect relationships have been established.

The assessment of endocrine disruption in crustaceans can be approached either from the perspective of the molecules suspected to cause endocrine disruption, *i.e.*, effects of established EDCs, or from the perspective of the endocrine targets of EDCs, *i.e.*, crustacean endocrinology. Environmental chemicals that have been classified as EDCs, are, for the most part, compounds that interfere with the vertebrate hormone system. Strenuous effort has been made to demonstrate possible endocrine disrupting effects of such EDCs in crustaceans (20–30). Although effects on growth and reproduction are often reported, most studies failed to demonstrate that endocrine mechanisms were involved. The generally high concentrations that are necessary to produce negative consequences for growth or reproduction suggest that the observed effects were merely a result of overt toxicity (*e.g.*, (31, 32). More specific assays are being developed that use elements of the crustacean endocrine system, such as reporter assays for the ecdysteroid and methyl farnesoate receptors, measurement of 20-hydroxyecdysone (20E) titers, or assays for chitobiase activity (33–38). Nevertheless, establishing reliable testing protocols for endocrine disruption in crustaceans remains challenging and widely ignores the importance of neurohormonal regulation for the control of many physiological functions in crustaceans.

This review argues in favor of a more arthropod specific approach to endocrine disruption in crustaceans.

EVOLUTION OF THE INVERTEBRATE ENDOCRINE SYSTEM

Endocrine systems are key features of evolution reflecting metazoan diversification (39). Metazoan endocrine systems have evolved from a common bilaterian ancestor before the divergence of protostomes and deuterostomes more than 600 million years ago (40, 41). Specialized neurosecretory cells were already present in the pre-bilaterian cnidarians and neurohormonal signaling persists as a major endocrine component in both, the protostome and deuterostome lineages (42–44). The arthropods diverged within the protostome lineage some 500 million years ago (45). Unique aspects to the physiology of the arthropods, including crustaceans, required the development of unique endocrine pathways to regulate these physiological processes. For example, arthropods lost the capacity to synthesize cholesterol (41, 46). This loss of cholesterol synthesis may have limited opportunities for the evolution of steroid hormones, which utilize cholesterol as a precursor. However, this loss may have also promoted the evolution of methyl farnesoate (MF) in crustaceans and juvenile hormone in insects, which do not utilize cholesterol, into functional hormones (41). The divergence of the arthropod endocrine system has been deepened further by the evolution of an exoskeleton in arthropods, which requires moulting for growth and reproduction (47). Endocrine signaling processes were required to regulate moulting and coordinate this process with those operative in growth and reproduction.

While the endocrine systems of the two major arthropod taxons, crustaceans and insects, share many commonalities, divergences also occurred. For example, both groups possess the capacity to produce MF. However, insects possess a cytochrome P450 monooxygenase, which epoxidates MF to form juvenile hormone III (48). This latter hormone regulates many of the processes in insects that are under the control of methyl farnesoate in crustaceans. Crustaceans produce a family of hormones known as crustacean hyperglycemic hormones (CHHs) (49, 50). These hormones regulate a myriad of processes including aspects of moulting, reproduction, and energy generation. Only a single member of this family, the ion transport peptide, is known to exist in insects. This insect hormone controls ion transport (51, 52).

The presence or absence of nuclear receptors, *i.e.*, ligand-regulated transcription factors, reflects the separation of steroid hormone signaling within the endocrine systems of crustaceans and vertebrates. The evolution of these receptors was shaped by whole genome duplications and losses combined with the evolution of neofunctionalization or subfunctionalization among duplicate receptors (39, 53–55). Importantly, arthropods lack receptors of the steroid receptor subfamily 3, which include the estrogen and androgen receptors. This may represent the loss of the progenitor of this subfamily (56, 57). However, subfamily 3 receptors are also absent in the ascidian *Cionia intestinalis*, a deuterostome invertebrate distantly related to vertebrates (55, 58). This latter observation suggests that subfamily 3 nuclear receptors evolved later in chordate evolution, long after protostomes and deuterostomes diverged (59, 60). This hypothesis is supported by the appearance of sex steroid receptors, including the estrogen receptor, in the cephalochordate *Amphioxus* (61, 62). The ecdysteroid receptor (EcR) of arthropods does not belong to the subfamily 3 nuclear receptors, but is an ortholog of the vertebrate liver X and farnesoid X receptors, which are members of the subfamily 1 nuclear receptors (63).

The loss and gain of functions and elements of the endocrine system, such as nuclear receptors or neuropeptide hormones in arthropods is likely to be related to the invention of a new body plan with an exoskeleton (64). The exoskeleton constrains growth and the impermeable cuticle limits gas and ion exchange with the environment. Moulting solves the first problem, while the second problem requires organs for gas (and ion) exchange, such as the gills in crustaceans or the tracheae in insects, both of which have similar organogenetic origins. Sanchez-Higueras et al. (65), demonstrated that trachea develop as serial homologues to the ectodermal prothoracic gland and the *corpora allata*, which have their counterparts in the Y-organ and the mandibular organ of crustaceans (see also (43)). These endocrine glands produce ecdysone and juvenile hormone/MF, respectively, *i.e.*, insect/crustacean hormones related to moulting and metamorphosis. Hence, these findings link the evolution of arthropod hormones and endocrine organs with the evolutionary innovation of an exoskeleton. As a matter of consequence, the homology of endocrine organs and gills provides evidence for the integration of environmental cues into physiological responses, such as respiration, osmoregulation and growth by an endocrine system specific to arthropods.

Crustaceans and vertebrates share the principal concept of connecting neural, neurosecretory, and endocrine components (58). Yet, the endocrine systems of arthropods and vertebrates have evolved independently and differently since more than 540 million years ago when crustaceans and deuterostomes appeared in the early Cambrian (66, 67). As a matter of consequence, they have little in common. The fundamental difference between arthropod and vertebrate endocrine systems has implications for determining endocrine disruption. Exogenous substances that alter functions of the endocrine system are, for the most part, likely to be different for crustaceans and vertebrates. Substances designed to interfere with the insect endocrine system (*i.e.*, insect growth regulating insecticides) by their design have significant potential to interfere with the crustacean endocrine system, but are much less likely to interfere with the endocrine system of vertebrates. Conversely, steroid hormone functional analogs are highly likely to disrupt endocrine regulated processes in vertebrates, but are much less likely to disrupt endocrine signaling in crustaceans. The most conserved elements associated with the endocrine regulation of physiological functions shared by both, arthropods and vertebrates are the upstream control of neurosecretory processes by biogenic amines. Besides their function as neurotransmitters and neuromodulators, biogenic amines, such as serotonin, can also serve as neurohormones circulating in the blood stream and affecting peripheral organs like ovaries.

ENDOCRINE REGULATION OF MOULTING

The monophyly of arthropods is based on a sclerotized exoskeleton (68). To allow for growth, the cuticle has to be shed and renewed periodically. Moulting, *i.e.*, ecdysis, is a distinctive characteristic of the crustacean life cycle (69), which involves a complex interplay of numerous neuropeptide and steroid hormones (**Figure 1**), thereby covering key features of the endocrine system of crustaceans. As such it is an endpoint par excellence for endocrine disruption in crustaceans. In many cases, moulting in crustaceans is also related to reproductive periods by alternating cycles of moulting and reproduction, as in *Daphnia* (80, 81), so that perturbations of ecdysis, may also affect reproductive phases.

The crustacean moult cycle is divided into five major stages comprising numerous substages [**Figure 1**; (69, 82)]. During the intermoult stage (C_4), the neuropeptide moult-inhibiting hormone (MIH) represses ecdysteroid synthesis. The proecdysial period begins with the apolysis of the old exoskeleton, during which the membrane layer and the endocuticle are degraded and their building materials are partially resorbed (D_1–D_3). Simultaneously, the new exoskeleton is synthesized. A surge of ecdysone during premoult triggers downstream events that lead to the extrication of

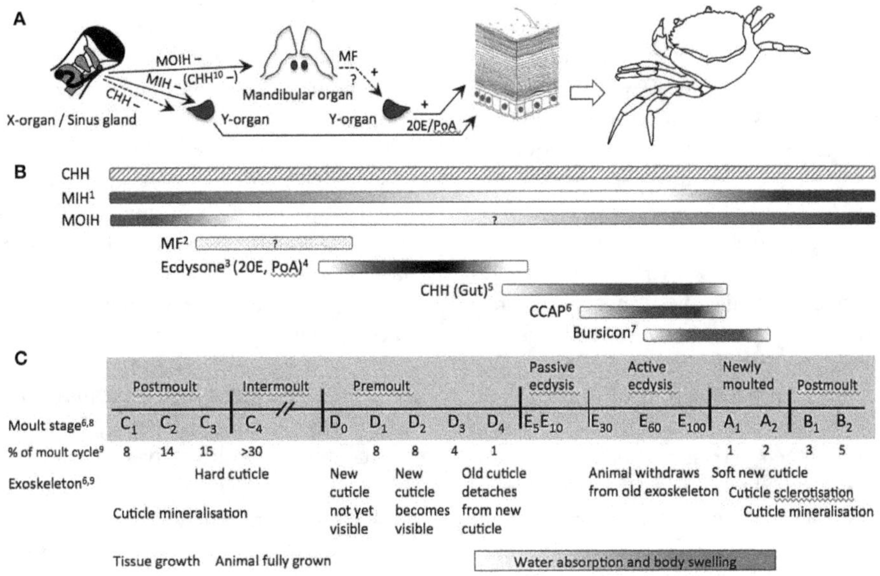

FIGURE 1 | Endocrine control of moulting in decapod crustaceans (Malacostraca). **(A)** Organs directly involved in the control of moulting (release of CCAP and bursicon by the central nervous system and/or the pericardial organ as well as release of CHH by paraneurons of the fore- and hindgut not shown): MIH and CHH from the X-organ/sinus gland-complex negatively inhibit the synthesis of ecdysone by the moulting gland (Y-organ); MOIH (and in some species CHH) negatively inhibit the synthesis of MF, the stimulatory activity for ecdysteroid synthesis has been reported in several studies; ecdysteroids of the major forms 20E and PoA stimulate the epidermis *via* its corresponding EcR to decalcify and to lyse the membrane layer and the old cuticle by proteases, chitinase and chitobiase, and to synthesize material for the new cuticle. **(B)** Dynamic hemolymph titres of (neuro-)hormones involved in the control and/or physiological processes during moulting and ecdysis over an entire moult cycle. **(C)** Moult stages and main modifications of exoskeleton and growth (non-proportional presentation with respect to duration of each period). Abbreviations: CCAP, crustacean cardioactive peptide; CHH, crustacean hyperglycemic hormone; EcR, ecdysteroid receptor; MF, methyl farnesoate; MIH, moult-inhibiting hormone; MOIH, mandibular organ-inhibiting hormone; 20E, 20-hydroxyecdysone; PoA, ponasterone **(A)** [1] (70); [2] (71); [3] (72); [4] (73); [5] (74); [6] (75); [7] (76); [8] (77); [9] (78); [10] (79).

the animal from its carapace (E). Despite the long history of endocrine research in crustaceans, the hormonal regulation of these events still lacks precise knowledge of some factors, such as homologs of ecdysis-triggering hormone (ETH) and eclosion hormone (EH). The function of these neuropeptides is well described for insects, but awaits further elucidation in crustaceans. More recent work also suggests a yet unknown role for corazonin in the control of moulting (83). Eventually, CHH and crustacean cardioactive peptide (CCAP) are tightly linked, respectively, with ecdysial water uptake and the onset of the behavioral motor program by which the animal extricates from its carapace. Tanning and sclerotization of the new cuticle are under the control of bursicon, another neuropeptide hormone. At large, the complex control of moulting described in the following, which involves many other hormones beyond MIH and ecdysone, provides various targets for endocrine disruption in crustaceans.

Neuro-Endocrine Regulation

Almost 70 years after Passano (84) proposed the existence of MIH secreted by the major neurohemal organ in decapod crustaceans, the X-organ/sinus gland (XO/SG) complex of the eyestalk (reviewed in (85, 86)) and the characterization of the respective neuropeptide by Webster and Keller in 1986 (87), the main features of neuroendocrine moult control are generally accepted for decapods. According to this regulatory model, the activity of the moulting gland (*i.e.*, Y-organ) is inhibited by MIH during intermoult, thus subjecting ecdysteroid signaling to the negative control by neuropeptides from the XO/SG (**Figure 1**) (69, 72, 88–90). Evidence is provided by experiments removing eyestalks or XO/SGs, which results in shortened moult intervals and higher moult frequency (72). This inhibition of ecdysis in eyestalk/XO/SG-ablated animals can be restored with extracts from the SG. Dynamic variations of MIH during the moult cycle as well as decreases of MIH stored in the SGs and circulating MIH in the hemolymph during pro- and postecdysis further corroborated the role of MIH in neuro-endocrine regulation of ecdysis (70, 88, 90, 91). Furthermore, Techa and Chung (70) suggest a feedback control by which elevated ecdysteroid concentrations in the hemolymph stimulate *mih*-expression, but inhibit MIH-secretion. As a matter of consequence, high amounts of MIH are stored in the SG during ecdysis and released during post-moult, resulting in low ecdysteroid titers. Hence, any perturbation of synthesis, storage and release of MIH from the XO/SG could result in modifications of Y-organ inhibition, ecdysone synthesis and the resulting circulation of ecdysteroid levels (*e.g.*, (92)).

MIH is not the only factor controlling ecdysteroid secretion from the Y-organ. During proecdysis, the Y-organ becomes progressively less sensitive toward MIH-mediated inhibition of ecdysteroid production (88, 89, 93, 94), most likely due to modifications in intracellular signaling cascades following binding of MIH to its G-protein coupled receptor. Little attention has been given to the role of CHH in the inhibition of ecdysone synthesis. Albeit, CHH is 10-fold less effective in inhibiting the Y-organ, its levels are roughly 10-fold higher than those of MIH. Chung and Webster (88), therefore, argued that CHH could have an equivalent role to MIH in the negative control of ecdysteroid synthesis. The situation is further complicated by the implication of other neurohormones in moulting (**Figure 1**). Notably, CCAP displays considerable dynamics during ecdysis (75) and increases massively during late ecdysis when the animals actively exuviate. Phlippen et al. (75) explain this surge of CCAP by its mytropic action, thus potentiating muscle contraction while the animals withdraw from their old exoskeleton, and by its effect on cardiovascular functions regulating hemolymph flow and pressure. Interestingly, CHH released from paraneurons of the fore- and hindgut rises about 100-fold during ecdysis, followed by the surge of CCAP, both reaching their maximum at late ecdysis and decreasing rapidly in newly moulted animals (74) (**Figure 1**). Injections of CHH at physiological concentrations were able to initiate ecdysis through swelling as a result of isosmotic water uptake by the hindgut, suggesting a role of CHH in ion and water uptake during moulting, similar to the function of the homologous ion transport peptides in the hindgut of insects (74). Eventually, bursicon, another neuropeptide hormone produced by the central nervous system overlapping with CCAP is massively released from the pericardial organ into the hemolymph when ecdysis is completed and remains significantly elevated during early postmoult (76) (**Figure 1**). Its consistent presence throughout the moult cycle at about one quarter of its concentration during ecdysis gives rise to further cuticle-associated functions of bursicon during moulting (95).

Interestingly, the nature of hindgut CHH, CCAP, and bursicon and their role in ecdysis bear resemblance to neuropeptides involved in the ecdysis of insects. Because any spontaneous release of, notably, CCAP could be excluded, the existence of yet non-identified ecdysis-inducing factors similar to ETH and EH of insects would complete the overall picture of ecdysis in crustaceans (75). Indeed, analyses of the *Daphnia pulex* genome, suggest that such factors may exist in crustaceans (96, 97). More recently, carcikinin, an ortholog of ETH was identified in *Carcinus maenas* (98) and ETH genes were found in several crustacean transcriptomes [see (99) for references]. Injection of ETH into the crayfish *Cherax quadricarinatus* prolonged the moult period, suggesting a role in the control of the moult cycle in decapod crustaceans (99). Similarly, EH was identified in the shrimp *Exopalaemon carinicauda*, and displayed highest expression levels during premoult, while gene-silencing lead to a delay in moulting and reduced rates of ecdysis (100). Furthermore, the virtually exclusive expression of a G-protein coupled receptor for corazonin in the Y-organ indicates a role for this neuropeptide in the control of ecdysis (83). Despite these promising results, the roles of ETH, EH, and corazonin in crustacean ecdysis await further characterization.

Ecdysteroids

Ecdysteroids are the predominant hormones responsible for moulting and other processes in crustaceans. Ecdysteroid metabolism is relatively well understood owing to advances in insect biochemistry and conserved pathways between insects and crustaceans. While crustacean ecdysteroids and their nuclear receptors are similar to those of insects, they differ in the number of hormones and in the number and structure of the receptor isoforms (101).

The concentrations of ecdysteroid hormones circulating within crustaceans vary during the moult cycle, and depending on the species, either gradually or quite rapidly spike to start a period of ecdysis or moulting (**Figure 1**) (102). Ecdysteroids and the enzymes responsible for breakdown of the chitin skeleton have been measured through various molecular and cellular assays targeting gene expression and/or enzyme synthesis, respectively.

Enzyme Synthesis and Inactivation

Ecdysteroid biosynthesis is divided into two stages (103). The first stage involves the conversion of cholesterol, derived from diet, to 5β-diketol and the second stage converts 5β-diketol to secreted products. Depending on the species, four major secreted products are ecdysone, 3-dehydroecdysone (3DE), 25-deoxyecdysone (25dE), and 3-dehydro-25-deoxyecdysone (3D25dE) (103). A large number of ecdysteroidogenic enzymes and associated genes have been identified in insects and other arthropods (104) with a large degree of conservation in the crustaceans (105, 106). For example, orthologs of *nmg/sro*, *spo*, *phm*, *dib*, *sad*, and *shd* have been identified in the *D. pulex* genome (46, 107, 108).

Both the increase and subsequent rapid decline in ecdysteroid titers are critical to moulting. The cytochrome P450 hydroxylase cyp18a1 is primarily responsible for the inactivation of the hormone, rendering it susceptible to further modification and elimination (103, 109).

The inhibition of cytochrome P450s by chemical compounds is a widespread mechanism (110), which could interfere with the multiple hydroxylation reactions catalyzed by the cytochrome P450s encoded by the "Halloween genes" (104). For instance, several classes of fungicides function by inhibiting cytochrome P450-mediated demethylation of sterols that are critical components of fungal cell membranes. Some of these compounds are also capable of inhibiting cytochrome P450s of non-target organisms that are involved in steroid biosynthesis. Exposure of *Daphnia magna* to the demethylase inhibiting fungicides fenarimol, pyrifenox, prochloraz, triadimefon, and propiconazole delayed moulting and/or caused developmental abnormalities in neonates (111, 112). Mechanistic studies revealed that fenarimol exposure reduced ecdysteroid levels in daphnids and that co-exposure with 20E protected against the delay in moulting and developmental abnormalities caused by this fungicide (113). These results are consistent with the hypothesis that fenarimol elicited toxicity by inhibiting cytochrome P450s involved in ecdysteroid synthesis.

Receptor-Mediated Activation

Ecdysteroid hormones, such as the major forms 20E and ponasterone A (PoA), bind to the ligand-binding domain of the EcR and activate the expression of primary early ecdysteroid responsive genes, such as E75 and E74 and early late genes such as HR3 and HR4 (114, 115) (see also reviews by (116, 117)). These transcriptional regulators drive the "late genes" responsible for metamorphosis, moulting, and/or ovarian development (114, 118–120). For ligand binding, the EcR forms a heterodimer with the retinoid-X-receptor (RXR), the ortholog of the insect ultraspiracle (121). The RXR contributes to DNA-binding and helps to stabilize the EcR-ligand binding pocket and allows for flexibility in ligand binding (122, 123). Unliganded EcR-RXR is a repressor of transcription (123).

An account of the transcriptional activities of some of these late genes during premoult and ecdysis is given by Li et al. (124). Notably, genes involved glucosamine synthesis, corresponding to the formation of material for a new cuticle, were upregulated during the premoult, whereas genes encoding chitin synthase and several chitinases were upregulated during ecdysis and postmoult stages. Consequently, enzymes such chitobiase (125), N-acetyl-β-glucosaminidase (126) or chitin synthase (127) can be used as biomarkers for EcR-induced late genes provided that the xenobiotic concentrations are low and act *via* EcR-signaling rather than inhibiting the enzyme itself or exerting non-specific effects on gene-expression. Furthermore, enzyme-expression and activity have to be put in the perspective of the precise moulting stage (127, 128).

Disruption of Ecdysteroid Signaling

Several targets exist at which environmental chemicals might interfere with ecdysteroid signaling. These include disruptions in ecdysteroid synthesis, ecdysteroid inactivation, and interactions with the EcR. The neuroendocrine regulation of ecdysteroid signaling also may provide targets of disruption, though few definitive examples of such disruption exist. Overall, the XO/SG-Y-organ-EcR axis of malacostracan crustaceans offers an endocrine signaling cascade similar to the mammalian hypothalamus-pituitary-gonadal-ER axis.

Modulation of Ecdysteroid Levels

Studies have reported on the ability of environmental chemicals to alter the expression of ecdysteroid biosynthetic or biotransformation enzymes. For example, exposure of the copepod *Tigriopus japonicas* to 20 mg·L^{-1} atrazine resulted in a reduction of mRNA transcripts for several enzymes involved in ecdysteroid biosynthesis and biotransformation (129). Unfortunately, impacts on ecdysteroid levels were not established. A generalized reduction in relevant gene expression levels suggest that atrazine may have disrupted common neuro-endocrine control of these genes, or that the high concentration of atrazine used resulted in overt toxicity presented as an overall decrease in transcription.

Exposure of the Chinese mitten crab, *Eriocheir sinensis*, to the pharmaceutical carbamazepine reduced hemolymph ecdysteroid levels and epidermal chitobiase activity. Carbamazepine exposure also increased *chh* and *mih*-expression; while, decreasing EcR and RXR mRNA levels. Taken together, these effects suggest that carbamazepine may have perturbed the neuroendocrine control of ecdysteroid synthesis resulting in a decrease in ecdysteroid levels and a down-regulation of ecdysteroid-regulated genes. These perturbations in the ecdysteroid-signaling pathway also resulted in delayed moulting (130).

Ecdysteroid Receptor Agonists/Antagonists

Plants produce compounds with ecdysteroidal activity, presumably to serve as an endocrine-disrupting defense against invading insects (*e.g.*, (131)). Similarly, EcR-agonist activity has been exploited as a mode of action of some next-generation non-steroidal insecticides (132). The insecticidal EcR-agonist tebufenozide only weakly activated the *D. magna* EcR in a reporter two-hybrid assay (133). Similarly, tebufenozide, along with the related diacylhydrazines halofenozide and methoxyfenozide were weak agonists in a reporter assay containing the shrimp *Neocaridina davidi*-EcR (34). De Wilde et al. (33), however, could not confirm accommodation of tebufenozide into the ligand binding pocket of the shrimp *Neomysis integer* and found no effect of 100 µg tebufenozide·L^{-1} on nymphal development and moulting. Taken together, these results are consistent with the manufacturer's report that the diacylhydrazine insecticides exhibit low specificity for EcRs of non-target arthropods (132). They may, however, displace 20E and/or PoA from the binding site by competitive binding (34).

A recent *in silico* study by (134) identified 274 potential non-steroidal EcR-ligands. Furthermore, the screening of 8795 compounds listed in the US EPA's ToxCast chemical library revealed 34 potential agonists including the diacylhydrazines insecticides and numerous pharmaceuticals, such as non-steroidal anti-inflammatory drugs containing pyrazolone derivatives, or members of the amphenicol antibiotic family. Using the *Drosophila melanogaster* B_{II} cell assay, Dinan et al. (135) detected no EcR-agonist activity among 80 environmental chemicals. Bisphenol A, diethylphthalate, some polycyclic aromatic hydrocarbons, naphthalenes, pesticides, and pharmaceuticals were weak antagonists in this assay. Notably, estradiol, progesterone, and testosterone as well as synthetic steroids neither displayed agonist, nor antagonist activity, except for two compounds, 4-androstene-3,17-dione and 17α-ethinylestradiol, which were weak antagonists.

Despite the lack of anti-ecdysteroidal activity associated with testosterone reported by Dinan et al. (135), weak EcR-antagonist activity of testosterone was reported in daphnids (136). Exposure of *D. magna* to micromolar concentrations of testosterone caused a concentration-dependent delay in moulting and an increase in developmental abnormalities among neonates. Co-exposure with 20E protected against this toxicity of testosterone. Testosterone did not lower endogenous 20E-levels, but rather appeared to antagonize the EcR, based upon competition assays between testosterone and 20E in ecdysone-responsive *Drosophila* Kc cells. While these results suggest that testosterone is anti-ecdysteroidogenic in daphnids, the results have little environmental relevance to environmental androgens due to the high concentrations required to elicit a response.

Gene Product Changes

Several studies have reported on the impacts of exposure to pollutants, pharmaceuticals, and vertebrate hormones on expression profiles of mRNAs or proteins along the ecdysteroid signaling pathway. Expression of *ecr* was elevated from exposure of prawns, *Macrobrachium potiuna*, to glyphosate-based herbicides, ethinylestradiol (estrogen), 4-hydroxytamoxifen (anti-estrogen), 17α-methyltestosterone (androgen), and cyproterone acetate (anti-androgen) (30, 137). Exposure of the intertidal mud crab *Macrophthalmus japonicas* to bisphenol A and di-(2-ethylhexyl) phthalate significantly elevated *ecr* expression levels (138). Studies, such as these are indicative of exposure to potential endocrine disrupting chemicals. However, whether the exposure actually results in apical disruption remains equivocal in the absence of demonstrated consequences of the molecular alterations.

Conversely, several studies have reported on effects of chemical exposure on apical endpoints, such as moulting. Zou (139) identified 33 compounds that have been shown to delay, impede, or advance moulting in crustaceans. While such studies inform on the toxicity of the chemicals to crustaceans, they do not provide insight on whether the effects elicited are actually due to endocrine disruption.

Neurohormone Activity Modulation

The negative control of ecdysteroid synthesis by MIH and by CHH is under the control of biogenic amines, notably, serotonin (5-hydroxytryptamine, 5-HT). Evidence suggests that the hyperglycemic action of 5-HT is due to the direct stimulation of CHH neurons (50, 140, 141). Indeed, 5-HT-immunopositive efferent axons to the *medulla terminalis* and the XO-neuropile have been demonstrated (142). The excitatory role of 5-HT on these XO-neurons was shown by Sáenz et al. (143). Therefore, serotoninergic stimulation of the release of neurohormones from the XO/SG-complex is likely to be a general phenomenon that applies to CHH as well as to MIH or mandibular organ inhibiting hormone (MOIH). The effects of fluoxetine on ecdysteroid levels in *C. maenas* demonstrated that fluoxetine, a selective serotonin reuptake inhibitor, significantly decreased 20E-levels at 0.5 and 0.75 μM after 8 and 4 h, respectively (92). Because, this effect was even more rapid and more pronounced with 0.5 μM 5-HT, but no effect of 5-HT or fluoxetine on 20E-levels could be observed in eyestalk-ablated animals, it was concluded that the mechanism leading to reduced 20E would be the inhibition of ecdysteroid synthesis by 5-HT-stimulated release of MIH. Interestingly, low ecdysteroid levels appeared to relate to an increased *mih*-expression in this study.

To date, only few studies examined the effects of pollutants on neuroendocrine processes that control moulting in crustaceans and only recently has MIH been proposed as a biomarker of endocrine disruption in crustaceans (30). This may be explained by the difficulties to quantify MIH-levels in the hemolymph, due to its 10 times lesser concentrations as compared to CHH and because of the pulsatory release of these neuropeptides from the SG (88, 144). Thus, *mih*-expression has been used to evaluate the effects of EDCs on the neuroendocrine regulation of moulting (30, 92, 137). Gismondi (30) and de Melo et al. (137) found an over-expression of *mih* in response to estrogen agonists and antagonists as well as antiandrogenic and androgenic compounds and a glyphosate-based herbicide. Because 20E equally increased *mih*-expression in the study of Gismondi (30), probably by the feedback control described by Techa and Chung (70), it was concluded that EDCs interfering with vertebrate steroid hormone signaling could affect *mih*-expression *via* an ecdysteroid related pathway, but without any further mechanistic explanation. The fact that very different compounds, which either activate or block the estrogen receptor or interact with other steroid receptors and even glyphosate all stimulated *mih*- as well as *ecr*-expression rather points to other, non-specific effects. Nevertheless, increased expression of *mih* may lead to an increased synthesis and release of this neuropeptide with the potential to modulate ecdysis.

Vertebrate-Type Sex Steroids

Whether or not crustaceans utilize estrogen, androgen, and progestogen signaling pathways has been debated for decades (145). Evidence in support of these signaling pathways is based largely upon observational studies; while, evidence against the existence of these signaling pathways is supported by genomic investigations and evolutionary biology. Interaction with the EcR is often cited as a mechanism by which vertebrate-type sex steroids function in crustaceans. However, as discussed above such interactions typically occur at high, non-physiologic levels.

Evidence in Support

Presence of the Hormones

The detection of vertebrate-type sex steroids in crustaceans was often cited in earlier literature as evidence that these hormones are of physiological significance in these organisms (146, 147). These include 17β-estradiol and testosterone in amphipods (148) and crayfish (149), pregnenolone in brine shrimp (150), and progesterone in shrimp (151). Several studies report that vertebrate-type steroid levels vary with the ovarian development cycle suggesting some functionality related to this process (discussed in (152)). However, the mere presence of a hormone in an organism does not indicate that the chemical possesses a signaling role in that organism. The hormone may be present as a consequence of dietary uptake or as a non-functional intermediate or metabolite of a biosynthetic pathway (153–156).

Responses to Exogenous Steroids

Many studies have demonstrated physiological responses of crustaceans to exogenously administered steroid hormones. For example, administration of 17β-estradiol advanced ovarian development (29) and stimulated vitellogenesis in female decapods (28). This compound also suppressed vitellogenesis-inhibiting hormone gene-expression, which was presumably responsible for the effects on ovarian development (28). While 17β-estradiol administration to crayfish stimulated vitellogenin-mRNA accumulation in the hepatopancreas, progesterone administration increased vitellogenin protein levels in the hemolymph of crayfish (157).

The provision of exogenous 17β-estradiol and progesterone support suggestions of a role for these hormones in crustacean reproduction. Some studies, however, indicate that estrogens downregulate monoamine oxidase activity (158–160) and may, therefore, increase 5-HT-levels that directly influence ovarian development. Furthermore, administration of testosterone has largely resulted in detrimental effects. Administration of testosterone to water fleas suppressed embryo development (136) and decreased lipid storage (161). These effects were attributed to the ability of testosterone to elicit anti-ecdysteroidal activity.

Responses to Endocrine Disruptors

Several investigators have reported on the negative effects of estrogenic and anti-androgenic compounds on crustaceans. Estrogenic compounds, such as diethylstilbestrol, endosulfan, Aroclor 1242, and diethylphthalate delayed moulting in *D. magna* (162, 163). Studies that have shown neuroendocrine disruption by some of these compounds [**Table 1**; (172, 173, 176–178)] may provide an explanation for these observations and would situate their effects upstream of ecdysteroid signaling.

The anti-androgen cyproterone acetate severely reduced growth of *D. magna* without eliciting any discernible effect on moult frequency (145). Effects of several anti-androgens (cyproterone acetate, linuron, vinclozolin, p,p'-DDE) on the reproductive system of copepods revealed varied effects, although consistent among the treatments were degeneration of spermatocytes and deformed spermatophores (163).

Evidence Against

Lack of a Critical Enzyme for Estrogen Biosynthesis

Aromatase (CYP19) is responsible for the metabolic conversion of androstenedione to estrone and testosterone to estradiol. It is thus critical to the synthesis of estrogens. CYP19 is a product of chordate evolution (187) and has not been detected among the protostome invertebrates. Notably, CYP19 is absent from the *D. pulex* genome (159, 188). While it is possible that estrogens are synthesized in crustaceans *via* an alternative metabolic pathway, we are aware of no support for this premise.

Lack of Sex Steroid Receptors

Arguably, the greatest evidence against a role of vertebrate-type sex steroids in crustaceans and other Ecdysozoans is the lack of sex steroid hormone receptors (see Section 2). Immunochemical studies have suggested the presence of estrogen receptor α in *Gammarus fossarum* (27), androgen and estrogen receptors in the mud crab (189), and progesterone and estrogen receptors in crayfish (190). However, immunochemical assays are prone to false positive results due to cross-reactivities or non-specific binding to abundant proteins (191). In the latter studies, putative estrogen receptor co-localized with the other receptor evaluated (progesterone receptor in crayfish and androgen receptor in crab) indicating that antibodies in the same studies may have all been binding to the same abundant protein. Further, results from these studies were inconsistent with estrogen receptor detected in the cytosol from crayfish and membranes of the crab.

We are aware of no reports of the identification of high-affinity sex-steroid binding proteins, indicative of receptors, in crustaceans. Importantly, no sex steroid receptor genes were found in the genome of *D. pulex* (57). Similarly, the sequenced genomes of the ecdyzoans *D. melanogaster* and *Caenorhabditis elegans* revealed no androgen, estrogen, or progesterone receptors [discussed in (27)]. The dominant consensus among researchers is that sex steroid receptors were lost in the lineage leading to the evolution of arthropods (54) and are not present in crustaceans.

High Exposure Concentrations of Hormones and EDCs Are Typically Required to Elicit a Response

Steroid, and similar acting, hormones regulate physiological processes such as development, growth, metabolism, and reproduction. Thus, the action of these chemicals, *via* receptor-mediated signal transduction, typically does not result in rapid, overt responses by the organism (*e.g.*, acute responses). Rather, acute responses to these chemicals are largely the consequence of some ancillary response to high exposure concentrations of the chemical (*e.g.*, membrane disruption). In contrast, receptor-mediated responses to the chemical present as long-term consequences, such as alterations in development or reproduction (*e.g.*, chronic responses). These chronic responses are often, though not always, elicited at exposure concentrations significantly below those that elicit acute responses. The magnitude of the difference between concentrations of a chemical that elicit acute *versus* chronic responses is a function, in part, of the binding affinity of the agonist to responsive receptor protein. Hormones bind their receptors with high affinity and, thus, chronic responses to the hormone are typically elicited at concentrations orders-of-magnitude below concentrations that elicit acute toxicity (*e.g.*, high acute/chronic ratio; see **Table 2**, 20E).

Compounds known to be endocrine active in crustaceans typically elicit an acute/chronic ratio of 10–1,000 (**Table 2A**). The chronic responses listed in **Table 2A** are due to disruption of ecdysteroid and MF-signaling. Compounds known to act in vertebrates *via* estrogen and androgen signaling pathways, typically elicit acute/chronic ratios in crustaceans of <10 (**Table 2B**). The latter suggests that chronic responses of crustaceans to these vertebrate EDCs are not elicited through interaction with a hormone receptor.

The strongest evidence for the susceptibility of crustaceans to vertebrate sex steroid agonists are those studies that have shown effects of 17β-estradiol on reproductive system development. Studies cited above reported stimulatory effects of 17β-estradiol on crustacean vitellogenesis (28, 157). However, 17β-estradiol treatments also have been shown to have a negative effect or no effect on crustacean vitellogenesis (194). Exposure of daphnids to the estrogens diethylstilbestrol and bisphenol A had no effect on vitellogenin mRNA levels (195). 17β-Estradiol has been shown to interact with the ecdysteroid receptor at sufficiently high concentrations (196), thus some effects of estrogen injection, the common mode of administration in these studies, may have been the consequence of low affinity interaction of the estrogenic hormone with the ecdysteroid receptor.

ENDOCRINE REGULATION OF COLOR CHANGE

Neuro-Endocrine Regulation

Active color changes are termed "morphological" in the case of slow color changes established over weeks and months, whereas the rapid type that can take place in minutes to hours is termed "physiological" (197, 198). In arthropods, coloration and

TABLE 1 | Disruption of neuroendocrine pathways in crustaceans.

Species	Chemical	Concentration*	Effect	Endpoint	Reference
Procamburus clarkii	$CdCl_2$	5 $mg{\cdot}L^{-1}$	Stimulation of CHH release; reduction of CHH responsiveness	Glycaemia	(164)
Uca pugilator	$CdCl_2$	10 $mg{\cdot}L^{-1}$	Inhibition of PDH synthesis	Color change	(165)
U. pugilator	$CdCl_2$	10 $mg{\cdot}L^{-1}$	Reduction of NE-mediated PDH release from SG	Distal pigment migration	(166)
P. clarkii	$CdCl_2$ $HgCl_2$	0.5 µg/g body weight (injection)	Inhibition of 5-HT mediated VSH release	Ovarian growth	(167)
U. pugilator	$CdCl_2$	1 $mg{\cdot}L^{-1}$	Increase of VIH secretion from SG	Ovarian growth	(168)
Chasmagnathus granulata	$CdCl_2$ $CuCl_2$	0.5 $mg{\cdot}L^{-1}$ 0.1 $mg{\cdot}L^{-1}$	Reduction of VIH secretion from SG	Ovarian growth	(169)
Palaemon elegans	$CuCl_2$	0.1 + 0.5 $mg{\cdot}L^{-1}$	5-HT mediated increase of CHH release from SG	Glycaemia	(170, 171)
Barytelphusa guerini	DDT	2 $mg{\cdot}L^{-1}$ (injection)	Increase of CHH release from SG	Glycaemia	(172)
U. pugilator	PCB	8 $\mu g{\cdot}L^{-1}$ (Aroclor1242)	Reduction of NE-mediated PDH release from SG	Color change	(173)
Oziotelphusa senex senex	Fenitrothion	0.1 $mg{\cdot}L^{-1}$	Increase of VIH secretion from SG	Ovarian growth	(174)
		0.5, 1, 2 $mg{\cdot}L^{-1}$	Increase of CHH release from SG	Glycaemia	(175)
U. pugilator	Naphthalene	10 $mg{\cdot}L^{-1}$	Inhibition of VSH release	Ovarian growth	(176)
U. pugilator	Naphthalene	2.54, 7.83, 9.98 $mg{\cdot}L^{-1}$	Inhibition of NE-mediated melanin dispersion	Color change	(177, 178)
U. pugilator	Fluoxetine Fluvoxamine	20 µg/animal 20 µg/animal	Increased 5-HT mediated red pigment dispersion, reduced red pigment concentration	Color change	(179)
U. pugilator	Reserpine Bretylium	20 µg/animal 20 µg/animal	Increased NE-mediated melanin concentration, reduced melanin dispersion	Color change	(180)
U. pugilator, P. clarkii	Opioids	10^{-10} –10^{-8} mol/animal	Increase of VIH secretion from SG Inhibition of VSH release	Ovarian growth	(181, 182)
Daphnia magna	Fluoxetine	40 $\mu g{\cdot}L^{-1}$	Increase of offspring production under limiting food conditions *via* 5-HT signaling	Reproductive output	(183)
Carcinus maenas	Fluoxetine	0.5 nM (injection)	Stimulation of CHH (and MIH) release from SG	Glycaemia, ecdysteroids	(92)
C. maenas	Fluoxetine	0.5–1nM (inject.)	5-HT mediated activation of heart and-scaphognathites	Cardioventilatory activity	(184)
Erichoeir sinensis	Carbamazepine	0.01–10 $\mu g{\cdot}L^{-1}$	Increase of *chh* and *mih*-expression	Ecdysteroids, moulting	(130)
Daphnia pulex	Fluoxetine Citalopram	1 µM 1 µM	Increase of male production under short-day photo-period *via* glutamate/monoamine signaling	Male sex determination	(185)
Crangon crangon	Fluoxetine	0.1, 10, 100 $ng{\cdot}L^{-1}$	Increased 5-HT mediated red pigment dispersion	Color change	(186)

**All concentrations correspond to waterborne exposures unless otherwise stated.*

CHH, crustacean hyperglycemic hormone; MIH, moult inhibiting hormone; NE, norepinephrine; PDH, pigment dispersing hormone; SG, sinus gland; VIH, vitellogenesis inhibiting hormone; VSH, vitellogenesis stimulating hormone; 5-HT, 5-hydroxytryptamine, serotonin.

reversible color change have evolved together with the development of an exoskeleton (197). Hence, color may be produced by pigments embedded in the pigmented layer of the endocuticle, or by pigment-containing cells in the epidermis (199). Accordingly, morphological color changes are related to moulting, notably, in terms of ontogenetic color changes (200, 201), whereas physiological color changes are produced by chromatophores.

Rapid color changes in most crustaceans rely on the dispersion and aggregation of pigments within stellate cells containing pigment granules. Generally, monochromatic chromatophores, *i.e.*, black-brown melanophores, red erythrophores, yellow xanthophores, and white leucophores, are intimately arranged in clusters called chromatosomes so as to produce a wide variety of colors (197, 198, 202–204). The dispersion of pigment granules, *i.e.*, their migration from the cell center into the ramifications of the chromatophores renders the coloration more intense, whereas the opposite is the case when the pigment granules aggregate within the center of the cell. Dispersion and aggregation of pigment granules can be completed within half an hour in *Crangon* up to 2 h in *Carcinus* or *Macrobrachium* (83, 205–208). Aggregation and dispersion are regulated by an antagonistic system of neuropeptide hormones composed of red pigment concentrating hormone (RPCH, or simply PCH) and pigment dispersing hormone (PDH) with its isoforms α- and β-PDH (198, 203). Notably, RPCH represents a highly conserved neuropeptide, which, in all decapods so far investigated, has an identical sequence (209, 210).

The antagonistic neurosecretory control of rapid color changes belongs to the best-studied hormonal systems in crustaceans [reviewed in (198, 202, 203)]. Indeed, RPCH and PDH have been the first neuropeptides to be characterized in crustaceans (211, 212). It has been established long ago that the eyestalk of decapod crustaceans is the source of hormones regulating color change in crustaceans (202). This was confirmed by Mangerich et al. (213), who localized the main perikarya of RPCH-secreting cells adjacent to or within the XO of *C. maenas* and *Orconectes limosus*, respectively. More recently, Alexander et al. (83) confirmed the presence of about 30 perikarya located in the XO, which project into the SG. A similar situation was shown for PDH, with the majority of PDH-perikarya located between the *medulla interna* and the

TABLE 2 | Acute and chronic toxicity values for crustaceans exposed to **(A)** compounds that disrupt ecdysteroid or methyl farnesoate signaling and **(B)** compounds that disrupt estrogen or androgen signaling.

Species	Chemical	EC50 (mg·L^{-1})[1]	MATC (mg·L^{-1})[1]	Acute/chronic ratio	Chronic endpoint
A. Endocrine active chemicals in crustaceans					
Water flea (*Daphnia magna*)	Tributyltin	1.67	0.14	11.9	Reproduction
Opossum shrimp (*Americamysis bahia*)	Tributyltin	2.2	0.37	5.9	Growth/reproduction
Water flea (*Daphnia magna*)	Methoprene	340	15.7	21.6	Development
Opossum shrimp (*Neomysis integer*)	Methoprene	320	10	32	Moulting
Water flea (*Daphnia magna*)	Pyriproxyfen	80	0.070	1,143	Reproduction
Opossum shrimp (*Neomysis integer*)	Pyriproxyfen	65	–		
Scud (*Gammarus fossarum*)	Pyriproxyfen	–	1.5	43[2]	Reproduction
Water flea (*Daphnia magna*)	Ponasterone	175[3]	<12.5[3]	>14	Moulting
Water flea (*Daphnia magna*)	20-Hydroxyecdysone	2,457[3]	88[3]	28	Moulting
Water flea (*Daphnia magna*)	Azadirachtin	680	82	8.3	Reproduction
Water flea (*Daphnia magna*)	Tebufenozide	17,370	62	280	Reproduction
Opossum shrimp (*Americamysis bahia*)	Tebufenozide	10,000	138	>72	Growth
B. Endocrine active chemicals in vertebrates					
Water flea (*Daphnia magna*)	Bisphenol A	1,336	540	2.5	Reproduction
Water louse (*Asellus aquaticus*)	Bisphenol A	9,500	224	42	Moulting
Water flea (*Daphnia magna*)	Diethylstilbestrol	1,550[4]	350[5]	4.4	Moulting
Water flea (*Daphnia magna*)	4-Nonylphenol	130	35	3.7	Reproduction
Scud (*Hyalella azteca*)	4-Nonylphenol	38	7.0	5.4	Survival
Water flea (*Daphnia magna*)	Atrazine	54,000	6,900	7.8	Reproduction
Copepod (*Amphiascus tenuiremis*)	Atrazine	>1000	86	>11.6	Reproduction
Water flea (*Daphnia magna*)	Cyproterone acetate	–	353[6]	–	Growth/reproduction
Water flea (*Daphnia magna*)	Butyl benzyl phthalate	3,700	444	8.3	Reproduction
Opossum shrimp (*Americamysis bahia*)	Butyl benzyl phthalate	900	113	8.0	Reproduction

[1]Acute (EC50) and chronic toxicity values derived from the EPA EcoTox database (https://cfpub.epa.gov/ecotox/) unless indicated otherwise in comments. Chronic values (CVs) represent the square root of the no observed effect concentration (NOEC) X the lowest observed effect concentration (LOEC)). The NOEC or LOEC was used as a surrogate for the CV where both values were not available. [2]Value was determined using EC50 with Neomysis and maximum acceptable toxicant concentration (MATC) with Gammarus. [3] (192), [4] (193), [5] (20), [6] (145)

medulla lateralis of the eyestalks of *C. maenas* and *O. limosus* (214), the axon terminals of which may project into the SG. Hence the major neurosecretory structures of RPCH and PDH are located within the eyestalk from where these neurohormones are released into hemolymph that transports them to the respective epithelial target cells. Because pigment dispersion and aggregation in eyestalk ablated animals could be observed, extra-eyestalk sources of RPCH and PDH have been considered. Indeed, RPCH-cells were found in small numbers in the brain, the thoracic ganglia and the circumoesophageal commissure as well as PDH-cells in the thoracic and connective ganglia (83, 213, 215). However RPCH and PDH of some of these cells may rather serve as a neurotransmitter instead of being implied in color change [*e.g.*, (216)].

A model for signal transduction and intracellular signaling cascades upon binding of RPCH to a G-protein coupled receptor has been proposed for the freshwater shrimp *Macrobrachium olfersii* (207, 217). In this model, RPCH activates cyclic guanosine monophosphate (cGMP) and Ca^{2+} second messenger cascades, which in turn stimulate a protein kinase to phosphorylate a myosin II molecular motor. As a result, pigment aggregation is effectuated by the movement of pigment granules along actin filaments in the chromatophore [for details see (198, 218)]. More recently, highly specific RPCH receptors (RPCHR) have been cloned and functionally deorphanized in *D. pulex* and *C. maenas* (83, 210). The RPCHR of *C. maenas* bound RPCH at doses lower than 0.001 nM (EC50 0.02nM). A dose of as low as 0.1 pmol effectively induced pigment aggregation in erythrophores *in vivo* within 5 min and the effect was stronger and longer lasting when the concentrations of RPCH were increased to 1 and 10 pmol, respectively (83). The RPCHR of *D. pulex*, on the other hand, bound *Daphnia*-RPCH at an EC_{50} of 0.065 nM, but binding of crustacean RPCH was at least two orders of magnitude less efficient. Insect adipokinetic hormone did equally activate the *Daphnia*-RPCHR in a dose-dependent and only slightly less efficient manner than *Daphnia*-RPCH (210).

Potential Sites of Endocrine Disruption

The capacity to change color and to adapt to the surrounding luminance may be impaired by pollutants as different as metals, such cadmium or mercury (165), organic chlorine compounds, like PCBs and naphthalene (173, 177), or drugs that affect the levels of biogenic amines (179, 180, 219) (**Table 1**). In spite of the high concentrations that were employed in these studies, the authors could exclude toxicity and plausibly demonstrate that the respective compounds caused neuroendocrine disruption by affecting the neurotransmitters responsible for the release of, notably, PDH, or the synthesis of the latter. For instance, Aroclor 1242 appeared to reduce norepinephrine (NE) titers in the XO-neuropile (173), thereby reducing the dispersion of black pigment in the chromatophores. Similar observations were made for naphthalene (177). In both studies, the authors took care to verify that neither the chromatophores were affected, which were still able to respond to extracts from the eyestalk containing PDH, nor was the neural tissue damaged. In the case of cadmium, rather the amount of PDH stored in the SG was affected, putatively by inhibiting the synthesis of PDH (165). Fingerman et al. also showed that drugs that deplete monoamine levels, such as reserpine or bretylium, hamper pigment dispersion when fiddler crabs, *Uca pugliator*, were transferred from a white background with concentrated pigments to a black background, whereas fluoxetine enhanced pigment dispersion by increasing 5-HT-levels (179, 180, 219). Therefore, these early studies pointed to the possibility of psychoactive drugs targeting monoamine levels to interfere with the neurohormonal regulation of color change. This was confirmed by recent studies using more environmentally realistic concentrations of waterborne antidepressants (186). Color change in the sand shrimp, *Crangon crangon*, was affected by fluoxetine in the range of 10–1,000 ng·L^{-1} when exposed for 1 day or 1 week (186), suggesting enhanced dark adaptation following fluoxetine exposure (**Table 1**).

ENDOCRINE REGULATION OF SEXUAL DIFFERENTIATION

Vertebrates typically utilize a variety of genetic sex-determining strategies including sex-determining genes assembled on sex-chromosomes where females are the heterogametic sex, and sex-determining genes assembled on sex-chromosomes where males are the heterogametic sex (220), and autosomal sex-determining genes whose expression are environmentally controlled (221). Common to these sex-determining strategies, sex steroids (androgens, estrogens) are ultimately responsible for sexual differentiation. Indeed, androgens and estrogens from exogenous sources can sometimes circumvent genetic sex-determination (222).

Similarly, crustaceans possess diversity in sex determining mechanisms. Some decapods utilize sex chromosome where female are the heterogametic sex [*Penaeus monodon* (223); *Penaeus japonicus* (224)], while male are the heterogametic sex in others [*Orchestia cavimana* and *Orchestia gammarellus*, (225)]. Among branchiopods, clam shrimp *Eulimnadia texana* consists of monogametic males and heterogametic hermaphrodites (226), and brine shrimp *Artemia franciscana* consist of monogametic males and heterogametic females (227). In contrast, the female and male genomes of *D. pulex* are identical (228). A major distinction between vertebrates and crustaceans is that crustaceans have evolved strategies for sexual differentiation that do not involve steroidal androgens and estrogens.

Malacostracans

Evidence for an underlying genetic component to sex-determination in malacostracan crustaceans has come from a series of ablation/implantation experiments followed by cross breeding. The chromosomal system for these crustaceans is often referred to as ZW males and WW females. Using isopods (*Armadillidium vulgare*), Suzuki and Yamasaki (229) were able to transform males into functional females through the ablation of the androgenic gland (AG) and females into functional males through the implantation of the AG. The reciprocal crosses of "genetic" males with converted females and "genetic" females with converted females results in single sex broods. Similar experiments have been done with a variety of other crustaceans including prawns, crayfish, and hermit crabs (230–232). Further evidence of a genetic and potential chromosomal basis to sex-determination has come from breeding experiments with intersex crayfish. When intersex crayfish, *Cherax quadricarinatus*, that are functionally males were crossed with females the result was a 1:3 (male:female) sex ratio (232). Subsequent crossbreeding between female (WW) crayfish with normal males resulted in an all-female progeny 0:1 (male: female), leading the authors to conclude that the intersex specimens must have been genetic females (WZ). While the evidence for a genetic component to sex- determination remains strong, sex determination in Crustacea can also show degrees of plasticity. Therefore, it is most likely controlled also by epigenetic factors including environmental variables such as light and temperature (233, 234), parasites (235), and even diet (236).

Androgenic Gland Hormone

Male secondary sex characteristics in malacostracan crustaceans are under the control of androgenic gland hormone (AGH), which is produced by the ductless AG (237–239). The AG is usually situated on the paired testes or *vas deferens* in crustaceans. Its important role was discovered through a series of ablation and implantation experiments in the 1950's (240–243). Removal of AG results in the cessation of spermatogenesis and the demasculinization of male secondary sexual characteristics [(244) and references within]. Complete andrectomy in some species leads to the conversion of testicular to ovarian tissues that have the capacity to accumulate yolk proteins (245). Similarly, implantation of AGs into female crustaceans results in the conversion from ovarian to testicular tissues and the development of male sexual characteristics. Suzuki (230) was also able to demonstrate through a series of these ablation and implantation experiments at different maturation stages within the isopods that AGH was a sex- differentiating, but not a sex-determining factor in these organisms.

First purifications by Hasegawa et al. and Martin et al. have identified the AGH (246–248). The full insulin like peptide structure, consisting of B chain, A chain, and C peptide and the gene sequence of AGH have been characterised in the late 1990s for the isopod *A. vulgare* (249–251). Immunohistochemistry has shown that antibodies raised from AGH-peptides display relatively strong species specificity (252), which is not surprising as sexual characteristics are under strong selection pressures. Unfortunately, this makes developing immuno-histochemistry based bioassays for endocrine disrupter studies more problematic. The cDNA sequence for the insulin-like androgenic gland (IAG) gene has now been reported by several species including crayfish, and several prawn/shrimp and crabs (253). This allows for RNA interference (RNAi) techniques to be used to demasculinize and sex reverse aquaculture species with an AG-specific IAG peptide-encoding transcript (254, 255).

Potential Targets of Endocrine Disruption

Currently, it is not known whether environmental pollutants can impact the development of the AG development, or the synthesis of AGH. A number of studies correlated pollutants with increased incidences of intersexuality in crustaceans or male crustaceans displaying certain degrees of feminization or de-masculinization (18). These phenotypic changes in field collected animals mirror the physiological changes caused by feminizing parasite infection, AG ablation or RNAi silencing the AG leading authors to hypothesize whether chemicals can directly or indirectly interfere with the AG or AGH (18, 244). These hypotheses require further testing. In the light of an endocrine axis between the XO/SG, the AG and the male reproductive system, which has been confirmed for decapods (256), a disruption of the neuroendocrine regulation of AGH synthesis and spermatogenesis is conceivable. Indeed, specific CHH-isoforms appear to regulate AGH-expression (257) and its has been demonstrated that metal and organic pollution has the potential to affect CHH-synthesis or -secretion (92, 164, 170–172) (**Table 1**).

Branchiopods

Sexual differentiation in branchiopods has been extensively studied in *Daphnia*. Daphnids do not possess sex chromosomes (258, 259) and sexual differentiation of offspring is regulated by environmental cues (32). Under environmental conditions that favor rapid population growth, daphnids reproduce parthenogenetically (diploid oocytes) with all offspring being largely female (260). Maternal organisms produce broods, often consisting of dozens of offspring, every few days. These female offspring then mature in a matter of days and begin producing broods of female offspring. As a result, the population expands at an exponential rate. Under conditions that foretell adversity to population sustainability (exhaustion of resources, impending temperature extremes associated with summer or winter), females introduce male offspring to the population. Males mate with females that are producing haploid oocytes (260). The resulting embryo has undergone genetic exchange, which helps to purge deleterious mutations (261). The embryo is in a resting state of diapause to wait out the period of adversity, and is encased in a protective ephippium, which withstands desiccation and freezing. The ephippium is also hydrophobic, which facilitates transport on transient biota (*e.g.*, aquatic birds) or dispersal in air currents. This facilitates dispersal of the organisms to new habitats (262).

Environmental Regulation

The role of photoperiod and temperature in male sex differentiation of daphnids has been well characterized. Photoperiod and temperature function in concert to regulate sex ratios in *D. pulex* and *D. magna* populations (263). Under a long-day, summer-like photoperiod, daphnids produced only female offspring, regardless of temperature (range evaluated was 16-22°C). However, under a short-day, autumn-like photoperiod, daphnids became susceptible to temperature-dependent sex-determination. The different species exhibited different temperature optima for male sex-determination, probably relating to the geographic locations at which the populations used in the study were originally derived. Other environmental factors that have been implicated in male sex-determination include food restriction (264) and crowding (265).

Neuroendocrine Regulation

Exposure of daphnids to environmental conditions that stimulate the production of male offspring resulted in increased mRNA levels for various components of glutamate signaling based upon gene ontology (GO) terms (266). Further, Camp et al. (185) demonstrated that environmental stimulation of male sex determination resulted in increased mRNA levels of the subunit 2 of the N-methyl-D receptor (NMDAR) while having no effect on the NDMAR-a subunit. This change in the abundance of a single subunit of the receptor would result in alterations in subunit composition of the receptors, which has been shown to be responsible for plasticity in receptor function in vertebrates (267, 268). Conceivable, a reduction in the NMDAR-a/NMDAR-b subunit ratio may prompt glutamate signaling leading to male sex differentiation.

A role for the NMDAR in male sex-differentiation was further indicated by the observation that exposure of maternal daphnids to the NMDAR antagonists MK-801 and desipramine significantly increased the number of male offspring (185). Toyota et al. (266) also observed an effect of MK-801 on male sex differentiation; however, these investigators reported that the NMDAR antagonist suppressed male offspring production (266). Differences in results between these two research teams may reflect differences in experimental design. Where Camp et al. (185) reported the number of male and female offspring produced per female over six broods, Toyota et al. (266) reported the percentage of 30-day-old females that produced males, presumably in a single brood.

MK-801 also inhibits 5-HT, NE, and dopamine reuptake transporters, while desipramine inhibits noradrenergic reuptake transporters (269, 270). Therefore, Camp et al. (185) investigated the potential role of these neurotransmitter-signaling pathways in male sex differentiation. The mRNA levels of the serotonin reuptake transporter *SERT-a* and the α-adrenergic-like octopamine receptor *OctaR-A* were significantly elevated in daphnids reared upon a short-day photoperiod as compared to those reared under a long-day photoperiod. Two selective serotonin reuptake inhibitors fluoxetine hydrochloride and citalopram hydrobrimide increased offspring male sex determination, although the effect of fluoxetine hydrochloride was not statistically significant ($p=0.08$). These results suggest that in addition to glutamate signaling other neurotransmitters may be operative in male sex differentiation.

Methyl Farnesoate

Farnesyl units (C15), derived from acetate serve as building blocks for several important biomolecules, such as cholesterol and steroid hormones. In crustaceans, and other arthropods, farnesyl units also are used for the synthesis of farnesoic acid. Crustaceans utilize farnesoic acid as the substrate for MF. MF is a major sesquiterpenoid hormone in crustaceans, akin to juvenile hormone in insects (271).

Male-sex differentiation depends on MF (272, 273). During late stages of maturation MF programs oocytes to differentiate into males. In the absence of methyl farnesoate, offspring differentiate into females (272). MF is responsible for the induction of the doublesex gene (*dsx1*) during oocyte susceptibility to sex differentiation (274). The doublesex gene product is transcriptionally upregulated in males and is responsible for orchestrating male sex-differentiation (274, 275). Sexually dimorphic expression of the double sex gene also has been shown in other Branchiopod crustaceans including *D. magna*, *Ceriodaphnia dubia*, and *Moina macrocopa* (276).

Synthesis and Degradation

In insects, MF is a product of the mevalonate biosynthetic pathway (277), as is likely the case in crustaceans. Two enzymes along this pathway were identified in lobster that were induced commensurate with MF synthesis (278). 3-Hydroxy-3-methyl-glutaryl-coenzyme A reductase (HMGCR) activity increased within 24 h of eye-stalk ablation, which increased MF hemolymph levels, while farnesoic acid O-methyl transferase (FAMeT) activity was increased substantially two weeks after ablation. The reduction of HMGCR is the final step in the biosynthesis of mevalonate; while, methylation of farnesoic acid is the final step in the synthesis of MF. The authors surmised that increased production of mevalonate *via* heightened HMGCR reductase activity was responsible for the immediate increase in MF-production following eyestalk ablation, while prolonged increased synthesis of MF was due to elevation in FAMT activity.

In insects, MF is susceptible to metabolism and inactivation through ester hydrolysis and conjugation to polar molecules (279). These inactivation processes are operative in crustaceans as well (276, 280).

The location of synthesis in branchiopod crustaceans has not been established. In decapod crustaceans, MF is synthesized in the mandibular organ, which is under the negative control of mandibular organ inhibiting hormone (281, 282) (**Figure 1**). MF functions in some aspects of masculinization in decapods, such as the development of the male reproductive morphotype of the spider crab, *Libinia emarginata*. Abraded males (have not moulted in about a year or more) characteristically have high hemolymph MF-levels, large reproductive organs, and aggressive mating behavior (283).

Receptor-Mediated Activation

The regulatory activity of MF is mediated primarily through interaction with the bHLH-PAS protein methoprene-tolerant (MET) (284, 285). MET derives its name from the discovery that resistance of *Drosophila* to the insecticidal MF-analog, methoprene, was associated with a functional mutation in this gene (286). MF-activated MET recruits the bHLH-PAS protein, steroid receptor coactivator (SRC) (37). Together, this MET-SRC complex comprises the activated MF- receptor (MfR) in crustaceans.

Other suggested receptors for MF in crustaceans include the RXR and hormone receptor 97g (HR97g). RXR is a member of the nuclear receptor superfamily that has been identified in several crustacean species including the American lobster *Homarus americanus* (287), the fiddler crab *Uca pugilator* (288), the tropical land crab *Gecarinus lateralis* (289), the crayfish *Procambarus clarkii* (290), the amphipod *G. fossarum* (291) and the water fleas (*D. magna, D. pulex*) (58, 292). While MF was unable to activate daphnid RXR in a luciferase reporter assay, its co-administration with 20E to a reporter system consisting of RXR and EcR, resulted in activation greater than that observed with 20E alone (293). This apparent synergistic interaction between activated EcR and activated RXR was also observed *in vivo* using tributyltin as the RXR agonist (294). These results suggest that MF, through interaction with RXR, may function in concert with 20E to regulate crustacean moulting.

Nuclear receptor HR97g, isolated from *D. pulex*, was mildly activated by MF and the MF-analog pyriproxyfen in a luciferase reporter assay (295). This crustacean receptor was first identified in *D. pulex* (57), and has since been identified in the spiny lobster *Panulirus ornatus* (296). The physiological significance of the receptor as a ligand-activated regulator of crustacean physiology remains unknown.

Known Targets of Disruption

The MfR is the best-demonstrated target of disruption of this regulatory pathway by environmental chemicals. Compounds that elicit insecticidal activity as juvenile hormone analogs also typically bind and activate the MfR (37, 285). This activity is responsible for the high sensitivity of crustaceans to this class of insecticides (273, 297, 298). However, the MfR appears to have high ligand recognition specificity. We are aware of no demonstrations that compounds, other than juvenile hormone analogs, are capable of activating the MfR at environmentally relevant exposure levels (37).

Potential Targets of Disruption

Alterations in MF levels due to toxicant-mediated effects on biosynthetic or inactivating hormones is a plausible mechanism of endocrine disruption. The herbicide atrazine reportedly increased male offspring production in *Daphnia pulicaria* (299). However, atrazine did not interact with the MfR (37), suggesting that if atrazine did indeed activate this pathway, it may have been due atrazine increasing endogenous MF. Such an effect may have been the consequence of competition between atrazine and MF at a site of inactivation or elimination. Alternatively, atrazine disrupts endocrine function in mammals by increasing dopamine and reducing NE levels in the hypothalamus (300). These neuromediators are operative in the regulation of MF and sex determination in daphnids (185). Thus, disruption of these upstream signaling components may be responsible for the effects of atrazine on the MF-signaling pathway.

FUTURE DIRECTIONS OF RESEARCH ON ENDOCRINE DISRUPTION IN CRUSTACEANS

In 1998, a workshop was held in the Netherlands to address the issue of endocrine disruption in invertebrates sponsored by The Society of Environmental Toxicology and Chemistry (SETAC).

The proceedings of this workshop were subsequently published (301) and made a number of recommendations. Recently, Ford and LeBlanc conducted a survey of experts to reflect on the progress made in endocrine disruptor studies with invertebrates over the past few decades (302). The majority of participants in that survey believed endocrine disruption was an issue for invertebrates that needed to be addressed, but were mixed over the relative progress that had been made. Strikingly, many of the recommendations provided in this recent survey mirrored those made back in 1998 indicating that the field had not significantly progressed.

A major impediment to advancing research on endocrine disruption in crustaceans has been attempts to detect endocrine effects using chemicals known to be endocrine disruptors in vertebrate species along with endpoints known to be indicative of endocrine disruption in vertebrates. This conclusion has recently been acknowledged by several researchers (303, 304). For example, many studies focus upon the effects of estrogens on crustaceans (18) and use biomarkers of feminization, such as vitellogenin induction, in crustaceans (305). Elevated vitellogenin levels following chemical exposure or in field-collected samples has often been interpreted as an estrogenic effect (306). However, unlike vertebrates, vitellogenin is not regulated by estrogens in crustaceans (195). Despite existing knowledge on the endocrine regulation of vitellogenesis in crustaceans, the precise molecular mechanisms by which vitellogenesis and ovarian maturation are controlled require further elucidation (307). Given the lack of clear understanding of seasonal or developmental fluctuations in normal vitellogenin levels and overall susceptibility of vitellogenin production to non-endocrine stressors, associations between altered vitellogenin levels and endocrine disruption in crustaceans are tenuous at best.

One area where progress has been made is the onset of more affordable "omic" technologies allowing for the high-throughput sequencing of genomes, transcriptomes, peptidomes, and metabolomes (19, 139, 304). These omics-techniques offer a rich opportunity for discovering conserved molecular and biochemical pathways, which can applied to the development of adverse outcome pathways (308). These in turn provide opportunities for further advancing our mechanistic understanding of crustacean endocrinology from which to develop appropriate biomarkers of disruption. Zou (139) in a recent review identified over 30 compounds that have either inhibited or stimulated moulting in crustaceans. However, in the absence of mechanistic linkages between exposure and effect, endocrine disruption cannot be invoked as responsible for these effects on moulting. The identification of appropriate biomarkers will facilitate establishing whether an effect on moulting, or some other endocrine-regulated process, is due to specific disruption of the endocrine system or due to some non-specific toxicity.

We hope to have advocated strongly that a "crab is not a fish" and therefore toxicity evaluations using crustaceans require appropriate endpoints to determine whether current and newly licensed chemical compounds might target endocrine processes in this ecologically important group. While significant progress has been made in our understanding of crustacean endocrinology, application of this knowledge to the study of endocrine disruption in crustaceans is lagging. Where, in the past, we were limited in our ability to develop the tools to confirm whether a substance was an endocrine disruptor, these limitations have been largely overcome with affordable omics-technologies. We now have the ability to develop high throughput screenings using key crustacean-relevant endocrine targets. Given the number of crustacean species incorporated into national toxicity programs, such tools are sorely needed.

AUTHOR CONTRIBUTIONS

TK, GL, and AF have developed the concept of this review and have contributed to the writing. All authors contributed to the article and approved the submitted version.

FUNDING

This work was financially supported by the European Union through the Interreg France (Channel) England program. TK and AF worked on this article in the framework of the Project "Reduction of Pollution by endocrine disrupting compounds at source: innovative products for the commercial lab market" (RedPol; Interreg 5 a, # 185).

ACKNOWLEDGMENTS

We gratefully acknowledge H. Dircksen for encouraging us to write this article and T. Monsinjon for help with the bibliography.

REFERENCES

1. Bergman ÅWorld Health Organization and United Nations Environment Programme. *State of the science of endocrine disrupting chemicals - 2012: an assessment of the state of the science of endocrine disruptors prepared by a group of experts for the United Nations Environment Programme and World Health Organization.* Genève; Nairobi: WHO; UNEP (2012).
2. Hutchinson TH. Small is useful in endocrine disrupter assessment—four key recommendations for aquatic invertebrate research. *Ecotoxicology* (2007) 16:231–8. doi: 10.1007/s10646-006-0107-z
3. Song Y, Villeneuve DL, Toyota K, Iguchi T, Tollefsen KE. Ecdysone receptor agonism leading to lethal molting disruption in arthropods: review and adverse outcome pathway development. *Environ Sci Technol* (2017) 51:4142–57. doi: 10.1021/acs.est.7b00480
4. Martin J, Davis G. Historical trends in crustacean systematics. *Crustaceana* (2006) 79:1347–68. doi: 10.1163/156854006779277321
5. Van Hook AM, Patel NH. Crustaceans. *Curr Biol* (2008) 18:R547–50. doi: 10.1016/j.cub.2008.05.021
6. Ahyong ST. "Evolution and radiation of crustacea," In: Poore GC and Thiel M, editors. *The Natural History of the Crustacea: Evolution and Biogeographyof the Crustacea.* USA: Oxford University Press USA. (2020) 8:53–79.
7. Penn JW, Caputi N, de Lestang S, Johnston D, Kangas M, Bopp J. "Crustacean Fisheries," In: Cochran JK, Bokuniewicz HJ and Yager PL,

editors. *Encyclopedia of Ocean Sciences (Third Edition)*. Oxford: Academic Press (2019). p. 324–37. doi: 10.1016/B978-0-12-409548-9.09577-4

8. Reid AJ, Carlson AK, Creed IF, Eliason EJ, Gell PA, Johnson PT. Emerging threats and persistent conservation challenges for freshwater diversity. *Biol Rev* (2019) 94:849–73. doi: 10.1111/brv.12480
9. Maity S, Jannasch A, Adamec J, Watkins JM, Nalepa T, Höök TO, et al. Elucidating causes of diporeia decline in the Great Lakes via metabolomics: Physiological responses after exposure to different stressors. *Physiol Biochem Zool* (2013) 86:213–23. doi: 10.1086/669132
10. Auer MT, Auer NA, Urban NR, Auer T. Distribution of the amphipod *Diporeia* in lake Superior: the ring of fire. *J Gt Lakes Res* (2013) 39:33–46. doi: 10.1016/j.jglr.2012.12.020
11. Matafonov DV, Bazova NV. Decline of *Gammarus lacustris* Sars (Crustacea: Amphipoda) population in the delta of the Selenga River. *Biol Bull* (2014) 41:168–75. doi: 10.1134/S1062359014020071
12. Lipcius RN. Stockhausen WT Concurrent decline of the spawning stock, recruitment, larval abundance, and size of the blue crab *Callinectes sapidus* inChesapeake Bay. *Mar Ecol Prog Ser* (2002) 226:45–61. doi:10.3354/meps226045
13. States Greffe. *Draft sea fisheries (minimum size limits) (amendment n°7) (Jersey)*. Ministry of Environment, Sates of Jersey. (2019). https://statesassembly.gov.je/assemblypropositions/2019/p.41-2019.pdf.
14. Moore CG, Stevenson JM. The occurrence of intersexuality in harpacticoid copepods and its relationship with pollution. *Mar Pollut Bull* (1991) 22:72–4. doi: 10.1016/0025-326X(91)90139-J
15. Ford AT, Fernandes TF, Rider SA, Read PA, Robinson CD, Davies IM. Endocrine disruption in a marine amphipod? Field observations of intersexuality and de-masculinisation. *Mar Environ Res* (2004) 58:169–73. doi: 10.1016/j.marenvres.2004.03.013
16. Mazurová E, Hilscherová K, Šídlová-Štěpánková T, Köhler H-R, Triebskorn R, Jungmann D, et al. Chronic toxicity of contaminated sediments on reproduction and histopathology of the crustacean *Gammarus fossarum* and relationship with the chemical contamination and *in vitro* effects. *J Soils Sediments* (2010) 10:423–33. doi: 10.1007/s11368-009-0166-x
17. Stentiford GD. Histological intersex (ovotestis) in the European lobster*Homarus gammarus* and a commentary on its potential mechanisticbasis. *Dis Aquat Organ* (2012)100:185–90. doi:10.3354/dao02455
18. Ford AT. Intersexuality in Crustacea: An environmental issue? *Aquat Toxicol* (2012) 108:125–9. doi: 10.1016/j.aquatox.2011.08.016
19. Short S, Yang G, Guler Y, Green Etxabe A, Kille P, Ford AT. Crustacean intersexuality is feminization without demasculinization: Implications for environmental toxicology. *Environ Sci Technol* (2014) 48:13520–9. doi: 10.1021/es5050503
20. Baldwin WS, Milam DL, Leblanc GA. Physiological and biochemical perturbations in *Daphnia magna* following exposure to the model environmental estrogen diethylstilbestrol. *Environ Toxicol Chem* (1995) 14:945–52. doi: 10.1002/etc.5620140604
21. Zou E, Fingerman M. Effects of estrogenic xenobiotics on molting of the water flea, *Daphnia magna*. *Ecotoxicol Environ Saf* (1997) 38:281–5. doi: 10.1006/eesa.1997.1589
22. Bechmann RK. Effect of the endocrine disrupter nonylphenol on the marine copepod *Tisbe battagliai*. *Sci Total Environ* (1999) 233:33–46. doi: 10.1016/S0048-9697(99)00177-1
23. Breitholtz M, Bengtsson B-E. Oestrogens have no hormonal effect on the development and reproduction of the harpacticoid copepod *Nitocra spinipes*. *Mar Pollut Bull* (2001) 42:879–86. doi: 10.1016/S0025-326X(01)00046-7
24. Vandenbergh GF, Adriaens D, Verslycke T, Janssen CR. Effects of 17α-ethinylestradiol on sexual development of the amphipod *Hyalella azteca*. *Ecotoxicol Environ Saf* (2003) 54:216–22. doi: 10.1016/S0147-6513(02)00030-1
25. Lye CM, Bentley MG, Clare AS, Sefton EM. Endocrine disruption in the shore crab *Carcinusmaenas*—a biomarker for benthic marine invertebrates? *Mar EcolProg Ser* (2005) 288:221–32.doi: 10.3354/meps288221
26. Gunamalai V, Kirubagaran R, Subramoniam T. Vertebrate steroids and the control of female reproduction in two decapod crustaceans, *Emerita asiatica* and *Macrobrachium rosenbergii*. *Curr Sci* (2006) 90:119–23.
27. Köhler H-R, Kloas W, Schirling M, Lutz I, Reye AL, Langen J-S, et al. Sex steroid receptor evolution and signalling in aquatic invertebrates. *Ecotoxicology* (2007) 16:131–43. doi: 10.1007/s10646-006-0111-3
28. Li GL, Chen HP, Deng SP, Ye M, Jiang S, Chan SF, et al. *In vivo* and *in vitro* inhibitory action of 17β-estradiol and environmental estrogen. *Genet Mol Res* (2015) 14:14056–65. doi: 10.4238/2015.October.29.25
29. Lu Y, Liu M, Gong J, Cheng Y, Wu X. Effect of exogenous estrogen on the ovarian development and gene expression in the female swimming crab *Portunus trituberculatus* (Miers, 1876) (Decapoda: Brachyura: Portunidae). *J Crustac Biol* (2018) 38:367–73. doi: 10.1093/jcbiol/ruy013
30. Gismondi E. Identification of molt-inhibiting hormone and ecdysteroid receptor cDNA sequences in *Gammarus pulex*, and variations after endocrine disruptor exposures. *Ecotoxicol Environ Saf* (2018) 158:9–17. doi: 10.1016/j.ecoenv.2018.04.017
31. Segner H, Caroll K, Fenske M, Janssen CR, Maack G, Pascoe D, et al. Identification of endocrine-disrupting effects in aquatic vertebrates and invertebrates: report from the European IDEA project. *Ecotoxicol Environ Saf* (2003) 54:302–14. doi: 10.1016/S0147-6513(02)00039-8
32. LeBlanc GA. Crustacean endocrine toxicology: a review. *Ecotoxicology* (2007) 16:61–81. doi: 10.1007/s10646-006-0115-z
33. De Wilde R, Swevers L, Soin T, Christiaens O, Rougé P, Cooreman K, et al. Cloning and functional analysis of the ecdysteroid receptor complex in the opossum shrimp *Neomysis integer* (Leach, 1814). *Aquat Toxicol* (2013) 130–131:31–40. doi: 10.1016/j.aquatox.2012.12.011
34. Chan YH, Chu KH, Chan KM. Ecdysteroid-mimicking compounds act as both agonists and antagonists to the crustacean ecdysone receptor. *Chemosphere* (2019) 237:124551. doi: 10.1016/j.chemosphere.2019.124551
35. Abe R, Watanabe H, Yamamuro M, Iguchi T, Tatarazako N. Establishment of a short-term, *in vivo* screening method for detecting chemicals with juvenile hormone activity using adult *Daphnia magna*. *J Appl Toxicol* (2015) 35:75–82. doi: 10.1002/jat.2989
36. Lafontaine A, Gismondi E, Boulangé-Lecomte C, Geraudie P, Dodet N, Caupos F, et al. Effects of chlordecone on 20-hydroxyecdysone concentration and chitobiase activity in a decapod crustacean, *Macrobrachium rosenbergii*. *Aquat Toxicol* (2016) 176:53–63. doi: 10.1016/j.aquatox.2016.04.006
37. Medlock Kakaley EK, Eytcheson SA, LeBlanc GA. Ligand-mediated receptor assembly as an end point for high-throughput chemical toxicity screening. *Environ Sci Technol* (2017) 51:9327–33. doi: 10.1021/acs.est.7b02882
38. Song Y, Evenseth LM, Iguchi T, Tollefsen KE. Release of chitobiase as an indicator of potential molting disruption in juvenile *Daphnia magna* exposed to the ecdysone receptor agonist 20-hydroxyecdysone. *J Toxicol Environ Health A* (2017) 80:954–62. doi: 10.1080/15287394.2017.1352215
39. Bonett RM. Analyzing endocrine system conservation and evolution. *Gen Comp Endocrinol* (2016) 234:3–9. doi: 10.1016/j.ygcen.2016.03.011
40. Erwin DH, Davidson EH. The last common bilaterian ancestor. *Dev Camb Engl* (2002) 129:3021–32.
41. Loof AD, Lindemans M, Liu F, Groef BD, Schoofs L. Endocrine archeology: Do insects retain ancestrally inherited counterparts of the vertebrate releasing hormones GnRH, GHRH, TRH, and CRF? *Gen Comp Endocrinol* (2012) 177:18–27. doi: 10.1016/j.ygcen.2012.02.002
42. Marco HG. Unity and diversity in chemical signals of arthropods: the role of neuropeptides in crustaceans and insects. *Int Congr Ser* (2004) 1275:126–33. doi: 10.1016/j.ics.2004.08.053
43. Hartenstein V. The neuroendocrine system of invertebrates: a developmental and evolutionary perspective. *J Endocrinol* (2006) 190:555–70. doi: 10.1677/joe.1.06964
44. Elphick MR, Mirabeau O, Larhammar D. Evolution of neuropeptide signalling systems. *J Exp Biol* (2018) 221:jeb151092. doi: 10.1242/jeb.151092
45. Ayala FJ, Rzhetsky A, Ayala FJ. Origin of the metazoan phyla: Molecular clocks confirm paleontological estimates. *Proc Natl Acad Sci* (1998) 95:606. doi: 10.1073/pnas.95.2.606
46. Markov GV, Tavares R, Dauphin-Villemant C, Demeneix BA, Baker ME, Laudet V. Independent elaboration of steroid hormone signaling pathways in metazoans. *Proc Natl Acad Sci USA* (2009) 106:11913–8. doi: 10.1073/pnas.0812138106
47. Jegla T. Evidence for ecdysteroids as molting hormones in Chelicerata, Crustacea, and Myriapoda. In: Gupta A, editor. *"Morphogenetic Hormones of Arthropods"*. London: Rutgers Univ. Press (1990).
48. Defelipe LA, Dolghih E, Roitberg AE, Nouzova M, Mayoral JG, Noriega FG, et al. Juvenile hormone synthesis: "esterify then epoxidize" or "epoxidize

then esterify"? Insights from the structural characterization of juvenile hormone acid methyltransferase. *Insect Biochem Mol Biol* (2011) 41:228–35. doi: 10.1016/j.ibmb.2010.12.008

49. Mercier J, Doucet D, Retnakaran A. Molecular physiology of crustacean and insect neuropeptides. *J Pestic Sci* (2007) 32:345–59. doi: 10.1584/jpestics.R07-04
50. Webster SG, Keller R, Dircksen H. The CHH-superfamily of multifunctional peptide hormones controlling crustacean metabolism, osmoregulation, moulting, and reproduction. *Gen Comp Endocrinol* (2012) 175:217–33. doi: 10.1016/j.ygcen.2011.11.035
51. Dircksen H. Insect ion transport peptides are derived from alternatively spliced genes and differentially expressed in the central and peripheral nervous system. *J Exp Biol* (2009) 212:401–12. doi: 10.1242/jeb.026112
52. Gáliková M, Dircksen H, Nässel DR. The thirsty fly: Ion transport peptide (ITP) is a novel endocrine regulator of water homeostasis in *Drosophila*. *PloS Genet* (2018) 14:e1007618. doi: 10.1371/journal.pgen.1007618
53. Sandve SR, Rohlfs RV, Hvidsten TR. Subfunctionalization versus neofunctionalization after whole-genome duplication. *Nat Genet* (2018) 50:908–9. doi: 10.1038/s41588-018-0162-4
54. Thornton JW, Need E, Crews D. Resurrecting the ancestral steroid receptor: ancient origin of estrogen signaling. *Science* (2003) 301:1714–7. doi: 10.1126/science.1086185
55. Escriva H, Bertrand S, Laudet V. The evolution of the nuclear receptor superfamily. *Essays Biochem* (2004) 40:11–26. doi: 10.1042/bse0400011
56. Bertrand S, Brunet FG, Escriva H, Parmentier G, Laudet V, Robinson-Rechavi M. Evolutionary genomics of nuclear receptors: from twenty-five ancestral genes to derived endocrine systems. *Mol Biol Evol* (2004) 21:1923–37. doi: 10.1093/molbev/msh200
57. Thomson SA, Baldwin WS, Wang YH, Kwon G, LeBlanc GA. Annotation, phylogenetics, and expression of the nuclear receptors in *Daphnia pulex*. *BMC Genomics* (2009) 10:500. doi: 10.1186/1471-2164-10-500
58. Campbell RK, Satoh N, Degnan BM. Piecing together evolution of the vertebrate endocrine system. *Trends Genet* (2004) 20:359–66. doi: 10.1016/j.tig.2004.06.005
59. Baker ME. Evolution of adrenal and sex steroid action in vertebrates: a ligand-based mechanism for complexity. *BioEssays News Rev Mol Cell Dev Biol* (2003) 25:396–400. doi: 10.1002/bies.10252
60. Baker ME. Trichoplax, the simplest known animal, contains an estrogen-related receptor but no estrogen receptor: Implications for estrogen receptor evolution. *Biochem Biophys Res Commun* (2008) 375:623–7. doi: 10.1016/j.bbrc.2008.08.047
61. Bridgham JT, Brown JE, Rodríguez-Marí A, Catchen JM, Thornton JW. Evolution of a new function by degenerative mutation in cephalochordate steroid receptors. *PloS Genet* (2008) 4:e1000191. doi: 10.1371/journal.pgen.1000191
62. Baker ME. Steroid receptors and vertebrate evolution. *Mol Cell Endocrinol* (2019) 496:110526. doi: 10.1016/j.mce.2019.110526
63. Bonneton F, Zelus D, Iwema T, Robinson-Rechavi M, Laudet V. Rapid divergence of the ecdysone receptor in *Diptera* and *Lepidoptera* suggests coevolution between ECR and USP-RXR. *Mol Biol Evol* (2003) 20:541–53. doi: 10.1093/molbev/msg054
64. Grillo M, Casanova J, Averof M. Development: a deep breath for endocrine organ evolution. *Curr Biol* (2014) 24:R38–40. doi: 10.1016/j.cub.2013.11.033
65. Sánchez-Higueras C, Sotillos S, Castelli-Gair Hombría J. Common origin of insect trachea and endocrine organs from a segmentally repeated precursor. *Curr Biol* (2014) 24:76–81. doi: 10.1016/j.cub.2013.11.010
66. Siveter DJ, Williams M, Waloszek D. A phosphatocopid crustacean with appendages from the lower Cambrian. *Science* (2001) 293:479–81. doi: 10.1126/science.1061697
67. Han J, Morris SC, Ou Q, Shu D, Huang H. Meiofaunal deuterostomes from the basal Cambrian of Shaanxi (China). *Nature* (2017) 542:228–31. doi: 10.1038/nature21072
68. Richter S, Wirkner CS. What the ur-crustacean lookedlike. Poore G and Thiel M (eds). *Evolution and Biogeography (Volume 8 in the Series The Natural History of the Crustacea)*. Oxford University Press (2020). pp. 1–20.
69. Skinner DM, Graham DE, Holland CH, Mykles DL, Soumoff C, Yamaoka LH. "Control of molting incrustacea," In: Wenner AM. *Crustacean Issues 3: factors in adult growth*. Rotterdam: A.A. Balkema Publishers (1985). p. 3–14. doi: 10.1201/9781315140681
70. Techa S, Chung JS. Ecdysteroids regulate the levels of Molt-Inhibiting Hormone (MIH) expression in the blue crab, *Callinectes sapidus*. *PloS One* (2015) 10:e0117278. doi: 10.1371/journal.pone.0117278
71. Nagaraju GPC, Reddy PR, Reddy PS. *In vitro* methyl farnesoate secretion by mandibular organs isolated from different molt and reproductive stages of the crab *Oziotelphusa senex senex*. *Fish Sci* (2006) 72:410–4. doi: 10.1111/j.1444-2906.2006.01164.x
72. Chang ES, Mykles DL. Regulation of crustacean molting: A review and our perspectives. *Gen Comp Endocrinol* (2011) 172:323–30. doi: 10.1016/j.ygcen.2011.04.003
73. Chung JS. Hemolymph ecdysteroids during the last three molt cycles of the blue crab, *Callinectes sapidus*: quantitative and qualitative analyses and regulation. *Arch Insect Biochem Physiol* (2010) 73:1–13. doi: 10.1002/arch.20327
74. Chung JS, Dircksen H. Webster SG. A remarkable, precisely timed release of hyperglycemic hormone from endocrine cells in the gut is associated with ecdysis in the crab *Carcinus maenas*. *Proc Natl Acad Sci USA* (1999) 96:13103–7. doi: 10.1073/pnas.96.23.13103
75. Phlippen MK, Webster SG, Chung JS, Dircksen H. Ecdysis of decapod crustaceans is associated with a dramatic release of crustacean cardioactive peptide into the haemolymph. *J Exp Biol* (2000) 203:521–36.
76. Webster SG, Wilcockson DC, Mrinalini, Sharp JH. Bursicon and neuropeptide cascades during the ecdysis program of the shore crab, *Carcinus maenas*. *Gen Comp Endocrinol* (2013) 182:54–64. doi: 10.1016/j.ygcen.2012.11.018
77. Drach P. Mue et cycle d'intermue chez les crustaces decapodes. *Ann Inst Ocean Monaco* (1939) 19:103–391.
78. Kuballa A, Elizur A. Novel molecular approach to study moulting in crustaceans. *Bull-Fish Res Agency Jpn* (2007) 20:53.
79. Liu L, Laufer H. Isolation and characterization of sinus gland neuropeptides with both mandibular organ inhibiting and hyperglycemic effects from the spider crab *Libinia emarginata*. *Arch Insect Biochem Physiol* (1996) 32:375–85. doi: 10.1002/(SICI)1520-6327(1996)32:3/4<375::AID-ARCH10>3.0.CO;2-9
80. Martin-Creuzburg D, Westerlund SA, Hoffmann KH. Ecdysteroid levels in *Daphnia magna* during a molt cycle: Determination by radioimmunoassay (RIA) and liquid chromatography–mass spectrometry (LC–MS). *Gen Comp Endocrinol* (2007) 151:66–71. doi: 10.1016/j.ygcen.2006.11.015
81. Sumiya E, Ogino Y, Miyakawa H, Hiruta C, Toyota K, Miyagawa S, et al. Roles of ecdysteroids for progression of reproductive cycle in the fresh water crustacean *Daphnia magna*. *Front Zool* (2014) 11:60. doi: 10.1186/s12983-014-0060-2
82. Drach P, Tchernigovtzeff C. Sur la méthode de détermination des stades d'intermue et son application générale aux crustacés. *Vie Milieu* (1967) 18A:595–610.
83. Alexander JL, Oliphant A, Wilcockson DC, Audsley N, Down RE, Lafont R, et al. Functional characterization and signaling systems of corazonin and red pigment concentrating hormone in the green shore crab, *Carcinus maenas*. *Front Neurosci* (2018) 11:752. doi: 10.3389/fnins.2017.00752
84. Passano L. Neurosecretory control of molting in crabs by the X-organ sinus gland complex. *Physiol Comp Oecol* (1953) 3:5–1.
85. Brown FA. Hormones in the crustacea: Their sources and activities. *Q Rev Biol* (1944) 19:32–46. doi: 10.1086/394686
86. Knowles SFGW, Carlisle DB. Endocrine control in the crustacea. *Biol Rev* (1956) 31:396–467. doi: 10.1111/j.1469-185X.1956.tb01556.x
87. Webster SG, Keller R. Purification, characterisation and amino acid composition of the putative moult-inhibiting hormone (MIH) of *Carcinus maenas* (Crustacea, Decapoda). *J Comp Physiol B* (1986) 156:617–24. doi: 10.1007/BF00692738
88. Chung JS, Webster SG. Moult cycle-related changes in biological activity of moult-inhibiting hormone (MIH) and crustacean hyperglycaemic hormone (CHH) in the crab, *Carcinus maenas*. From target to transcript. *Eur J Biochem* (2003) 270:3280–8. doi: 10.1046/j.1432-1033.2003.03720.x
89. Chung JS, Webster SG. Dynamics of *in vivo* release of molt-inhibiting hormone and crustacean hyperglycemic hormone in the shore crab, *Carcinus maenas*. *Endocrinology* (2005) 146:5545–51. doi: 10.1210/en.2005-0859

90. Nakatsuji T, Keino H, Tamura K, Yoshimura S, Kawakami T, Aimoto S, et al. Changes in the amounts of the Molt-Inhibiting Hormone in sinus glands during the molt cycle of the American crayfish, *Procambarus clarkii. Zoolog Sci* (2000) 17:1129–36. doi: 10.2108/zsj.17.1129
91. Watson RD, Lee KJ, Shihong Q, Ming L, Heidi RU, Robert DR, et al. Molecular cloning, expression, and tissue distribution of crustacean Molt-Inhibiting Hormone. *Am Zool* (2001) 41:407–17. doi: 10.1093/icb/41.3.407
92. Robert A, Monsinjon T, Delbecque J-P, Olivier S, Poret A, Foll FL, et al. Neuroendocrine disruption in the shore crab *Carcinus maenas*: Effects of serotonin and fluoxetine on *chh*- and *mih*-gene expression, glycaemia and ecdysteroid levels. *Aquat Toxicol* (2016) 175:192–204. doi: 10.1016/j.aquatox.2016.03.025
93. Sefiani M, Caer J-PL, Soyez D. Characterization of hyperglycemic and molt-inhibiting activity from sinus glands of the penaeid shrimp, *Penaeus vannamei. Gen Comp Endocrinol* (1996) 103:41–53. doi: 10.1006/gcen.1996.0092
94. Nakatsuji T, Sonobe H. Regulation of ecdysteroid secretion from the Y-organ by molt-inhibiting hormone in the American crayfish, *Procambarus clarkii. Gen Comp Endocrinol* (2004) 135:358–64. doi: 10.1016/j.ygcen.2003.11.001
95. Chung JS, Katayama H, Dircksen H. New functions of arthropod bursicon: inducing deposition and thickening of new cuticle and hemocyte granulation in the blue crab, *Callinectes sapidus. PloS One* (2012) 7(9):e46299. doi: 10.1371/journal.pone.0046299
96. Christie AE, McCoole MD, Harmon SM, Baer KN, Lenz PH. Genomic analyses of the *Daphnia pulex* peptidome. *Gen Comp Endocrinol* (2011) 171:131–50. doi: 10.1016/j.ygcen.2011.01.002
97. Dircksen H, Neupert S, Predel R, Verleyen P, Huybrechts J, Strauss J, et al. Genomics, transcriptomics, and peptidomics of *Daphnia pulex* neuropeptides and protein hormones. *J Proteome Res* (2011) 10:4478–504. doi: 10.1021/pr200284e
98. Oliphant A, Alexander JL, Swain MT, Webster SG, Wilcockson DC. Transcriptomic analysis of crustacean neuropeptide signaling during the moult cycle in the green shore crab, *Carcinus maenas. BMC Genomics* (2018) 19:711. doi: 10.1186/s12864-018-5057-3
99. Nhut TM, Mykles DL, Elizur A, Ventura T. Ecdysis triggering hormone modulates molt behaviour in the redclawcrayfish *Cherax quadricarinatus*, providing a mechanistic evidence for conservedfunction in molt regulation across Pancrustacea. *Gen Comp Endocrinol* (2020) 298:113556. 10.1016/j.ygcen.2020.113556
100. Zhou L, Li S, Wang Z, Li F, Xiang J. An eclosion hormone-like gene participates in the molting process of Palaemonid shrimp *Exopalaemon carinicauda. Dev Genes Evol* (2017) 227:189–99. 10.1007/s00427-017-0580-9
101. Hopkins PM. "Crustacean ecdysteroids and their receptors," In: Smagghe G, editor. *Ecdysone: Structures and Functions.* Dordrecht: Springer Netherlands (2009). p. 73–97. doi: 10.1007/978-1-4020-9112-4_3
102. Soumoff C, Skinner DM. Ecdysteroid titers during the molt cycle of the blue crab resemble those of other crustacea. *Biol Bull* (1983) 165:321–9. doi: 10.2307/1541372
103. Mykles DL. Ecdysteroid metabolism in crustaceans. *J Steroid Biochem Mol Biol* (2011) 127:196–203. doi: 10.1016/j.jsbmb.2010.09.001
104. Schumann I, Kenny N, Hui J, Hering L, Mayer G. Halloween genes in panarthropods and the evolution of the early moulting pathway in ecdysozoa. *R Soc Open Sci* (2018) 5:180888. doi: 10.1098/rsos.180888
105. Niwa R, Niwa YS. Enzymes for ecdysteroid biosynthesis: their biological functions in insects and beyond. *Biosci Biotechnol Biochem* (2014) 78:1283–92. doi: 10.1080/09168451.2014.942250
106. Hosamani N, Reddy S, Reddy R. Crustacean molting: regulation and effects of environmentaltoxicants. *J Mar Sci Res Dev* (2017) 7:2. 10.4172/2155-9910.1000236
107. Rewitz KF, Gilbert LI. *Daphnia* Halloween genes that encode cytochrome P450s mediating the synthesis of the arthropod molting hormone: Evolutionary implications. *BMC Evol Biol* (2008) 8:60. doi: 10.1186/1471-2148-8-60
108. Niwa R, Namiki T, Ito K, Shimada-Niwa Y, Kiuchi M, Kawaoka S, et al. Non-molting glossy shroud encodes a short-chain dehydrogenase/reductase that functions in the 'Black Box' of the ecdysteroid biosynthesis pathway. *Development* (2010) 137:1991. doi: 10.1242/dev.045641
109. Sumiya E, Ogino Y, Toyota K, Miyakawa H, Miyagawa S, Iguchi T. Neverland regulates embryonic moltings through the regulation of ecdysteroid synthesis in the water flea *Daphnia magna*, and may thus act as a target for chemical disruption of molting. *J Appl Toxicol* (2016) 36:1476–85. doi: 10.1002/jat.3306
110. Fontana E, Dansette PM, Poli SM. Cytochrome p450 enzymes mechanism based inhibitors: common sub-structures and reactivity. *Curr Drug Metab* (2005) 6:413–54. doi: 10.2174/138920005774330639
111. Hassold E, Backhaus T. Chronic toxicity of five structurally diverse demethylase-inhibiting fungicides to the crustacean *Daphnia magna*: A comparative assessment. *Environ Toxicol Chem* (2009) 28:1218–26. doi: 10.1897/08-339.1
112. Kast-Hutcheson K, Rider CV, LeBlanc GA. The fungicide propiconazole interferes with embryonic development of the crustacean *Daphnia magna. Environ Toxicol Chem* (2001) 20:502–9. doi: 10.1002/etc.5620200308
113. Mu X, LeBlanc GA. Environmental antiecdysteroids alter embryo development in the crustacean *Daphnia magna. J Exp Zool* (2002) 292:287–92. doi: 10.1002/jez.10020
114. Bonneton F, Chaumot A, Laudet V. Annotation of *Tribolium* nuclear receptors reveals an increase in evolutionary rate of a network controlling the ecdysone cascade. *Insect Biochem Mol Biol* (2008) 38:416–29. doi: 10.1016/j.ibmb.2007.10.006
115. Hannas BR, LeBlanc GA. Expression and ecdysteroid responsiveness of the nuclear receptors HR3 and E75 in the crustacean *Daphnia magna. Mol Cell Endocrinol* (2010) 315:208–18. doi: 10.1016/j.mce.2009.07.013
116. Riddiford LM, Cherbas P, Truman JW. Ecdysone receptors and their biological actions. *Vitam Horm* (2000) 60:1–73. doi: 10.1016/S0083-6729(00)60016-X
117. Hill RJ, Billas IML, Bonneton F, Graham LD, Lawrence MC. Ecdysone receptors: From the Ashburner model to structural biology. *Annu Rev Entomol* (2013) 58:251–71. doi: 10.1146/annurev-ento-120811-153610
118. Baehrecke EH. Ecdysone signaling cascade and regulation of Drosophilametamorphosis. *Arch Insect Biochem Physiol* (1996) 33:231–44. doi: 10.1002/(SICI)1520-6327(1996)33:3/4<231::AID-ARCH5>3.0.CO;2-V
119. Belles X, Piulachs M-D. Ecdysone signalling and ovarian development in insects: from stem cells to ovarian follicle formation. *Biochim Biophys Acta* (2015) 1849:181–6. doi: 10.1016/j.bbagrm.2014.05.025
120. Gong J, Ye H, Xie Y, Yang Y, Huang H, Li S, et al. Ecdysone receptor in the mud crab *Scylla paramamosain*: a possible role in promoting ovarian development. *J Endocrinol* (2015) 224:273–87. doi: 10.1530/JOE-14-0526
121. Yao T-P, Forman BM, Jiang Z, Cherbas L, Chen J-D, McKeown M, et al. Functional ecdysone receptor is the product of EcR and Ultraspiraclegenes. *Nature* (1993) 366:476–9. doi: 10.1038/366476a0
122. Billas IML, Iwema T, Garnier J-M, Mitschler A, Rochel N, Moras D. Structural adaptability in the ligand-binding pocket of the ecdysone hormone receptor. *Nature* (2003) 426:91–6. doi: 10.1038/nature02112
123. Hu X, Cherbas L, Cherbas P. Transcription activation by the Ecdysone Receptor (EcR/USP): Identification of activation functions. *Mol Endocrinol* (2003) 17:716–31. doi: 10.1210/me.2002-0287
124. Li J, Sun J, Dong X, Geng X, Qiu G. Transcriptomic analysis of gills provides insights into the molecular basis of molting in Chinese mitten crab (*Eriocheir sinensis*). *PeerJ* (2019) 7:e7182–2. doi: 10.7717/peerj.7182
125. Zou E, Fingerman M. Chitobiase activity in the epidermis and hepatopancreas of the fiddler crab *Uca pugilator* during the molting cycle. *Mar Biol* (1999) 133:97–101. doi: 10.1007/s002270050447
126. Meng Y, Zou E. Impacts of molt-inhibiting organochlorine compounds on epidermal ecdysteroid signaling in the fiddler crab, *Uca pugilator, in vitro. Comp Biochem Physiol Part C Toxicol Pharmacol* (2009) 150:436–41. doi: 10.1016/j.cbpc.2009.06.009
127. Qian Z, He S, Liu T, Liu Y, Hou F, Liu Q, et al. Identification of ecdysteroid signaling late-response genes from different tissues of the Pacific white shrimp, *Litopenaeus vannamei. Comp Biochem Physiol A Mol Integr Physiol* (2014) 172:10–30. doi: 10.1016/j.cbpa.2014.02.011
128. Espie PJ, Roff JC. A biochemical index of duration of the molt cycle for planktonic crustacea based on the chitin-degrading enzyme, chitobiase. *Limnol Oceanogr* (1995) 40:1028–34. doi: 10.4319/lo.1995.40.6.1028
129. Yoon D-S, Park JC, Park HG, Lee J-S, Han J. Effects of atrazine on life parameters, oxidative stress, and ecdysteroid biosynthetic pathway in the

marine copepod *Tigriopus japonicus*. *Aquat Toxicol* (2019) 213:105213. doi: 10.1016/j.aquatox.2019.05.015

130. Chen H, Gu X, Zeng Q, Mao Z, Liang X, Martyniuk CJ. Carbamazepine disrupts molting hormone signaling and inhibits molting and growth of *Eriocheir sinensis* at environmentally relevant concentrations. *Aquat Toxicol* (2019) 208:138–45. doi: 10.1016/j.aquatox.2019.01.010
131. Dinan L, Whiting P, Girault J-P, Lafont R, Dhadialla ST, Cress ED, et al. Cucurbitacins are insect steroid hormone antagonists acting at the ecdysteroid receptor. *Biochem J* (1997) 327:643–50. doi: 10.1042/bj3270643
132. Dhadialla TS, Carlson GR, Le DP. New insecticides with ecdysteroidal and juvenile hormone activity. *Annu Rev Entomol* (1998) 43:545–69. doi: 10.1146/annurev.ento.43.1.545
133. Kato Y, Kobayashi K, Oda S, Tatarazako N, Watanabe H, Iguchi T. Cloning and characterization of the ecdysone receptor and ultraspiracle protein from the water flea *Daphnia magna*. *J Endocrinol* (2007) 193:183–94. doi: 10.1677/JOE-06-0228
134. Mellor CL, Tollefsen KE, LaLone C, Cronin MTD, Firman JW. *In silico* identification of chemicals capable of binding to the ecdysone receptor. *Environ Toxicol Chem* (2020) 39:1438–50. doi: 10.1002/etc.4733
135. Dinan L, Bourne P, Whiting P, Dhadialla TS, Hutchinson TH. Screening of environmental contaminants for ecdysteroid agonist and antagonist activity using the *Drosophila melanogaster* BII cell *in vitro* assay. *Environ Toxicol Chem* (2001) 20:2038–46. doi: 10.1002/etc.5620200924
136. Mu X, LeBlanc GA. Developmental toxicity of testosterone in the crustacean *Daphnia magna* involves anti-ecdysteroidal activity. *Gen Comp Endocrinol* (2002) 129:127–33. doi: 10.1016/S0016-6480(02)00518-X
137. de Melo MS, Nazari EM, Joaquim-Justo C, Muller YMR, Gismondi E. Effects of low glyphosate-based herbicide concentrations on endocrine-related gene expression in the decapoda *Macrobrachium potiuna*. *Environ Sci Pollut Res* (2019) 26:21535–45. doi: 10.1007/s11356-019-05496-1
138. Park K, Kim W-S, Kwak I-S. Characterization and transcriptional response of ecdysone receptor gene in the mud crab *Macrophthalmus japonicus*: Effects of osmotic stress and endocrine disrupting chemicals. *Ocean Sci J* (2019) 54:611–20. doi: 10.1007/s12601-019-0029-3
139. Zou E. Invisible endocrine disruption and its mechanisms: A current review. *Gen Comp Endocrinol* (2020) 293:113470. doi: 10.1016/j.ygcen.2020.113470
140. Keller R, Beyer J. Zur hyperglykämischen Wirkung von Serotonin und Augenstielextrakt beim Flusskrebs *Orconectes limosus*. *Z Vgl Physiol* (1968) 59:78–85. doi: 10.1007/BF00298812
141. Lee CY, Yang PF, Zou HS. Serotonergic regulation of crustacean hyperglycemic hormone secretion in the crayfish, *Procambarus clarkii*. *Physiol Biochem Zool* (2001) 74:376–82. doi: 10.1086/320430
142. Alvarado-Alvarez R, Aréchiga H, García U. Serotonin activates a Ca(2+)-dependent K(+) current in identified peptidergic neurons from the crayfish. *J Exp Biol* (2000) 203:715–23.
143. Sáenz F, García U, Aréchiga U. Modulation of electrical activity by 5-hydroxytryptamine in crayfish neurosecretory cells. *J Exp Biol* (1997) 200:3079–90.
144. Webster SG. High-affinity binding of putative moult-inhibiting hormone (MIH) and crustacean hyperglycaemic hormone (CHH) to membrane-bound receptors on the Y-organ of the shore crab *Carcinus maenus*. *Proc R Soc Lond B Biol Sci* (1993) 251:53–9. doi: 10.1098/rspb.1993.0008
145. LeBlanc GA, McLachlan JB. Molt-independent growth inhibition of *Daphnia magna* by a vertebrate antiandrogen. *Environ Toxicol Chem* (1999) 18:1450–5. doi: 10.1002/etc.5620180715
146. DeLoof A, DeClerk D, Andriesm JC, Dhainaut A. Vertebrate-type steroids in arthropods: Identification, concentrations and possible functions. In: Porchet M, editor. *"Advances in Invertebrate Reproduction"*, vol. 4. Amsterdam: Elsevier (1986).
147. Jeng SS, Wan WC-M, Chang CF. Existence of an estrogen-like compound in the ovary of the shrimp *Parapenaeus fissurus*. *Gen Comp Endocrinol* (1978) 36:211–4. doi: 10.1016/0016-6480(78)90024-2
148. Lewis SE, Freund JG, Riddell GE, Wankowski JL, Dick JTA, Baldridge MG. Interspecific comparison of estrogen and testosterone concentrations in three species of amphipods (*Gammarus duebeni celticus*, *G. pseudolimnaeus*, and *G. pulex*). *J Crustac Biol* (2015) 35:789–92. doi: 10.1163/1937240X-00002379
149. Mackevieciene G, Chibisova N. Concentration of steroid hormones at different stages of the intermoult cycle in the crayfish *Astacus astacus* and *Pacifastacus leniusculus*. *Freshw Crayfish* (1995) 10:267–73.
150. Novak F, Van Beek E, Lambert J, De Loof A. Pregnenolone and estradiol identification in the brine shrimp,*Artemia sp.*, by means of gas chromatographical-mass spectrometricalanalysis. *Comp Biochem Physiol Part B Comp Biochem* (1990) 95:565–9. 10.1016/0305-0491(90)90022-L
151. Merlin JR, Mohanlal DL, Balasubramanian CP, Vijayan KK, Subramoniam T, Tomy S, et al. Vertebrate-type steroid profile in different tissues of wild and endocrinologically manipulated female brood stocks of *Penaeus monodon*. *Curr Sci* (2016) 111:1194–200.
152. Subramoniam T. Steroidal control of vitellogenesis in Crustacea: a newunderstanding for improving shrimp hatchery production. *Proc Indian Natl SciAcad* (2017) 83:595–610. 10.16943/ptinsa/2017/48969
153. Young NJ, Quinlan PT, Goad LJ. Progesterone metabolism *in vitro* in the decapod crustacean, *Penaeus monodon*. *Gen Comp Endocrinol* (1992) 87:300–11. doi: 10.1016/0016-6480(92)90035-I
154. Burns BG, Sangalang GB, Freeman HC, McMenemy M. Bioconversion of steroids by the testes of the American lobster, *Homarus americanus, in vitro*. *Gen Comp Endocrinol* (1984) 54:422–8. doi: 10.1016/0016-6480(84)90157-6
155. Baldwin WS, LeBlanc GA. *In vivo* biotransformation of testosterone by phase I and II detoxication enzymes and their modulation by 20-hydroxyecdysone in *Daphnia magna*. *Aquat Toxicol* (1994) 29:103–17. doi: 10.1016/0166-445X(94)90051-5
156. Depledge MH, Billinghurst Z. Ecological significance of endocrine disruption in marine invertebrates. *Mar Pollut Bull* (1999) 39:32–8. doi: 10.1016/S0025-326X(99)00115-0
157. Coccia E, Lisa ED, Cristo CD, Cosmo AD, Paolucci M. Effects of estradiol and progesterone on the reproduction of the freshwater crayfish *Cherax albidus*. *Biol Bull* (2010) 218:36–47. doi: 10.1086/BBLv218n1p36
158. Zhang Z, Chen K, Shih JC, Teng CT. Estrogen-related receptors-stimulated monoamine oxidase B promoter activity is down-regulated by estrogen receptors. *Mol Endocrinol* (2006) 20:1547–61. doi: 10.1210/me.2005-0252
159. Chakravorty SG, Halbreich U. The influence of estrogen on monoamine oxidase activity. *Psychopharmacol Bull* (1997) 33:229–33.
160. Ma Z-Q, Violani E, Villa F, Picotti GB, Maggi A. Estrogenic control of monoamine oxidase A activity in human neuroblastoma cells expressing physiological concentrations of estrogen receptor. *Eur J Pharmacol* (1995) 284:171–6. doi: 10.1016/0014-2999(95)00387-Z
161. Jordão R, Campos B, Piña B, Tauler R, Soares AMVM, Barata C. Mechanisms of action of compounds that enhance storage lipid accumulation in *Daphnia magna*. *Environ Sci Technol* (2016) 50:13565–73. doi: 10.1021/acs.est.6b04768
162. Zou E, Fingerman M. Synthetic estrogenic agents do not interfere with sex differentiation but do inhibit molting of the cladoceran *Daphnia magna*. *Bull Environ Contam Toxicol* (1997) 58:596–602. doi: 10.1007/s001289900376
163. Watermann BT, Albanis TA, Galassi S, Gnass K, Kusk KO, Sakkas VA, et al. Effects of anti-androgens cyproterone acetate, linuron, vinclozolin, and p,p'-DDE on the reproductive organs of the copepod *Acartia tonsa*. *J Environ Sci Health Part A* (2016) 51:1111–20. doi: 10.1080/10934529.2016.1199769
164. Reddy PS, Devi M, Sarojini R, Nagabhushanam R, Fingerman M. Cadmium chloride induced hyperglycemia in the red swamp crayfish, *Procambarus clarkii*: Possible role of crustacean hyperglycemic hormone. *Comp Biochem Physiol C Pharmacol Toxicol Endocrinol* (1994) 107:57–61. doi: 10.1016/1367-8280(94)90010-8
165. Reddy PS, Fingerman M. Effect of cadmium chloride on physiological color changes of thefiddler crab. *Uca Pugilator Ecotoxicol Environ Saf* (1995) 31:69–75. doi: 10.1006/eesa.1995.1045
166. Reddy PS, Nguyen LK, Obih P, Fingerman M. Effect of cadmium chloride on the distal retinal pigment cells of the fiddler crab, *Uca pugilator*. *Bull Environ Contam Toxicol* (1997) 58:504–10. doi: 10.1007/s001289900363
167. Reddy PS, Tuberty SR, Fingerman M. Effects of cadmium and mercury on ovarian maturation in the red swamp crayfish, *Procambarus clarkii*. *Ecotoxicol Environ Saf* (1997) 37:62–5. doi: 10.1006/eesa.1997.1523
168. Rodríguez EM, Greco LSL, Fingerman M. Inhibition of ovarian growth by cadmium in the fiddler crab, *Uca pugilator* (Decapoda, Ocypodidae). *Ecotoxicol Environ Saf* (2000) 46:202–6. doi: 10.1006/eesa.1999.1896

169. Medesani DA, Greco LSL, Rodrıguez EM. Interference of cadmium and copper with the endocrine control of ovarian growth, in the estuarine crab *Chasmagnathus granulata*. *Aquat Toxicol* (2004) 69:165–74. doi: 10.1016/j.aquatox.2004.05.003
170. Lorenzon S, Edomi P, Giulianini PG, Mettulio R, Ferrero EA. Variation of crustacean hyperglycemic hormone (cHH) level in the eyestalk and haemolymph of the shrimp *Palaemon elegans* following stress. *J Exp Biol* (2004) 207:4205–13. doi: 10.1242/jeb.01264
171. Lorenzon S, Edomi P, Giulianini PG, Mettulio R, Ferrero EA. Role of biogenic amines and cHH in the crustacean hyperglycemic stress response. *J Exp Biol* (2005) 208:3341–7. doi: 10.1242/jeb.01761
172. Fingerman M, Hanumate MM, Deshpande UD, Nagabhushanam R. Increase in the total reducing substances in the hemolymph of the freshwater crab, *Barytelphusa guerini*, produced by a pesticide (DDT) and an indolealkylamine (serotonin). *Experientia* (1981) 37:178–9. doi: 10.1007/BF01963219
173. Hanumante MM, Fingerman SW, Fingerman M. Antagonism of the inhibitory effect of the polychlorinated biphenyl preparation, Aroclor 1242, on color changes of the fiddler crab, *Uca pugilator*, by norepinephrine and drugs affecting noradrenergic neurotransmission. *Bull Environ Contam Toxicol* (1981) 26:479–84. doi: 10.1007/BF01622123
174. Reddy PS, Bhagyalakshmi A, Ramamurthi R. Effect of sumithion on ovarian growth of a fresh water rice field crab (*Oziotelphusa senex senex* Fabricius). *Toxicol Lett* (1983) 18:273–6. doi: 10.1016/0378-4274(83)90106-6
175. Bhagyalakshmi A, Reddy PS, Ramamurthi R. Changes in hemolymph glucose, hepatopancreas glycogen, total carbohydrates, phosphorylase and amino transferases of sumithion-stressed freshwater rice-field crab (*Oziotelphusa senex senex*). *Toxicol Lett* (1983) 18:277–84. doi: 10.1016/0378-4274(83)90107-8
176. Sarojini R, Nagabhushanam R, Fingerman M. A possible neurotransmitter-neuroendocrine mechanism in naphthalene-induced atresia of the ovary of the red swamp crayfish, *Procambarus clarkii*. *Comp Biochem Physiol C Pharmacol Toxicol Endocrinol* (1994) 108:33–8. doi: 10.1016/1367-8280(94)90085-X
177. Staub GC. Fingerman M. A mechanism of action for the inhibition of black pigment dispersion in the fiddler crab, *Uca pugilator*, by naphthalene. *Comp Biochem Physiol Part C Comp Pharmacol* (1984) 79:447–53. doi: 10.1016/0742-8413(84)90229-9
178. Staub GC, Fingerman M. Effect of naphthalene on color changes of the sand fiddler crab, *Uca pugilator*. *Comp Biochem Physiol Part C Comp Pharmacol* (1984) 77:7–12. doi: 10.1016/0742-8413(84)90123-3
179. Fingerman M, Hanumante MM, Fingerman SW. The effects of biogenic amines on color changes of the fiddler crab, *Uca pugilator*: Further evidence for roles of 5-hydroxytryptamine and dopamine as neurotransmitters triggering release of erythrophorotropic hormones. *Comp Biochem Physiol Part C Comp Pharmacol* (1981) 68:205–11. doi: 10.1016/0306-4492(81)90017-4
180. Hanumante MM, Fingerman M. Further evidence for norepinephrine as a neurotransmitter stimulating release of melanin-dispersing hormone in the fiddler crab, *Uca pugilator*: The changes in the melanophores of the crabs following reserpine, 6-hydroxydopamine and bretylium administration. *Gen Pharmacol Vasc Syst* (1982) 13:99–103. doi: 10.1016/0306-3623(82)90063-5
181. Sarojini R, Nagabhushanam R, Fingerman M. Evidence for opioid involvement in the regulation of ovarian maturation of the fiddler crab, *Uca pugilator*. *Comp Biochem Physiol A Physiol* (1995) 111:279–82. doi: 10.1016/0300-9629(94)00214-E
182. Sarojini R, Nagabhushanam R, Fingerman M. *In vivo* assessment of opioid agonists and antagonists on ovarian maturation in the red swamp crayfish, *Procambarus clarkii*. *Comp Biochem Physiol C Pharmacol Toxicol Endocrinol* (1996) 115:149–53. doi: 10.1016/S0742-8413(96)00108-9
183. Campos B, Rivetti C, Kress T, Barata C, Dircksen H. Depressing antidepressant: Fluoxetine affects serotonin neurons causing adverse reproductive responses in *Daphnia magna*. *Environ Sci Technol* (2016) 50:6000–7. doi: 10.1021/acs.est.6b00826
184. Robert A, Monsinjon T, Péden R, Rasoamampianina V, Le Mével J-C, Knigge T. *In vivo* effects of serotonin and fluoxetine on cardio-ventilatory functions in the shore crab *Carcinus maenas* (L. 1758). *Aquat Toxicol* (2019) 207:132–41. doi: 10.1016/j.aquatox.2018.12.004
185. Camp AA, Yun J, Chambers SA, Haeba MH, LeBlanc GA. Involvement of glutamate and serotonin transmitter systems in male sex determination in *Daphnia pulex*. *J Insect Physiol* (2020) 121:104015. doi: 10.1016/j.jinsphys.2020.104015
186. Ford AT, Feuerhelm E. Effects of the antidepressant fluoxetine on pigment dispersion in chromatophores of the common sand shrimp, *Crangon crangon*: repeated experiments paint an inconclusive picture. *Ecotoxicology* (2020) 29:1368–76. doi: 10.1007/s10646-020-02272-7
187. Nelson DR, Goldstone JV, Stegeman JJ. The cytochrome P450 genesis locus: the origin and evolution of animal cytochrome P450s. *Philos Trans R Soc B Biol Sci* (2013) 368:20120474. doi: 10.1098/rstb.2012.0474
188. Baldwin WS, Marko PB, Nelson DR. The cytochrome P450 (CYP) gene superfamily in *Daphnia pulex*. *BMC Genomics* (2009) 10:169. doi: 10.1186/1471-2164-10-169
189. Ye H, Huang H, Li S, Wang G. Immunorecognition of estrogen and androgen receptors in the brain and thoracic ganglion mass of mud crab, *Scylla paramamosain*. *Prog Nat Sci* (2008) 18:691–5. doi: 10.1016/j.pnsc.2007.12.012
190. Paolucci M, Cristo CD, Cosmo AD. Immunological evidence for progesterone and estradiol receptors in the freshwater crayfish *Austropotamobius pallipes*. *Mol Reprod Dev* (2002) 63:55–62. doi: 10.1002/mrd.10158
191. Gilda JE, Ghosh R, Cheah JX, West TM, Bodine SC, Gomes AV. Western blotting inaccuracies with unverified antibodies: Need for a Western Blotting Minimal Reporting Standard (WBMRS). *PloS One* (2015) 10:e0135392. doi: 10.1371/journal.pone.0135392
192. Baldwin WS, Bailey R, Long KE, Klaine S. Incomplete ecdysis is an indicator of ecdysteroid exposure in *Daphnia magna*. *Environ Toxicol Chem* (2001) 20:1564–9. doi: 10.1002/etc.5620200721
193. Brennan SJ, Brougham CA, Roche JJ, Fogarty AM. Multi-generational effects of four selected environmental oestrogens on *Daphnia magna*. *Chemosphere* (2006) 64:49–55. doi: 10.1016/j.chemosphere.2005.11.046
194. Tsukimura B. Crustacean vitellogenesis: Its role in oocyte development. *Am Zool* (2015) 41:465–76. doi: 10.1093/icb/41.3.465
195. Hannas BR, Wang YH, Thomson S, Kwon G, Li H, LeBlanc GA. Regulation and dysregulation of vitellogenin mRNA accumulation in daphnids (*Daphnia magna*). *Aquat Toxicol* (2011) 101:351–7. doi: 10.1016/j.aquatox.2010.11.006
196. Swetha CH, Girish BP, Reddy PS. Elucidation of the role of estradiol and progesterone in regulating reproduction in the edible crab, *Oziothelphusa senex senex*. *RSC Adv* (2016) 6:24959–67. doi: 10.1039/C5RA23637A
197. Umbers KDL, Fabricant SA, Gawryszewski FM, Seago AE, Herberstein ME. Reversible colour change in Arthropoda. *Biol Rev Camb Philos Soc* (2014) 89:820–48. doi: 10.1111/brv.12079
198. McNamara JC, Milograna SR. Adaptive color change and the molecular endocrinology of pigmenttranslocation in crustacean chromatophores. In: Chang ES and Thiel M (Eds). *Nat Hist Crust Vol 4* (2015) 4:68–102. Physiology. Oxford University Press: Oxford, England ISBN: 9780199832415
199. Noël P, Chassard-Bouchaud C. "Chromatophores et pigmentation," In: *Traité de zoologie: anatomie, systématique, biologie: VII Crustacés: 1. Morphologie, physiologie, reproduction, systématique*. Paris: Masson (1994). p. 145–60.
200. Detto T, Hemmi JM, Backwell PRY. Colouration and colour changes of the fiddler crab, *Uca capricornis*: a descriptive study. *PloS One* (2008) 3:e1629. doi: 10.1371/journal.pone.0001629
201. Wade NM, Melville-Smith R, Degnan BM, Hall MR. Control of shell colour changes in the lobster, *Panulirus cygnus*. *J Exp Biol* (2008) 211:1512–9. doi: 10.1242/jeb.012930
202. Fingerman M. Chromatophores. *Physiol Rev* (1965) 45:296–339. 10.1152/physrev.1965.45.2.296
203. Rao KR. Crustacean pigmentary-effector hormones: Chemistry and functions of RPCH, PDH, and related peptides. *Am Zool* (2001) 41:364–79. doi: 10.1093/icb/41.3.364
204. Davie PJ, Guinot D, Ng PK. Anatomy and functional morphology ofBrachyura. In: Castro P, Davie PJF, Guinot D, Schram F and Von Vaupel Klein C, eds. *Treatise on Zoology-Anatomy, Taxonomy, Biology. The Crustacea*, Volume 9 Part C (2 vols). Leiden: E.J. Brill. p. 11–163.

205. O'Halloran M-J. Color control in shrimp. *Test Stud Lab Teach* (1990) 111990:15–26.
206. Stevens M, Lown AE, Wood LE. Camouflage and individual variation in shore crabs (*Carcinus maenas*) from different habitats. *PloS One* (2014) 9: e115586. doi: 10.1371/journal.pone.0115586
207. Milograna SR, Bell FT, McNamara JC. Signal transduction, plasma membrane calcium movements, and pigment translocation in freshwater shrimp chromatophores. *J Exp Zool* (2010) 313A:605–17. doi: 10.1002/jez.633
208. Siegenthaler A, Mastin A, Dufaut C, Mondal D, Benvenuto C. Background matching in the brown shrimp *Crangon crangon*: adaptive camouflage and behavioural-plasticity. *Sci Rep* (2018) 8:3292. doi: 10.1038/s41598-018-21412-y
209. Gaus G, Kleinholz LH, Kegel G, Keller R. Isolation and characterization of red-pigment-concentrating hormone (RPCH) from six crustacean species. *J Comp Physiol B* (1990) 160:373–9. doi: 10.1007/BF01075668
210. Marco HG, Verlinden H, Vanden Broeck J, Gäde G. Characterisation and pharmacological analysis of a crustacean G protein-coupled receptor: the red pigment-concentrating hormone receptor of *Daphnia pulex*. *Sci Rep* (2017) 7:6851. doi: 10.1038/s41598-017-06805-9
211. Fernlund P, Josefsson L. Crustacean color-change hormone: Amino acid sequence and chemical synthesis. *Science* (1972) 177:173–5. doi: 10.1126/science.177.4044.173
212. Fernlund P. Structure of a light-adapting hormone from the shrimp, *Pandalus borealis*. *Biochim Biophys Acta* (1976) 439:17–25. doi: 10.1016/0005-2795(76)90155-0
213. Mangerich S, Keller R, Dircksen H. Immunocytochemical identification of structures containing putative red pigment-concentrating hormone in two species of decapod crustaceans. *Cell Tissue Res* (1986) 245:377–86. doi: 10.1007/BF00213945
214. Mangerich S, Keller R, Dircksen H, Rao KR, Riehm JP. Immunocytochemical localization of pigment-dispersing hormone (PDH) and its coexistence with FMRFamide-immunoreactive material in the eyestalks of the decapod crustaceans *Carcinus maenas* and *Orconectes limosus*. *Cell Tissue Res* (1987) 250:365–75. doi: 10.1007/BF00219081
215. Löhr J, Klein J, Webster S, Dircksen H. Quantification, immunoaffinity purification and sequence analysis of a pigment-dispersing hormone of the shore crab, *Carcinus maenas* (L.). *Comp Biochem Physiol B* (1993) 104:699—706. doi: 10.1016/0305-0491(93)90200-o
216. Sarojini R, Nagabhushanam R, Fingerman M. A neurotransmitter role for red-pigment-concentrating hormone in ovarian maturation in the red swamp crayfish *Procambarus clarkii*. *J Exp Biol* (1995) 198:1253–7.
217. Milograna SR, Bell FT, McNamara JC. Signaling events during cyclic guanosine monophosphate-regulated pigment aggregation in freshwater shrimp chromatophores. *Biol Bull* (2012) 223:178–91. doi: 10.1086/BBLv223n2p178
218. Milograna SR, Ribeiro MR, Bell FT, McNamara JC. Pigment translocation in caridean shrimp chromatophores: Receptor type, signal transduction, second messengers, and cross talk among multiple signaling cascades. *J Exp Zool Part Ecol Genet Physiol* (2016) 325:565–80. doi: 10.1002/jez.2052
219. Hanumante MM, Fingerman M. 5-Hydroxytryptaminergic control of red pigment-dispersing hormone release in the fiddler crab, *Uca pugilator*: Effects of a 5-hydroxytryptamine uptake inhibitor and a 5-hydroxytryptamine receptor blocker on 5-hydroxytryptamine-induced and iproniazid-induced red pigment dispersion. *Gen Comp Endocrinol* (1981) 45:395–401. doi: 10.1016/0016-6480(81)90080-0
220. Bull JJ. Sex determining mechanisms: An evolutionary perspective. *Experientia* (1985) 41:1285–96. doi: 10.1007/BF01952071
221. Hattori RS, Gould RJ, Fujioka T, Saito T, Kurita J, Strüssmann CA, et al. Temperature-dependent sex determination in Hd-rR medaka *Oryzias latipes*: Gender sensitivity, thermal threshold, critical period, and DMRT1 expression profile. *Sex Dev* (2007) 1:138–46. doi: 10.1159/000100035
222. Piferrer F. Endocrine sex control strategies for the feminization of teleost fish. *Reprod Biotechnol Finfish Aquac* (2001) 197:229–81. doi: 10.1016/S0044-8486(01)00589-0
223. Staelens J, Rombaut D, Vercauteren I, Argue B, Benzie J, Vuylsteke M. High-density linkage maps and sex-linked markers for the black tiger shrimp (*Penaeus monodon*). *Genetics* (2008) 179:917. doi: 10.1534/genetics.107.080150
224. Li Y, Dierens L, Byrne K, Miggiano E, Lehnert S, Preston N, et al. QTL detection of production traits for the Kuruma prawn *Penaeus japonicus* (Bate) using AFLP markers. *Aquaculture* (2006) 258:198–210. doi: 10.1016/j.aquaculture.2006.04.027
225. Juchault P, Rigaud T. Evidence for female heterogamety in two terrestrial crustaceans and the problem of sex chromosome evolution in isopods. *Heredity* (1995) 75:466–71. doi: 10.1038/hdy.1995.163
226. Weeks SC, Benvenuto C, Sanderson TF, Duff RJ. Sex chromosome evolution in the clam shrimp, *Eulimnadia texana*. *J Evol Biol* (2010) 23:1100–6. doi: 10.1111/j.1420-9101.2010.01963.x
227. De Vos S, Bossier P, Van Stappen G, Vercauteren I, Sorgeloos P, Vuylsteke M. A first AFLP-based genetic linkage map for brine shrimp *Artemia franciscana* and its application in mapping the sex locus. *PloS One* (2013) 8:e57585. doi: 10.1371/journal.pone.0057585
228. Kvist J, Athanàsio CG, Pfrender ME, Brown JB, Colbourne JK, Mirbahai L. A comprehensive epigenomic analysis of phenotypically distinguishable, genetically identical female and male *Daphnia pulex*. *BMC Genomics* (2020) 21:17. doi: 10.1186/s12864-019-6415-5
229. Suzuki S, Yamasaki K. Sex-reversal of male *Armadillidium vulgare* (Isopoda, Malacostraca, Crustacea) following andrectomy and partial gonadectomy. *Gen Comp Endocrinol* (1991) 83:375–8. doi: 10.1016/0016-6480(91)90142-S
230. Suzuki S. Androgenic gland hormone is a sex-reversing factor but cannot be a sex-determining factor in the female crustacean isopod *Armadillidium vulgare*. *Gen Comp Endocrinol* (1999) 115:370–8. doi: 10.1006/gcen.1999.7324
231. Aflalo ED, Hoang TTT, Nguyen VH, Lam Q, Nguyen DM, Trinh QS, et al. A novel two-step procedure for mass production of all-male populations of the giant freshwater prawn *Macrobrachium rosenbergii*. *Aquaculture* (2006) 256:468–78. doi: 10.1016/j.aquaculture.2006.01.035
232. Parnes S, Khalaila I, Hulata G, Sagi A. Sex determination in crayfish: are intersex *Cherax quadricarinatus* (Decapoda, Parastacidae) genetically females? *Genet Res* (2003) 82:107–16. doi: 10.1017/S0016672303006372
233. Dunn AM, Hogg JC, Kelly A, Hatcher MJ. Two cues for sex determination in *Gammarus duebeni*: Adaptive variation in environmental sex determination? *Limnol Oceanogr* (2005) 50:346–53. doi: 10.4319/lo.2005.50.1.0346
234. Guler Y, Short S, Green Etxabe A, Sherhod CM, Kille P, Ford AT. Impacts of a newly identified behaviour-altering trematode on its host amphipod: from the level of gene expression to population. *Parasitology* (2015) 142:1469–80. doi: 10.1017/S0031182015000918
235. Bulnheim H. Microsporidian infections of amphipods with special reference to host-parasite relationships: a review. *Mar Fish Rev* (1975) 37:39–45.
236. Zupo V, Messina P. How do dietary diatoms cause the sex reversal of the shrimp *Hippolyte inermis* Leach (Crustacea, Decapoda). *Mar Biol* (2007) 151:907–17. doi: 10.1007/s00227-006-0524-9
237. Charniaux-Cotton H. Discovery in an amphipod crustacean (*Orchestia gammarella*) of an endocrine gland responsible for the differentiation of primary and secondary male sex characteristics. *C R Acad Sci Paris* (1954) 239:780–2.
238. Charniaux-Cotton H. Vitellogenesis and its control in Malacostracan crustacea. *Am Zool* (1985) 25:197–206. doi: 10.1093/icb/25.1.197
239. Sagi A, Snir E, Khalaila I. Sexual differentiation in decapod crustaceans: role of the androgenic gland. *Invertebr Reprod Dev* (1997) 31:55–61. doi: 10.1080/07924259.1997.9672563
240. Charniaux-Cotton H. Surgical castration in an amphipod crustacean (*Orchestia gammarella*) and determination of the secondary sexual characteristics: first results. *CR Acad Sci Paris* (1952) 234:2570–2.
241. Charniaux-Cotton H. Etude du déterminisme des caractères sexuels secondaires par castration chirurgicale et implantation d'ovaire chez un Crustacé Amphipode (*Orchestia gammarella*). *C R Acad Sci Paris* (1953) 236:141–3.
242. Charniaux-Cotton H. Contrôle hormonal de la différenciation du sexe et de la reproduction chez les Crustacés supérieurs. *Bull Soc Zool* (1958) 82:314–36.
243. Charniaux-Cotton H, Payen G. Sexual differentiation. In: Bliss DE and Mantel LH, editors. *The Biology of Crustacea, Volume 9*. New York: Academic Press (1985).
244. Ford AT. Can you feminise a crustacean? *Aquat Toxicol* (2008) 88:316–21. doi: 10.1016/j.aquatox.2008.04.013

245. Barki A, Karplus I, Manor R, Sagi A. Intersexuality and behavior in crayfish: The de-masculinization effects of androgenic gland ablation. *Horm Behav* (2006) 50:322–31. doi: 10.1016/j.yhbeh.2006.03.017
246. Hasegawa Y, Haino-Fukushima K, Katakura Y. Isolation and properties of androgenic gland hormone from the terrestrial isopod, *Armadillidium vulgare. Gen Comp Endocrinol* (1987) 67:101–10. doi: 10.1016/0016-6480(87)90209-7
247. Martin G, Juchault P, Sorokine O, Van Dorsselaer A. Purification and characterization of androgenic hormone from the terrestrial isopod *Armadillidium vulgare* Latr. (Crustacea, Oniscidea). *Gen Comp Endocrinol* (1990) 80:349–54. doi: 10.1016/0016-6480(90)90183-M
248. Okuno A, Hasegawa Y, Nagasawa H. Purification and properties of androgenic gland hormone from the terrestrial isopod *Armadillidium vulgare. Zool Sci* (1997) 14:837–42. doi: 10.2108/zsj.14.837
249. Martin G, Sorokine O, Moniatte M, Van Dorsselaer A. The androgenic hormone of the crustacean isopod *Armadillidium vulgare. Ann N Y Acad Sci* (1998) 839:111–7. doi: 10.1111/j.1749-6632.1998.tb10741.x
250. Martin G, Sorokine O, Moniatte M, Bulet P, Hetru C, Van Dorsselaer A. The structure of a glycosylated protein hormone responsible for sex determination in the isopod, *Armadillidium vulgare. Eur J Biochem* (1999) 262:727–36. doi: 10.1046/j.1432-1327.1999.00442.x
251. Okuno A, Hasegawa Y, Ohira T, Katakura Y, Nagasawa H. Characterization and cDNA cloning of androgenic gland hormone of the terrestrial isopod *Armadillidium vulgare. Biochem Biophys Res Commun* (1999) 264:419–23. doi: 10.1006/bbrc.1999.1522
252. Martin G, Juchault P. Androgenic hormone specificity in terrestrial isopods (Oniscidea): Systematic involvements. *J Crustac Biol* (1999) 19:684–9. doi: 10.1163/193724099X00402
253. Guo Q, Li S, Lv X, Xiang J, Sagi A, Manor R, et al. A putative insulin-like androgenic gland hormone receptor gene specifically expressed in male chinese shrimp. *Endocrinology* (2018) 159:2173–85. doi: 10.1210/en.2017-03253
254. Ventura T, Manor R, Aflalo ED, Weil S, Raviv S, Glazer L, et al. Temporal silencing of an androgenic gland-specific insulin-like gene affecting phenotypical gender differences and spermatogenesis. *Endocrinology* (2009) 150:1278–86. doi: 10.1210/en.2008-0906
255. Ventura T, Manor R, Aflalo ED, Weil S, Rosen O, Sagi A. Timing sexual differentiation: Full functional sex reversal achieved through silencing of a single insulin-like gene in the prawn, *Macrobrachium rosenbergii. Biol Reprod* (2012) 86 86(3):90,1-6. doi: 10.1095/biolreprod.111.097261
256. Khalaila I, Manor R, Weil S, Granot Y, Keller R, Sagi A. The eyestalk–androgenic gland–testis endocrine axis in the crayfish *Cherax quadricarinatus. Gen Comp Endocrinol* (2002) 127:147–56. doi: 10.1016/S0016-6480(02)00031-X
257. Guo Q, Li S, Lv X, Xiang J, Manor R, Sagi A, et al. Sex-biased CHHs and their putative receptor regulate the expression of IAG gene in the shrimp *Litopenaeus vannamei. Front Physiol* (2019) 10:1525. doi: 10.3389/fphys.2019.01525
258. Cristescu MEA, Colbourne JK, Radivojac J. Lynch M. A microsatellite-based genetic linkage map of the waterflea, *Daphnia pulex*: On the prospect of crustacean genomics. *Genomics* (2006) 88:415–30. doi: 10.1016/j.ygeno.2006.03.007
259. Routtu J, Jansen B, Colson I, De Meester L, Ebert D. The first-generation *Daphnia magna* linkage map. *BMC Genomics* (2010) 11:508. doi: 10.1186/1471-2164-11-508
260. Hebert PDN. The adaptive significance of cyclomorphosis in *Daphnia*: more possibilities. *Freshw Biol* (1978) 8:313–20. doi: 10.1111/j.1365-2427.1978.tb01452.x
261. Paland S, Lynch M. Transitions to asexuality result in excess amino acid substitutions. *Science* (2006) 311:990–2. doi: 10.1126/science.1118152
262. Brendonck L, De Meester L. Egg banks in freshwater zooplankton: evolutionary and ecological archives in the sediment. *Hydrobiologia* (2003) 491:65–84. doi: 10.1023/A:1024454905119
263. Camp AA, Haeba MH, LeBlanc GA. Complementary roles of photoperiod and temperature in environmental sex determination in *Daphnia spp. J Exp Biol* (2019) 222:jeb195289. doi: 10.1242/jeb.195289
264. Kleiven OT, Larsson P, Hobæk A. Sexual reproduction in *Daphnia magna* requires three stimuli. *Oikos* (1992) 65:197–206. doi: 10.2307/3545010
265. Hobaek A, Larsson P. Sex Determination in *Daphnia magna. Ecology* (1990) 71:2255–68. doi: 10.2307/1938637
266. Toyota K, Miyakawa H, Yamaguchi K, Shigenobu S, Ogino Y, Tatarazako N, et al. NMDA receptor activation upstream of methyl farnesoate signaling for short day-induced male offspring production in the water flea, *Daphnia pulex. BMC Genomics* (2015) 16:186. doi: 10.1186/s12864-015-1392-9
267. Traynelis SF, Wollmuth LP, McBain CJ, Menniti FS, Vance KM, Ogden KK, et al. Glutamate Receptor Ion Channels: Structure, Regulation, and Function. *Pharmacol Rev* (2010) 62:405. doi: 10.1124/pr.109.002451
268. Paoletti P, Bellone C, Zhou Q. NMDA receptor subunit diversity: impact on receptor properties, synaptic plasticity and disease. *Nat Rev Neurosci* (2013) 14:383–400. doi: 10.1038/nrn3504
269. Nishimura M, Sato K, Okada T, Schloss P, Shimada S, Tohyama M. MK-801 blocks monoamine transporters expressed in HEK cells. *FEBS Lett* (1998) 423:376–80. doi: 10.1016/S0014-5793(98)00126-4
270. Brunello N, Mendlewicz J, Kasper S, Leonard B, Montgomery S, Nelson JC, et al. The role of noradrenaline and selective noradrenaline reuptake inhibition in depression. *Eur Neuropsychopharmacol* (2002) 12:461–75. doi: 10.1016/S0924-977X(02)00057-3
271. Hui JHL, Hayward A, Bendena WG, Takahashi T, Tobe SS. Evolution and functional divergence of enzymes involved in sesquiterpenoid hormone biosynthesis in crustaceans and insects. *Peptides* (2010) 31:451–5. doi: 10.1016/j.peptides.2009.10.003
272. Olmstead AW, LeBlanc GA. Juvenoid hormone methyl farnesoate is a sex determinant in the crustacean *Daphnia magna. J Exp Zool* (2002) 293:736–9. doi: 10.1002/jez.10162
273. Tatarazako N, Oda S, Watanabe H, Morita M, Iguchi T. Juvenile hormone agonists affect the occurrence of male *Daphnia. Chemosphere* (2003) 53:827–33. doi: 10.1016/S0045-6535(03)00761-6
274. Kato Y, Kobayashi K, Watanabe H, Iguchi T. Environmental sex determination in the branchiopod crustacean *Daphnia magna*: deep conservation of a Doublesex gene in the sex-determining pathway. *PloS Genet* (2011) 7:e1001345. doi: 10.1371/journal.pgen.1001345
275. Nong QD, Mohamad Ishak NS, Matsuura T, Kato Y, Watanabe H. Mapping the expression of the sex determining factor Doublesex1 in *Daphnia magna* using a knock-in reporter. *Sci Rep* (2017) 7:13521. doi: 10.1038/s41598-017-13730-4
276. Toyota K, Kato Y, Sato M, Sugiura N, Miyagawa S, Miyakawa H, et al. Molecular cloning of doublesex genes of four cladocera (water flea) species. *BMC Genomics* (2013) 14:239. doi: 10.1186/1471-2164-14-239
277. Bellés X, Martín D, Piulachs M-D. The mevalonate pathway and the synthesis of juvenile hormone in insects. *Annu Rev Entomol* (2004) 50:181–99. doi: 10.1146/annurev.ento.50.071803.130356
278. Li S, Friesen JA, Holford KC, Borst DW. Methyl farnesoate synthesis in the lobster mandibular organ: The roles of HMG-CoA reductase and farnesoic acid O-methyltransferase. *Comp Biochem Physiol A Mol Integr Physiol* (2010) 155:49–55. doi: 10.1016/j.cbpa.2009.09.016
279. White AF. Metabolism of the juvenile hormone analogue methyl farnesoate 10, 11-epoxide in two insect species. *Life Sci* (1972) 11:201–10. doi: 10.1016/0024-3205(72)90110-5
280. Homola E, Chang ES. Assay methods for methyl farnesoate esterases in crustaceans. *Arch Insect Biochem Physiol* (1997) 36:115–28. doi: 10.1002/(SICI)1520-6327(1997)36:2<115::AID-ARCH4>3.0.CO;2-U
281. Wainwright G, Webster SG, Wilkinson MC, Chung JS, Rees HH. Structure and significance of mandibular organ-inhibiting hormone in the crab, *Cancer pagurus* involvement in multihormonal regulation of growth and reproduction. *J Biol Chem* (1996) 271:12749–54. doi: 10.1042/bj3340651
282. Wainwright G, Webster SG, Rees HH. Neuropeptide regulation of biosynthesis of the juvenoid, methyl farnesoate, in the edible crab, *Cancer pagurus. Biochem J* (1998) 334:651–7. doi: 10.1042/bj3340651
283. Laufer H, Landau M, Homola E, Borst DW. Methyl farnesoate: Its site of synthesis and regulation of secretion in a juvenile crustacean. *Insect Biochem* (1987) 17:1129–31. doi: 10.1016/0020-1790(87)90134-X
284. LeBlanc GA, Wang YH, Holmes CN, Kwon G, Medlock EK. A transgenerational endocrine signaling pathway in Crustacea. *PloS One* (2013) 8:e61715. doi: 10.1371/journal.pone.0061715

285. Miyakawa H, Toyota K, Hirakawa I, Ogino Y, Miyagawa S, Oda S, et al. A mutation in the receptor Methoprene-tolerant alters juvenile hormone response in insects and crustaceans. *Nat Commun* (2013) 4:1856. doi: 10.1038/ncomms2868
286. Wilson TG. Fabian J. A *Drosophila melanogaster* mutant resistant to a chemical analog of juvenile hormone. *Dev Biol* (1986) 118:190–201. doi: 10.1016/0012-1606(86)90087-4
287. Tiu SH-K, Hult EF, Yagi KJ, Tobe SS. Farnesoic acid and methyl farnesoate production during lobster reproduction: Possible functional correlation with retinoid X receptor expression. *Gen Comp Endocrinol* (2012) 175:259–69. doi: 10.1016/j.ygcen.2011.11.016
288. Durica DS, Wu X, Anilkumar G, Hopkins PM, Chung AC-K. Characterization of crab EcR and RXR homologs and expression during limb regeneration and oocyte maturation. *Mol Cell Endocrinol* (2002) 189:59–76. doi: 10.1016/S0303-7207(01)00740-7
289. Kim H-W, Lee SG, Mykles DL. Ecdysteroid-responsive genes, RXR and E75, in the tropical land crab, *Gecarcinus lateralis*: Differential tissue expression of multiple RXR isoforms generated at three alternative splicing sites in the hinge and ligand-binding domains. *Mol Cell Endocrinol* (2005) 242:80–95. doi: 10.1016/j.mce.2005.08.001
290. Dai T-H, Sserwadda A, Song K, Zang Y-N, Shen H-S. Cloning and Expression of Ecdysone Receptor and Retinoid X Receptor from *Procambarus clarkii*: Induction by Eyestalk Ablation. *Int J Mol Sci* (2016) 17(10):1739. doi: 10.3390/ijms17101739
291. Gouveia D, Bonneton F, Almunia C, Armengaud J, Quéau H, Degli-Esposti D, et al. Identification, expression, and endocrine-disruption of three ecdysone-responsive genes in the sentinel species *Gammarus fossarum*. *Sci Rep* (2018) 8:3793. doi: 10.1038/s41598-018-22235-7
292. Wang YH, Wang G, LeBlanc GA. Cloning and characterization of the retinoid X receptor from a primitive crustacean *Daphnia magna*. *Gen Comp Endocrinol* (2007) 150:309–18. doi: 10.1016/j.ygcen.2006.08.002
293. Wang YH, LeBlanc GA. Interactions of methyl farnesoate and related compounds with a crustacean retinoid X receptor. *Mol Cell Endocrinol* (2009) 309:109–16. doi: 10.1016/j.mce.2009.05.016
294. Wang YH, Kwon G, Li H, LeBlanc GA. Tributyltin synergizes with 20-hydroxyecdysone to produce endocrine toxicity. *Toxicol Sci* (2011) 123:71–9. doi: 10.1093/toxsci/kfr154
295. Li Y, Ginjupalli GK, Baldwin WS. The HR97 (NR1L) group of nuclear receptors: A new group of nuclear receptors discovered in *Daphnia species*. *Gen Comp Endocrinol* (2014) 206:30–42. doi: 10.1016/j.ygcen.2014.07.022
296. Hyde CJ, Fitzgibbon QP, Elizur A, Smith GG, Ventura T. Transcriptional profiling of spiny lobster metamorphosis reveals three new additions to the nuclear receptor superfamily. *BMC Genomics* (2019) 20:531. doi: 10.1186/s12864-019-5925-5
297. Wang HY, Olmstead AW, Li H, LeBlanc GA. The screening of chemicals for juvenoid-related endocrine activity using the water flea *Daphnia magna*. *Aquat Toxicol* (2005) 74:193–204. doi: 10.1016/j.aquatox.2005.05.010
298. Olmstead AW, LeBlanc GA. Insecticidal juvenile hormone analogs stimulate the production of male offspring in the crustacean *Daphnia magna*. *Environ Health Perspect* (2003) 111:919–24. doi: 10.1289/ehp.5982
299. Dodson SI, Merritt CM, Shannahan J-P, Shults CM. Low exposure concentrations of atrazine increase male production in *Daphnia pulicaria*. *Environ Toxicol Chem* (1999) 18:1568–73. doi: 10.1002/etc.5620180732
300. Cooper RL, Stoker TE, Tyrey L, Goldman JM, McElroy WK. Atrazine disrupts the hypothalamic control of pituitary-ovarian function. *Toxicol Sci* (2000) 53:297–307. doi: 10.1093/toxsci/53.2.297
301. DeFur PL, Crane M, Ingersoll C, Tattersfield L. *Endocrine disruption in invertebrates: endocrinology, testing, andassessment*. Pensacola: SETAC technical publication series. SETAC press (1999).
302. Ford AT, LeBlanc GA. Endocrine disruption in invertebrates: A survey of research progress. *Environ Sci Technol* (2020) 54:13365–9. doi: 10.1021/acs.est.0c04226
303. Katsiadaki I. Are marine invertebrates really at risk from endocrine-disrupting chemicals? *Curr Opin Environ Sci Health* (2019) 11:37–42. doi: 10.1016/j.coesh.2019.06.005
304. Cuvillier-Hot V, Lenoir A. Invertebrates facing environmental contamination by endocrine disruptors: Novel evidences and recent insights. *Mol Cell Endocrinol* (2020) 504:110712. doi: 10.1016/j.mce.2020.110712
305. Short S, Yang G, Kille P, Ford AT. Vitellogenin is not an appropriate biomarker of feminisation in a Crustacean. *Aquat Toxicol* (2014) 153:89–97. doi: 10.1016/j.aquatox.2013.11.014
306. Matozzo V, Gagné F, Marin MG, Ricciardi F, Blaise C. Vitellogenin as a biomarker of exposure to estrogenic compounds in aquatic invertebrates: A review. *Environ Int* (2008) 34:531–45. doi: 10.1016/j.envint.2007.09.008
307. Jayasankar V, Tomy S, Wilder M. Insights on molecular mechanisms of ovarian development in decapod crustacea: Focus on vitellogenesis-stimulating factors and pathways. *Front Endocrinol* (2020) 11:577925. doi: 10.3389/fendo.2020.577925
308. Villeneuve DL, Crump D, Garcia-Reyero N, Hecker M, Hutchinson TH, LaLone CA, et al. Adverse Outcome Pathway (AOP) development I: Strategies and principles. *Toxicol Sci* (2014) 142:312–20. doi: 10.1093/toxsci/kfu199

10

Parasites and steroid hormones: Corticosteroid and sex steroid synthesis, their role in the parasite physiology and development

Marta C. Romano[1], Pedro Jiménez[2], Carolina Miranda-Brito[1] and Ricardo A. Valdez[1]*

[1] Departamento de Fisiología, Biofísica y Neurociencias, CINVESTAV del IPN, Mexico city, Mexico, [2] Centro de Investigación en Reproducción Animal, CINVESTAV-UAT, Tlaxcala, Mexico

Edited by:
Hubert Vaudry,
University of Rouen, France

Reviewed by:
Rafael Vazquez-Martinez,
University of Cordoba, Spain
Yves Tremblay,
Laval University and Centre Hospitalier Universitaire de Québec, Canada

****Correspondence:***
Marta C. Romano,
Departamento de Fisiología, Biofísica y Neurociencias, CINVESTAV del IPN,
Apdo. Postal 14-745,
07360 Mexico city, Mexico
mromano@fisio.cinvestav.mx

In many cases parasites display highly complex life cycles that include the penetration and permanence of the larva or adults within host organs, but even in those that only have one host, reciprocal, intricate interactions occur. Evidence indicates that steroid hormones have an influence on the development and course of parasitic infections. The host gender's susceptibility to infection, and the related differences in the immune response are good examples of the host-parasite interplay. However, the capacity of these organisms to synthesize their own steroidogenic hormones still has more questions than answers. It is now well-known that many parasites synthesize ecdysteroids, but limited information is available on sex steroid and corticosteroid synthesis. This review intends to summarize some of the existing information in the field. In most, but not all parasitosis the host's hormonal environment determines the susceptibility, the course, and severity of parasite infections. In most cases the infection disturbs the host environment, and activates immune responses that end up affecting the endocrine system. Furthermore, sex steroids and corticosteroids may also directly modify the parasite reproduction and molting. Available information indicates that parasites synthesize some steroid hormones, such as ecdysteroids and sex steroids, and the presence and activity of related enzymes have been demonstrated. More recently, the synthesis of corticosteroid-like compounds has been shown in *Taenia solium* cysticerci and tapeworms, and in *Taenia crassiceps* WFU cysticerci. In-depth knowledge of the parasite's endocrine properties will contribute to understand their reproduction and reciprocal interactions with the host, and may also help designing tools to combat the infection in some clinical situations.

Keywords: parasites, steroid synthesis, sex steroids, corticosteroids, steroidogenic enzymes, *Taenias*, cysticerci

Parasites and Host Interplay: Steroid Hormones Influence Parasite Development and Survival

Progesterone, androgens, and estrogens are present and have critical roles in the vertebrate reproduction and metabolism, but the influence and occurrence of steroid hormones in invertebrates had received less attention (Lafont, 2000) the interplay between the parasite and the host defines the intensity of parasite infections. In many cases, the presence of parasites in the host changes its endocrine equilibrium due to the activation of the immune system response, which finally affects the endocrine system through the influence of cytokines and growth factors released by the immune cells. It is now widely accepted that corticosteroids and sex-related hormones influence the immune response (Roberts et al., 2001; Coutinho and Chapman, 2011; Reyes-Hernandez et al., 2013), thereafter any endocrine perturbation initiated by an infection will change the neuroendocrine equilibrium. These hormonal changes resulting from a spontaneous or experimental infection, affect the parasitic charge, the course of the infection and the parasite's survival (Barthelemy et al., 2004). On the other hand, some parasite infections disrupt the host endocrine system, in a noteworthy example, the dromedary bull, *Camelus dromedarius*, parasitized with *Tripanosoma evansi*, presents changes in the sexual steroid plasmatic concentrations, as well as in the semen characteristics (Al Qarawi, 2005). Furthermore, the male Fence Lizard (*Sceloporus occidentalis*) infected with the malarial parasite *Plasmodium mexicanum* shows several reproductive pathologies, such as fewer courtship and decreased testosterone levels (Dunlap and Schall, 1995) and the *Toxoplasma gondee* infection enhances testicular steroidogenesis in rats (Lim et al., 2013). Interestingly, it has been shown that the host hormonal environment determines the susceptibility, the course, and severity of many parasite infections, and therefore a clear dichotomy in infection susceptibility between males and females had been observed (Morales-Montor et al., 2004). A rich estrogen environment facilitates *Taenia crassiceps* cysticerci proliferation, blocking thus the P450-aromatase with fadrozole decreased parasite load (Morales-Montor et al., 2002). Parasites may also alter the host's reproductive behavior (Thompson and Kavaliers, 1994) as had been also shown in *Taenia crassiceps* ORF infected male mice (Morales et al., 1996).

Steroids and steroid synthesis inhibitors influence the fertility of *Schistosoma mansoni in vitro* (Morrison et al., 1986) while progesterone, makisterone, and ecdysone increased the length of the larvae *Ascaris suum*, a roundworm swine parasite (Fleming, 1985), while progesterone, 17β-estradiol, and testosterone added to the culture medium enhanced the number of *Plasmodium falciparum* gametocytes (Lingnau et al., 1993). Progesterone, but not testosterone decreased the *in vitro* molting process of *Trichinella spiralis* (Hernández-Bello et al., 2011) and *T. crassiceps* ORF cysticerci cell proliferation was increased by physiological concentrations of testosterone, and 17β-estradiol added to the culture media (Romano et al., 2003), while high concentrations inhibited its reproduction (Escobedo et al., 2004).

The Role of Corticosteroids in the Host-parasite Interplay

It is well-known that non-physiological stress situations, such as social isolation, infections, persecution, etc., increase serum corticosteroids levels with the consequent impairment of the immune response. The interplay host-parasite is not the exception, for example social stress caused by female isolation increased blood *Typanosoma cruzi* infection in the wild mouse *Calomys callosus*, which showed body weight loss and impaired immune response (Santos et al., 2008), whereas the hypothalamus-pituitary-interregnal axis of rainbow trout was altered by the parasite haemoflagelate *Cryptobia* infection (Madison et al., 2013). In addition, the infection with *Anguillicola novaezelandiae* affects cortisol levels in the European Eel (Dangel et al., 2014). Frequently, the host and the parasites are affected in the course of infection, as in Bluegill Sunfish (*Lepomis macrochirus*) infected with *Utterbackia imbecillis*, which results in plasma cortisol increment in the host, favoring thus the parasite juvenile metamorphosis (Dubansky et al., 2011). On the other hand, *in vivo* treatment of rats with cortisol increased the growth rate of the protozoan parasite *Toxoplasma gondii* in isolated peritoneal macrophages (Wang et al., 2014).

Direct Effects of Glucocorticoids on Parasite Growth

Aside from the influence of corticosteroids in the course of parasitic infections, it had been shown that these hormones directly influence parasite's growth. For instance, cortisol and dexamethasone increase the *in vitro* multiplication of the haemoflagellate *Cryptobia salmonistica*, possible by their interaction with glucocorticoid receptor-like protein (Li et al., 2013, 2014). In this regard, dehydroepiandrosterone (DHEA) addition to the culture media decreased, while cortisol increased the *in vitro* growth and viability of *Entamoeba histolytica* (Carrero et al., 2006). We had shown that corticosterone and dexamethasone increase the capacity of *T. crassiceps* WFU cysticerci to synthesize androgens and estrogens, hormones that favor the parasite reproduction (Hinojosa et al., 2011).

Parasites Synthesize Steroid Hormones

Lipids and Steroid Hormones

Lipids, and particularly cholesterol and their metabolites, are required and synthesized by some parasites. Bansal et al. (2005) reviewed the requirement for lipids, particularly cholesterol, by pathogens like protozoa (Leishmaniosis, Malaria, and Toxoplasmosis). It has recently been stated that cholesterol exerts many of its functions by maintaining a specialized type of membrane domain called "lipid rafts" in a functional state. These domains are rich in cholesterol and sphingolipids and could be involved in signal transduction and in the entry of pathogens to the host cells (Simons and Toomre, 2000).

The incorporation and utilization of arachidonic acid, linoleic acid, 3-sn-phosphatidycholine, tripalmitylglycerol,and cholesterol by adult *Schistosoma mansoni* was demonstrated by Rumjanek and Simpson (1980). These parasites exchange cholesterol and other metabolites during reproduction (Popiel and Basch, 1986; Silveria et al., 1986), while cholesterol is absorbed by the hydatid cysts of *Echinococcus granulosus* (Bahr et al., 1979). On the other hand, parasites like *Trypanosome cruzi* and some species of *Leishmania* cannot use cholesterol but they synthesize ergosterol and related

24-alkylated sterols. Furthermore, *Leishmania* has a strict requirement for ergosterol for their survival and growth (Urbina et al., 2002; Magaraci et al., 2003; Bazin et al., 2006).

Ecdysteroids

Several parasites synthesize ecdysteroids, steroid hormones that are essential for arthropod molting; the capacity to synthesize these hormones has been used to classify cestodes (de Loof and Huybrechts, 1998). However, the role of these steroids in parasites remains obscure. Ecdysterone production has been reported in a variety of helminth species, among them, the nematodes *Dirofilaria immitis, Brugia pahangi, Ascaris suum*, and *Anisakis simplex*, the cestodes: *Moniezia expansa, Echinococcus granulosus*, and *Hymenolepis diminuta* and the trematodes: *Fasciola hepatica* and *Schistosoma mansoni* (Mendis et al., 1983, 1984; Fleming, 1985; Cleator et al., 1987; Evershed et al., 1987; Mercer et al., 1987a,b, 1990; Foster et al., 1992). In male and female, *Dirofilaria immitis*, and in female, *Ascaris suum* ecdysteroids were concentrated in the reproductive system, whereas the presence of ecdysteroids in the eggs of *Schistosoma mansoni* suggests a regulatory role in embryogenesis (Mercer, 1985). Ecdysteroids have also been found in cestodes like the sheep parasite *Moniezia expansa* and in the rat tapeworm *Hymenolepis diminuta* (Mercer et al., 1987b). Ecdysterone can be detected in the sera of infected hosts parasitized by *Schistosoma*, a trematode that synthesizes and releases the steroid to the host's circulation (Mercer, 1985). Although the role of ecdysteroids during insect metamorphosis had been widely demonstrated, the function of these steroids in parasites remains obscure.

Sex Steroids

Evidence for the steroidogenic capacity of *Schistosoma mansoni* was provided years ago by data showing the conversion of steroid precursors to its metabolites by the parasite homogenate (Briggs, 1972). We had shown that cultured *Trypanosoma cruzi* trypomastigotes synthesize androgens and estrogens from androstenedione and DHEA (Vacchina et al., 2008). We had also investigated the steroidogenic capacity of the cysticerci and tapeworm from *Taenia solium* and *Taenia crassiceps* WFU. The adult worm of *Taenia solium* and *crassiceps* WFU tapeworms are attached to the host gut with hooks that surrounds their head, and develop reproductive units called proglottids, where testis and ovaries gradually differentiate, and finally contain spermatocytes and infective eggs (Willms et al., 2003). *Taenia solium* cysticerci is the larval stage of the parasite and is found in the brain or muscle of humans and pigs, whereas *Taenia crassiceps* WFU cysticerci constitute a useful laboratory model due to their reproduction by budding in the peritoneal cavity of mice. We had been exploring the capacity of cysticerci to synthesize sex steroids *in vitro* and found that *T. solium* and *T. crassiceps* ORF cysticerci transform steroid precursors such as progesterone, dehydroepiandrostenedione, and androstenedione to androgens and estrogens (Gómez et al., 2000; Jiménez et al., 2006; Valdez et al., 2006). Other experiments showed that drugs that block steroidogenic enzymes interfered the *in vitro* steroid synthesis, suggesting the existence of this enzymes in the parasites (Aceves-Ramos et al., 2013).

Because of the presence of testis and ovaries in tapeworm proglottids, we had investigated the *in vitro* steroidogenic capacity of experimental *Taenia crassiceps* WFU and *solium* tapeworms obtained from the intestine of infected hamsters. *Taenia crassiceps* WFU tapeworms were incubated in the presence of ^{3}H-DHEA and tritiated androstenediol and 17β-estradiol where recovered from the culture media, which strongly suggest the presence and activity of enzymes from the $\Delta 5$ steroid pathway in these tapeworms (Fernández Presas et al., 2008). *Taenia solium* tapeworms kept in culture also synthesized sex steroids (Valdez et al., 2014).

Corticosteroids

Since the above mentioned literature indicated that *Taenia solium* and *Taenia crassiceps* cysticerci and tapeworms synthesized sex steroid hormones, we thought these organisms could also synthesize corticosteroids. Thereafter, we had incubated *Taenia crassiceps* cysticerci in the presence of ^{3}H-progesterone and found an important transformation into deoxycorticosterone (Valdez et al., 2012), a steroid that has mineralocorticoid functions in vertebrates and also display some glucocorticoid properties. In addition, the parasites synthesized corticosterone, which was measured by radioimmunoassay in the culture media. More recently, we found corticosteroid-like synthesis in *Taenia solium* tapeworms (Valdez et al., 2014). It had been shown that in the adrenal reticular zone of mammals an excess of progesterone can be inactivated by 20HSD activity (Pelletier et al., 2005) and that cortisol and corticosterone can be inactivated by 11β-hydroxylase in the adrenal glomerulose zone (for a review see Odermatt and Atanasov, 2009) but to our knowledge these enzymes had not been investigated in *Taenia solium* or *crassiceps* WFU organisms. Besides their effects on the own parasite development and differentiation, the cysticerci, and tapeworm's steroidogenic capacity might play a role in the permanence of the parasites in muscle and brain tissues and in the host intestine.

Parasites Express Steroidogenic Enzymes

Some steroidogenic enzymes had been described in parasites. For instance, sterol-sterifying enzymes were found in *Toxoplasma gondee*, a protozoan incapable of cholesterol de novo synthesis (Lige et al., 2013). The presence of 3β-hydroxysteroid dehydrogenase in *Sarcocystis spp* had been shown by immunohistochemistry (Yarim et al., 2004); the enzyme is also present in *Taenia solium* cysticerci and tapeworms (Fernández Presas et al., 2008). Genes from the cholesterol synthesis pathway have been found and expressed in Giardia intestinalis (Hernandez and Wasserman, 2006). The parasite flatworm *Schistosoma japonicum* has a type 12 17-HSD that metabolizes estrone to estradiol (Zhou et al., 2009).

We have recently shown that *Taenia solium* cysticerci express the enzyme 17β-HSD that belongs to the short chain dehydrogenases/reductase family (Aceves-Ramos et al., 2014). Transient transfection of HEK293T cells with Tsol17β-HSD-pcDNA3.1 (+) induced expression of Tsol17β-HSD that transformed ^{3}H-androstenedione into testosterone. In contrast, ^{3}H-estrone was not significantly transformed into estradiol. Therefore, *Taenia solium* cysticerci express a 17β-HSD that catalyzes the androgen reduction and belongs to the short chain dehydrogenases/reductase (SDR) protein superfamily (Aceves-Ramos et al., 2014). Recently, a sequence (EmW000624600 which is available at: www.genedb.org/Homepage/Emultilocularis) with an identity of 84% with Tsol-17βHSD and a total coverage has been described for *E. multilocularis*, suggesting the presence of 17 HSD enzymes in this *Taeniid* family (Tsai et al., 2012). However, the expression level and enzyme activity has not been yet investigated.

Concluding Remarks

The knowledge of parasite endocrinology will contribute to our understanding of parasite biology and their interactions with the host. Sex steroids and corticosteroids are important hormones for the growth, differentiation, and performance in many species. Therefore, the synthesis of these hormones by parasites themselves may be critical for their own development and viability. In addition, it was shown that the production of steroids by parasites is regulated by corticosteroids and affected by steroidogenic inhibitors, which may be used as tools to combat the infection in some clinical situations. Furthermore, steroid synthesis by parasites may contribute to defend them from the attack of immune cells and therefore facilitate their survival in the host tissues.

References

Aceves-Ramos, A., de la Torre, P., Hinojosa, L., Ponce, A., García-Villegas, R., Laclette, J. P., et al. (2014). Cloning, characterization and functional expression of *Taenia solium* 17 beta-hydroxysteroid dehydrogenase. *Gen. Comp. Endocrinol.* 203, 186–192. doi: 10.1016/j.ygcen.2014.03.021

Aceves-Ramos, A., Valdez, R. A., Gaona, B., Willms, K., and Romano, M. C. (2013). Steroid synthesis by *Taenia crassiceps* WFU cysticerci is regulated by enzyme inhibitors. *Gen. Comp. Endocrinol.* 188, 212–217. doi: 10.1016/j.ygcen.2013.03.034

Al Qarawi, A. A. (2005). Infertility in the dromedary bull: a review of causes, relations and implications. *Anim. Reprod. Sci.* 87, 73–92. doi: 10.1016/j.anireprosci.2004.11.003

Bahr, J. M., Frayha, G. J., and Hajjar, J. J. (1979). Mechanism of cholesterol absorption by the hydatid cysts of *Echinococcus granulosus* (Cestoda). *Comp. Biochem. Physiol.* 62A, 485–490. doi: 10.1016/0300-9629(79)90090-2

Bansal, D., Bahatti, H. S., and Seghal, R. (2005). Role of cholesterol in parasitic infections. *Lipid. Health Dis.* 9, 4–10. doi: 10.1186/1476-511X-4-10

Barthelemy, M., Gabrion, C., and Petit, G. (2004). Reduction in testosterone concentration and its effect on the reproductive output of chronic malaria-infected male mice. *Parasitol. Res.* 93, 475–481. doi: 10.1007/s00436-004-1160-2

Bazin, M. A., Loiseau, P. M., Bories, C., Letoumeux, Y., Rault, S., and El Kihen, L. (2006). Synthesis of oxysterols and nitrogenous sterols with antileshmania and tripacidal activities. *Eur. J. Med. Chem.* 41, 1109–1116. doi: 10.1016/j.ejmech.2006.03.033

Briggs, M. H. (1972). Metabolism of steroid hormones by schistosomes. *Biochim. Biophys. Acta* 280, 480–485. doi: 10.1016/0005-2760(72)90256-1

Carrero, J. C., Cervantes, C., Moreno-Mendoza, N., Saavedra, E., and Morales-Montor, J. (2006). Dehydroepiandrosterone decreases while cortisol increases *in vitro* growth and viability of *Entamoeba histolytica*. *Microbes Infect.* 8, 323–331. doi: 10.1016/j.micinf.2005.06.030

Cleator, M., Delves, C. J., Howells, R. E., and Rees, H. H. (1987). Identity and tissue localization of free and conjugated edcysteroids in adults of *Dirofilaria immitis* and *Ascaris surum*. *Mol. Biochem. Parasitol.* 25, 93–105. doi: 10.1016/0166-6851(87)90022-3

Coutinho, A. E., and Chapman, K. E. (2011). The anti-inflammatory and immunosuppressive effects of glucocorticoids, recent developments and mechanistic insights. *Mol. Cell Endocrinol.* 335, 2–13. doi: 10.1016/j.mce.2010.04.005

Dangel, K. C., Keppel, M., Tabujew, K., and Sures, S. (2014). Effects of *Anguillicola novaezelandiae* on the levels of cortisol and hsp70 in the European Eel. *Parasitol. Res.* 113, 3817–3822. doi: 10.1007/s00436-014-4049-8

de Loof, A., and Huybrechts, R. (1998). "Insects do not have sex hormones": a myth? *Gen. Comp. Endocrinol.* 111, 245–260. doi: 10.1006/gcen.1998.7101

Dubansky, B., Whitaker, B., and Galvez, F. (2011). Influence of cortisol on the attachment and metamorphosis of larval *Utterbackia imbecillis* on Bluegill Sunfish (*Lepomis macrochirus*). *Biol. Bull.* 220, 97–106. doi: 10.2307/23046932

Dunlap, D. D., and Schall, J. J. (1995). Hormonal alterations and reproduction inhibition in male fence lizards (*Sceloporus occidentals*) infected with the malarial parasite *Plasmodium mexicanum*. *Physiol. Zool.* 68, 608–621.

Escobedo, G., Larralde, C., Chavarria, A., Cerbón, M. A., and Morales-Montor, J. (2004). Molecular mechanisms involved in the differential effects of sex steroids on the reproduction and infectivity of *Taenia crassiceps*. *J. Parasitol.* 6, 1235–1244. doi: 10.1645/GE-297R

Evershed, R. P., Mercer, J. G., and Rees, H. H. (1987). Capillary gas chromatography-mass spectrometry of ecdysteroids. *J. Chromatogr.* 390, 357–369. doi: 10.1016/S0021-9673(01)94387-0

Hernández-Bello, R., Ramirez-Nieto, R., Muñiz-Hernández, S., Nava-Castro, K., Pavón, L., Sánchez-Acosta, A. G., et al. (2011). Sex steroids effects on the molting process of the helminth human parasite *Trichinella spiralis*. *J. Biomed. Biotechnol.* 2011:625380. doi: 10.1155/2011/625380

Fernández Presas, A. M., Willms, K., and Romano, M. C. (2008). The key steroidogenic enzyme 3ß-hydroxysteroid dehydrogenase is present in the strobilae and larvae of *Taenia solium* and *T. crassiceps* WFU strain. *Parasitol. Res.* 103, 847–852. doi: 10.1007/s00436-008-1066-5

Fleming, M. W. (1985). *Ascaris suum;* role of ecdysteroids in molting. *Exp. Parasitol* 60, 207–210. doi: 10.1016/0014-4894(85)90024-4

Foster, J. M., Mercer, J. G., and Rees, H. H. (1992). Analysis of ecdysteroids in the trematodes, *Schistosoma mansoni* and *Fasciola hepatica*. *Trop. Med. Parasitol.* 43, 239–244.

Gómez, Y., Valdez, R. A., Larralde, C., and Romano, M. C. (2000). Sex steroids and parasitism. *Taenia crassiceps* cysticercus metabolizes exogenous androstenedione to testosterone *in vitro*. *J. Steroid. Biochem. Mol. Biol.* 74, 143–147. doi: 10.1016/S0960-0760(00)00099-6

Hernandez, P. C., and Wasserman, M. (2006). Do genes from the cholesterol pathway exist and express in *Giardia intestinalis*? *Parsitol. Res.* 98, 194–199. doi: 10.1007/s00436-005-0039-1

Hinojosa, L., Valdez, R. A., Salvador, V., Rodriguez, A. G., Willms, K., and Romano, M. C. (2011). The effect of corticosteroids on sex steroid synthesis in cultured *Taenia crassiceps* Wake Forest University (WFU) cysticerci. *J. Helminthol.* 86, 465–469. doi: 10.1017/S0022149X11000708

Jiménez, P., Valdéz, R. A., and Romano, M. C. (2006). Metabolism of steroid hormones by *Taenia solium* and *Taenia crassiceps* cysticerci. *J. Steroid Biochem. Mol.* 99, 203–208. doi: 10.1016/j.jsbmb.2006.01.002

Lafont, R. (2000). The endocrinology of invertebrates. *Ecotoxicology* 9, 41–57 doi: 10.1023/A:1008912127592

Li, M., Leatherland, J. F., and Woo, P. T. K. (2013). Cortisol and dexamethasone increase the *in vitro* multiplication of the haemoflagellate *Cryptobia salmonistica*, possible by interaction with glucocorticoid receptor-like protein. *Int. J. Parasitol.* 43, 353–360. doi: 10.1016/j.ijpara.2012.11.009

Li, M., Patrick, T. K., and Woo, P. T. K. (2014). Glucocorticoid receptors on and in a unicellular organism, *Cryptobia salmonistica. Int. J. Parasitol.* 44, 205–210. doi: 10.1016/j.ijpara.2013.10.006

Lige, B., Sampels, V., and Coppens, I. (2013). Characterization of a second sterol-esterfying enzyme in Toxoplama highlights the importance of cholesterol storage pathways for the parasite. *Mol. Microbiol.* 87, 951–967. doi: 10.1111/mmi.12142

Lim, A., Kumar, V., Hari Dass, S. A., and Vyas, A. (2013). *Toxoplasma gondee* infection enhances testicular steroidogenesis in rats. *Mol. Ecol.* 22, 102–110. doi: 10.1111/mec.12042

Lingnau, A., Margos, G., Maier, W. A., and Seitz, H. M. (1993). The effects of hormones on the gametocytogenesis of *Plasmodium falciparum in vitro. Appl. Parasitol.* 34, 153–160.

Madison, B. N., Woo, P. T., and Bernier, N. J. (2013). Duress without stress: cryptobia infection results in HPI disfunction in rainbow trout. *J. Endocrinol.* 218, 287–297. doi: 10.1530/JOE-13-0155

Magaraci, F., Jiménez, C. J., Rodrigues, C., Rodrígues, J. C., Braga, M. V., Yardley, V., et al. (2003). Azasterols as inhibitors of sterol 24-methyltransferase in *Leishmania* species and *Tryposoma cruzi. J. Med. Chem.* 46, 4714–4727. doi: 10.1021/jm021114j

Mendis, A. H., Rees, H. H., and Gooswin, T. W. (1984). The occurrence of ecdysteroid in the cestode. *Monieza expansa. Mol. Biochem. Parasitol.* 10, 123–138. doi: 10.1016/0166-6851(84)90001-X

Mendis, A. H., Rose, M. E., Rees, H. H., and Goodwin, T. W. (1983). Ecdysteroids in adults of the nematode, *Dirofilaria immitis. Mol. Biochem. Parasitol.* 9, 209–226. doi: 10.1016/0166-6851(83)90098-1

Mercer, J. G. (1985). Developmental hormones in parasitic helminths. *Parasitol. Today* 1, 96–100.

Mercer, J. G., Barker, G. C., Howells, R. E., and Rees, H. H. (1990). Investigation of ecdysteroid excretion by adult *Dirofilaria immitis* and *Brugia pahangi. Mol. Biochem. Parasitol.* 38, 89–95. doi: 10.1016/0166-6851(90)90208-4

Mercer, J. G., Munn, A. E., and Rees, H. H. (1987a). *Echinococcus granulosus*: occurrence of ecdcysteroids in protoscoleces and hydatid cyst fluid. *Mol. Biochem. Parasitol.* 24, 203–214. doi: 10.1016/0166-6851(87)90107-1

Mercer, J. G., Munn, A. E., and Rees, H. H. (1987b). Analysis of ecdsysteroids in different developmental stages of *Hymenolepis diminuta. Mol. Biochem. Parasitol.* 25, 61–71. doi: 10.1016/0166-6851(87)90019-3

Morales, J., Larralde, C., Arteaga, M., Govezensky, T., Romano, M. C., and Moralí, G. (1996). Inhibition of sexual behavior in male mice infected with *Taenia Crassiceps* cysticerci. *J. Parasitol.* 82, 689–693. doi: 10.2307/3283875

Morales-Montor, J., Chavarria, A., de Leon, M. A., del Castillo, L. I., Escobedo, E. G., Sanchez, E. N., et al. (2004). Host gender in parasitic infections of mammals: an evaluation of the female host supremacy paradigm. *J. Parasitol.* 90, 531–546. doi: 10.1645/GE-113R3

Morales-Montor, J., Hallal-Caballeros, C., Romano, M. C., and Damian, R. T. (2002). Inhibition of P450-aromatase prevents feminization and induces protection during cisticercosis. *Int. J. Parasitol.* 32, 1379–1387. doi: 10.1016/S0020-7519(02)00130-3

Morrison, D. D., Vandee Waa, E., and Bennett, J. L. (1986). Effects of steroids and steroid synthesis inhibitors on fecundity of *Schistosoma mansoni in vitro. J. Chem. Ecol.* 12, 1901–1908. doi: 10.1007/BF01022391

Odermatt, A., and Atanasov, A. G. (2009). Mineralocorticoid receptors: emerging complexity and functional diversity. *Steroids* 74, 163–171. doi: 10.1016/j.steroids.2008.10.010

Pelletier, G., Luu-The, V., Li, S., and Labrie, F. (2005). Localization of type 5 17β-hydroxysteroid dehydrogenase mRNA in mouse tissues as studied by *in situ* hybridization. *Cell Tissue Res.* 320, 393–398. doi: 10.1007/s00441-005-1105-9

Popiel, I., and Basch, P. F. (1986). *Schistosoma mansoni* colesterol uptake by paired and unpaired worms. *Exp. Parasitol.* 61, 343–347. doi: 10.1016/0014-4894(86)90189-X

Reyes-Hernandez, J. L., Leung, G., and McKay, D. M. (2013). Cestode regulation of inflammation and inflammatory research. *Int. J. Parasitol.* 43, 233–243. doi: 10.1016/j.ijpara.2012.09.005

Roberts, C. W., Walker, W., and Alexander, J. (2001). Sex-associated hormones and immunity of protozoan parasites. *Clin. Microbiol. Rev.* 14, 476–488. doi: 10.1128/CMR.14.3.476-488.2001

Romano, M. C., Valdez, R. A., Cartas, A. L., Gómez, Y., and Larralde, C. (2003). Steroid hormone production by parasites: the case of *Taenia crassiceps* and *Taenia solium* cysticerci. *J. Steroid Biochem. Mol. Biol.* 85, 221–225. doi: 10.1016/S0960-0760(03)00233-4

Rumjanek, F. D., and Simpson, A. J. G. (1980). The incorporation and utilization of radiolabelled lipids by adult *Schistosoma mansoni in vitro. Mol. Biochem. Parasitol.* 1, 31–44.

Santos, C. D., Toldo, M. P., Levy, A. M., and Prado, J. C. Jr. (2008). *Trypanosoma cruzi*: effects of social stress in *Calomys callosus* a natural reservoir of infection. *Exp. Parasitol.* 119, 197–201. doi: 10.1016/j.exppara.2008.01.011

Silveria, A. M., Friche, A. A., and Rumjanek, F. D. (1986). Transfer of (14C) cholesterol and its metabolities between adult male and female worms of *schistosoma mansoni. Comp. Biochem. Physiol. B* 85, 851–857. doi: 10.1016/0305-0491(86)90186-0

Simons, K., and Toomre, D. (2000). Lipids rafts signal transduction. *Nat. Rev.* 1, 31–39. doi: 10.1038/35036052

Thompson, S. N., and Kavaliers, M. (1994). Physiological basis for parasite induced alterations of host behavior. *Parasitology* 109, S119–S138. doi: 10.1017/S0031182000085139

Tsai, I. J., Zarowiecki, M., Holroyd, N., Garciarrubio, A., Sanchez-Flores, A., Brooks, K. L., et al. (2012). The genomes of four tapeworm species reveal adaptations to parasitism. *Nature* 496, 57–63. doi: 10.1038/nature 12031

Urbina, J. A., Conception, J. L., Rangel, S., Visval, G., and Lira, R. (2002). Mol. Squalene synthase as a chemotherapeutic target in *Tripsosoma cruzi* and *Leishmania mexicana. Biochem. Parasitol.* 125, 35–45. doi: 10.1016/S0166-6851(02)00206-2

Vacchina, P., Valdez, R. A., Revelli, S., and Romano, M. C. (2008). Steroidogenic capacity of *Trypanosome cruzi* trypomastigotes. *J. Steroid Biochem. Mol. Biol.* 111, 282–286. doi: 10.1016/j.jsbmb.2008.06.016

Valdez, R. A., Hinojosa, L., Gómez, Y., Willms, K., and Romano, M. C. (2012). *Taenia crassiceps* WFU cysticerci synthesize corticosteroids *in vitro*: metyrapone regulates the production. *Comp. Endocrinol.* 176, 409–414. doi: 10.1016/j.ygcen.2012.01.015

Valdez, R. A., Jiménez, P., Cartas, A. L., Gómez, Y., and Romano, M. C. (2006). *Taenia solium* cysticerci synthesize androgens and estrogens *in vitro. Parasitol. Res.* 98, 472–476. doi: 10.1007/s00436-005-0095-6

Valdez, R. A., Jiménez, P., Fernández-Presas, A. M., Aguilar, L., Willms, K., and Romano, M. C. (2014). *Taenia solium* tapeworms synthesize corticosteroids and sex steroids *in vitro. Gen. Comp. Endocrinol.* 205, 62–67. doi: 10.1016/j.ygcen.2014.04.014

Wang, T., Gao, J.-M., Yi, S. Q., Geng, G. Q., Gao, X. J., Shen, J. L., et al. (2014). The growth rate of *Toxoplasma gondii*, a protozoan parasite, increased in the peritoneal macrophages of rats treated with glucocorticoids *in vivo. Parasitol. Res.* 113, 351–358. doi: 10.1007/s00436-013-3661-3

Willms, K., Caro, J. A., and Robert, L. (2003). Ultrastructure of spermatogonia and spermatocyte lobules in *Taenia solium* strobilac (Cestoda, *Cyclophyllidea, Taeniidae*) from golden hamsters. *Parasitol. Res.* 90, 479–488. doi: 10.1007/s00436-003-0897-3

Yarim, M., Yildiz, K., and Kabakci, N. (2004). Immunohistochemical localization of 3β-hydroxysteroid dehydrogenase in Sarcocystis sp. *Parasitol. Res.* 93, 457–460. doi: 10.1007/s00436-004-1152-2

Zhou, Y., Zheng, H., Chen, Y., Zhang, L., Wang, K., Guo, J., Huang, Z., et al. (2009). The *Schistosoma japonicum* genome reveals features of host-parasite interplay. *Nature* 460, 345–351. doi: 10.1038/nature08140

11

ESR1 mutations are not a common mechanism of endocrine resistance in patients with estrogen receptor–positive breast cancer treated with neoadjuvant aromatase inhibitor therapy

Tomás Reinert[1,2,3], Susana Ramalho[4], Vivian Castro Antunes de Vasconcelos[4], Leonardo Roberto Silva[4], Ana Elisa Ribeiro da Silva[4], Camila Annicchino de Andrade[4], Maria Beatriz de Paula Leite Kraft[4], Guilherme Portela Coelho[5], Jovana Mandelli[5], Monique Binotto[2], Cesar Cabello[4], Geisilene Russano de Paiva Silva[6], José Bines[7], Carlos H. Barrios[3], Matthew J. Ellis[8] and Marcia Silveira Graudenz[1]*

[1] Postgraduate Program in Medical Sciences, Universidade Federal Do Rio Grande Do Sul (UFRGS), Porto Alegre, Brazil, [2] Centro de Pesquisa da Serra Gaucha (CEPESG), Caxias Do Sul, Brazil, [3] Latin American Cooperative Oncology Group (LACOG), Porto Alegre, Brazil, [4] Department of Obstetrics and Gynecology, Faculty of Medical Sciences, State University of Campinas (UNICAMP), Campinas, Brazil, [5] Diagnose Patologia e Biologia Molecular, Caxias Do Sul, Brazil, [6] Laboratory of Molecular and Investigative Pathology – LAPE, Faculty of Medical Sciences, State University of Campinas (UNICAMP), Campinas, Brazil, [7] Instituto Nacional Do Câncer (INCA – HCIII), Rio de Janeiro, Brazil, [8] Lester and Sue Smith Breast Cancer Center, Baylor College of Medicine, Houston, TX, United States

Edited by:
Carmine De Angelis, University of Naples Federico II, Italy

Reviewed by:
Luca Gelsomino, University of Calabria, Italy
Alessandro Igor Cavalcanti Leal, Johns Hopkins Medicine, United States

***Correspondence:**
Tomás Reinert
tomasreinert@hotmail.com

Introduction: Mutations in the *ESR1* gene (*ESR1*m) are important mechanisms of resistance to endocrine therapy in estrogen receptor–positive (ER+) metastatic breast cancer and have been studied as a potential therapeutic target, as well as a predictive and prognostic biomarker. Nonetheless, the role of *ESR1*m as a possible mechanism of primary endocrine resistance, as well as whether it also occurs in tumors that are resistant to ET administered in early-stage disease as (neo)adjuvant, has not been adequately studied. In this study, we evaluated the prevalence of *ESR1*m in tumor samples from patients with ER+ breast cancer resistant to neoadjuvant aromatase inhibitor therapy.

Methods: We followed a prospective cohort of patients with ER+ HER2− stages II and III breast cancer treated with neoadjuvant endocrine therapy (NET). Tumor samples from patients with a pattern of primary endocrine resistance [defined as a Preoperative Endocrine Prognostic Index (PEPI) score of ≥4] were identified and analyzed for the presence of *ESR1*m.

Results: One hundred twenty-seven patients were included in the cohort, of which 100 (79%) had completed NET and underwent surgery. Among these patients, the PEPI score ranged from 0 to 3 in 70% (70/100), whereas 30% (30/100) had a PEPI score of 4 or more. Twenty-three of these patients were included in the analysis. *ESR1* mutations were not identified in any of the 23 patients with early-stage ER+ breast cancer resistant to NET.

Discussion: Growing evidence supports the notion that there are different mechanisms for primary and secondary endocrine resistance. Our study suggests that *ESR1* mutations do not evolve rapidly and do not represent a common mechanism of primary endocrine resistance in the neoadjuvant setting. Therefore, *ESR1*m should be considered a mechanism of acquired endocrine resistance in the context of advanced disease. Further research should be conducted to identify factors associated with intrinsic resistance to ET.

Keywords: breast cancer, endocrine therapy, *ESR1*, *ESR1* mutations, neoadjuvant, aromatase inhibitors

INTRODUCTION

Estrogen receptor-positive (ER+) breast cancer is the most prevalent breast cancer subtype. Endocrine therapy (ET) remains the mainstay of treatment in all stages of the disease (1). Nevertheless, endocrine resistance associated with disease progression remains an important challenge (2, 3). Mutations of the *ESR1* gene, which encodes the ER protein, have been increasingly identified as one of the most important mechanisms of endocrine resistance (4).

Breast tumors are known to undergo genomic evolution, and *ESR1* mutations (*ESR1*m) have been identified in 9–40% of patients with metastatic ER+ breast cancer resistant to aromatase inhibitors (AIs) (3–7). In Brazilian patients with visceral metastasis of ER+ HER2-negative breast cancer, our group reported the presence of *ESR1*m in 25% of the cases (8). In the metastatic setting, the presence of *ESR1*m is a biomarker of a worse prognosis. The function of *ESR1*m as a potential therapeutic target, as well as a predictive and prognostic biomarker, is being studied (9). However, the role of *ESR1*m as a possible mechanism of ET resistance in the early-stage disease is unclear. Regardless of the extensive research that is being conducted in this field, several questions remain unanswered about *ESR1*m, such as whether it is associated with endocrine resistance to AIs used with a curative intent treatment in the (neo)adjuvant setting.

Neoadjuvant endocrine therapy (NET) is a therapeutic approach that is being increasingly explored, not only to allow less extensive surgery but also as a scientific tool (10). The Preoperative Endocrine Prognostic Index (PEPI) is a surrogate of endocrine sensitivity and identifies a subgroup of patients with primary resistance to NET (11, 12).

The objective of this study was to evaluate the potential role of *ESR1*m as a mechanism of resistance in postmenopausal patients with breast cancer treated with NET with a high PEPI score as a surrogate for primarily endocrine-resistant biology.

METHODS

We conducted a prospective cohort of patients with breast cancer treated with NET in two institutions. The population included postmenopausal women presenting with stages II and III ER+ Her2-negative breast cancer. Protocols of diagnosis, therapies, and follow-up of patients were standardized and based on major international guidelines. These procedures are not part of the study.

Eligible patients were treated with NET with anastrozole for a recommended period of at least 3 months, followed by surgery. Pathological and immunohistochemistry (IHC) protocols were standardized and followed American Society of Clinical Oncology/College of American Pathologists guidelines and the international consensus of pathologic assessment of the breast and axilla after preoperative therapy (13). For all patients who underwent surgery, the PEPI score was calculated (described in **Table 1**). All IHC assessments were reviewed by two pathologists. Tumor samples from patients with a pattern of primary endocrine-resistant tumors (defined as a PEPI score of ≥4) were selected and analyzed for the presence of *ESR1*m.

*ESR1*m were evaluated in formalin-fixed paraffin-embedded breast cancer tissue using real-time quantitative polymerase

TABLE 1 | The preoperative endocrine prognostic index (PEPI) score following 4–6 months of neoadjuvant AI or other endocrine therapy provides another strategy to identify endocrine-sensitive vs. endocrine-resistant tumors in the early-stage setting.

Surgical factors	RFS HR	PEPI score
TUMOR SIZE		
T1/T2	–	0
T3/T4	2.8	3
NODE STATUS		
Negative	–	0
Positive	3.2	3
Ki67 LEVEL		
0–2.7%	**-**	**0**
>2.7–7.3%	1.3	1
>7.3–19.7%	1.7	1
>19.7–53.1%	2.2	2
>53.1%	2.9	3
ER STATUS		
Negative	2.8	3
Positive	0	0

A PEPI score of 0 [pT1/2, node-negative (N0), Ki67$<$2.7%, estrogen receptor-positive (ER$^+$)] is being investigated prospectively as a surrogate of endocrine therapy-sensitive disease that does not need chemotherapy, and a PEPI of $>$0 identifies patients with an increased risk of relapse. The hazard ratio (HR) of each surgical factor for relapse-free survival (RFS) and assigned PEPI points based on the data from the P024 trial are shown in the table. Adapted from Ma et al. (3).

chain reaction (RT-qPCR). For each sample, the tumor area was identified and marked by the same pathologist, and this was followed by DNA extraction with the Wizard© Genomic DNA Purification kit (Promega, Madison, WI, USA). DNA was quantified using Qubit Fluorometric Quantitation (Thermo Fisher Scientific, Waltham, MA, USA), and 20 ng/μL was the threshold for the analysis of the mutation. The reactions were performed with the equipment 7500 Fast Real-Time PCR System using TaqMan Genotyping Master Mix, primers, and TaqMan© probes and followed all recommendations of the manufacturer. A TaqMan© reference probe was used to evaluate the presence of the mutations, followed by analysis in the 7500 Software v2.06 (Thermo Fisher Scientific). The analyzed mutations were Y537N, Y537C, Y537S, E380Q, and D538G. A description of the primer sequences used for RT-PCR can be found in **Supplementary Material**.

Statistical analysis was performed using Statistical Package for Social Sciences 22.0 (SPSS, Armonk, NY, USA). Categorical variables are described by frequencies and percentages. The primary endpoint is the prevalence of *ESR1*m. For the primary endpoint, the point estimate is presented together with the exact 95% confidence interval. Continuous variables are described by means and standard deviation or median, depending on Shapiro–Wilk test analysis. Correlations between categorical variables were analyzed using the χ^2 test. Differences between means are analyzed using the Student *t*-test. This project was reviewed and

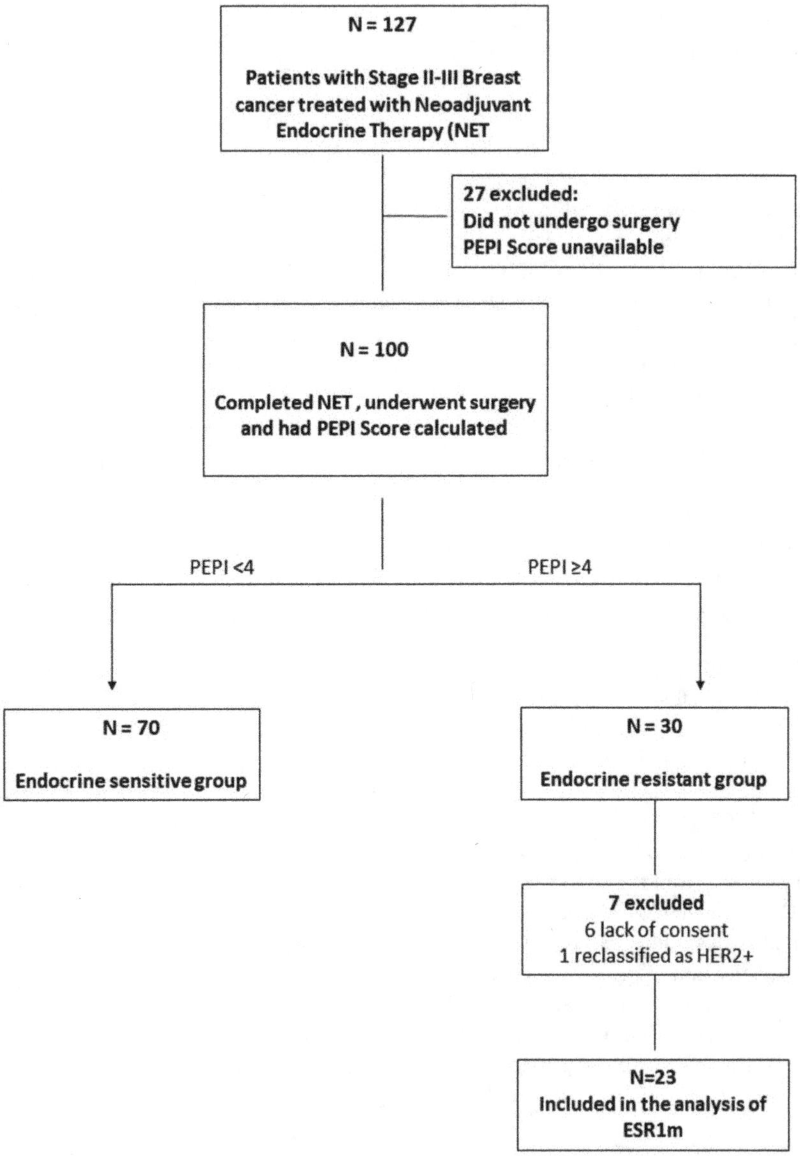

FIGURE 1 | Flowchart of patients with ER+ HER2− stages II and III breast cancer treated with neoadjuvant endocrine therapy (NET). Tumor samples from patients with a pattern of primary endocrine resistance [defined as a Preoperative Endocrine Prognostic Index (PEPI) score of 4] were identified and analyzed for the presence of *ESR1*m.

TABLE 2 | Patients characteristics, pathology and IHC results (initial biopsy sample) ($n = 23$).

Age	Median 70 years (54–84)
Histology	Ductal: 20 (86.9%) Lobular: 3 (13.1%)
Clinical tumor size	cT1/T2: 14 (60.8%) cT3/T4: 9 (39.2%)
Clinical lymph node status	Negative (cN–): 10 (43.4%) Positive (cN+): 13 (56.5%)
Ki67 level—baseline	<2.7%: 2 (8.6%) 2.8–7.3%: 1 (4.3%) 7.4–19.7%: 12 (52.1%) 19.8–53.1%: 8 (34.7%) >53.2%: 0
Duration of NET	Median 22 weeks (4–35)

TABLE 3 | PEPI Score, pathology and IHC results after NET (surgical sample).

PEPI score	4: 16 (69.5%) 5: 2 (8.6%) 6: 3 (13%) 7: 2 (8.6%)
Pathological tumor size—surgical specimen	ypT1/T2: 17 (73.9%) ypT3/T4: 6 (26%)
Pathological lymph node status	Negative (ypN–): 2 (8.6%) Positive (ypN+): 21 (91.3%)
ER status, Allred score	0–2: 1 (4.3%) 3–8: 22 (95.6%)
Ki67 level—surgical specimen	<2.7%: 5 (21.7%) 2.8–7.3%: 5 (21.7%) 7.4–19.7%: 11 (47.8%) 19.8–53.1%: 1 (4.3%) >53.2%: 1 (4.3%)

approved by the institutional review board (ethical committee) of both institutions.

RESULTS

One hundred twenty-seven patients were included in the cohort, of which 100 (79%) completed NET and surgery. Among these patients, the PEPI score ranged from 0 to 3 in 70% (70/100), and 30% (30/100) had a PEPI score of 4 or more and were selected. Twenty-three patients were included in the analysis (six did not consent or were lost to follow-up, and one was found to be HER2-positive in the surgical sample). These data are summarized in **Figure 1**.

Table 2 summarizes the most important characteristics of the patients and biopsy findings at the initial diagnosis. Tumors classified as primarily resistant to ET (PEPI score of four or more) were selected and had their tumors analyzed for *ESR1*m. In our analysis, the median age was 70 years. There was a predominance of ductal carcinoma (86.9%) and T1-T2 tumors (60.8%), and the majority of our patients had clinical positive axillary nodes (56.5%) before treatment and had a Ki67 index between 7.4 and 19.7%. **Table 3** describes the results in terms of PEPI score and pathological and IHC evaluation. On pathological analysis (after NET), most of the tumors were T1/T2 (73.9%), had a compromised axilla (91.3%), maintained ER positivity (95.6%), and had intermediate levels of Ki67.

The median duration of NET was 22 weeks (range, 4-35 weeks). All samples of tumor tissue from the surgical specimens after NET were evaluable. Quantification of DNA extraction and reference gene cycle threshold values confirmed that the material was adequate for the analysis. *ESR1* mutations were not identified in any of the 23 samples. Therefore, the prevalence of *ESR1*m in patients with early-stage ER+ HER2-negative breast cancer that were intrinsically resistant to NET is 0% (95% confidence interval, 0–12.2%).

DISCUSSION

Our study reports that differently than in AI-resistant metastatic breast cancer, *ESR1*m are not a common mechanism of resistance in tumors with primary endocrine resistance in the neoadjuvant setting. This finding may have implications for the future development of *ESR1*m as a biomarker and therapeutic target.

Estrogen receptor-positive tumors are the most common form of breast cancer and the major cause of mortality by this disease worldwide (14). The use of endocrine agents that interfere with the ER pathway such as tamoxifen and AIs remains the standard-of-care treatment both for patients with early-stage disease and for advanced disease when the use of ET is associated with objective response and disease control in a significant proportion of patients. Nevertheless, tumor evolution caused by a complex network of mechanisms of endocrine resistance continues to be an important challenge (14). In early-stage disease, a considerable proportion of patients will develop disease recurrence despite the use of curative-intent treatment with a combination of therapies such as surgery, chemotherapy, radiation, and adjuvant hormone therapy.

Estrogen receptor, a protein encoded by the *ESR1* gene, is expressed in the majority of breast cancers and is one of the key factors for disease classification and treatment definition. A significant body of research has confirmed the essential role of the ER pathway in physiological mammary gland development and also in tumorigenesis (15). Estrogen binding triggers several events, resulting in conformational changes in the ligand-binding domain (LBD), receptor activation, and allowing the ligand–receptor complex to bind to specific sequences of the genome and to interact with corepressor and coactivator proteins to regulate the transcription of estrogen-response elements (16). The most common molecular alterations in the *ESR1* gene found in breast tumors are mutations, most commonly missense mutations found in codons 380, 537, and 538. *ESR1*m are most commonly missense mutations clustered in codons 537 and 538 of the LBD (17). The most prevalent *ESR1* point mutations are Y537S and D538G, whereas others have been described at significantly lower frequencies (15). Additionally, *ESR1* is known to undergo amplifications and translocations that are potential mechanisms of resistance to ET (17–19).

*ESR1*m have been consistently associated with more aggressive disease, presence of visceral metastasis, and worst prognosis

(8, 15, 20). Extensive research addressing the potential role of *ESR1*m as a predictive biomarker to guide therapeutic decisions is ongoing (20). Additionally, the development of targeted therapies directed to tumor cells harboring *ESR1* mutations is a logical and appealing concept, and extensive preclinical research has been conducted in this field (4, 21), and promising work evaluating treatment with new generation endocrine agents is in progress (22, 23).

The role of *ESR1*m has been mostly studied in the metastatic setting in patients who had disease progression on first-line ET, usually presenting with a clinical pattern of acquired (secondary) ET resistance. Nevertheless, the potential role of *ESR1*m in patients with early-stage breast cancer treated with (neo)adjuvant ET has not been adequately studied. While *ESR1*m have been identified in advanced breast cancer, their presence in primary tumors is very low (24). Understanding mechanisms of intrinsic (acquired) endocrine resistance is of great importance, given that it could lead to the development of biomarkers and therapeutic agents that could be incorporated in the context of curative-intent treatment of breast cancer.

Historically, NET has been indicated as a clinical tool for tumor downstaging to allow breast-conserving surgery. Recently, NET is being used not only as a clinical tool but also as a scientific tool for the study of tumoral patterns of intrinsic endocrine sensitivity or resistance. Importantly, NET allows an *in vivo* observation of the response to estrogen deprivation therapies (25).

Preoperative Endocrine Prognostic Index, described in **Figure 1**, was created to distinguish tumors that are sensitive to NET from tumors that have an intrinsic degree of endocrine resistance (25). This tool is composed of four independent prognostic factors: pathological tumor size, lymph node status, level of ER expression, and Ki67 expression at the surgical sample following neoadjuvant AI therapy. The PEPI score was validated in samples from patients included in two NET clinical trials: the PO24 and IMPACT studies (11). In both trials, the rate of early relapse was very low in patients with a PEPI score of zero (25). The rate of PEPI-0 tumors in neoadjuvant AI therapy trials ranges from 17 to 37% (25). This population has a very favorable prognosis, and these patients could potentially receive adjuvant endocrine monotherapy and be spared from chemotherapy (3). Preoperative Endocrine Prognostic Index scores greater than zero were associated with an incremental increase in the risk of relapse, especially in patients with a score higher than 3 (12).

These findings were compared with a study from our group using the same methodology in patients with advanced disease where *ESR1* mutations were identified in 25% ($n = 32$) of cases with visceral metastasis of ER+ breast cancer resistant to ET (8). A statistically significant association of the presence of *ESR1*m in metastatic disease compared with tumors resistant to AIs used in the neoadjuvant setting was demonstrated ($p = 0.01$, Fisher exact test).

Therefore, the discovery of biomarkers associated with resistance to NET, as well as adjuvant ET, remains an unmet need. Our data reinforce the notion that mutations in the *ESR1* gene do not seem to evolve rapidly and are probably mechanisms of secondary resistance to ET. Ongoing studies are evaluating a variety of potential mechanisms of primary endocrine resistance, such as defects in the DNA repair machinery (26) and aberrant FGFR signaling (27).

Our study has limitations, and we understand that the detected prevalence of *ESR1*m can be underestimated given the fact that a PCR-based methodology analyzed only specific mutations in the most commonly mutated codons. Therefore, it is possible that cases with mutations in different codons of the *ESR1* gene potentially detectable with next-generation sequencing (NGS) technologies were not identified (28, 29). However, it is essential to emphasize that a robust body of literature clearly shows that *ESR1*m usually occurs in hotspots within the LBD, and the vast majority of the published data in this field reported mutations in the same codons we studied (15). Moreover, other studies showed that a specific real-time PCR assay does provide a rapid and reliable diagnostic tool for accurate detection of *ESR1*m (30).

We acknowledge that unidimensional biomarker analysis is not the best approach to investigate primary resistance and that NGS-based evaluation of whole-genome sequences, whole-exome sequencing, and even targeted gene panels could expand the identification of mechanisms of endocrine resistance. Nevertheless, the evaluation of the role of other mutations associated with endocrine resistance is beyond the scope of this article.

Additionally, and despite the challenge of conducting a prospective cohort of NET that includes more than 100 breast cancer patients, we acknowledge that the relatively low sample size of 23 cases of tumors with a PEPI score of 4 or more is a limitation and highlights the challenges of studying primary endocrine resistance. Furthermore, our patients were treated with a median 3 months of NET. Therefore, we cannot exclude that resistance documented after longer treatment durations (6–12 months) could not be related to receptor mutations. Still, in these cases, it would be expected that patients would have at least stable disease or a degree of response to allow for the continuation of treatment. These considerations would make it unlikely to relate *ESR1*m with primary resistance.

Among the strengths of our study, we highlight the conduction of a well-designed prospective cohort including 127 breast cancer patients who were treated with standard-of-care NET and whose tumors were evaluated with uniform procedures of pathology and IHC. Additionally, we used a validated methodology for *ESR1* determination, and we were able to perform a prespecified comparison in two different settings (neoadjuvant and metastatic). Despite the relatively low sample size, we demonstrated that the prevalence of *ESR1*m in NET-resistant tumors is very low (95% of chance of being inferior to 12%). Therefore, the chances that this molecular alteration will have a practical role for patient care in this setting are minimal.

Integrative approaches to evaluate the genetic and phenotypic heterogeneity of breast tumors with the use of a more comprehensive analysis of the genome, transcriptome, epigenetic regulators, and modern quantitative proteomics methods associated with advanced bioinformatics and statistical analysis may lead to advances that can potentially be translated into improved outcomes for cancer patients (31). Advances in the understanding of the molecular biology of ER+ breast cancer led to a revolution in this field with the development of a variety of therapeutic agents that are now being used in routine clinical care in patients with metastatic disease such as CDK4/6, PI3K, and mTOR inhibitors (1). However, a clinically useful biomarker to identify primary sensitivity and resistance to ET has not yet been developed and remains an unmet need.

CONCLUSION

Growing evidence supports the notion that there are different mechanisms of primary and secondary endocrine resistance. Our study suggests that *ESR1* mutations do not evolve rapidly and do not represent a common mechanism of primary endocrine resistance in the neoadjuvant setting. Therefore, *ESR1*m should be considered a mechanism of acquired endocrine resistance in the context of advanced breast cancer. Further research should be conducted to identify factors associated with intrinsic resistance to ET.

ETHICS STATEMENT

All procedures performed in studies involving human participants were in accordance with the ethical standards of the institutional and/or national research committee and with the 1964 Helsinki declaration and its later amendments or comparable ethical standards. Informed consent was obtained from all individual participants included in the study. This article does not contain any studies with animals performed by any of the authors.

AUTHOR CONTRIBUTIONS

TR, SR, CC, JB, CB, ME, and MG designed the study. TR, SR, VV, LS, CC, CA, AS, and MK were involved in the oncologic treatment of patients. GC, JM, GP, and MG did the pathologic and molecular biology evaluation. TR, SR, VV, and MB analyzed and interpreted the data. All authors read and approved the final manuscript.

REFERENCES

1. Cardoso F, Senkus E, Costa A, Papadopoulos E, Aapro M, André F, et al. 4th ESO-ESMO international consensus guidelines for advanced breast cancer (ABC 4)†. *Ann Oncol.* (2018) 29:1634–57. doi: 10.1093/annonc/mdy192
2. Osborne CK, Schiff R. Mechanisms of endocrine resistance in breast cancer. *Annu Rev Med.* (2011) 62:233–47. doi: 10.1146/annurev-med-070909-182917
3. Ma CX, Reinert T, Chmielewska I, Ellis MJ. Mechanisms of aromatase inhibitor resistance. *Nat Rev Cancer.* (2015) 15:261–75. doi: 10.1038/nrc3920
4. Jeselsohn R, Yelensky R, Buchwalter G, Frampton G, Meric-Bernstam F, Gonzalez-Angulo AM, et al. Emergence of constitutively active estrogen receptor-α mutations in pretreated advanced estrogen receptor-positive breast cancer. *Clin Cancer Res.* (2014) 20:1757–67. doi: 10.1158/1078-0432.CCR-13-2332
5. Kumar S, Lindsay D, Chen QB, Garrett AL, Tan XM, Anders CK, et al. Tracking plasma DNA mutation dynamics in estrogen receptor positive metastatic breast cancer with dPCR-SEQ. *NPJ Breast Cancer.* (2018) 4:39. doi: 10.1038/s41523-018-0093-3
6. Chu D, Paoletti C, Gersch C, VanDenBerg DA, Zabransky DJ, Cochran RL, et al. ESR1 mutations in circulating plasma tumor DNA from metastatic breast cancer patients. *Clin Cancer Res.* (2016) 22:993–9. doi: 10.1158/1078-0432.CCR-15-0943
7. Schiavon G, Hrebien S, Garcia-Murillas I, Cutts RJ, Pearson A, Tarazona N, et al. Analysis of ESR1 mutation in circulating tumor DNA demonstrates evolution during therapy for metastatic breast cancer. *Sci Transl Med.* (2015) 7:313ra182. doi: 10.1126/scitranslmed.aac7551
8. Reinert T, Coelho GP, Mandelli J, Zimermann E, Zaffaroni F, Bines J, et al. Association of ESR1 mutations and visceral metastasis in patients with estrogen receptor-positive advanced breast cancer from Brazil. *J Oncol.* (2019) 2019:1947215. doi: 10.1155/2019/1947215
9. Jeselsohn R, Buchwalter G, De Angelis C, Brown M, Schiff R. ESR1 mutations—a mechanism for acquired endocrine resistance in breast cancer. *Nat Rev Clin Oncol.* (2015) 12:573–83. doi: 10.1038/nrclinonc.2015.117
10. Ramalho S, Ramalh S, Gonçalves R, Barrios CH, Graudenz MS, Bines J. Multidisciplinary approach to neoadjuvant endocrine therapy in breast cancer: a comprehensive review. *Rev Bras Ginecol Obstet.* (2016) 38:615–22. doi: 10.1055/s-0036-1597579
11. Reinert T, Gonçalves R, Ellis MJ. Current status of neoadjuvant endocrine therapy in early stage breast cancer. *Curr Treat Options Oncol.* (2018) 19:23. doi: 10.1007/s11864-018-0538-9
12. Ellis MJ, Suman VJ, Hoog J, Goncalves R, Sanati S, Creighton CJ, et al. Ki67 proliferation index as a tool for chemotherapy decisions during and after neoadjuvant aromatase inhibitor treatment of breast cancer: results from the American college of surgeons oncology group Z1031 trial (alliance). *J Clin Oncol.* (2017) 35:1061–9. doi: 10.1200/JCO.2016.69.4406
13. Amoroso V, Generali D, Buchholz T, Cristofanilli M, Pedersini R, Curigliano G, et al. International expert consensus on primary systemic therapy in the management of early breast cancer: highlights of the fifth symposium on primary systemic therapy in the management of operable breast cancer, cremona, Italy (2013). *J Natl Cancer Inst Monogr.* (2015) 2015: 90–6. doi: 10.1093/jncimonographs/lgv023
14. Tryfonidis K, Zardavas D, Katzenellenbogen BS, Piccart M. Endocrine treatment in breast cancer: cure, resistance and beyond. *Cancer Treat Rev.* (2016) 50:68–81. doi: 10.1016/j.ctrv.2016.08.008
15. Reinert T, Saad ED, Barrios CH, Bines J. Clinical implications of ESR1 mutations in hormone receptor-positive advanced breast cancer. *Front Oncol.* (2017) 7:26. doi: 10.3389/fonc.2017.00026
16. Schiff R, Massarweh S, Shou J, Osborne CK. Breast cancer endocrine resistance: how growth factor signaling and estrogen receptor coregulators modulate response. *Clin Cancer Res.* (2003) 9(1 Pt 2):447S–54S. doi: 10.1158/1078-0432.ccr-031212
17. Fanning SW, Mayne CG, Dharmarajan V, Carlos KE, Martin TA, Novick SJ, et al. Estrogen receptor alpha somatic mutations Y537S and D538G confer breast cancer endocrine resistance by stabilizing the activating function-2 binding conformation. *Breast Cancer Treat.* (2017) 9: 462–8. doi: 10.7554/eLife.12792
18. Li S, Shen D, Shao J, Crowder R, Liu W, Prat A, et al. Endocrine-therapy-resistant ESR1 variants revealed by genomic characterization of breast-cancer-derived xenografts. *Cell Rep.* (2013) 4:1116–30. doi: 10.1016/j.celrep.2013.08.022
19. Holst F. Estrogen receptor alpha gene amplification in breast cancer: 25 years of debate. *World J Clin Oncol.* (2016) 7:160–73. doi: 10.5306/wjco.v7.i2.160
20. Jeselsohn R, De Angelis C, Brown M, Schiff R. The evolving role of the estrogen receptor mutations in endocrine therapy-resistant breast cancer. *Curr Oncol Rep.* (2017) 19:35. doi: 10.1007/s11912-017-0591-8
21. Spoerke JM, Gendreau S, Walter K, Qiu J, Wilson TR, Savage H, et al. Heterogeneity and clinical significance of ESR1 mutations in ER-positive metastatic breast cancer patients receiving

fulvestrant. *Nat Commun.* (2016) 7:11579. doi: 10.1038/ncomms11579

22. Weir HM, Bradbury RH, Lawson M, Rabow AA, Buttar D, Callis RJ, et al. AZD9496: an oral estrogen receptor inhibitor that blocks the growth of ER-positive and ESR1-mutant breast tumors in preclinical models. *Cancer Res.* (2016) 76:3307–18. doi: 10.1158/0008-5472.CAN-15-2357
23. Fanning SW, Jeselsohn R, Dharmarajan V, Mayne CG, Karimi M, Buchwalter G, et al. The SERM/SERD bazedoxifene disrupts ESR1 helix 12 to overcome acquired hormone resistance in breast cancer cells. *Elife.* (2018) 7:e37161. doi: 10.7554/eLife.37161
24. Bertucci, F, Ng CKY, Patsouris A, Droin N, Piscuoglio S, Carbuccia A, et al. Genomic characterization of metastatic breast cancer. *Nature.* (2019) 569:560–4. doi: 10.1038/s41586-019-1056-z
25. Ellis MJ, Tao Y, Luo J, A'Hern R, Evans DB, Bhatnagar AS, et al. Outcome prediction for estrogen receptor-positive breast cancer based on postneoadjuvant endocrine therapy tumor characteristics. *J Natl Cancer Inst.* (2008) 100:1380–8. doi: 10.1093/jnci/djn309
26. Haricharan S, Ellis MJ. Defects in mismatch repair: the achilles heel of estrogen receptor positive breast cancer with intrinsic endocrine therapy resistance? *Oncoscience.* (2017) 4:77–8. doi: 10.18632/oncoscience.363
27. Formisano L, Lu Y, Servetto A, Hanker AB, Jansen VM, Bauer JA, et al. Aberrant FGFR signaling mediates resistance to CDK4/6 inhibitors in ER+ breast cancer. *Nat Commun.* (2019) 10:1373. doi: 10.1038/s41467-019-09068-2
28. Shaw JA, Guttery DS, Hills A, Fernandez-Garcia D, Page K, Rosales BM, et al. Mutation analysis of cell-free DNA and single circulating tumor cells in metastatic breast cancer patients with high circulating tumor cell counts. *Clin Cancer Res.* (2017) 23:88–96. doi: 10.1158/1078-0432.CCR-16-0825
29. Jeselsohn R. Are we ready to use ESR1 mutations in clinical practice? *Breast Care.* (2017) 12:309–13. doi: 10.1159/000481428
30. Wang T, Liu JH, Zhang J, Wang L, Chen C, Dai PG, et al. A multiplex allele-specific real-time PCR assay for screening of ESR1 mutations in metastatic breast cancer. *Exp Mol Pathol.* (2015) 98:152–7. doi: 10.1016/j.yexmp.2015.03.004
31. Cieslik M, Chinnaiyan AM. Cancer transcriptome profiling at the juncture of clinical translation. *Nat Rev Genet.* (2018) 19:93–109. doi: 10.1038/nrg.2017.96

12

Gut melatonin in vertebrates: Chronobiology and physiology

*Sourav Mukherjee and Saumen Kumar Maitra**

Department of Zoology, Visva-Bharati University, Santiniketan, India

Edited by:
Hubert Vaudry,
University of Rouen, France

Reviewed by:
Etienne Challet,
Centre National de la Recherche Scientifique, France
Fabrice Morin,
University of Rouen, France

***Correspondence:**
Saumen Kumar Maitra,
Department of Zoology,
Visva-Bharati University,
Santiniketan – 731235, India
dgp_skmaitra@yahoo.co.in

Melatonin, following discovery in the bovine pineal gland, has been detected in several extra-pineal sources including gastrointestinal tract or gut. Arylalkylamine *N*-acetyltransferase (AANAT) is the key regulator of its biosynthesis. Melatonin in pineal is rhythmically produced with a nocturnal peak in synchronization with environmental light–dark cycle. A recent study on carp reported first that melatonin levels and intensity of a ~23 kDa AANAT protein in each gut segment also exhibit significant daily variations but, unlike pineal, show a peak at midday in all seasons. Extensive experimental studies ruled out direct role of light–dark conditions in determining temporal pattern of gut melatoninergic system in carp, and opened up possible role of environmental non-photic cue(s) as its synchronizer. Based on mammalian findings, physiological significance of gut-derived melatonin also appears unique because its actions at local levels sharing paracrine and/or autocrine functions have been emphasized. The purpose of this mini review is to summarize the existing data on the chronobiology and physiology of gut melatonin and to emphasize their relation with the same hormone derived in the pineal in vertebrates including fish.

Keywords: gut melatonin, AANAT, chronobiology, physiology

Introduction

Extensive research carried out in past 50 years have clearly depicted melatonin (5-methoxy-*N*-acetyltryptamine) as a potent chronobiotic molecule involved in the regulation of a variety of physiological functions (1). Following discovery in the bovine pineal gland (2), melatonin is detected in several non-pineal tissues/organs, such as retina, Harderian gland, and gastrointestinal tract (GIT) or gut. However, existing knowledge on melatonin has stemmed largely from the studies on pineal that too in mammals, leaving non-pineal tissues, especially in lower vertebrates, as an interesting topic of research. Though functional characterization of melatonin in gut, relative to that in retina and Harderian gland, has received serious attention, the studies are limited mostly to the mammals, especially rodents and pigs. Moreover, current knowledge on the cellular localization, distribution, and temporal pattern of gut melatonin is scarce and inconsistent as well. Thus, a brief review of the existing literature on gut melatonin appears meaningful for understanding its unique features in vertebrates.

Cellular Localization and Distribution

Localization of melatonin in the enterochromaffin cells (EC) of digestive mucosa of rat was followed by its quantitative estimation in gut tissues. At the sub-cellular level, strongest binding was noted in nuclear fraction, followed by microsomal, mitochondrial, and cytosolic fractions (3).

In mammals, melatonin-producing cells were found in submucosa and muscularis layer of esophagus, the glandular portion of the gastric wall and in the area of Lieberkühn's crypts and Brunner's glands of duodenum, and more specifically in EC of mucosal layer (3). As in birds and mammals, maximum immunoreactivity was noted at the outer margin of lamina propria in mucosal layer of intestinal villi in carp gut (4).

Generally, melatonin concentrations in gut tissues surpass the levels of melatonin in circulation by 10–100 times (3). Daytime levels of gut melatonin were measured in several species (5) of fish, e.g., sturgeon, rainbow trout, and carp (stomach ~102 pg/g, proximal gut or PG ~146 pg/g, and distal gut or DG ~141 pg/g); amphibians, e.g., axolotl (stomach and PG ~44 pg/g and DG ~92 pg/g), and bullfrog (esophagus ~73 pg/g, stomach ~78 pg/g, PG ~20 pg/g, and DG ~152 pg/g); and reptiles, e.g., red-sided garter snake (stomach ~1018 pg/g, PG ~328 pg/g, and DG ~511 pg/g). The midday values of melatonin in the anterior (~550 pg/g), middle (~538 pg/g), and posterior (~578 pg/g) segments of gut in a day-active carp (6) did not indicate any regional variations in its distribution in the same animal, but depicted species-specific variations in a particular gut segment (5). However, it remains obscure whether gut melatonin levels vary between the day-active and night-active animals.

Biosynthesis of Melatonin

The synthesis of melatonin in all the melatonin-synthesizing cells is a four-step phenomenon. First, the precursor L-tryptophan is taken up from the circulation (blood) and is converted to 5-hydroxy-tryptophan (5-HTP) in the mitochondria by Trp-5-mono-oxygenase/hydroxylase and is then decarboxylated in the cytosol by L-aromatic amino acid decarboxylase to form serotonin (5-hydroxytryptamine, 5-HT), that in turn is acetylated (*N*-acetylation) into *N*-acetyl serotonin by arylalkylamine-*N*-acetyltransferase (AANAT) (7), which is considered as the rate-limiting enzyme in melatonin biosynthetic pathway. Finally, *N*-acetyl serotonin is O-methylated by hydroxyindole-O-methyltransferase (HIOMT) to form melatonin (8).

Endogenous melatonin biosynthesis within the ECs of the digestive mucosa has been evident from the studies on the expression of genes for two key melatonin-synthesizing enzymes. The study of gut tissues detected mRNA expression of *Aanat* in rat (9) and *Hiomt* in quail (10) as well as goldfish (11). *Aanat*-2 expression, as noted in the gut of goldfish (11) and rainbow trout (12), was supported by densitometric analysis of AANAT protein in the carp gut (6). The study detected a ~23 kDa AANAT protein corresponding to AANAT in the pineal of pike, trout, and carp (13) in gut tissue homogenates and thereby ensured endogenous synthesis of melatonin in gut.

Chronobiology

Temporal Pattern of Gut Melatonin

Circulating profiles of melatonin in different vertebrates (14), including carp (15), exhibit precise diurnal rhythms with a peak during the dark phase and nadir during the photo phase and such rhythms are primarily generated by pineal AANAT (7). Until recently, comparable data on the temporal pattern of gut melatonin and its regulatory mechanisms were unknown for any vertebrates. A study on mice reported lower melatonin level during the day relative to nocturnal values only in the duodenum–jejunum segment of the GIT (16). In goldfish, though titers of melatonin were not measured, analysis of *Aanat*-2 mRNA expression revealed a daily rhythm in hindgut, but not in foregut (11). Importantly, the daily peak in the *Aanat*-2 mRNA expression persisted under continuous light as well as continuous darkness (11). Conversely, the study on carp by showing parallel changes in the levels of melatonin and AANAT density for the first time demonstrated that melatonin-synthesizing system in each gut segment, irrespective of seasons, undergoes significant daily variations with a peak at midday (6). Such findings also opened up a possibility that regulatory mechanism of melatonin synthesis in gut and pineal in the same animal species (**Figure 1**) is different (13).

Influence of Photoperiods on Rhythmicity in Gut Melatonin

The duration of light and thereby duration of darkness in a 24-h cycle is known to play a key role in the regulation of melatonin synthesis in the pineal (14). It is noteworthy that in fish, including carp (13), light acts directly on the pineal gland. By contrast, in mammals, light is detected by the retina and affects the pineal gland indirectly with a multisynaptic pathway (14). However, the question whether lighting conditions play a critical role of a synchronizer or regulator of gut melatonin was not duly addressed. Thus, a study was undertaken with carp (17), which due to its natural surface dwelling habit maintains close contact with environmental light and thereby is considered as an ideal model for the study of photo-response mechanisms in any melatonin-synthesizing tissue. Accordingly, the carp were held either under altered long (LP) or short photoperiods (SP) in a 24-h cycle, or under continuous light (LL) or darkness (DD) for equal duration. The results of the study indicated that none of the employed photo-regimens has any significant effect *per se* on the daily profiles of gut melatonin levels and AANAT protein density (17). Notably, an earlier study on the same carp demonstrated that diurnal rhythmicity in serum melatonin and pineal AANAT with a nocturnal peak (13) was lost when fish were held under LL or DD. Taken together, it is suggested that melatonin synthesis in gut, unlike pineal, is not a dark-dependent phenomenon, and environmental lighting conditions may not serve the role of external cue(s) in determining its rhythmic features in a daily cycle.

Influences of Food on Rhythmicity in Gut Melatonin

One of the periodic variables in the gut is the availability of food, which may serve as an important cue to determine daily periodicity of melatonin synthesis in gut (18). Notably, the study on the distribution of melatonin in different parts of the GIT in cow (poly-gastric) and pig (mono-gastric) revealed that cows had higher melatonin levels in stomach and ileum, but lower in cecum and colon (19). Accordingly, a relation between melatonin secretion and the digestive functions is sought. Depending on the meal frequency and timing of meals, several circulating metabolites and hormones undergo daily variations (20), and these variations

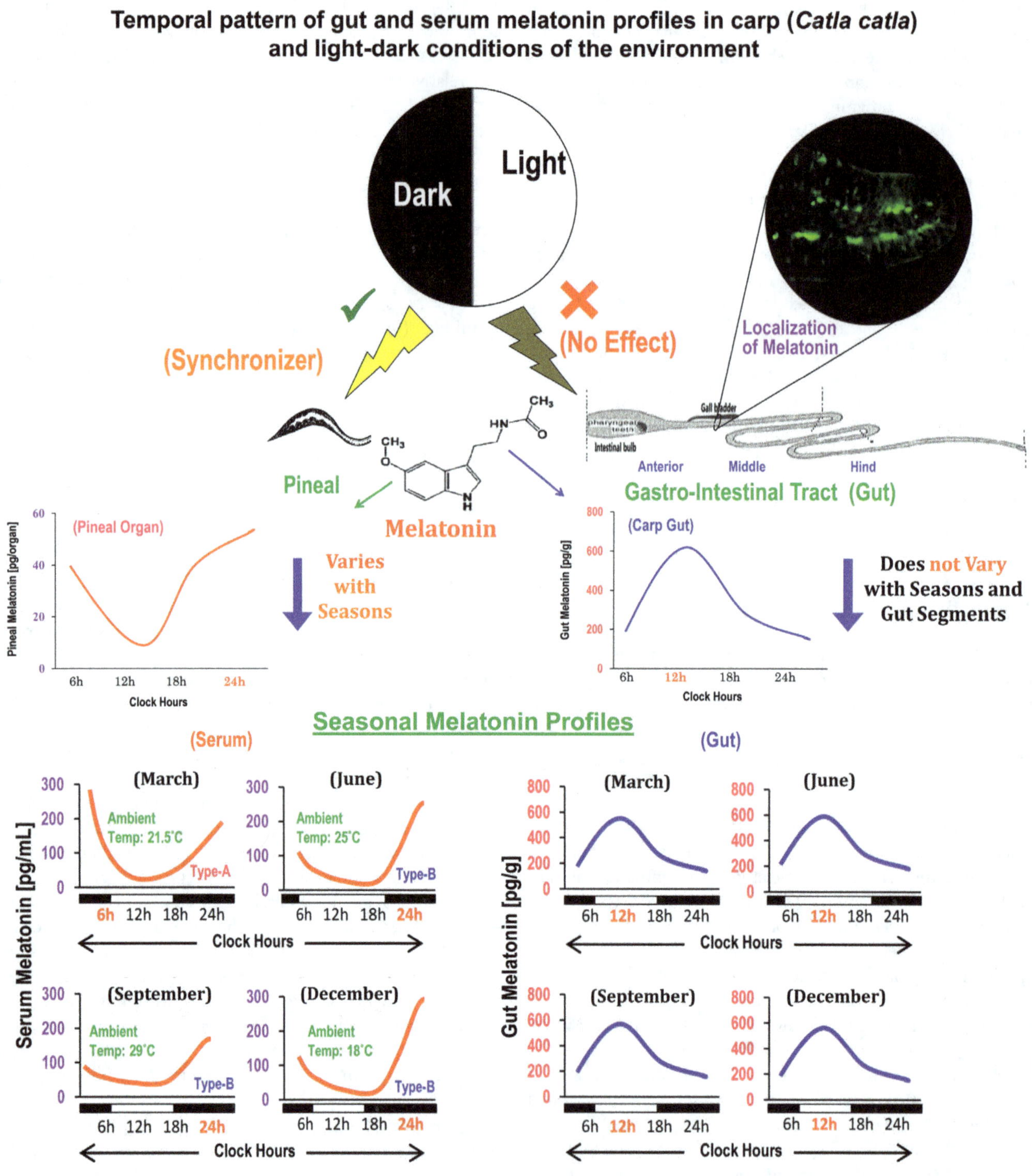

FIGURE 1 | Schematic presentation of the summary of existing information on the localization, distribution, and temporal organization of melatonin concentrations in different anatomical segments of gut in relation to the diurnal and seasonal profiles of serum melatonin in carp *Catla catla* and light–dark cycle in the environment.

are dependent on whether the animal is fed, fasted, or starved. Because timing of food intake is roughly opposite in phase between diurnal and nocturnal species, it is likely that synthesis of gut melatonin is correlated with feeding in various animals including fish species. However, any data from appropriate experimental studies that could support the hypothesis on a direct role of food availability and its timings on gut melatoninergic system in any animal species still remain unknown.

Physiology of Gut Melatonin

Melatonin is a lipophilic compound diffusing rapidly through biological membranes and actions in an endocrine and/or, paracrine and/or, autocrine manners. It is involved in the regulation of multiple functions, including the control of gastrointestinal system. Melatonin produced by EC may perform paracrine functions, while its action in the intestinal muscles may be either direct or it may act via the myenteric nervous system (3, 19).

A study on rainbow trout demonstrated that melatonin is released from gastrointestinal tissue and addition of L-tryptophan to the incubation medium stimulates melatonin synthesis and release (21). The presence of melatonin in intestinal villi indicated that melatonin might be involved in the transmembrane transport of electrolytes and ions. Moreover, melatonin increased water content in feces (22) and the topical application of melatonin stimulated short-circuit current in colonic cells (23). Experimental studies confirmed that melatonin also inhibited the contraction of smooth muscles in stomach, ileum, and colon (24). In rats, endogenous melatonin affected the electro-myogram of pre- and post-prandial motility, though such actions were observed only at night (25), when the concentration of melatonin in blood remained usually high. Perhaps, melatonin relaxes gastrointestinal muscles by specifically blocking nicotinic channels (26).

The assumption that melatonin may also interact with dopamine-sensitive, possibly Ca^{2+}-activated, K^+ channels (27) earned support from the study, in which inhibition of small-conductance K^+ channels attenuated melatonin-induced relaxation of gastric muscles (28). In addition to its relaxation effect presented in several *in vitro* studies, melatonin appeared to inhibit serotonin (5-HT) action also *in vivo*. Serotonin facilitated the "food transit time" (FTT) (the moment of food intake to the appearance of the first feces stained with food coloring), as compared to controls, whereas injection of melatonin to serotonin implanted mice significantly increased the FTT (19). In a similar study, small doses of melatonin relaxed the gut muscles and facilitated intestinal motility in rats (19). Further studies argued that a counterbalancing system exists between serotonin and melatonin which within the GIT melatonin functions as a physiological antagonist of serotonin (22). High dose of melatonin inhibited the spontaneous or serotonin-induced contraction of GIT muscles and induced intestinal elongation. Conversely, low doses of melatonin stimulated intestinal contraction, resulting in the shortening of gut (3).

Several mammalian studies indicated that melatonin may have a protective role against development of gastric ulcers (29, 30). It is proposed that the prevention of stress- or ethanol-induced gastric lesions in rats is probably due to the anti-serotoninergic effect of melatonin (29). The incidence and severity of spontaneously induced gastric ulcers are significantly reduced in pigs, which were fed with 5 mg melatonin/kg enriched food. The highest incidence of ulcers is observed in pigs with the lowest level of melatonin in their plasma and stomach tissues (30). Protection against stress-induced lesions might be due to a strong antioxidant action of melatonin and the restoration of microcirculation (31).

In addition to its antioxidant effect, melatonin action in the prevention or treatment of colitis (32) includes the stimulation of the immune system. Though direct evidence is lacking, indications are available to show that melatonin administration to rats significantly increased the number and size of Peyer's patches, the major immune tissue of the GIT (33). Melatonin treatment may improve irritable bowel symptoms (IBS) as well (34). Thus, over the decades, melatonin has been promoted as a "magic cure" for the treatment or prevention of several physiological disorders ranging from aging to aggression, depression to hypertension, suppressed immunity to oxidative stress, insomnia to jet lag (1). However, convincing data are yet to be known to prove that such actions are also ascribed to gut-derived melatonin.

Conclusion

The information gathered so far provides indications that environmental and neuroendocrine regulatory mechanisms of melatonin synthesis in the pineal and in the gut are different. Likewise, functional characteristics of pineal-derived and GIT-derived melatonin may not be identical, as the nature of release and function of this extra-pineal melatonin are not yet fully understood. There are reasons to argue that pineal melatonin mostly acts as an endocrine agent, whereas GIT melatonin performs not only endocrine functions but also in autocrine and paracrine manners (18). However, emergence of a general idea on the physiological significance of gut melatonin has suffered a major setback due to lack of data from studies on any non-mammalian species and thereby warrants further carefully controlled research under diverse experimental conditions using animals representing different groups of vertebrates.

Acknowledgments

Financial assistance from the Council of Scientific and Industrial Research [37(1390)/09/EMR-II] and the Department of Biotechnology (BT/PR11423/AAQ/03/421/2008), Govt. of India, New Delhi to SKM, and a Research Associateship (A/F/4S/2786/2015) by the Department of Biotechnology, and an international travel grant from the Department of Science and Technology (SB/ITS/02594/2014-15), Govt. of India to SM, are thankfully acknowledged. The authors are grateful to the editor and two reviewers for their critique and invaluable comments on the previous version of the manuscript.

References

1. Chowdhury I, Maitra SK. Chapter 1: melatonin in the promotion of health. In: Watson RR, editor. *Melatonin Time Line: From Discovery to Therapy*. Boca Raton, FL: Taylor and Francis (2012). p. 1–60.
2. Lerner AB, Case JD, Takahashi Y, Lee TH, Mori N. Isolation of melatonin, pineal factor that lightens melanocytes. *J Am Chem Soc* (1958) **80**:2587. doi:10.1021/ja01543a060
3. Bubenik GA. Gastrointestinal melatonin localization, function, and clinical relevance. *Dig Dis Sci* (2002) **47**:2336–48. doi:10.1023/A:1020107915919

4. Mukherjee S. *Gut Melatonin in Carp Catla catla: Distribution, Daily Profiles in Relation to Photoperiods, Food and Feeding Schedule*. Ph.D. thesis, Visva-Bharati, Santiniketan, India (2014).
5. Bubenik GA, Pang SF. Melatonin level in the gastrointestinal tissue of fish, amphibians, and a reptile. *Gen Comp Endocrinol* (1997) **106**:415–9. doi:10.1006/gcen.1997.6889
6. Mukherjee S, Moniruzzaman M, Maitra SK. Daily and seasonal profiles of gut melatonin and their temporal relationship with pineal and serum melatonin in carp *Catla catla* under natural photo-thermal conditions. *Biol Rhythm Res* (2014) **45**:301–15. doi:10.1080/09291016.2013.817139
7. Voisin P, Namboodiri MAA, Klein DC. Arylamine N-acetyltransferase and arylalkylamine *N*-acetyltransferase in the mammalian pineal gland. *J Biol Chem* (1984) **259**:10913–8.
8. Axelrod J, Weissbach H. Enzymatic O-methylation of N-acetylserotonin to melatonin. *Science* (1960) **131**:1312. doi:10.1126/science.131.3409.1312
9. Stefulj J, Hörtner M, Ghosh M, Schauenstein K, Rinner I, Wölfler A, et al. Gene expression of the key enzymes of melatonin synthesis in extrapineal tissues of the rat. *J Pineal Res* (2001) **30**:243–7. doi:10.1034/j.1600-079X.2001.300408.x
10. Hong GX, Pang SF. N-Acetyltransferase activity in the quail (*Cotornix coturnix jap*) duodenum. *Comp Biochem Physiol* (1995) **112**:251–5. doi:10.1016/0305-0491(95)00083-6
11. Velarde E, Cerdá-Reverter JM, Alonso-Gómez AL, Sánchez E, Isorna E, Delgado MJ. Melatonin-synthesizing enzymes in pineal, retina, liver, and gut of the goldfish (*Carassius*): mRNA expression pattern and regulation of daily rhythms by lighting conditions. *Chronobiol Int* (2010) **27**:1178–201. doi:10.3109/07420528.2010.496911
12. Fernández-Durán B, Ruibal C, Polakof S, Ceinos RM, Soengas JL, Míguez JM. Evidence for arylalkylamine N-acetyltransferase (AANAT2) expression in rainbow trout peripheral tissues with emphasis in the gastrointestinal tract. *Gen Comp Endocrinol* (2007) **152**:289–94. doi:10.1016/j.ygcen.2006.12.008
13. Seth M, Maitra SK. Importance of light in temporal organization of photoreceptor proteins and melatonin-producing system in the pineal of carp *Catla catla*. *Chronobiol Int* (2010) **27**:463–86. doi:10.3109/07420521003666416
14. Falcón J, Migaud H, Muñoz-Cueto JA, Carrillo M. Current knowledge on the melatonin system in teleost fish. *Gen Comp Endocrinol* (2010) **165**:469–82. doi:10.1016/j.ygcen.2009.04.026
15. Maitra SK, Chattoraj A, Bhattacharyya S. Implication of melatonin in oocyte maturation in Indian major carp *Catla catla*. *Fish Physiol Biochem* (2005) **31**:201–7. doi:10.1007/s10695-006-0025-2
16. Bubenik GA, Niles LP, Pang SF, Pentney PJ. Diurnal variation and binding characteristics of melatonin in the mouse brain and gastrointestinal tissues. *Comp Biochem Physiol* (1993) **104**:221–4.
17. Mukherjee S, Moniruzzaman M, Maitra SK. Impact of artificial lighting conditions on the diurnal profiles of gut melatonin in a surface dwelling carp (*Catla catla*). *Biol Rhythm Res* (2014) **45**:831–48. doi:10.1080/09291016.2014.923618
18. Vera LM, De Pedro N, Gómez-Milán E, Delgado MJ, Sánchez-Muros MJ, Madrid JA, et al. Feeding entrainment of locomotor activity rhythms, digestive enzymes and neuroendocrine factors in goldfish. *Physiol Behav* (2007) **90**:518–24. doi:10.1016/j.physbeh.2006.10.017
19. Bubenik GA. Thirty four years since the discovery of gastrointestinal melatonin. *J Physiol Pharmacol* (2008) **59**:33–51.
20. Boujard T, Leatherland JF. Circadian rhythms and feeding time in fishes. *Environ Biol Fish* (1992) **35**:109–31. doi:10.1007/BF00002186
21. Lepage O, Larson ET, Mayer I, Winberg S. Tryptophan affects both gastrointestinal melatonin production and interrenal activity in stressed and nonstressed rainbow trout. *J Pineal Res* (2005) **38**:264–71. doi:10.1111/j.1600-079X.2004.00201.x
22. Bubenik GA, Pang SF. The role of serotonin and melatonin in the gastrointestinal physiology: ontogeny, regulation of food intake and mutual 5-HT, melatonin feedbacks. *J Pineal Res* (1994) **16**:91–9. doi:10.1111/j.1600-079X.1994.tb00088.x
23. Chan H, Lui K, Wong W, Poon A. Effect of melatonin on chloride secretion by human colonic T_{84} cells. *Life Sci* (1998) **23**:2151–8. doi:10.1016/S0024-3205(98)00190-8
24. Harlow HJ, Weekly BL. Effect of melatonin on the force of spontaneous contractions of *in vitro* rat small and large intestines. *J Pineal Res* (1986) **3**:277–84. doi:10.1111/j.1600-079X.1986.tb00750.x
25. Merle A, Delagrange PH, Renard P, Lesieur D, Cuber JC, Roche M, et al. Effect of melatonin on motility pattern of small intestine in rats and its inhibition by melatonin receptor antagonist S 221152. *J Pineal Res* (2000) **29**:116–24. doi:10.1034/j.1600-079X.2000.290208.x
26. Barajas-Lopez C, Peres AL, Espinosa-Luna R, Reyes-Vazquez C, Prieto-Gomez B. Melatonin modulates cholinergic transmission by blocking nicotinic channels in the guineapig submucous plexus. *Eur J Pharmacol* (1996) **312**:319–25. doi:10.1016/0014-2999(96)00481-5
27. Reyes-Vasquez C, Naranjo-Rodriguez EB, Garcia-Segoviano JA, Trujillo-Santana J, Prieto-Gomez B. Apamin blocks the direct relaxant effect of melatonin on rat ileal smooth muscles. *J Pineal Res* (1997) **22**:1–8. doi:10.1111/j.1600-079X.1997.tb00295.x
28. Storr M, Schudziarra V, Allescher H-D. Inhibition of small conductance K^+ channels attenuated melatonin-induced relaxation of serotonin-contracted rat gastric fundus. *Can J Physiol Pharmacol* (2000) **78**:799–806. doi:10.1139/y00-059
29. Cho CH, Pang SF, Chen BW, Pfeiffer CJ. Modulating action of melatonin on serotonin-induced aggravation of ethanol ulceration and changes of mucosal blood flow in rat stomach. *J Pineal Res* (1989) **6**:89–97. doi:10.1111/j.1600-079X.1989.tb00406.x
30. Bubenik GA, Ayles HL, Ball RO, Friendship RM, Brown GM. Relationship between melatonin levels in plasma and gastrointestinal tissues and the incidence and severity of gastric ulcers in pigs. *J Pineal Res* (1998) **24**:62–6. doi:10.1111/j.1600-079X.1998.tb00367.x
31. Konturek PC, Brzozowski T, Konturek SJ. Gut clock: implication of circadian rhythms in the gastrointestinal tract. *J Physiol Pharmacol* (2011) **62**:139–50.
32. Pentney P, Bubenik GA. Melatonin reduces the severity of dextran-induced colitis in mice. *J Pineal Res* (1995) **19**:31–9. doi:10.1111/j.1600-079X.1995.tb00168.x
33. Yanagisawa M, Kachi T. Effects of the pineal hormone on Payer's patches in the small intestine. *Acta Anat Nippon* (1994) **69**:522–7.
34. Elsenbruch S. Melatonin: a novel treatment for IBS? *Gut* (2005) **10**:1353–4. doi:10.1136/gut.2005.074377

13

A positive affective neuroendocrinology approach to reward and behavioral dysregulation

*Keith M. Welker[1], June Gruber[1] and Pranjal H. Mehta[2]**

[1] Department of Psychology and Neuroscience, University of Colorado Boulder, Boulder, CO, USA, [2] Department of Psychology, University of Oregon, Eugene, OR, USA

Edited by:
Miriam Melis,
University of Cagliari, Italy

Reviewed by:
Liangsuo Ma,
University of Texas Health Science Center at Houston, USA
Kesong Hu,
Cornell University, USA

***Correspondence:**
Pranjal H. Mehta,
Department of Psychology, 1227 University of Oregon, Eugene, OR 97403, USA
mehta@uoregon.edu

Emerging lines of research suggest that both testosterone and maladaptive reward processing can modulate behavioral dysregulation. Yet, to date, no integrative account has been provided that systematically explains neuroendocrine function, dysregulation of reward, and behavioral dysregulation in a unified perspective. This is particularly important given specific neuroendocrine systems are potential mechanisms underlying and giving rise to reward-relevant behaviors. In this review, we propose a forward-thinking approach to study the mechanisms of reward and behavioral dysregulation from a positive affective neuroendocrinology (PANE) perspective. This approach holds that testosterone increases reward processing and motivation, which increase the likelihood of behavioral dysregulation. Additionally, the PANE framework holds that reward processing mediates the effects of testosterone on behavioral dysregulation. We also explore sources of potential sex differences and the roles of age, cortisol, and individual differences within the PANE framework. Finally, we discuss future prospects for research questions and methodology in the emerging field of affective neuroendocrinology.

Keywords: testosterone, cortisol, emotion, affect, reward, self-regulation, sex differences

Introduction

In recent decades, separate lines of research have investigated the psychological, neural, and neuroendocrine mechanisms of behavioral dysregulation, defined here as appetitive, risky behaviors, such as sexual risk-taking (e.g., unprotected sex), dangerous driving, risky financial decision making, and substance use. Two bodies of research of relevance have independently examined the hormonal mechanisms of behavioral dysregulation. One perspective investigates the hormonal predictors and mechanisms (particularly testosterone), while another has focused on reward dysregulation, defined by researchers as the pursuit of pleasurable feelings and stimuli and heightened responsiveness to positive, reward-related stimuli [e.g., Ref. (1–3)]. As we argue, these systems share overlapping psychological and physiological mechanisms, yet have not been simultaneously deployed to understand behavioral dysregulation. Thus, there is a need to integrate these disparate lines of work into a common theoretical framework. This framework should not only be consistent with extant findings but also make novel predictions to be tested in future research.

In this paper, we propose a forward-thinking approach to study reward motivation and behavioral dysregulation, referred to as the positive affective neuroendocrinology (PANE) approach. The PANE approach incorporates existing research in the hormonal mechanisms of behavioral dysregulation with research on reward dysregulation and related positive affectivity. This approach suggests that reward dysregulation underlies the established links between testosterone and behavioral dysregulation. The PANE approach also holds that testosterone increases reward processing – or neural activity in the reward-relevant regions of the brain – and reward motivation, which in turn increase the likelihood of behavioral dysregulation. More specifically, this framework posits that increases in reward mediate the effects of testosterone on behavioral dysregulation. In this paper, we provide a focused review of the roles of testosterone in modulating behavioral dysregulation and then discuss how reward dysregulation represents a crucial mechanism in this relationship. We also explore the potential sources of sex differences and the effects of age, cortisol, and individual differences within a PANE perspective. Finally, we close with a discussion of future research prospects in the emerging field of affective neuroendocrinology.

Evidence for PANE

What is the evidence for the PANE framework of reward and behavioral dysregulation? In the following sections, we discuss the evidence from three areas for why the association between testosterone and behavioral dysregulation may be mediated by elevated reward dysregulation: (1) evidence showing that testosterone is a predictor and mechanism of behavioral dysregulation, (2) evidence for how reward dysregulation is a critical mechanism of behavioral dysregulation, and (3) evidence that testosterone increases reward dysregulation.

Testosterone and Behavioral Dysregulation

Testosterone, a steroid hormone and end-product of the hypothalamic–pituitary–gonadal (HPG) axis, is of prime relevance to behavioral dysregulation. In men, testosterone is primarily produced in the testes, while women's testosterone is produced in smaller quantities by the ovaries and adrenal cortex (4). Testosterone also has a diurnal cycle, where testosterone is highest upon waking and decreases across the day, flattening in the afternoon (5). Researchers often distinguish between organizational effects of testosterone – the "permanent modification of brain structure and function during prenatal and early postnatal life due to exposure to testosterone" [Ref. (6), p. 15268] – and activational effects of testosterone – temporary, non-developmental moment-to-moment effects of testosterone that modulate affect, cognition, and behavior upon administration or release of testosterone.

Research on the dysregulatory behavioral effects and correlates of testosterone confirms both stable and dynamic, contextual psychological effects of the HPG axis. Studying the stable, trait-like elements of testosterone involves inferring stable levels of testosterone from either multiple samples at the same time of day [e.g., Ref. (7)], or taking a sample at one time of the day for all participants, after a period of neutral activity (8). Support for this approach comes from reports that testosterone concentrations are relatively stable when measured at the same time of day (9). Thus, baseline testosterone can be considered a trait-like index of testosterone. Large-scale studies have linked baseline testosterone to several dysregulatory behaviors in army veterans, such as substance use, previous juvenile delinquency, and law breaking [e.g., Ref. (10)]. Baseline testosterone is also positively associated with risky financial decision making and preferences [see Ref. (11), for a review; e.g., Ref. (12, 13)].

Collectively, there is a weak positive association between stable, trait-like testosterone concentrations and risk-taking, with some inconsistent findings. For instance, Stanton et al. (14) report a non-linear relationship between testosterone and risk-taking, suggesting that risk-taking is elevated in low and high testosterone individuals, but not those with middle-range testosterone concentrations. Additionally, Sapienza et al. (6) report a positive association between testosterone and risk-taking in women, but not men. Furthermore, Schipper (15) found a negative association between testosterone and risk-aversion for gains, but not losses, in men.

The lack of strong effects of baseline testosterone on risk-taking in humans may be due to the potential for testosterone concentrations to alter in response to social events. Although baseline testosterone may predict how individuals generally respond and act across a wide variety of contexts and self-reported psychological traits, a more fine-tuned assessment of testosterone may be needed for assessing situation-specific behaviors. For example, previous work has examined the behavioral effects of testosterone responses to competitions (16–19), opposite sex interactions (20), men's interactions with women (21, 22), social exclusion (23), holding dominant vs. submissive postures (24), and aggressive provocation (25). These dynamic effects of testosterone are theorized to be more robustly associated with context-specific social behaviors than baseline testosterone (26), and this notion is supported by several emerging studies [e.g., Ref. (16, 27, 28)] showing robust effects of testosterone changes predicting aggressive behavior in social contexts. This work is also bolstered by a recent study showing that acute changes in testosterone in response to monetary wins and losses also are associated with increased financial risk-taking in men (29). Collectively, these studies suggest that both baseline and dynamic changes in testosterone are positively related to a range of dysregulatory behaviors, particularly risk-taking.

Reward-Seeking and Behavioral Dysregulation

Theories of behavioral dysregulation (e.g., risk-taking) have distinguished between appetitive, approach-oriented, reward motivations based on achieving satisfaction and avoidance motivations based on reducing or avoiding negative consequences, such as pain, punishment, or losses [e.g., Ref. (30–32)]. Affective and motivational accounts of risk-taking specify reward dysregulation as a critical component [e.g., Ref. (33)]. Additionally, elevations in reward-seeking facilitate the heightened risk-taking behaviors associated with adolescence [see Ref. (34), for review] and underlie a host of dysregulatory behaviors, such as addictive gambling (35), substance abuse (36), traffic violations (37), and childhood obesity (38). In this work, both the elevated experience of positive emotions and the experience of excessive reward motivation are critical components to behavioral dysregulation.

The deleterious effects of reward motivation and excessive positive emotion also emerge in clinical disorders. Disorders associated with risk-taking behavior, such as bipolar disorder (BD), are characterized by elevated and abnormally persistent positive emotions (39), excessive reward pursuit and deficits in reward-related learning [e.g., Ref. (40)], and deficits in positive emotion regulation [e.g., Ref. (41–43)]. BD is often characterized by elevated risk-taking behaviors and impulsivity (44, 45), such as substance use (46), impulsive gambling behavior (47), aggressive behavior (48), and harmful substance use (46). Broadly, deficits in the behavioral approach system (BAS) are thought to characterize BD and elevated behavioral dysregulation (49).

The effects of positive emotion regulation and elevated, persistent positive affect on behavioral dysregulation are becoming increasingly known. When experiencing urgent positive emotions, people are more likely to engage in a variety of dysregulatory behaviors, such as substance use and risky-sexual behavior (50, 51). Elevated reward processing and positive affect have a robust association with risk-taking (52). Additionally, dysregulatory behaviors such as substance use, binge eating, and risky-sexual behavior, are more likely to occur in the context of positive emotions (50, 51). Elevated reward processing and positive affect have a robust association with risk-taking (52). Additionally, elevated reward-sensitivity uniquely characterizes a subpopulation of drug addicts that are motivated toward drug addiction through the presence of potential for rewards (53, 54).

Research on clinical disorders has also provided insights into the fundamental affective mechanisms of behavioral dysregulation. This research suggests that reward dysregulation is a critical component of behavioral dysregulation. Affective accounts of risk-taking specify reward dysregulation as a critical component [e.g., Ref. (33)]. Clinical disorders associated with risk-taking behavior, such as BD, are characterized by elevated and abnormally persistent positive emotions (39), excessive reward pursuits and deficits in reward-related learning [e.g., Ref. (40)], and deficits in positive emotion regulation [e.g., Ref. (3, 41, 42)]. BD is often characterized by elevated risk-taking behaviors and impulsivity (44, 45), such as substance use (46), impulsive gambling behavior (47), aggressive behavior (48), and harmful substance use (46). In addition to excessive positive emotion, this heightened irritability may also potentiate behavioral dysregulation, such as impulsive aggression (55).

Reward-Related Neural Function and Behavioral Dysregulation

In addition to elevated positive affect and reward motivation, neural structures related to positive affect and reward also predict behavioral dysregulation. The reward system has been broadly thought to be the neural basis of the BAS, which operates via the mesolimbic dopaminergic network (56, 57). Connectivity between these dopaminergic regions is theorized to form the basis of the neural circuits of reward and appetitive behavior [see Ref. (58) for a review]. Broadly, this reward system of the brain utilizes several key dopamine-linked structures, such as the ventral tegmental area (VTA) and nucleus accumbens (NAcc), the latter of which is nested in the ventral striatum (59–61). Within these regions, the VTA has numerous dopaminergic pathways with output to the hippocampus, amygdala, medial pre-frontal cortex (PFC) ventral pallidum, and of prime relevance, the NAcc [Ref. (62), for a review]. For example, dopaminergic neuron activation in the VTA that stimulates the NAcc aids in reinforcing responses to food and drugs used in substance abuse [see Ref. (63), for a review], as well as reward cues (64). The NAcc also plays a critical role in affect and appetitive motivation, reaction to novel stimuli, reward-related learning, responses to delayed reward, controlling feeding, and hedonic taste preferences [e.g., Ref. (65–70)]. More broadly, dopamine release in the ventral striatum is associated with self-reported euphoria in humans [e.g., Ref. (71)] and is thought to be a critical modulator of reward anticipation in mammals (72).

Dysregulation in the dopaminergic system has attracted considerable attention in researching behavioral dysregulation and related psychiatric disorders [see Ref. (59, 73), for a review]. For instance, the dopaminergic reward system and dopamine receptor polymorphisms have been linked to the crucial rewarding effects of substance abuse and addiction (74) and pathological gambling [e.g., Ref. (75–77)]. The dopamine system and receptors also modulate increased risky-decision making in humans [e.g., Ref. (78, 79)] and impulsive behavior in rodents [e.g., Ref. (80)]. Furthermore, neural theories of self-regulation (81, 82) hold that self-control is a function of the balance of activation and connectivity between the mesolimbic dopaminergic regions and regions of the PFC – a putative mechanism of self-control, inhibiting craving, and emotional control (74, 83–85). As we will discuss, testosterone modulates activity in these regions (see **Figure 1**).

Testosterone and Reward

Our evidence for testosterone's role in reward-seeking comes from three areas of research: testosterone and reward-seeking behavior, testosterone and reward-related affect, and testosterone and the neural circuitry of reward.

Testosterone and Reward-Seeking Behavior and Traits

Without involving affective and neural processes, testosterone is associated with increased reward-focused traits, sensation seeking, and impulsive behaviors in humans and animals [e.g., Ref. (86–92)]. Additionally, previous work suggests that exogenous testosterone administration can shift sensitivity from punishment

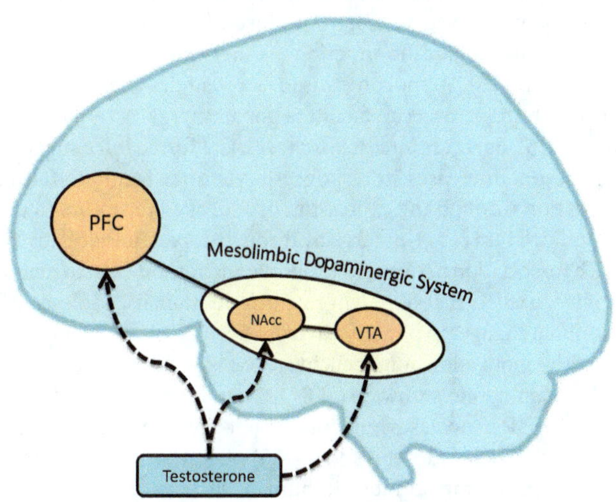

FIGURE 1 | Testosterone's effects on brain regions associated with reward dysregulation. PFC, prefrontal cortex; NAcc, nucleus accumbens; VTA, ventral tegmental area.

to reward dependency (93). Testosterone changes are also associated with increased monetary gains in stock traders (94). Broadly, this work suggests that testosterone increases motivation to seek rewards.

Testosterone and Reward-Related Affect

Testosterone may be related to reward-seeking behaviors, but is it associated with reward-related affect? Work using exogenously administered testosterone suggests that testosterone may shift focus away from withdrawal-related emotions to approach-related, reward-focused aggression (95, 96), and increase subjective and physiological measures of sexual-arousal (97). Testosterone may also be associated with approach-related positive affect. Indeed, testosterone increases are correlated with increased enjoyment of competition in decisive victories (98). Additionally, there is a well-established negative correlation between testosterone and depressive symptoms [see Ref. (99), for a review]. Previous work also suggests that exogenously administered testosterone can also decrease depression (100, 101) and increase manic symptoms (102). Furthermore, in women with BD, testosterone concentrations positively predict the number of manic episodes and suicide attempts (103).

Testosterone and Reward-Related Neural Function

Broadly, both testosterone's organizational and activational effects on the brain are associated with neural regions linked to increased dominance, reward, and approach behaviors [see Ref. (26, 104–106) for reviews; Ref. (107)]. Relevant to the current framework, an expansive literature suggests that testosterone is linked to reward-related neural function, both within animal and human literature. We summarize these associations in **Figure 1**. Animal research suggests testosterone modulates the dopaminergic system (108–110) and dopamine-linked sexual behaviors in rodents [e.g., Ref. (111, 112)], and has rewarding effects via the mesolimbic dopaminergic system [see Ref. (113), for a review]. For instance, rats show conditioned place preference for regions where they received testosterone injections, and this effect is mediated by dopamine function in the ventral striatum and NAcc (114, 115). Supporting this idea, research in hamsters also suggests testosterone can facilitate dopaminergic activity in the NAcc (116). Furthermore, research with California mice suggests testosterone increases in response to victories facilitate future aggression through the expression of androgen receptors in the ventral striatum (117), potentially through dopaminergic activity.

The association between testosterone and reward-related neural activity parallels that of rodent research. In humans, adolescents' hormonal changes in puberty have also been theorized to increase appetitive motivation by influencing reward-linked brain structures and dopaminergic pathways (118–122). In humans, testosterone administration increases functional connectivity in neural circuits linked with reduced depression (123). Additionally, exogenous testosterone administrations in humans increase ventral striatal responses to financial reward cues in adolescents and adults receiving monetary rewards (124, 125).

In summary, testosterone may increase reward motivation by acting directly on dopaminergic neural structures in the BAS. However, less work has focused on the effects of testosterone and the BAS beyond dopamine-dependent regions. Although some work suggests, for instance, that testosterone is associated with elevated dorsolateral pre-frontal cortex (DLPFC) activation during an anger control induction (126), other work has not revealed associations between testosterone and the DLPFC during aggressive interactions (127). Future research is needed to extend the specificity of the effects of testosterone beyond reward function to the BAS.

Reciprocal Associations Between Reward and Testosterone

Overall, the literature reviewed above suggests that testosterone can increase reward processing and dysregulation. However, there also may be a reciprocal effect of reward on testosterone increases. Reciprocal associations are consistent with existing neuroendocrine theories that posit hormones and behavior reciprocally affect each other through feedback loops [e.g., Ref. (128)]. Broadly, contexts that modulate testosterone responses, such as competitive outcomes and sexually attractive individuals, have rewarding properties. For instance, testosterone responses to competitive victories that facilitate aggressive and risk-taking behavior may occur because winning a competition is an enjoyable experience. Research supporting this possibility suggests a positive association between testosterone responses in winners of competitions and enjoyment of the competition (98). Additionally, the dynamic increases in testosterone following winning a competition and decreases following losing have been thought to facilitate changes in reward-dependent learning (129). However, to fully test this hypothesis, research experimentally manipulates reward in multiple contexts while measuring the effects on testosterone fluctuations is needed.

Critical Moderators

In the following section, we highlight potential critical moderators for within the PANE framework, including cortisol, sex, age, and individual differences linked to reward sensitivity and motivation.

Interactive Effects with Cortisol

Within the PANE framework, testosterone may interact with other hormones to predict behavioral dysregulation. Emerging work also suggests that cortisol – a glucocorticoid steroid hormone released as the end-product of the HPG axis – interacts with testosterone to modulate dysregulatory behavior [see Ref. (130), for a review]. From a neurobiological perspective, cortisol downregulates androgen receptors, inhibits HPG activity, and inhibits the effects of testosterone on specific tissues [e.g., Ref. (131–134)]. Additionally, the HPG and HPA axes are thought to have mutually inhibitory effects on each other (135). Therefore, it is possible that cortisol may also moderate the psychological and behavioral effects of testosterone. This notion is supported by psychological literature, finding that when cortisol levels are low, but not high, testosterone levels are positively associated with dominance (136), risk-taking (137), perceived status (138), violent crime (139, 140), and externalizing psychopathology in adolescents (141), although others did not find similar associations (10, 142). Recent research also suggests that acute testosterone changes are positively related to earnings in bargaining contexts when cortisol levels decrease, but not increase (143). In summary, not only do cortisol and testosterone have independent effects on costly behavioral dysregulation but these hormones may also co-regulate risk-taking behavior and impulsive traits. Future research is needed to further investigate the extent to which testosterone and cortisol jointly influence self-control related behaviors (144).

Sex Differences in the Psychoneuroendocrinology of Behavioral Dysregulation

A large literature suggests men are more impulsive, punishment insensitive, and sensation seeking than women [see Ref. (145), for a meta-analysis; Ref. (146)], and are on average, more risk-taking (147), although the effect sizes are small (148). Men also typically die earlier than women (149, 150), are more likely to die from violent deaths (151), are more aggressive [e.g., Ref. (152–155)], and are more likely to abuse alcohol (156). Additionally, relative to women, men have more psychopathological traits and disorders linked increased impulsivity (39, 157–160).

Sex differences in testosterone are thought to account for sex differences in risk-taking (6). Work by Sapienza and colleagues indicates that both the organizational functions of testosterone in prenatal development – indexed by the ratio of the second to fourth finger digits (161, 162) – and circulating levels of testosterone account for sex differences in risky-decision making. On the level of prenatal exposure to testosterone, previous work has found physiological indicators of prenatal testosterone exposure can alter children's social and empathic abilities (163). Although numerous cultural and social factors explain gender differences in behavioral dysregulation, both organizational and activational effects of testosterone likely explain a portion of this variability. It is important, however, not to rule out social and cultural factors facilitating differences in behavioral dysregulation between men and women. Gender roles often guide behavior through social pressures and conformity [see Ref. (164, 165), for reviews]. To explain sex differences in dysregulatory impulsivity and risk-taking, it is necessary to account for not only both the nature and nurture, but the interaction between the two (164–166).

The effects of dynamic changes in testosterone on behavior may be specific to men. For example, Carré et al. (16) find that testosterone reactivity mediates the effect of competitive outcomes on aggressive behavior specifically in men but not women. Although several studies investigating the effects of testosterone reactivity on dysregulatory behaviors have primarily focused on samples of men [e.g., Ref. (23, 28)], future research is needed to establish whether the dynamic effects of testosterone on dysregulatory behavior are sex-specific. This work does not imply, however, that testosterone cannot have behavioral and psychological effects in women. Several testosterone administration studies, for example, have produced behavioral and psychological effects of testosterone in samples of exclusively women [e.g., Ref. (167–170)]. Additionally, previous work has identified interactive effects of testosterone and cortisol in samples of both men and women (136, 137).

Several factors may additionally explain smaller psychological and behavioral effects of testosterone in women. First, animal research suggests that females may have less androgen sensitivity compared to males. Although exogenous androgens can influence sexual mounting behaviors in female hamsters, female hamsters are less responsive to the effects of androgens on neuroendocrine function and sexual behavior than males (171, 172). Females have also been found to have decreased androgen receptor immunoreactivity and density compared to males in several regions of the brain (173). Second, compared men, women produce far less testosterone and have less variability in testosterone. This restricted range reduces the statistical power to detect testosterone's psychological and behavioral effects (174) and this may hinder the detection of these effects in women. Additionally, the type of methodology used to measure testosterone can have sensitivity at different ranges (175) and may not always be well-suited for measuring the decreased concentrations of testosterone in women.

In summary, testosterone explains both intersex and intrasex variability in dysregulatory behavior. Researchers have several obstacles in measuring testosterone, which hopefully will be curtailed with the advent of greater precision in measurement and the accumulation of more data. Further exploring the role of testosterone in reward dysregulation within men and women would advance the study of the psychological effects of testosterone.

Age

Another potential moderator of the PANE framework is age. Post-adolescence aging coincides with decreases in testosterone [e.g., Ref. (176)], decline in neural reward-related function [e.g., Ref. (177)], increased preferences for delayed rewards (178), and decreased risk-taking behavior [e.g., Ref. (147)]. Furthermore, developmental researchers have proposed that pubertal increases in sex hormones including testosterone are linked to elevated risk-taking in adolescents (179, 180). Additionally, research on risk-taking suggest that both male and female adolescents engage in more risk-taking compared to adults [e.g., Ref. (181, 182)], leaving greater potential for testosterone to explain risk-taking in adolescents compared to adults. Thus, it is possible that age may moderate associations in the PANE framework and also modulate differences in the mechanisms of testosterone, reward function, and behavioral dysregulation.

Individual Differences

Although work on individual differences moderators of testosterone, reward, and behavioral dysregulation is preliminary, the associations in the PANE framework may be modulated by individual differences. For instance, Norman et al. (183) found that trait anxiety moderates the association between testosterone dynamics and impulsive aggression, while Schultheiss and colleagues (184, 185) report that implicit power motive can modulate testosterone responses to competitive contexts. Additionally, the mechanisms in PANE may also be affected by other individual differences related to reward motivation, such as the behavioral inhibition and activation scales [BIS/BAS; (186)] or regulatory focus (187).

The PANE Framework – A Summary

The PANE framework provides an organizing framework of existing research showing that the association between testosterone and behavioral dysregulation is mediated by increased reward motivation and reward dysregulation (see **Figure 2**). Specifically, the PANE approach primarily holds that both stable, trait-like levels and moment-to-moment dynamic changes in testosterone

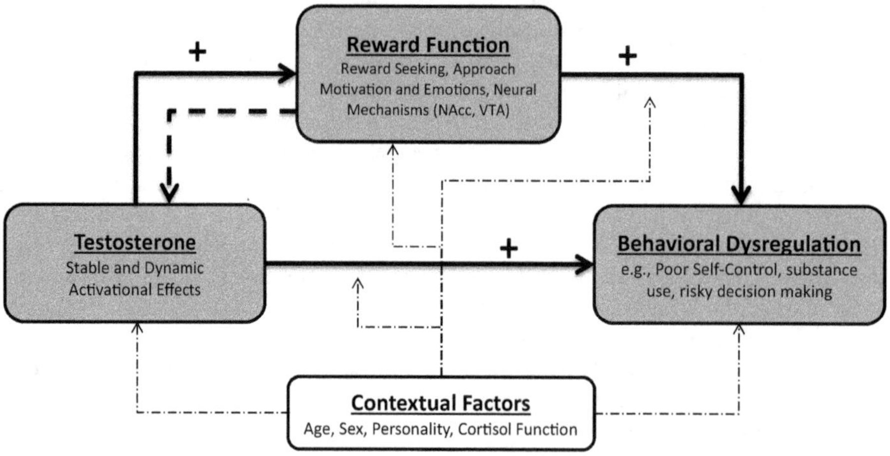

FIGURE 2 | The PANE framework of reward and behavioral dysregulation. The PANE framework specifies that elevated stable levels and dynamic increases of testosterone facilitate increased reward function. This increased reward function then facilitates behavioral dysregulation and behaviors indicative of excessive reward pursuit. This perspective also allows for the possibility that reward function can increase testosterone.

can increase reward dysregulation. Enhanced reward processing – a psychological and neural mechanism of behavioral dysregulation – then increases the likelihood of behavioral dysregulation. Because reward function is affected by testosterone and also serves as a key mechanism of behavioral dysregulation, we argue that reward function is a prime candidate for a mediator of the association between testosterone and behavioral dysregulation. Consistent with contemporary accounts of mediation (188), by specifying reward function as a mediator of the association between testosterone and behavioral dysregulation, we mean that reward function is a causal mechanism in this association. As we review above, testosterone and reward function and motivation modulate a common set of reward-dependent behaviors, and well-established causal directions among testosterone, reward, and behavioral dysregulation suggest that this network of relations is mediated.

The PANE approach is currently at a preliminary state in understanding neuroendocrine function, reward-dysfunction, and behavioral dysregulation. The current paper provides a rationale for why reward function may mediate the association between testosterone and behavioral dysregulation. However, as a whole, this mediation is untested by empirical articles. Future work is needed for researchers to test the overall mediation proposed by the PANE framework. This framework can be measured and tested in numerous forms and contexts, including using both human and animal samples, experimental manipulations of reward, pharmacological testosterone manipulations, testosterone modulating experimental paradigms (e.g., competitive outcomes), and multiple measures of behavioral dysregulation (e.g., poor financial decision making, substance abuse, risky-sexual behaviors). This flexibility allows for the PANE model to be tested and applied by researchers from many backgrounds.

It is necessary to note where the PANE approach differs from other neuroendocrine accounts of behavior. Previous accounts of testosterone and social behavior often indicate testosterone as a biomarker and mechanism of dominance and reproductive behaviors [e.g., Ref. (189, 190)], while recent research has also linked testosterone to threat-based neural function [e.g., Ref. (191)]. It is clear that testosterone modulates these psychological functions in addition to purely reward-related function. However, the literature we review suggests that dominance and sexual behavior are not the only variables regulated by testosterone. As we reviewed, testosterone is related to reward-related neural function, affect, and behaviors, as well as multiple phenotypes of behavioral dysregulation more distal to sexual behavior and dominance, such as substance use, risky-decision making, and sensation seeking. Thus, these behaviors are unlikely to be guided completely by the dominance and sexual behavior-related functions of testosterone. It is possible, instead, that rewards of status-seeking and sexual behavior may actually be a function of the reward-related function of testosterone, but future work is needed to test this possibility. At this point, the PANE framework is designed to be an additive perspective of the effects of testosterone on behavior in addition to other existing accounts.

Future Directions for Research on Reward Dysregulation, Testosterone, and Behavioral Dysregulation

Although the PANE approach proposes that reward function is a critical mediator in the association of testosterone and dysregulatory behaviors, this research can be developed in several ways. In the following sections, we also propose additional ways the PANE perspective can be expanded: (1) the role of social functioning, (2) translational work in psychiatric populations, (3) integration with neuroendocrine models of aggressive behavior, (4) the positive effects of behavioral dysregulation, and (5) integration with other systems of behavioral dysregulation.

Decreased Social Functioning

Testosterone may also increase risk-taking by decreasing social connections with others. It has been long known that socially isolated or disconnected individuals are more likely to engage in reckless behaviors, such as aggression, violence, and drug use (192, 193). This idea is consistent with recent reports suggesting a robust association between having social connections and decreased risk-taking. For instance, having better quality peer and family relationships is associated with decreased risk-taking in adolescents (194, 195) and higher levels of social support are linked with decreased risk-taking in stigmatized sexual minorities [e.g., Ref. (196, 197)]. Additionally, self-regulation has been found to be impaired by social exclusion (198). Socially excluded people are also more likely to engage in financial risk-taking (199).

How might testosterone decrease social relationship quality? Broadly, low testosterone is associated with nurturant, pro-social, relationship-promoting behavior (200–202). Basal testosterone is positively associated with having an avoidant, disconnected interpersonal approach, and greater loneliness (203). Testosterone is also positively related to decreased relationship satisfaction and commitment in couples, in both individuals and their romantic partners (204). Additionally, exogenous testosterone can decrease empathy and trust (168, 205), which may impair social relations. Furthermore, the increased risk-taking associated with testosterone function may also in turn decrease relationship quality, further impairing this process.

In summary, by decreasing the quality of social relationships, testosterone may increase the likelihood individuals engage in dysregulatory behaviors, such as maladaptive substance use to cope with poor social relationships [e.g., Ref. (206)]. We additionally suggest this association may be mediated by other processes we previously reviewed. For instance, research suggests having more meaningful family relationships can decrease risk-taking through neural activation indicative of decreased reward sensitivity and increased cognitive control [dorsolateral pre-frontal cortex, Ref. (194)]. Likewise, decreased empathy – an emergent property of reward and positive emotions (207, 208) – may also be related to the association between testosterone and reward processing.

Translational Implications for Psychiatric Illnesses

Numerous psychological disorders are characterized by trait impulsivity and behavioral dysregulation, such as BD, borderline personality disorder, and attention deficit hyperactivity disorder (39). From the PANE perspective, targeting hormones and affective states leading to behavioral dysregulation presents a novel, translational approach to understanding and treating these disorders. In particular, BD is a prime candidate to investigate the PANE approach. BD is characterized by increased reward sensitivity and difficulties down-regulating reward (2, 41), which may be of particular interest and application for the PANE approach. A chronic, severe, and often fatal psychiatric illness, BD ranks in the top 10 leading causes of worldwide disability by the World Health Organization. The core diagnostic criterion for BD involves periods of abnormally and persistently elevated positive mood (39) and impairments in reward processing have been proposed as a putative endophenotype for BD (209).

Three lines of evidence suggest that BD is a target population for studying testosterone and reward function. First, BD is associated with increased reward sensitivity. For example, people with BD exhibit increased reward reactivity (2, 210, 211), excessive pursuits aimed at obtaining rewards (1, 212), and impairments in reward-related learning (213). Second, empirical models of BD stress the importance of reward dysregulation in the causes and course of the disorder (1, 2, 210–212). Troubles with reward processing persist in BD, even during periods of symptom remission. For example, remitted BD patients report trouble decreasing or down-regulating reward (42), and engage in maladaptive strategies that amplify reward-relevant responses (43, 214), compared with healthy controls. Third, increased reward sensitivity is associated with clinical impairment in BD. Sensitivity to reward predicts increases in manic symptoms over time in BD (215).

Preliminary evidence also suggests that testosterone is important factor for understanding the course and symptom severity in BD. For instance, heightened testosterone levels are associated with significant increases in mania symptoms and severity in BD (103, 216), and oral administration of testosterone has been causally linked to the onset of manic symptoms (102). Future research is needed to understand the hormonal and reward-related mechanisms of BD and other disorders.

Integration with Theories of Aggressive Behavior

Much of research and theory links aggressive behavior to negative affective systems and threat processing [e.g., Ref. (217–221); see Ref. (26), for a review]. However, the reward systems are also implicated in aggressive behavior [e.g., Ref. (117, 222)]. A model of aggressive behavior accounting for reward and threat-processing may help explain mixed evidence for testosterone and aggressive behavior in neuroendocrine research. Although threat-function and negative affective systems undoubtedly play a critical role in facilitating aggressive behavior, a PANE approach to aggression may help enhance neuroendocrine models of aggressive behavior beyond just accounting for negative affect.

Exploring the "Light Side" of Behavioral Dysregulation

So far, the primary discussion of the PANE approach to impulsive behavioral dysregulation has focused on impulsive behaviors. However, just as calculated, non-impulsive behaviors can have antisocial consequences, not all impulsive acts have negative effects and many can be generous or pro-social to others [e.g., Ref. (223, 224)]. Emerging research suggests testosterone is positively associated with pro-social acts of fairness, cooperation, and reciprocity (205, 225, 226). Because positive emotionality has been found to be linked to pro-social behavior and because neural systems linked to reward are also related to pro-social behavior (227), the PANE approach may also explain the how testosterone can increase pro-social behaviors through positive emotions and reward motivation. Future research is needed to uncover further associations between testosterone, positive emotions, and pro-social behavior.

Integration with Other Systems of Behavioral Dysregulation

Although the PANE perspective specifies reward processing as a central mediator to the association between testosterone and behavioral dysregulation, reward is likely not the only mechanism. For example, one potential mechanism of increased risk-taking and impulsive behavior implicated are the pre-frontal regions of the brain linked to impulse control and self-regulation, such as the orbitofrontal cortex (OFC), which is related to risky-decision making [Ref. (228); see Ref. (179), for a review]. Although the literature suggesting testosterone can modulate the OFC is not as expansive as the testosterone-reward literature, the association testosterone has with aggression and risk-taking has been in part explained by decreased OFC activation (127) and volume in males (179). Furthermore, research suggests testosterone decreases connectivity between the OFC and subcortical areas like the amygdala (229, 230).

The effects of testosterone on the reward and self-control systems fit well with established dual-systems models of self-control. Hofmann et al. (231) specify that two systems modulate self-control: an impulsive associate system that automatically triggers impulsive responses to the environment and a reflective system providing executive control of overriding impulses and implementing strategic plans for goal pursuit. Based on what is known of the neural effects of testosterone, testosterone changes may modulate the activation of both impulsive and reflective systems. As more research emerges, one broad goal of the PANE perspective and surrounding research will be to integrate more with other mechanisms and perspectives of behavioral dysregulation, such as the dual-systems approach.

Conclusion

The PANE perspective is designed to organize the work on testosterone, reward dysregulation, and behavioral dysregulation into one coherent framework to stimulate research on behavioral dysregulation. The endocrine mechanisms discussed in this paper may also influence behavioral dysregulation through other mechanisms than reward [such as self-control systems and the OFC, Ref. (127)]. However, the evidence is clear that reward dysregulation is a principal mechanism modulating dysregulatory behaviors and it is necessary to unify this work into a larger framework. Broadly, researchers need to identify mediating psychological and neural mechanisms for the association between testosterone and behavioral dysregulation, and to unify these processes in an elegant, unified model. Together, both neuroendocrine and reward motivation accounts of behavioral dysregulation may hold promise in explaining poor self-control and impulsive behaviors across a wide range of clinical, health, and social contexts.

References

1. Alloy LB, Abramson LA. The role of the behavioral approach system (BAS) in bipolar spectrum disorders. *Curr Dir Psychol Sci* (2010) **19**(3):189–94. doi:10.1177/0963721410370292
2. Gruber J. Can feeling too good be bad? Positive emotion persistence (PEP) in bipolar disorder. *Curr Dir Psychol Sci* (2011) **20**(4):217–21. doi:10.1177/0963721411414632
3. Johnson SL, Gruber J, Eisner L. Emotion in bipolar disorder. In: Rottenberg J, Johnson SL, editors. *Emotion and Psychopathology: Bridging Affective and Clinical Science.* Washington, DC: American Psychological Association (APA) Books (2007). p. 123–50.
4. Nelson RJ. Chapter 2: the endocrine system. 3rd ed. *An Introduction to Behavioral Endocrinology.* Sunderland, MA: Sinauer Associates (2005). p. 37–88.
5. Dabbs JM. Salivary testosterone measurements: reliability across hours, days, and weeks. *Physiol Behav* (1990) **48**:83–6. doi:10.1016/0031-9384(90)90265-6
6. Sapienza P, Zingales L, Maestripieri D. Gender differences in financial risk aversion and career choices are affected by testosterone. *Proc Natl Acad Sci U S A* (2009) **106**(36):15268–73. doi:10.1073/pnas.0907352106
7. Glenn AL, Raine A, Schug RA, Gao Y, Granger DA. Increased testosterone-to-cortisol ratio in psychopathy. *J Abnorm Psychol* (2011) **120**(2):389. doi:10.1037/a0021407
8. Josephs RA, Telch MJ, Hixon JG, Evans JJ, Lee H, Knopik VS, et al. Genetic and hormonal sensitivity to threat: testing a serotonin transporter genotype × testosterone interaction. *Psychoneuroendocrinology* (2012) **37**(6):752–61. doi:10.1016/j.psyneuen.2011.09.006
9. Liening SH, Stanton SJ, Saini EK, Schultheiss OC. Salivary testosterone, cortisol, and progesterone: two-week stability, interhormone correlations, and effects of time of day, menstrual cycle, and oral contraceptive use on steroid hormone levels. *Physiol Behav* (2010) **99**(1):8–16. doi:10.1016/j.physbeh.2009.10.001
10. Mazur A, Booth A. Testosterone is related to deviance in male army veterans, but relationships are not moderated by cortisol. *Biol Psychol* (2014) **96**:72–6. doi:10.1016/j.biopsycho.2013.11.015
11. Apicella CL, Carré JM, Dreber A. Testosterone and economic risk taking: a review. *Adapt Human Behav Physiol* (2015):1–28. doi:10.1007/s40750-014-0020-2
12. Evans KL, Hampson E. Does risk-taking mediate the relationship between testosterone and decision-making on the Iowa gambling task? *Pers Individ Differ* (2014) **61**:57–62. doi:10.1016/j.paid.2014.01.011
13. Stanton SJ, Liening SH, Schultheiss OC. Testosterone is positively associated with risk taking in the Iowa gambling task. *Horm Behav* (2011) **59**(2):252–6. doi:10.1016/j.yhbeh.2010.12.003
14. Stanton SJ, Mullette-Gillman OA, McLaurin RE, Kuhn CM, LaBar KS, Platt ML, et al. Low- and high-testosterone individuals exhibit decreased aversion to economic risk. *Psychol Sci* (2011) **22**(4):447–53. doi:10.1177/0956797611401752
15. Schipper BC. *Sex Hormones and Choice Under Risk* (2012). doi:10.2139/ssrn.2046324
16. Carré JM, Campbell JA, Lozoya E, Goetz SMM, Welker KM. Changes in testosterone mediate the effect of winning on subsequent aggressive behaviour. *Psychoneuroendocrinology* (2013) **38**(10):2034–41. doi:10.1016/j.psyneuen.2013.03.008
17. Maner JK, Miller SL, Schmidt NB, Eckel LA. Submitting to defeat social anxiety, dominance threat, and decrements in testosterone. *Psychol Sci* (2008) **19**(8):764–8. doi:10.1111/j.1467-9280.2008.02154.x
18. Welker KM, Carré JM. Individual differences in testosterone predict persistence in men. *Eur J Pers* (2015) **29**:83–9. doi:10.1002/per.1958
19. Zilioli S, Mehta PH, Watson NV. Losing the battle but winning the war: uncertain outcomes reverse the usual effect of winning on testosterone. *Biol Psychol* (2014) **103**:54–62. doi:10.1016/j.biopsycho.2014.07.022
20. Ronay R, von Hippel W. The presence of an attractive woman elevates testosterone and physical risk taking in young men. *Soc Psychol Pers Sci* (2010) **1**(1):57–64. doi:10.1177/1948550609352807
21. Roney J, Mahler S, Maestripieri D. Behavioural and hormonal responses of men to brief interactions with women. *Evol Hum Behav* (2003) **24**:365–75. doi:10.1016/s1090-5138(03)00053-9
22. Roney J, Lukaszewski A, Simmons Z. Rapid endocrine responses of young men to social interactions with young women. *Horm Behav* (2007) **52**:326–33. doi:10.1016/j.yhbeh.2007.05.008
23. Geniole SN, Carré JM, McCormick CM. State, not trait, neuroendocrine function predicts costly reactive aggression in men after social exclusion and inclusion. *Biol Psychol* (2011) **87**(1):137–45. doi:10.1016/j.biopsycho.2011.02.020
24. Carney DR, Cuddy AJC, Yap AJ. Power posing: brief nonverbal displays affect neuroendocrine levels and risk tolerance. *Psychol Sci* (2010) **21**(10):1363–8. doi:10.1177/0956797610383437
25. Carré JM, Iselin AR, Welker KM, Hariri AR, Dodge KA. Testosterone reactivity to provocation mediates the effect of early intervention on aggressive behavior. *Psychol Sci* (2014) **25**(5):1140–6. doi:10.1177/0956797614525642
26. Carré JM, McCormick CM, Hariri AR. The social neuroendocrinology of human aggression. *Psychoneuroendocrinology* (2011) **36**(7):935–44. doi:10.1016/j.psyneuen.2011.02.001
27. Carré JM, Putnam SK, McCormick CM. Testosterone responses to competition predict future aggressive behaviour at a cost to reward

in men. *Psychoneuroendocrinology* (2009) **34**:561–70. doi:10.1016/j.psyneuen.2008.10.018

28. Carré JM, Baird-Rowe CD, Hariri AR. Testosterone responses to competition predict decreased trust ratings of emotionally neutral faces. *Psychoneuroendocrinology* (2014) **49**:79–83. doi:10.1016/j.psyneuen.2014.06.011
29. Apicella CL, Dreber A, Mollerstrom J. Salivary testosterone change following monetary wins and losses predicts future financial risk-taking. *Psychoneuroendocrinology* (2014) **39**:58–64. doi:10.1016/j.psyneuen.2013.09.025
30. Atkinson JW. Motivational determinants of risk-taking behavior. *Psychol Rev* (1957) **64**(6):359–72. doi:10.1037/h0043445
31. Gray JA. Précis of the neuropsychology of anxiety: an enquiry into the functions of the septo-hippocampal system. *Behav Brain Sci* (1982) **5**:469–534. doi:10.1017/s0140525x00013066
32. Gray JA. Perspectives on anxiety and impulsivity: a commentary. *J Res Pers* (1987) **21**(4):493–509. doi:10.1016/0092-6566(87)90036-5
33. Mason L, El-Deredy W, Richard B. Reward dysfunction in mania: neural correlates of risk and impulsivity in individuals vulnerable to bipolar disorder. *Int Clin Psychopharmacol* (2011) **26**:e46. doi:10.1097/01.yic.0000405710.14232.bf
34. Steinberg L. A social neuroscience perspective on adolescent risk-taking. *Dev Rev* (2008) **28**(1):78–106. doi:10.1016/j.dr.2007.08.002
35. Loxton NJ, Nguyen D, Casey L, Dawe S. Reward drive, rash impulsivity and punishment sensitivity in problem gamblers. *Pers Individ Differ* (2008) **45**(2):167–73. doi:10.1016/j.paid.2008.03.017
36. Dawe S, Gullo MJ, Loxton NJ. Reward drive and rash impulsiveness as dimensions of impulsivity: implications for substance misuse. *Addict Behav* (2004) **29**(7):1389–405. doi:10.1016/j.addbeh.2004.06.004
37. Castellà J, Pérez J. Sensitivity to punishment and sensitivity to reward and traffic violations. *Accid Anal Prev* (2004) **36**(6):947–52. doi:10.1016/j.aap.2003.10.003
38. Van den Berg L, Pieterse K, Malik JA, Luman M, van Dijk KW, Oosterlaan J, et al. Association between impulsivity, reward responsiveness and body mass index in children. *Int J Obes (Lond)* (2011) **35**(10):1301–7. doi:10.1038/ijo.2011.116
39. American Psychiatric Association. *Task Force on DSM-IV. Diagnostic and Statistical Manual of Mental Disorders: DSM-IV-TR*. Washington, DC: American Psychiatric Association (2000).
40. Gruber J, Gilbert KE, Youngstrom EA, Kogos Youngstrom J, Feeny NC, Findling RL. Reward dysregulation and mood symptoms in an adolescent outpatient sample. *J Abnorm Child Psychol* (2013) **41**(7):1053–65. doi:10.1007/s10802-013-9746-8
41. Gruber J. A review and synthesis of positive emotion and reward disturbance in bipolar disorder. *Clin Psychol Psychother* (2011) **18**(5):356–65. doi:10.1002/cpp.776
42. Gruber J, Harvey AG, Purcell A. What goes up can come down? A preliminary investigation of emotion reactivity and emotion recovery in bipolar disorder. *J Affect Disord* (2011) **133**(3):457–66. doi:10.1007/s10802-013-9746-8
43. Johnson SL, McKenzie G, McMurrich S. Ruminative responses to negative and positive affect among students diagnosed with bipolar disorder and major depressive disorder. *Cognit Ther Res* (2008) **32**(5):702–13. doi:10.1007/s10608-007-9158-6
44. Giovanelli A, Hoerger M, Johnson SL, Gruber J. Impulsive responses to positive mood and reward are related to mania risk. *Cogn Emot* (2013) **27**(6):1091–104. doi:10.1080/02699931.2013.772048
45. Reddy LF, Lee J, Davis MC, Altshuler L, Glahn DC, Miklowitz DJ, et al. Impulsivity and risk taking in bipolar disorder and schizophrenia. *Neuropsychopharmacology* (2013) **39**:456–63. doi:10.1038/npp.2013.218
46. Kathleen HM, Bearden CE, Barguil M, Fonseca M, Serap Monkul E, Nery FG, et al. Conceptualizing impulsivity and risk taking in bipolar disorder: importance of history of alcohol abuse. *Bipolar Disord* (2009) **11**(1):33–40. doi:10.1111/j.1399-5618.2009.00720.x
47. McIntyre RS, McElroy SL, Konarski JZ, Soczynska JK, Wilkins K, Kennedy SH. Problem gambling in bipolar disorder: results from the Canadian community health survey. *J Affect Disord* (2007) **102**(1):27–34. doi:10.1016/j.jad.2006.12.005
48. Garno JL, Gunawardane N, Goldberg JF. Predictors of trait aggression in bipolar disorder. *Bipolar Disord* (2008) **10**(2):285–92. doi:10.1111/j.1399-5618.2007.00489.x
49. Urošević S, Abramson LY, Harmon-Jones E, Alloy LB. Dysregulation of the behavioral approach system (BAS) in bipolar spectrum disorders: review of theory and evidence. *Clin Psychol Rev* (2008) **28**(7):1188–205. doi:10.1016/j.cpr.2008.04.004
50. Cyders MA, Smith GT. Clarifying the role of personality dispositions in risk for increased gambling behavior. *Pers Individ Differ* (2008) **45**(6):503–8. doi:10.1016/j.paid.2008.06.002
51. Cyders MA, Smith GT. Emotion-based dispositions to rash action: positive and negative urgency. *Psychol Bull* (2008) **134**(6):807–28. doi:10.1037/a0013341
52. Isen AM, Patrick R. The effect of positive feelings on risk taking: when the chips are down. *Organ Behav Human Perform* (1983) **31**(2):194–202. doi:10.1016/0030-5073(83)90120-4
53. Bechara A. Risky business: emotion, decision-making, and addiction. *J Gambl Stud* (2003) **19**(1):23–51. doi:10.1023/A:1021223113233
54. Bechara A, Damasio H. Decision-making and addiction (part I): impaired activation of somatic states in substance dependent individuals when pondering decisions with negative future consequences. *Neuropsychologia* (2002) **40**(10):1675–89. doi:10.1016/S0028-3932(02)00015-5
55. Stanford MS, Greve KW, Dickens TJ. Irritability and impulsiveness: relationship to self-reported impulsive aggression. *Pers Individ Differ* (1995) **19**:757–60. doi:10.1016/0191-8869(95)00144-u
56. Depue RA, Collins PF. Neurobiology of the structure of personality: dopamine, facilitation of incentive motivation, and extraversion. *Behav Brain Sci* (1999) **22**(3):491–517. doi:10.1017/S0140525X99002046
57. Pickering AD, Gray JA. The neuroscience of personality. In: Pervin LA, John SP, editors. *Handbook of Personality: Theory and Research*. New York: Guilford Publications (1999). p. 277–99.
58. Grace AA, Floresco SB, Goto Y, Lodge DJ. Regulation of firing of dopaminergic neurons and control of goal-directed behaviors. *Trends Neurosci* (2007) **30**(5):220–7. doi:10.1016/j.tins.2007.03.003
59. Chau DT, Roth RM, Green AI. The neural circuitry of reward and its relevance to psychiatric disorders. *Curr Psychiatry Rep* (2004) **6**:391–9. doi:10.1007/s11920-004-0026-8
60. Gregorios-Pippas L, Tobler PN, Schultz W. Short-term temporal discounting of reward value in human ventral striatum. *J Neurophysiol* (2009) **101**(3):1507–23. doi:10.1152/jn.90730.2008
61. Trantham-Davidson H, Neely LC, Lavin A, Seamans JK. Mechanisms underlying differential D1 versus D2 dopamine receptor regulation of inhibition in prefrontal cortex. *J Neurosci* (2004) **24**(47):10652–9. doi:10.1523/jneurosci.3179-04.2004
62. Pierce RC, Kumaresan V. The mesolimbic dopamine system: the final common pathway for the reinforcing effect of drugs of abuse? *Neurosci Biobehav Rev* (2006) **30**:215–38. doi:10.1016/j.neubiorev.2005.04.016
63. Wise RA. Addictive drugs and brain stimulation reward. *Annu Rev Neurosci* (1996) **19**:319–40. doi:10.1146/annurev.neuro.19.1.319
64. Schultz W, Apicella P, Scarnati E, Ljungberg T. Neuronal activity in monkey ventral striatum related to the expectation of reward. *J Neurosci* (1992) **12**(12):4595–610. doi:10.1016/j.neures.2009.09.526
65. Berridge KC, Robinson TE. Parsing reward. *Trends Neurosci* (2003) **26**:507–13. doi:10.1016/s0166-2236(03)00233-9
66. Cardinal RN, Parkinson JA, Hall J, Everitt BJ. Emotion and motivation: the role of the amygdala, ventral striatum, and prefrontal cortex. *Neurosci Biobehav Rev* (2002) **26**:321–52. doi:10.1016/s0149-7634(02)00007-6
67. Di Chiara G. Nucleus accumbens shell and core dopamine: differential role in behavior and addiction. *Behav Brain Res* (2002) **137**:75–114. doi:10.1016/s0166-4328(02)00286-3
68. Kelley AE. Ventral striatal control of appetitive motivation role in ingestive behavior and reward-related learning. *Neurosci Biobehav Rev* (2004) **27**:765–76. doi:10.1016/j.neubiorev.2003.11.015
69. Kelley AE, Bakshi VP, Haber SN, Steininger TL, Will MJ, Zhang M. Opiod modulation of taste hedonics within the ventral striatum. *Physiol Behav* (2002) **76**:365–77. doi:10.1016/s0031-9384(02)00751-5
70. Rebec GV, Grabner CP, Johnson M, Pierce RC, Bardo MT. Transient increases in catecholaminergic activity in medial prefrontal cortex and nucleus accumbens shell during novelty. *Neuroscience* (1997) **76**:707–14. doi:10.1016/s0306-4522(96)00382-x
71. Drevets WC, Gautier C, Price JC, Kupfer DJ, Kinahan PE, Grace AA, et al. Amphetamine-induced dopamine release in human ventral striatum correlates with euphoria. *Biol Psychiatry* (2001) **49**:81–96. doi:10.1016/S0006-3223(00)01038-6
72. Ikemoto S, Panksepp J. The role of nucleus accumbens dopamine in motivated behavior: a unifying interpretation with special reference to reward-seeking. *Brain Res Brain Res Rev* (1999) **31**:6–41. doi:10.1016/S0165-0173(99)00023-5

73. Berk M, Dodd S, Kauer-Sant'Anna M, Malhi GS, Bourin M, Kapczinski F, et al. Dopamine dysregulation syndrome: implications for a dopamine hypothesis of bipolar disorder. *Acta Psychiatr Scand* (2007) **116**(s434):41–9. doi:10.1111/j.1600-0447.2007.01058.x
74. Volkow ND, Wang GJ, Fowler JS, Tomasi D, Telang F. Addiction: beyond dopamine reward circuitry. *Proc Natl Acad Sci U S A* (2011) **108**(37):15037–42. doi:10.1073/pnas.1010654108
75. Fiorillo CD, Tobler PN, Schultz W. Discrete coding of reward probability and incertainty by dopamine neurons. *Science* (2003) **299**:1898–902. doi:10.1126/science.1077349
76. Joutsa J, Johansson J, Niemelä S, Ollikainen A, Hirvonen MM, Piepponen P, et al. Mesolimbic dopamine release is linked to symptom severity in pathological gambling. *Neuroimage* (2012) **60**(4):1992–9. doi:10.1016/j.neuroimage.2012.02.006
77. Kohno M, Ghahremani DG, Morales AM, Robertson CL, Ishibashi K, Morgan AT, et al. Risk-taking behavior: dopamine D2/D3 receptors, feedback, and frontolimbic activity. *Cereb Cortex* (2013) **25**:236–45. doi:10.1093/cercor/bht218
78. Mitchell MR, Weiss VG, Beas BS, Morgan D, Bizon JL, Setlow B. Adolescent risk taking, cocaine self-administration, and striatal dopamine signaling. *Neuropsychopharmacology* (2014) **39**(4):955–62. doi:10.1038/npp.2013.295
79. Norbury A, Manohar S, Rogers RD, Husain M. Dopamine modulates risk-taking as a function of baseline sensation-seeking trait. *J Neurosci* (2013) **33**(32):12982–6. doi:10.1523/jneurosci.5587-12.2013
80. Pattij T, Schetters D, Schoffelmeer AN. Dopaminergic modulation of impulsive decision making in the rat insular cortex. *Behav Brain Res* (2014) **270**:118–24. doi:10.1016/j.bbr.2014.05.010
81. Heatherton TF, Wagner DD. Cognitive neuroscience of self-regulation failure. *Trends Cogn Sci* (2011) **15**(3):132–9. doi:10.1016/j.tics.2010.12.005
82. Baler RD, Volkow ND. Drug addiction: the neurobiology of disrupted self-control. *Trends Mol Med* (2006) **12**(12):559–66. doi:10.1016/j.molmed.2006.10.005
83. Hare TA, Camerer CF, Rangel A. Self-control in decision-making involves modulation of the vmPFC valuation system. *Science* (2009) **324**(5927):646–8. doi:10.1126/science.1168450
84. Hester R, Garavan H. Executive dysfunction in cocaine addiction: evidence for discordant frontal, cingulate, and cerebellar activity. *J Neurosci* (2004) **24**(49):11017–22. doi:10.1523/JNEUROSCI.3321-04.2004
85. Van Honk J, Harmon-Jones E, Morgan BE, Schutter DJ. Socially explosive minds: the triple imbalance hypothesis of reactive aggression. *J Pers* (2010) **78**(1):67–94. doi:10.1111/j.1467-6494.2009.00609.x
86. Aluja A, García LF. Sensation seeking, sexual curiosity and testosterone in inmates. *Neuropsychobiology* (2005) **51**(1):28–33. doi:10.1159/000082852
87. Alvergne A, Jokela M, Faurie C, Lummaa V. Personality and testosterone in men from a high-fertility population. *Pers Individ Differ* (2010) **49**:840–4. doi:10.1016/j.paid.2010.07.006
88. Bayless DW, Darling JS, Daniel JM. Mechanisms by which neonatal testosterone exposure mediates sex differences in impulsivity in prepubertal rats. *Horm Behav* (2013) **64**(5):764–9. doi:10.1016/j.yhbeh.2013.10.003
89. Campbell BC, Dreber A, Apicella CL, Eisenberg DT, Gray PB, Little AC, et al. Testosterone exposure, dopaminergic reward, and sensation-seeking in young men. *Physiol Behav* (2010) **99**(4):451–6. doi:10.1016/j.physbeh.2009.12.011
90. Coccaro EF, Beresford B, Minar P, Kaskow J, Geracioti T. CSF testosterone: relationship to aggression, impulsivity, and venturesomeness in adult males with personality disorder. *J Psychiatr Res* (2007) **41**(6):488–92. doi:10.1016/j.jpsychires.2006.04.009
91. Daitzman R, Zuckerman M. Disinhibitory sensation seeking, personality and gonadal hormones. *Pers Individ Differ* (1980) **1**(2):103–10. doi:10.1016/0191-8869(80)90027-6
92. Määttänen I, Jokela M, Hintsa T, Firtser S, Kähönen M, Jula A, et al. Testosterone and temperament traits in men: longitudinal analysis. *Psychoneuroendocrinology* (2013) **38**(10):2243–8. doi:10.1016/j.psyneuen.2013.04.009
93. Van Honk J, Schutter DJ, Hermans EJ, Putman P, Tuiten A, Koppeschaar H. Testosterone shifts the balance between sensitivity for punishment and reward in healthy young women. *Psychoneuroendocrinology* (2004) **29**:937–43. doi:10.1016/j.psyneuen.2003.08.007
94. Coates JM, Herbert J. Endogenous steroids and financial risk taking on a London trading floor. *Proc Natl Acad Sci U S A* (2008) **105**(16):6167–72. doi:10.1073/pnas.0704025105
95. Van Honk J, Peper JS, Schutter DJ. Testosterone reduces unconscious fear but not consciously experienced anxiety: implications for the disorders of fear and anxiety. *Biol Psychiatry* (2005) **58**(3):218–25. doi:10.1016/j.biopsych.2005.04.003
96. Van Honk J, Schutter DJ. Vigilant and avoidant responses to angry facial expressions. In: Harmon-Jones E, Vinkielman P, editors. *Social Neuroscience: Integrating Biological and Psychological Explanations of Social Behavior*. New York, NY: Guilford Press (2007). p. 197–223.
97. Tuiten A, Van Honk J, Verbaten R, Laan E, Everaerd W, Stam H. Can sublingual testosterone increase subjective and physiological measures of laboratory-induced sexual arousal? *Arch Gen Psychiatry* (2002) **59**(5):465–6. doi:10.1001/archpsyc.59.5.465
98. Mehta PH, Snyder NA, Knight EL, Lassetter B. Close versus decisive victory moderates the effect of testosterone change on competitive decisions and task enjoyment. *Adapt Human Behav Physiol* (2014). doi:10.1007/s40750-014-0014-0
99. Ebinger M, Sievers C, Ivan D, Schneider HJ, Stalla GK. Is there a neuroendocrinological rationale for testosterone as a therapeutic option in depression? *J Psychopharmacol* (2009) **23**:841–53. doi:10.1177/0269881108092337
100. Amanatkar HR, Chibnall JT, Seo B, Manepalli JN, Grossberg GT. Impact of exogenous testosterone on mood: a systematic review and meta-analysis of randomized placebo-controlled trials. *Ann Clin Psychiatry* (2014) **26**:19–32. doi:10.1016/S0084-4071(08)70175-1
101. Zarrouf FA, Artz S, Griffith J, Sirbu C, Kommor M. Testosterone and depression: systematic review and meta-analysis. *J Psychiatr Pract* (2009) **15**(4):289–305. doi:10.1097/01.pra.0000358315.88931.fc
102. Pope HG, Kouri EM, Hudson JI. Effects of supraphysiologic doses of testosterone on mood and aggression in normal men a randomized controlled trial. *Arch Gen Psychiatry* (2000) **57**(2):133–40. doi:10.1001/archpsyc.57.2.133
103. Sher L, Grunebaum MF, Sullivan GM, Burke GM, Cooper TB, Mann JJ, et al. Testosterone levels in suicide attempters with bipolar disorder. *J Psychiatr Res* (2012) **46**:1267–71. doi:10.1016/j.jpsychires.2012.06.016
104. Mehta PH, Goetz SM, Carré JM. Genetic, hormonal, and neural underpinnings of human aggressive behavior. *Handbook of Neurosociology*. Springer (2013). p. 47–65.
105. Terburg D, Van Honk J. Approach-avoidance versus dominance-submissiveness: a multilevel neural framework on how testosterone promotes social status. *Emot Rev* (2013) **5**(3):296–302. doi:10.1177/1754073913477510
106. Van Honk J, Bos PA, Terburg D. Testosterone and dominance in humans: behavioral and brain mechanisms. *New Frontiers in Social Neuroscience*. Springer International Publishing (2014). p. 201–14.
107. Lombardo MV, Ashwin E, Auyeung B, Chakrabarti B, Lai MC, Taylor K, et al. Fetal programming effects of testosterone on the reward system and behavioral approach tendencies in humans. *Biol Psychiatry* (2012) **72**(10):839–47. doi:10.1016/j.biopsych.2012.05.027
108. Aubele T, Kritzer MF. Androgen influence on prefrontal dopamine systems in adult male rats: localization of cognate intracellular receptors in medial prefrontal projections to the ventral tegmental area and effects of gonadectomy and hormone replacement on glutamate-stimulated extracellular dopamine level. *Cereb Cortex* (2011) **22**:1799–812. doi:10.1093/cercor/bhr258
109. Bell MR, Sisk CL. Dopamine mediates testosterone-induced social reward in male Syrian hamsters. *Endocrinology* (2013) **154**:1225–34. doi:10.1210/en.2012-2042
110. Hernandez L, Gonzalez L, Murzi E, Páez X, Gottberg E, Baptista T. Testosterone modulates mesolimbic dopaminergic activity in male rats. *Neurosci Lett* (1994) **171**(1):172–4. doi:10.1016/0304-3940(94)90632-7
111. Hull EM, Du J, Lorrain DS, Matuszewich L. Testosterone, preoptic dopamine, and copulation in male rats. *Brain Res Bull* (1997) **44**(4):327–33. doi:10.1016/j.yhbeh.2003.06.006
112. Szczypka MS, Zhou QY, Palmiter RD. Dopamine-stimulated sexual behavior is testosterone dependent in mice. *Behav Neurosci* (1998) **112**(5):1229–35. doi:10.1037//0735-7044.112.5.1229
113. Wood RI. Anabolic-androgenic steroid dependence? Insights from animals and humans. *Front Neuroendocrinol* (2008) **29**:490–506. doi:10.1016/j.yfrne.2007.12.002
114. Packard MG, Cornell AH, Alexander GM. Rewarding affective properties of intra-nucleus accumbens injections of testosterone. *Behav Neurosci* (1997) **111**(1):219. doi:10.1037//0735-7044.111.1.219
115. Packard MG, Schroeder JP, Alexander GM. Expression of testosterone conditioned place preference is blocked by peripheral or intra-accumbens injection of α-flupenthixol. *Horm Behav* (1998) **34**(1):39–47. doi:10.1006/hbeh.1998.1461
116. DiMeo AN, Wood RI. ICV testosterone induces Fos in male Syrian hamster brain. *Psychoneuroendocrinology* (2006) **31**(2):237–49. doi:10.1016/j.psyneuen.2005.08.001

117. Fuxjager MJ, Forbes-Lorman RM, Coss DJ, Auger CJ, Auger AP, Marler CA. Winning territorial disputes selectively enhances androgen sensitivity in neural pathways related to motivation and social aggression. *Proc Natl Acad Sci U S A* (2010) **107**(27):12393–8. doi:10.3410/f.4098956.4799055
118. Blakemore SJ, Burnett S, Dahl RE. The role of puberty in the developing adolescent brain. *Hum Brain Mapp* (2010) **31**:926–33. doi:10.1002/hbm.21052
119. Forbes E, Dahl R. Pubertal development and behavior: hormonal activation of social and motivational tendencies. *Brain Cogn* (2010) **72**:66–72. doi:10.1016/j.bandc.2009.10.007
120. Graber J, Nichols T, Brooks-Gunn J. Putting pubertal timing in developmental context: implications for prevention. *Dev Psychobiol* (2010) **52**:254–62. doi:10.1002/dev.20438
121. Nelson E, Lieibenluft E, McClure E, Pine DS. The social re-orientation of adolescence: a neuroscience perspective on the process and its relation to psychopathology. *Psychol Med* (2005) **35**:163–74. doi:10.1017/S0033291704003915
122. Wahlstrom D, Collins P, White T, Luciana M. Developmental changes in dopamine neurotransmission in adolescence: behavioral implications and issues in assessment. *Brain Cogn* (2010) **72**:146–59. doi:10.1016/j.bandc.2009.10.013
123. Schutter DJ, Peper JS, Koppeschaar HP, Kahn RS, Van Honk J. Administration of testosterone increases functional connectivity in a cortico-cortical depression circuit. *J Neuropsychiatry Clin Neurosci* (2005) **17**(3):372–7. doi:10.1176/appi.neuropsych.17.3.372
124. Hermans EJ, Bos PA, Ossewaarde L, Ramsey NF, Fernández G, Van Honk J. Effects of exogenous testosterone on the ventral striatal BOLD response during reward anticipation in healthy women. *Neuroimage* (2010) **52**(1):277–83. doi:10.1016/j.neuroimage.2010.04.019
125. Op de Macks ZA, Moor BG, Overgaauw S, Güroğlu B, Dahl RE, Crone EA. Testosterone levels correspond with increased ventral striatum activation in response to monetary rewards in adolescents. *Dev Cogn Neurosci* (2011) **1**(4):506–16. doi:10.1016/j.dcn.2011.06.003
126. Denson TF, Ronay R, von Hippel W, Schira MM. Endogenous testosterone and cortisol modulate neural responses during induced anger control. *Soc Neurosci* (2013) **8**(2):165–77. doi:10.1080/17470919.2012.655425
127. Mehta PH, Beer J. Neural mechanisms of the testosterone-aggression relation: the role of orbitofrontal cortex. *J Cogn Neurosci* (2010) **22**(10):2357–68. doi:10.1162/jocn.2009.21389
128. Mazur A, Booth A. Testosterone and dominance in men. *Behav Brain Sci* (1998) **21**(3):353–97. doi:10.1017/S0140525X98001228
129. Schultheiss OC, Wirth MM, Torges CM, Pang JS, Villacorta MA, Welsh KM. Effects of implicit power motivation on men's and women's implicit learning and testosterone changes after social victory or defeat. *J Pers Soc Psychol* (2005) **88**(1):174. doi:10.1037/0022-3514.88.1.174
130. Mehta PH, Prasad S. The dual-hormone hypothesis: a brief review and future research agenda. *Curr Opin Behav Sci* (2015) **3**:163–68. doi:10.1016/j.cobeha.2015.04.008
131. Chen SY, Wang J, Yu GQ, Liu W, Pearce D. Androgen and glucocorticoid receptor heterodimer formation: a possible mechanism for mutual inhibition of transcriptional activity. *J Biol Chem* (1997) **272**(22):14087–92. doi:10.1074/jbc.272.22.14087
132. Johnson EO, Kamilaris TC, Chrousos GP, Gold PW. Mechanisms of stress: a dynamic overview of hormonal and behavioral homeostasis. *Neurosci Biobehav Rev* (1992) **16**(2):115–30. doi:10.1016/s0149-7634(05)80175-7
133. Smith RG, Syms AJ, Nag A, Lerner S, Norris JS. Mechanism of the glucocorticoid regulation of growth of the androgen-sensitive prostate-derived R3327H-G8-A1 tumor cell line. *J Biol Chem* (1985) **260**(23):12454–63. doi:10.1002/pros.2990090305
134. Tilbrook AJ, Turner AI, Clarke IJ. Effects of stress on reproduction in non-rodent mammals: the role of glucocorticoids and sex differences. *Rev Reprod* (2000) **5**(2):105–13. doi:10.1530/revreprod/5.2.105
135. Viau V. Functional cross-talk between the hypothalamic-pituitary-gonadal and -adrenal axes. *J Neuroendocrinol* (2002) **14**:506–13. doi:10.1046/j.1365-2826.2002.00798.x
136. Mehta PH, Josephs RA. Testosterone and cortisol jointly regulate dominance: evidence for a dual-hormone hypothesis. *Horm Behav* (2010) **58**(5):898–906. doi:10.1016/j.yhbeh.2010.08.020
137. Mehta PH, Welker KM, Zilioli S, Carré JM. Testosterone and cortisol jointly modulate risk-taking. *Psychoneuroendocrinology* (2015) **56**:88–99. doi:10.1016/j.psyneuen.2015.02.023
138. Edwards DA, Casto KV. Women's intercollegiate athletic competition: cortisol, testostorone, and the dual-hormone hypothesis as it relates to status among teammates. *Horm Behav* (2013) **64**:153–60. doi:10.1016/j.yhbeh.2013.03.003
139. Dabbs JM, Jurkovic GJ, Frady RL. Salivary testosterone and cortisol among late adolescent male offenders. *J Abnorm Child Psychol* (1991) **19**(4):469–78. doi:10.1007/bf00919089
140. Popma A, Vermeiren R, Geluk CA, Rinne T, van den Brink W, Knol DL, et al. Cortisol moderates the relationship between testosterone and aggression in delinquent male adolescents. *Biol Psychiatry* (2007) **61**(3):405–11. doi:10.1016/j.biopsych.2006.06.006
141. Tackett JL, Herzhoff K, Harden KP, Page-Gould E, Josephs RA. Personality×hormone interactions in adolescent externalizing psychopathology. *Personal Disord* (2014) **5**(3):235. doi:10.1037/per0000075
142. Welker KM, Lozoya E, Campbell JA, Carré JM, Neumann C. Testosterone, cortisol, and psychopathic traits in men and women. *Physiol Behav* (2014) **129**:230–6. doi:10.1016/j.physbeh.2014.02.057
143. Mehta PH, Mor S, Yap AJ, Prasad S. Dual-hormone changes are related to bargaining performance. *Psychol Sci* (2015) **26**(6):866–76. doi:10.1177/0956797615572905
144. Carré JM, Mehta PH. Importance of considering testosterone-cortisol interactions in predicting human aggression and dominance. *Aggress Behav* (2011) **37**:1–3. doi:10.1002/ab.20407
145. Cross CP, Copping LT, Campbell A. Sex differences in impulsivity: a meta-analysis. *Psychol Bull* (2011) **137**(1):97. doi:10.1037/a0021591
146. Zuckerman M, Kuhlman DM. Personality and risk-taking: common biosocial factors. *J Pers* (2000) **68**:999–1029. doi:10.1111/1467-6494.00124
147. Byrnes JP, Miller DC, Schafer WD. Gender differences in risk taking: a meta-analysis. *Psychol Bull* (1999) **125**(3):367. doi:10.1037/0033-2909.125.3.367
148. Nelson JA. Are women really more risk-averse than men? *SSRN Electron J* (2012). doi:10.2139/ssrn.2158950
149. Kruger DJ, Nesse RM. An evolutionary life-history framework for understanding sex differences in human mortality rates. *Hum Nat* (2006) **17**(1):74–97. doi:10.1007/s12110-006-1021-z
150. Pampel FC. Gender equality and the sex differential in mortality from accidents in high income nations. *Popul Res Policy Rev* (2001) **20**:397–421. doi:10.1023/A:1013307620643
151. Maxim PS, Keane C. Gender, age, and the risk of violent death in Canada, 1950-1986. *Can Rev Sociol* (1992) **29**(3):329–45. doi:10.1111/j.1755-618x.1992.tb02442.x
152. Archer J. Sex differences in aggression in real-world settings: a meta-analytic review. *Rev Gen Psychol* (2004) **8**(4):291. doi:10.1037/1089-2680.8.4.291
153. Bettencourt B, Miller N. Gender differences in aggression as a function of provocation: a meta-analysis. *Psychol Bull* (1996) **119**(3):422. doi:10.1037/0033-2909.119.3.422
154. Eagly AH, Steffen VJ. Gender and aggressive behaviour: a meta-analytic review of the social psychological literature. *Psychol Bull* (1986) **100**(3):309. doi:10.1037/0033-2909.100.3.309
155. Knight GP, Guthrie IK, Page MC, Fabes RA. Emotional arousal and gender differences in aggression: a meta-analysis. *Aggress Behav* (2002) **28**(5):366–93. doi:10.1002/ab.80011
156. Hill EM, Chow K. Life-history theory and risky drinking. *Addiction* (2002) **97**(4):401–13. doi:10.1046/j.1360-0443.2002.00020.x
157. Frank E, editor. *Gender and Its Effects on Psychopathology*. Arlington, VA: American Psychiatric Press (2000).
158. Gershon J, Gershon J. A meta-analytic review of gender differences in ADHD. *J Atten Disord* (2002) **5**:143–54. doi:10.1177/108705470200500302
159. Moffitt TE, editor. *Sex Differences in Antisocial Behaviour: Conduct Disorder, Delinquency, and Violence in the Dunedin Longitudinal Study*. Cambridge: Cambridge University Press (2001).
160. Rutter M, Caspi A, Moffitt TE. Using sex differences in psychopathology to study causal mechanisms: unifying issues and research strategies. *J Child Psychol Psychiatry* (2003) **44**(8):1092–115. doi:10.1111/1469-7610.00194
161. Manning JT. *Digit Ratio: A Pointer to Fertility, Behavior, and Health*. New Brunswick, NJ: Rutgers University Press (2002).
162. Manning JT, Bundred PE, Newton DJ, Flanigan BF. The second to fourth digit ratio and variation in the androgen receptor gene. *Evol Hum Behav* (2003) **24**:399–405. doi:10.1016/s1090-5138(03)00052-7
163. Knickmeyer R, Baron-Cohen S, Raggatt P, Taylor K, Hackett G. Fetal testosterone and empathy. *Horm Behav* (2006) **49**:282–92. doi:10.1016/j.yhbeh.2005.08.010

164. Wood W, Eagly AH. Biosocial construction of sex differences and similarities in behavior. *Adv Exp Soc Psychol* (2012) **46**:55. doi:10.1016/b978-0-12-394281-4.00002-7
165. Wood W, Eagly AH. Biology or culture alone cannot account for human sex differences and similarities. *Psychol Inq* (2013) **24**(3):241–7. doi:10.1080/1047840x.2013.815034
166. Eagly AH, Wood W. The nature-nurture debates 25 years of challenges in understanding the psychology of gender. *Perspect Psychol Sci* (2013) **8**(3):340–57. doi:10.1177/1745691613484767
167. Bos PA, Terburg D, Van Honk J. Testosterone decreases trust in socially naive humans. *Proc Natl Acad Sci U S A* (2010) **107**(22):9991–5. doi:10.1073/pnas.0911700107
168. Bos PA, Panksepp J, Bluthé RM, Honk JV. Acute effects of steroid hormones and neuropeptides on human social-emotional behavior: a review of single administration studies. *Front Neuroendocrinol* (2012) **33**(1):17–35. doi:10.1016/j.yfrne.2011.01.002
169. Terburg D, Aarts H, Van Honk J. Testosterone affects gaze aversion from angry faces outside of conscious awareness. *Psychol Sci* (2012) **23**(5):459–63. doi:10.1177/0956797611433336
170. Van Honk J, Tuiten A, Hermans E, Putnam P, Koppeschaar H, Thijssen J, et al. A single administration of testosterone induces cardiac accelerative responses to angry faces in healthy young women. *Behav Neurosci* (2001) **115**(1):238. doi:10.1037/0735-7044.115.1.238
171. DeBold JF, Clemens LG. Aromatization and the induction of male sexual behavior in male, female, and androgenized female hamsters. *Horm Behav* (1978) **11**:401–13. doi:10.1016/0018-506x(78)90040-5
172. Yellon SM, Hutchison JS, Goldman BD. Sexual differentiation of the steroid feedback mechanism regulating follicle-stimulating hormone secretion in the Syrian hamster. *Biol Reprod* (1989) **40**:7–14. doi:10.1095/biolreprod41.1.7
173. Wood RI, Newman SW. Androgen receptor immunoreactivity in the male and female Syrian hamster brain. *J Neurobiol* (1999) **39**(3):359–70. doi:10.1002/(SICI)1097-4695(19990605)39:3<359::AID-NEU3>3.0.CO;2-W
174. Cohen J. *Statistical Power Analysis for the Behavioral Sciences*. 2nd ed. Hillsdale, NJ: Erlbaum (1988).
175. Rosner W, Auchus RJ, Azziz R, Sluss PM, Raff H. Utility, limitations, and pitfalls in measuring testosterone: an endocrine society position statement. *J Clin Endocrinol Metab* (2007) **92**(2):405–13. doi:10.1210/jc.2006-1864
176. Kaufman JM, Vermeulen A. The decline of androgen levels in elderly men and its clinical and therapeutic implications. *Endocr Rev* (2005) **26**(6):833–76. doi:10.1210/er.2004-0013
177. Dreher JC, Meyer-Lindenberg A, Kohn P, Berman KF. Age-related changes in midbrain dopaminergic regulation of the human reward system. *Proc Natl Acad Sci U S A* (2008) **105**(39):15106–11. doi:10.1073/pnas.0802127105
178. Mischel W, Metzner R. Preference for delayed reward as a function of age, intelligence, and length of delay interval. *J Abnorm Soc Psychol* (1962) **64**(6):425. doi:10.1037/h0045046
179. Peper JS, Koolschijn PCM, Crone EA. Development of risk taking: contributions from adolescent testosterone and the orbito-frontal cortex. *J Cogn Neurosci* (2013) **25**(12):2141–50. doi:10.1162/jocn_a_00445
180. Somerville LH, Jones RM, Casey BJ. A time of change: behavioral and neural correlates of adolescent sensitivity to appetitive and aversive environmental cues. *Brain Cogn* (2010) **72**(1):124–33. doi:10.1016/j.bandc.2009.07.003
181. Figner B, Mackinlay RJ, Wilkening F, Weber EU. Affective and deliberative processes in risky choice: age differences in risk taking in the Columbia card task. *J Exp Psychol Learn Mem Cogn* (2009) **35**(3):709. doi:10.1037/a0014983
182. Figner B, Weber EU. Who takes risks when and why? Determinants of risk taking. *Curr Dir Psychol Sci* (2011) **20**(4):211–6. doi:10.1177/0963721411415790
183. Norman RE, Moreau BJP, Welker KM, Carré JM. Trait anxiety moderates the relationship between testosterone responses to competition and aggressive behavior. *Adapt Human Behav Physiol* (2014). doi:10.1007/s40750-014-0016-y
184. Schultheiss OC, Campbell KL, McClelland DC. Implicit power motivation moderates men's testosterone responses to imagined and real dominance success. *Horm Behav* (1999) **36**:234–41. doi:10.1006/hbeh.1999.1542
185. Schultheiss OC, Rhode W. Implicit power motivation predicts men's testosterone changes and implicit learning in a contest situation. *Horm Behav* (2002) **41**:195–202. doi:10.1006/hbeh.2001.1745
186. Carver CS, White TL. Behavioral inhibition, behavioral activation, and affective responses to impending reward and punishment: the BIS/BAS scales. *J Pers Soc Psychol* (1994) **67**(2):319. doi:10.1037/0022-3514.67.2.319
187. Crowe E, Higgins ET. Regulatory focus and strategic inclinations: promotion and prevention in decision-making. *Organ Behav Hum Decis Process* (1997) **69**(2):117–32. doi:10.1006/obhd.1996.2675
188. Hayes AF. *Introduction to Mediation, Moderation, and Conditional Process Analysis: A Regression-based Approach*. New York: Guilford Press (2013).
189. Mazur A. A biosocial model of status in face-to-face primate groups. *Soc Forces* (1985) **64**(2):377–402. doi:10.1093/sf/64.2.377
190. Wingfield JC, Hegner RE, Dufty AM Jr, Ball GF. The "challenge hypothesis": theoretical implications for patterns of testosterone secretion, mating systems, and breeding strategies. *Am Nat* (1990) **136**:829–46. doi:10.1086/285134
191. Goetz SM, Tang L, Thomason ME, Diamond MP, Hariri AR, Carré JM. Testosterone rapidly increases neural reactivity to threat in healthy men: a novel two-step pharmacological challenge paradigm. *Biol Psychiatry* (2014) **76**(4):324–31. doi:10.1016/j.biopsych.2014.01.016
192. Cohen AK. *Delinquent Boys: The Culture of the Gang*. Glencoe, IL: Free Press of Glencoe (1955).
193. Hirschi T. *Causes of Delinquency*. Berkeley, CA: University of California Press (2011).
194. Telzer EH, Fuligni AJ, Lieberman MD, Galván A. Meaningful family relationships: neurocognitive buffers of adolescent risk taking. *J Cogn Neurosci* (2013) **25**(3):374–87. doi:10.1162/jocn_a_00331
195. Telzer EH, Fuligni AJ, Lieberman MD, Miernicki M, Galván A. The quality of adolescents' peer relationships modulates neural sensitivity to risk taking. *Soc Cogn Affect Neurosci* (2014) **10**:389–98. doi:10.1093/scan/nsu064
196. Kapadia F, Siconolfi DE, Barton S, Olivieri B, Lombardo L, Halkitis PN. Social support network characteristics and sexual risk taking among a racially/ethnically diverse sample of young, urban men who have sex with men. *AIDS Behav* (2013) **17**(5):1819–28. doi:10.1007/s10461-013-0468-2
197. Kimberly JA, Serovich JM. The role of family and friend social support in reducing risk behaviors among HIV-positive gay men. *AIDS Educ Prev* (1999) **11**(6):465–75.
198. Baumeister RF, DeWall CN, Ciarocco NJ, Twenge JM. Social exclusion impairs self-regulation. *J Pers Soc Psychol* (2005) **88**(4):589. doi:10.1037/e501232006-005
199. Duclos R, Wan EW, Jiang Y. Show me the honey! Effects of social exclusion on financial risk-taking. *J Consum Res* (2013) **40**(1):122–35. doi:10.1086/668900
200. Harris JA, Rushton JP, Hampson E, Jackson DN. Salivary testosterone and self-report aggressive and pro-social personality characteristics in men and women. *Aggress Behav* (1996) **22**:321–31. doi:10.1002/(SICI)1098-2337(1996)22:5<321::AID-AB1>3.0.CO;2-M
201. van Anders SM, Goldey KL, Kuo PX. The steroid/peptide theory of social bonds: integrating testosterone and peptide responses for classifying social behavioral contexts. *Psychoneuroendocrinology* (2011) **36**:1265–75. doi:10.1016/j.psyneuen.2011.06.001
202. van Anders SM, Tolman RM, Volling BL. Baby cries and nurturance affect testosterone in men. *Horm Behav* (2012) **61**:31–6. doi:10.1016/j.yhbeh.2011.09.012
203. Turan B, Guo J, Boggiano MM, Bedgood D. Dominant, cold, avoidant, and lonely: basal testosterone as a biological marker for an interpersonal style. *J Res Pers* (2014) **50**:84–9. doi:10.1016/j.jrp.2014.03.008
204. Edelstein RS, van Anders SM, Chopik WJ, Goldey KL, Wardecker BM. Dyadic associations between testosterone and relationship quality in couples. *Horm Behav* (2014) **65**(4):401–7. doi:10.1016/j.yhbeh.2014.03.003
205. Boksem MA, Mehta PH, Van den Bergh B, van Son V, Trautmann ST, Roelofs K, et al. Testosterone inhibits trust but promotes reciprocity. *Psychol Sci* (2013) **24**(11):2306–14. doi:10.1177/0956797613495063
206. Grunbaum JA, Tortolero S, Weller N, Gingiss P. Cultural, social, and intrapersonal factors associated with substance use among alternative high school students. *Addict Behav* (2000) **25**(1):145–51. doi:10.1016/s0306-4603(99)00006-4
207. Devlin HC, Zaki J, Ong DC, Gruber J. Not as good as you think? Trait positive emotion is associated with increased self-reported empathy, but decreased empathic performance. *PLoS One* (2014) **9**(10):e110470. doi:10.1371/journal.pone.0110470
208. Forgas JP, East R. On being happy and gullible: mood effects on skepticism and the detection of deception. *J Exp Soc Psychol* (2008) **44**:1362–7. doi:10.1016/j.jesp.2008.04.010
209. Hasler G, Drevets WC, Gould TD, Gotteseman II, Manji HK. Toward constructing an endophenotype strategy for bipolar disorders. *Biol Psychiatry* (2006) **60**(2):93–105. doi:10.1590/S1516-44462006000200003

210. Meyer B, Johnson SL, Winters R. Responsiveness to threat and incentive in bipolar disorder: relations of the BIS/BAS scales with symptoms. *J Psychopathol Behav Assess* (2001) **23**:133–43. doi:10.1023/A:1010929402770
211. Nusslock R, Almeida JRC, Forbes EE, Versace A, Frank E, LaBarbara EJ, et al. Waiting to win: elevated striatal and orbitofrontal cortical activity during reward anticipation in euthymic bipolar disorder adults. *Bipolar Disord* (2012) **14**:249–60. doi:10.1111/j.1399-5618.2012.01012.x
212. Johnson SL. Mania and dysregulation in goal pursuit: a review. *Clin Psychol Rev* (2005) **25**(2):241–62. doi:10.1016/j.cpr.2004.11.002
213. Pizzagalli DA, Goetz E, Ostacher M, Iosifescu DV, Perlis RH. Euthymic patients with bipolar disorder show decreased reward learning on a probabilistic reward task. *Biol Psychiatry* (2008) **64**(2):162–8. doi:10.1016/j.biopsych.2007.12.001
214. Gruber J, Eidelman P, Johnson SL, Smith B, Harvey AG. Hooked on a feeling: rumination about positive and negative emotion in inter-episode bipolar disorder. *J Abnorm Psychol* (2011) **120**(4):956–61. doi:10.1037/a0023667
215. Gruber J, Culver JL, Johnson SL, Nam J, Keller KL, Ketter TK. Do positive emotions predict symptomatic change in bipolar disorder? *Bipolar Disord* (2009) **11**:330–6. doi:10.1111/j.1399-5618.2009.00679.x
216. Weiss EL, Bowers MB, Mazure CM. Testosterone-patch-induced psychotic mania. *Am J Psychiatry* (1999) **156**(6):969–969. doi:10.1176/ajp.156.6.969
217. Coccaro EF, McCloskey MS, Fitzgerald DA, Phan KL. Amygdala and orbitofrontal reactivity to social threat in individuals with impulsive aggression. *Biol Psychiatry* (2007) **62**(2):168–78. doi:10.1016/j.biopsych.2006.08.024
218. Josephs RA, Sellers JG, Newman ML, Mehta PH. The mismatch effect: when testosterone and status are at odds. *J Pers Soc Psychol* (2006) **90**(6):999. doi:10.1037/0022-3514.90.6.999
219. Newman ML, Sellers JG, Josephs RA. Testosterone, cognition, and social status. *Horm Behav* (2005) **47**(2):205–11. doi:10.1016/j.yhbeh.2004.09.008
220. Mehta PH, Jones AC, Josephs RA. The social endocrinology of dominance: basal testosterone predicts cortisol changes and behavior following victory and defeat. *J Pers Soc Psychol* (2008) **94**(6):1078. doi:10.1037/0022-3514.94.6.1078
221. Zilioli S, Watson NV. Winning isn't everything: mood and testosterone regulate the cortisol response in competition. *PLoS One* (2013) **8**(1):e52582. doi:10.1371/journal.pone.0052582
222. Schlüter T, Winz O, Henkel K, Prinz S, Rademacher L, Schmaljohann J, et al. The impact of dopamine on aggression: an [18F]-FDOPA PET Study in healthy males. *J Neurosci* (2013) **33**(43):16889–96. doi:10.1523/jneurosci.1398-13.2013
223. O'Sullivan SS, Evans AH, Quinn NP, Lawrence AD, Lees AJ. Reckless generosity in Parkinson's disease. *Mov Disord* (2010) **25**(2):221–3. doi:10.1002/mds.22687
224. Taute H, McQuitty S. Feeling good! Doing good! An exploratory look at the impulsive purchase of the social good. *J Mark Theory Pract* (2004) **12**:16–27. doi:10.1086/662199
225. Eisenegger C, Naef M, Snozzi R, Heinrichs M, Fehr E. Prejudice and truth about the effect of testosterone on human bargaining behaviour. *Nature* (2009) **463**(7279):356–9. doi:10.1038/nature08711
226. Van Honk J, Montoya ER, Bos PA, van Vugt M, Terburg D. New evidence on testosterone and cooperation. *Nature* (2012) **485**(7399):E4–5. doi:10.1038/nature11136
227. Mikulincer ME, Shaver PR. *Prosocial Motives, Emotions, and Behavior: The Better Angels of Our Nature*. Washington, DC: American Psychological Association (2010).
228. Eshel N, Nelson EE, Blair RJ, Pine DS, Ernst M. Neural substrates of choice selection in adults and adolescents: development of the ventrolateral prefrontal and anterior cingulate cortices. *Neuropsychologia* (2007) **45**(6):1270–9. doi:10.1016/j.neuropsychologia.2006.10.004
229. Spielberg JM, Forbes EE, Ladouceur CD, Worthman CM, Olino TM, Ryan ND, et al. Pubertal testosterone influences threat-related amygdala-orbitofrontal coupling. *Soc Cogn Affect Neurosci* (2014) **10**:408–15. doi:10.1093/scan/nsu062
230. van Wingen G, Mattern C, Verkes RJ, Buitelaar J, Fernández G. Testosterone reduces amygdale – orbitofrontal cortex coupling. *Psychoneuroendocrinology* (2010) **35**(1):105–13. doi:10.1093/scan/nsu062
231. Hofmann W, Friese M, Strack F. Impulse and self-control from a dual-systems perspective. *Perspect Psychol Sci* (2009) **4**(2):162–76. doi:10.1111/j.1745-6924.2009.01116.x

14

Molecular cloning, sequencing and tissue expression of vasotocin and isotocin precursor genes from Ostariophysian catfishes: phylogeny and evolutionary considerations in teleosts

Putul Banerjee [1], Radha Chaube [2] and Keerikkattil P. Joy [1]*

[1] Department of Zoology, Centre of Advanced Study, Banaras Hindu University, Varanasi, India, [2] Zoology Department, Mahila Mahavidhylaya, Banaras Hindu University, Varanasi, India

Edited by:
Hubert Vaudry, University of Rouen, France

Reviewed by:
Hervé Tostivint, Natural History Museum, France
Leo T. O. Lee, The University of Hong Kong, China

***Correspondence:**
Keerikkattil P. Joy, Department of Zoology, Centre of Advanced Study, Faculty of Science, Banaras Hindu University, Varanasi 221005, India
kpjoybhu@gmail.com

Basic and neutral neurohypophyseal (NH) nonapeptides have evolved from vasotocin (VT) by a gene duplication at the base of the gnathostome lineage. In teleosts, VT and IT are the basic and neutral peptides, respectively. In the present study, VT and IT precursor genes of *Heteropneustes fossilis* and *Clarias batrachus* (Siluriformes, Ostariophysi) were cloned and sequenced. The channel catfish *Icatalurus punctatus* NH precursor sequences were obtained from EST database. The catfish NH sequences were used along with the available Acanthopterygii and other vertebrate NH precursor sequences to draw phylogenetic inference on the evolutionary history of the teleost NH peptides. Synteny analysis of the NH gene loci in various teleost species was done to complement the phylogenetic analysis. In *H. fossilis,* the NH transcripts were also sequenced from the ovary. The cloned genes and the deduced precursor proteins showed conserved characteristics of the NH nonapeptide precursors. The genes are expressed in brain and ovary (follicular envelope) of *H. fossilis* with higher transcript abundance in the brain. The addition of the catfish sequences in the phylogenetic analysis revealed that the VT and IT precursors of the species-rich superorders of teleosts have a distinct phylogenetic history with the Acanthopterygii VT and IT precursors sharing a less evolutionary distance and the Ostariophysi VT and IT having a greater evolutionary distance. The genomic location of VT and IT precursors, and synteny analysis of the NH loci lend support to the phylogenetic inference and suggest a footprint of fish- specific whole genome duplication (3R) and subsequent diploidization in the NH loci. The VT and IT precursor genes are most likely lineage-specific paralogs resulting from differential losses of the 3R NH paralogs in the two superorders. The independent yet consistent retention of VT and IT in the two superorders might be directed by a stringent ligand-receptor selectivity.

Keywords: catfish, cloning, phylogeny, vasotocin-isotocin precursors, synteny analysis

Introduction

The neurohypophyseal (NH) nonapeptides are an evolutionarily old family which is believed to have originated much before the vertebrates, as one of the first neurotransmitters in the archetype metazoan nervous system (Grimmelikhuijzen et al., 2002). Starting from the most primitive metazoan- the cnidarians, the presence of nonapeptide homologs has been documented in several nonvertebrate phyla (Grimmelikhuijzen et al., 1982; Cruz et al., 1987; Proux et al., 1987; Satake et al., 1999; Takuwa-Kwodo et al., 2003; Kawada et al., 2008; Stafflinger et al., 2008). In vertebrates, studies are relatively extensive and the nonapeptide precursor genes have been cloned from several vertebrate groups: cyclostomes (Lane et al., 1988; Suzuki et al., 1995; Gwee et al., 2009), cartilaginous fish (Hyodo et al., 2004; Gwee et al., 2009), teleosts (Heierhorst et al., 1989; Morley et al., 1990; Hyodo et al., 1991; Suzuki et al., 1992; Venkatesh and Brenner, 1995; Warne et al., 2000), lungfishes (Hyodo et al., 1997), coelacanth (Gwee et al., 2008), amphibians (Nojiri et al., 1987; Searcy et al., 2009), reptiles (Montefiano et al., 2001), and birds (Hamann et al., 1992). This has complemented earlier works of characterization of peptide principles of the neurohypophysis by chromatographic methods and has provided useful insights into the distribution of the peptides in different vertebrate species, their precursor structure and evolution. The nonapeptides are synthesized as part of a large precursor molecule that undergo post-translational processing to release the nine amino acid hormone with two half cysteine residues at the first and sixth positions forming a disulphide bridge, and a cysteine- rich protein called neurophysin (Acher, 1996). Neurophysin aids in proper folding of the precursor and its sorting into secretory vesicles (de Bree et al., 2000). In vertebrates, about 15 nonapeptides are known till date. They are classified into two families on the basis of the amino acid at the 8th position, as the basic and neutral peptide families. Each vertebrate possesses at least two peptides, one each from the two families except cyclostomes, where only the basic peptide representative vasotocin (VT) is documented (Gwee et al., 2009). This has led to a widely accepted theory that the VT precursor gene is the ancestor of all vertebrate nonapeptide precursor genes, and has given rise to the two lineages following an event of duplication early in the vertebrate evolution probably at the base of the gnathostome lineage. Evolutionarily too, the two peptide families follow distinct lineages with VT representing the common basic peptide in all nonmammalian vertebrates to be replaced by vasopressin (VP) in mammals, while isotocin (IT) is the neutral peptide in teleosts, mesotocin (MT) in lobe-finned fishes and noneutherian tetrapods, and oxytocin (OT) in eutherians. In elasmobranchs, a host of different neutral peptide homologs has been reported which is in contrast with the remarkable stability in the type and numbers of nonapeptides in any other group of Vertebrata (Acher, 1996). Presence of more than two neurohypophyseal peptides has been reported from groups like elasmobranchs, amphibians, and metatherians (Chauvet et al., 1983, 1984, 1985; Rouille et al., 1988, 1989; Parry et al., 2000; Hyodo et al., 2004). In teleosts, VT and IT have been reported as the basic and neutral hormone representatives, respectively. Larhammar et al. (2009) emphasized the need for simplifying the nomenclature with the original names VP for the basic peptides and OT for all neutral peptides.

The two evolutionary lines of basic and neutral nonapeptides across vertebrates represent a contrasting picture in the frequency of substitutions in the 9 amino acid (aa) hormone. In the basic lineage, there have been lesser substitutions than that in the neutral line, as evident from the distribution of the peptides in vertebrates. In fact, the number of cognate receptors for the two peptide families is also contrasting. While the stable basic nonapeptide line has a diverse repertoire of at least five types of cognate receptors (V1A, V1B, V2A, V2B, and V2C), the neutral nonapeptide series has a single type (OTR) in all vertebrate groups (Ocampo Daza et al., 2012; Yagamuchi et al., 2012; Lagman et al., 2013). All types of receptors are present in the early gnathostomes, the cartilaginous fish (Yagamuchi et al., 2012) suggesting that the ligand-receptor selectivity might have been established very early in the vertebrate evolution and it is the co-evolution of the hormone with its cognate receptors which has maintained the two families of basic and neutral nonapeptides, and allowed only a basic amino acid substitution at the 8th position in the basic line and a neutral amino acid substitution at the 8th position in the neutral line. While, the ligand- receptor selectivity might have directed the evolution only in the 9 aa hormone part; the larger neurophysin region is not under this evolutionary pressure. Therefore, to know the evolutionary history of the NH precursors especially in the light of recurrent local and global duplication events occurring throughout the vertebrate history, there is a need to do a phylogenetic study over the entire precursor rather than considering the distribution of peptides in different vertebrate groups.

Teleosts had undergone a third round of whole genome duplication, (3R) (Meyer and Schartl, 1999; Christoffels et al., 2004; Jaillon et al., 2004) in addition to the two vertebrate-specific whole genome duplications. After the 3R in teleosts, there was diploidization by the loss of 3R paralogs. These losses of the 3R paralogs were different in various groups of teleosts (Garcia de la serrana et al., 2014). Even in such a scenario, the consistency in the number and type of nonapeptides in teleosts is noteworthy. However, the teleost NH precursors available in the public database are mostly sequences from the species-rich superorder Acanthopterygii while only few nonapeptide precursor sequences from the other species-rich group, the superorder Ostariophysi are available. The Acanthopterygii and Ostariophysi have undergone independent adaptive radiations (Santini et al., 2009), and are known to have suffered differential losses of 3R paralogs. Therefore, it is pertinent to have sequence information from more species representing all groups in Teleostei, particularly the superorder Ostariophysi to understand the evolution of the NH precursor genes in teleosts.

Previous studies from our laboratory have shown a well-developed and highly organized VT system in the Asian air-breathing catfish *Heteropneustes fossilis*. VT was characterized in both brain and ovary of the catfish with seasonal changes (Singh and Joy, 2008), and has been shown to be involved in reproductive functions such as steroidogenesis, oocyte maturation, oocyte hydration, ovulation and prostaglandin secretion (Singh and Joy, 2009b, 2010, 2011; Joy and Singh,

2013). IT is less effective in influencing these events. Three VT receptors have been cloned from the catfish V1a1 (accession no.KF434615.1), V1a2 (accession no.KF434616.1), and V2A (accession no.KF434617.1), which display a wide tissue distribution (Rawat et al., 2015). All the three receptors are expressed in the brain and ovary, which are the two major sites of VT production.

The catfish *H. fossilis* holds an important phylogenetic position as it is believed to be the sole survivor of an old clade that went extinct at the K-T (Cretaceous-Tertiary transition period) boundary (Jansen et al., 2006) when a major extinction event took place due to severe volcanic activity (Deccan traps) in the Asian region. This might have severely polluted and deoxygenated the inland water bodies and only fish with air-breathing apparatus survived. Air-breathing habit also demands a shift in osmoregulation and fluid homeostasis in which apart from other systems, the NH nonapeptides play a key role. In view of the important taxonomic and phylogenetic position of *H. fossilis* and its air-breathing habit, molecular characterization of the NH peptide genes as a follow on of earlier anatomical and physiological studies on VT has been attempted in the present work. The sequence information was also extended to *Clarias batrachus,* another air- breathing catfish, and used in the phylogenetic analysis. The catfish NH precursor sequence information from the present study will add to the information pool of teleost nonapeptides from a group other than the superorder Acanthopterygii and allow discussing the phylogeny of the vertebrate NH nonapeptides in the light of 3R and subsequent diploidization in teleosts. A tissue distribution profile for these genes was also carried out since VT was described in the catfish ovary earlier.

Materials and Methods

Animal Collection and Acclimation

Adult *H. fossilis* (40–50 g) were collected from local fish markets in Varanasi. They were maintained in the laboratory for 48 h under natural photoperiod (13.0 L: 11.0 D) and temperature (25 ± 2°C) to overcome stress due to transportation and fed daily with goat liver *ad libitum*. Adult *C. batrachus* were obtained in the resting phase for the cloning work. The fish were weighed and sacrificed by decapitation. All experiments were performed in accordance with the guidelines of the Animal Ethics Committee, Banaras Hindu University, Varanasi.

Chemicals and Reagents

Guanidine thiocyanate—phenol solution (Qiagen), Revert-Aid H Minus First Strand cDNA Synthesis Kit (Fermentas), 2X PCR Master Mix (Fermentas), DNase (Ambion) and veriquest SYBR green qPCR master mix (affymetrix) were purchased through local suppliers. Agarose, Tris base, Glacial acetic acid, EDTA–Na2 and other chemicals were of molecular grade, purchased from E-Merck, India. LB broth, LB Agar, ampicillin, X-Gal and IPTG were purchased from Himedia, India. Hyaluronidase type IV was purchased from Sigma-Aldrich, India. The primers used were synthesized by Integrated DNA Technology, India.

Cloning of VT and IT genes from *H. fossilis* and *C. batrachus*

For cloning of VT, an approach of first isolating partial VT cDNA using degenerate PCR (polymerase chain reaction) followed by 3′ and 5′ Rapid Amplification of cDNA ends (RACE) to obtain the full length VT cDNA sequence was applied. Total RNA from the brain of acclimatized female catfish in the resting phase of the reproductive cycle was prepared by the single-step method of RNA isolation (Chomczynski and Sacchi, 1987) by acid guanidium thiocyanate-phenol-chloroform extraction using Qiazol (Qiagen) as the monophasic lysis buffer. Five μg total RNA was reverse- transcribed using random hexamer primers and Revert Aid M-MuLV reverse transcriptase in a 20 μL reaction volume (first strand cDNA synthesis kit, Fermantas) using the manufacturer's protocol. One μL of the resulting cDNA was used to amplify partial VT cDNA in 25 μL reaction volume using 2 X PCR master mix (Fermentas) and VT degenerate forward primer and VT degenerate reverse primer in a cycling condition of one cycle of 95°C, 5 min; then 35 cycles of 95°C, 30 s; 57°C, 30 s; 72°C, 1 min; and a final 7-min elongation at 72°C. The degenerate primers were designed using the software iCODEHOP (COnsensus-DEgenerate Hybrid Oligonucleotide Primers), in which teleost VT precursor sequences were used as inputs (**Table 1**). The resulting 145 bp partial VT amplicon was purified using Nucleo-pore PCR clean- up gel extraction kit (Genetix) and sequenced taking services of Eurofin genomics, Bangalore, India. For obtaining full length sequence, 3′ RACE was done for which total RNA from the brain was reverse-transcribed using oligo dT anchor primer and Revert Aid M-MuLV reverse transcriptase. One μL of the resulting cDNA was amplified using a VT H FP (corresponding to the hormone moiety), designed from the partial sequence and anchor primer to obtain a 700 bp 3′ RACE amplicon, which was cloned and sequenced. This sequence was utilized for designing two gene-specific nested reverse primers to do 5′ RACE. Total RNA from the brain was reverse-transcribed using the outer gene specific VT RP and Revert Aid M-MuLV reverse transcriptase. The resulting cDNA was purified using the Nucleo-pore PCR clean- up gel extraction kit (Genetix) to remove residual dNTPs. The purified cDNA was dA tailed using dATP and terminal transferase. The dA tailed cDNA was used for PCR amplification using the nested RP 2 primer and oligo dT anchor primer. The 5′ RACE amplicon was purified, cloned and sequenced. Full length VT cDNA sequence was submitted to the GenBank with the accession no. JX035928.1

For cloning IT precursor cDNA, total RNA from the brain was reverse-transcribed using an oligo dT anchor primer and Revert Aid M-MuLV reverse transcriptase. One μL of the resulting cDNA was PCR amplified using a sense or forward primer IT H FP designed from the IT hormone moiety and anchor primer, following the 3′ RACE protocol. The resulting 700 bp amplicon was sequenced taking services from Eurofin genomics. To get the 5′ end of the precursor cDNA, 5′ RACE was done. Total RNA from the brain was reverse- transcribed using an outer reverse or antisense primer, RP1 (designed over a conserved region of the neurohypophyseal peptide neurophysin) and Revert Aid M-MuLV reverse transcriptase. The resulting cDNA was

TABLE 1 | List of primers used for cloning and qPCR of vasotocin and isotocin precursors.

Primers	Sequences
VT d FP	TCCGCTTGTTACATCCARAAYTGYCC
VT d RP	ACATCCCAGTCCCTCTCCRCARCDAT
VT H FP	GTTACATCCAGAACTGCCCCAGA
VT FP	TGTTACATCCAGAACTGCCCCAGA
VT RP	CAGCCCAGTCCTTCTCCACAGCA
RP1	TTTATCTCCAGGACCGCAAG
RP2	CAGGACCGCAAGACATACAC
VT UTR FP	GTCCAGTGAGAGACAGACCTCCGG
IT H FP	ACATCTCCAACTGTCCCATC
IT UTR FP	CATCAGCTACTGAAGCTACTGATTCGT
Oligo dT anchor primer	GACCACGCGTATCGATGTCGACTTTTTTTTTTTTTTTTV
Anchor primer	GACCACGCGTATCGATGTCGAC
IT FP	TCAATCTTCTGCATGCTGTGTCT
IT RP	CACACGCCATGCACTGTCTATTG
β actin FP	TGGCCGTGACCTGACTGAC
β actin RP	CCTGCTCAAAGTCAAGAGCGAC

purified and dA tailed. The dA tailed cDNA was used for PCR amplification using an overlapping and nested antisense primer RP2 and oligodT anchor primer. The resulting 200 bp 5′ RACE amplicon was ligated into pGEMT vector (promega kit), following the manufacturer's protocol and transformed into the *E. coli* DH5 α competent cells. Transformed cells were plated into LB Agar solid medium containing ampicillin, X- Gal and IPTG to select positive transformants and blue-white screening was done for recombinant colonies. Plasmids from white colonies (colonies transformed with recombinant plasmids) were extracted by alkaline lysis method and sequenced. Sequence information from the IT precursor containing inserts (as known by *in silico* translation of the insert sequences) was used to design a sense primer from the 5′ UTR region (IT UTR FP), followed by 3′ RACE with this primer to obtain the entire IT precursor sequence, which was submitted to the GenBank with the accession no. JX669009.1.

Partial sequences of *C. batrachus* VT and IT precursors were obtained by 3′ RACE with the forward primers VT H FP and IT H FP (the same used for *H. fossilis*), to obtain a sequence read from the hormone region till the 3′ untranslated region. The primer details are given (**Table 1**).

Sequencing of VT and IT Transcripts from Ovary

Since the VT and IT transcripts are less abundant in the ovarian follicles, a semi-nested 3′ RACE was done to get a single, sharp amplification of the gene transcripts. Briefly, it included a primary PCR using VT UTR FP, IT UTR FP spanning the 5′ UTR region of VT and IT genes, respectively and anchor primer to amplify 1 μL of follicular cDNA (made by reverse transcription of RNA using oligodT anchor primer), followed by a secondary PCR using VT H FP, IT H FP and anchor primer to amplify1 μL of the primary PCR product. The amplicons from the secondary PCR was purified and sequenced.

Data Mining for Phylogenetic Analysis

The NH nonapeptide precursor sequences of species representing most vertebrate classes were tried to be included in the phylogenetic analysis. The sequences were procured from the GenBank. Details of the sequences of the species with accession numbers are given in Supplementary Table 1. For procuring the NH precursors of *Ictalurus punctatus*, a BLAST search against the *Ictalurus* EST database (Lu et al., 2010) was done using the *H. fossilis* VT and IT sequences as queries. The identities of the putative VT and IT precursor mRNAs obtained were confirmed by *in silico* translation of the sequences. The spotted gar *Lepisosteus oculatus*, Holostei is a basal actinopterygian species representing a pre 3R genome. The neurohypophyseal nonapeptide precursor sequences of this species were procured by BLAST searches in its Nucleotide database and analyzed.

Phylogenetic Analysis

Phylogenetic trees were constructed using the Neighbor- Joining (NJ) and Maximum-Likelihood (ML) method. Evolutionary distances were computed using the Poisson correction method for rate of amino acid substitution. All phylogenetic studies were done using the software MEGA 6 (Tamura et al., 2013). In addition to the calculation of evolutionary distance of precursor sequences within and between species, the sequences were grouped according to the taxonomic units for calculation of evolutionary distance between groups (**Table 2**). Keeping in view of the enormous species diversity, the teleost sequences of the two superorders Acanthopterygii and Ostariophysi were independently treated. Multiple sequence alignment used for the tree construction and distance calculation was the same and was done in MEGA6 using Clustal W parameters. Gonnet protein weight matrix with gap opening and gap extension penalties of 10 and 0.2 respectively was used for the alignment. The alignment is provided in a Supplementary data sheet 1.

Analysis of VT and IT Genomic Location and Synteny Analysis

The nonapeptide gene-containing chromosome blocks of spotted gar and representative teleost species were obtained from the NCBI and Ensembl genome browser. Fugu, medaka, tilapia, and stickleback belong to the teleost superorder Acanthopterygii, and zebrafish and cavefish belong to the superorder Ostariophysi. The selection of the chromosome blocks from Ensembl database was based both on searching the genome assemblies for the nonapeptide genes by named searches as well as BLAST searches using teleost nonapeptides as queries. This is to ensure that nonapeptide loci are obtained even in the species where the genes are not annotated. The chromosome blocks were obtained from the NCBI database mostly by navigating the genomic context of the genes. Blocks obtained from both Ensembl and NCBI were tallied for each species and a consensus assembly of genes on the blocks was arrived at by filling in for the nonannotated genes in one of the databases from information obtained from the other. Apart from the nonapeptide genes, the assemblies were also searched for the genes linked with the nonapeptide genes and the additional chromosomal blocks harboring these genes (paralogous to the linked genes), if distinct from the

TABLE 2 | Details of the taxonomic groups and the species included in each for the phylogenetic distance calculation between groups.

S. No	Taxonomic group	Species
1	Cyclostome VT	*Lethenteron camtschaticum*, *Eptatretus burgeri*
2	Acanthopterygii VT	*Thalassoma bifasciatum*, *Parajulis poecilepterus*, *Halichoeres trimaculatus*, *Sparus aurata*, *Takifugu rubripes*, *Platichthys flesus*, *Epinephelus coioides*, *Amphiprion melanopus*, *Oryzias latipes*, *Cyprinodon variegates*, *Haplochromis burtoni*
3	Ostariophysi VT	*Heteopneustes fossilis*, *Clarias batrachus* and *Ictalurus punctatus*, *Danio rerio*, *Astyanas mexicanus* (LOC103042813, LOC103030472)
5	Cartilaginous fish VT	*Triakis scyllium*, *Callorhinchus milli*
6	Lungfish VT	*Neoceratodus forsteri*, *Protopterus annactens*
7	Coelacanth VT	*Latimeria menadoensis*
8	Acanthopterygii IT	*Platichthys flesus*, *Sparus aurata*, *Halichoeres trimaculatus*, *Parajulis poecilepterus*, *Takifugu rubripes*, *Oryzias latipes*, *Xiphophorus maculatus*, *Amphiprion melanopus*, *Haplochromis burtoni*
8	Ostariophysi IT	*Heteopneustes fossilis*, *Clarias batrachus*, *Ictalurus punctatus*, *Danio rerio*, *Asatyanax mexicanus* (LOC103043649, LOC103044969)
10	Cartilaginous fish neutral hormone precursors	*Triakis scyllium phasitocin*, *Triakis scyllium asvatocin*, *Torpedo marmorata isotocin*, *Callorhinchus milii oxytocin*
11	Lungfish MT	*Neoceratodus forsteri*, *Protopterus annectens*
12	Coelacanth MT	*Latimeria menadoensis*
12	Amphibian VT	*Bufo japonicus*, *Plethodon shermani*, *Taricha granulosa*, *Typhlonectes natans*
13	Amphibian MT	*Bufo japonicus*, *Typhlonectes natans*, *Taricha granulosa*
14	Reptilian VT	*Podarcis siculus*
15	Reptile MT	*Podarcis siculus*
16	Avian VT	*Taeniopygia guttata*, *Coturnix coturnix*, *Gallus gallus*
17	Avian MT	*Taeniopygia guttata*
18	Mammalian VP	*Homo sapiens*, *Rattus norvegicus*
19	Mammalian OT	*Homo sapiens*, *Rattus norvegicus*

The accession numbers of the sequences are given in Supplementary Table 1.

nonapeptide loci. Additionally, the loci of the linked genes in human were obtained and used as a reference tetrapod assembly for comparison of conserved synteny.

Analysis of VT and IT Precursor Gene Expression

A two step qPCR was conducted to show tissue and seasonal expression of VT and IT genes. For tissue expression profile, various tissues viz. brain, gills, liver, muscle, kidney, and gonads were collected. For the ovarian tissue sample, the follicles were collected from the post-vitellogenic ovary and the follicular layer was separated from oocyte using hyaluronidase treatment (Mishra and Joy, 2006). Briefly, the protocol included treatment of a batch of about 500 follicles with 0.3% hyaluronidase (Type IV) for 5 min. The isolated follicular envelope (granulosa and theca cells) and the denuded oocytes were used for the expression studies. For seasonal expression, brain and ovary was collected during the different reproductive phases, resting (November–January), preparatory (February–April), pre-spawning (May–June), spawning (July–August) and post-spawning (September–October). About 100 mg tissues were used for extraction of total RNA by the single-step method of RNA isolation. To remove genomic DNA contamination from the preparation, DNAase (Ambion) treatment (2 units/10 μg RNA) was given and subsequently DNAase was heat inactivated at 75°C in presence of EDTA. RNA purity was checked by A_{260}/A_{280} ratio. Samples having a ratio above 1.8 were only considered for reverse transcription. Two μg of the total RNA was reverse-transcribed using random hexamer primers and Revert Aid M-MuLV reverse transcriptase in a 20 μL reaction volume (first strand cDNA synthesis kit, Fermantas) using the manufacturer's protocol. The resulting cDNA was diluted 10 times and 1 μL was used in a PCR reaction of 20 μL containing veriquest SYBR green 2X master mix and VT/IT FP and IT FP/ RP using manufacturer's protocol in an Applied Biosystem 7500 machine with a thermal condition of 50°C for 2 min, 95°C for 10 min, followed by 40 cycles of 95°C for 15 s and 60°C for 1 min. The specificity of the PCR product was checked by dissociation curve analysis of the amplicon and was also checked by agarose gel electrophoresis. The relative gene expression in different tissues and across different reproductive seasons was expressed using the comparative CT method with the catfish β-actin (accession number FJ409641.2), used as the endogenous control. The resting phase brain cDNA was taken as the calibrator sample for relative quantity calculation (Livak and Schmittgen, 2001). Each reaction was set up in duplicate and the average CT value was taken for calculation. Graphs were plotted with the mean RQ (relative quantity) values ($2^{-\Delta\Delta CT}$) of five fish and represented as mean ± SEM. The results were analyzed by One-Way ANOVA ($p < 0.001$), followed by Newman-Keuls' test ($p < 0.05$) for statistical significance.

Results

Sequence Analysis of VT and IT Precursors from *H. fossilis*

The isolated full length cDNA of the HfVT precursor is 618 bp long with a cds from 60 to 524 bp and encodes a VT precursor of 155 amino acids (aa; **Figure 1**; Supplementary Figure 1A). The deduced VT precursor codes for a signal peptide (1–20 aa), a 9 aa hormone moiety (21–29 aa), a 3 aa enzymatic processing site (30–32 aa) and a 122 aa neurophysin (34–155 aa). The central part of the neurophysin (40–118 aa) is highly conserved and belongs to the hormone_5 superfamily (NCBI CDD accession *pfam00184*) of the neurohypophyseal hormones (NCBI CDD accession *smart00003*). There are 14 cysteine residues in this region (42, 45, 53, 59, 60, 66, 76, 86, 93, 100, 106, 107, 112, and 118). The C- terminal part of the neurophysin (119–155 aa) is poorly conserved except for the presence of a leucine-rich region "LLLRILH" (141–146 aa) (**Figure 1**) that is conserved across all vertebrate groups. All these features conform to the typical features of the neurohypophyseal hormones. There is no putative site for N- linked glycosylation in C-terminal domain corresponding to copeptin, making it akin to other teleost neurohypophyseal hormone precursors, unlike lungfish and tetrapod hormone precursors.

The isolated HfIT precursor cDNA is of 708 bp long with a cds from 56 to 508 bp and encodes the hormone precursor of 151 aa (**Figure 1**; Supplementary Figure 1B). Similar to the VT precursor, the putative IT precursor encodes for a signal peptide (1–20 aa), a hormone moiety of 9 aa (21–29 aa), enzymatic processing signal (30–32 aa) and a 118 aa neurophysin (34–151 aa). Further, the central part of neurophysin (40–118 bp) is highly conserved and belongs to the hormone_5 superfamily (NCBI CDD accession pfam00184) of the neurohypophyseal hormones (NCBI CDD accession smart 00003) and there are 14 cystine residues in this region (42, 45, 53, 59, 60, 66, 76, 86, 93, 100, 106, 107, 112, 118) (**Figure 1**). The presence of an extended C-terminal part homologous to the C- terminal part of the VT precursors and the mammalian vasopressin-associated copeptin makes it similar to other IT precursor but dissimilar to other neutral peptide precursors like MT and OT precursors and other cartilaginous fish neutral hormone precursors which lack an extended C-terminal region. The C- terminal part of the neurophysin (119–151 aa) is poorly conserved except for the presence of a leucine- rich region "LLKLLHL" (138–144 aa), which is a signature of the C-terminal region of the neurohypophyseal hormone precursors. There is neither a dibasic cleavage site nor putative site for N- linked glycosylation in this region similar to the VT precursor.

Sequence Analysis of Other Catfish VT and IT Precursors

The cloned partial sequences of *C. batrachus* (Cb) VT and IT cDNA extend from the N-terminal neurophysin coding region to the 3′ UTR (Supplementary Figures 1C,D). The putative precursors, like the *H. fossilis* precursors, have all the essential features of the neurohypophyseal precursor proteins, with a

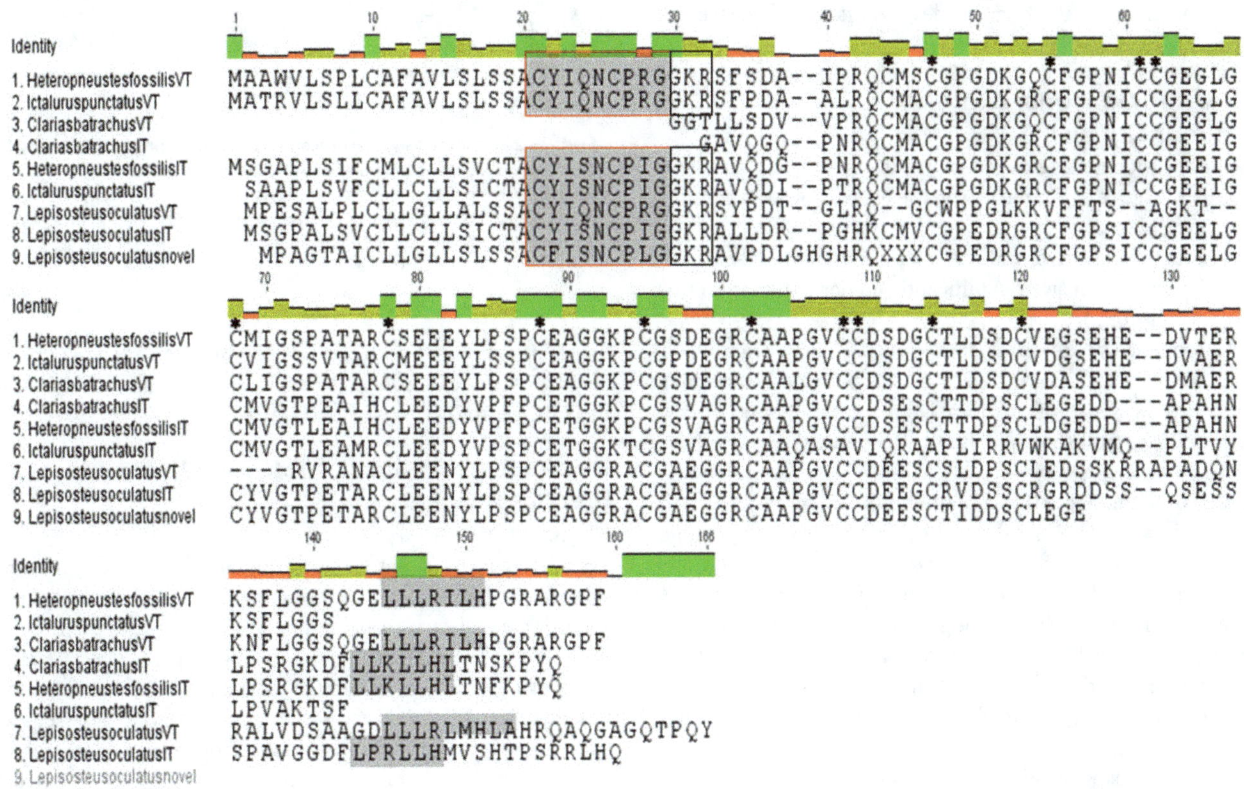

FIGURE 1 | Multiple sequence alignment of predicted structures of VT and IT precursors of *H. fossilis, C. batrachus, I. punctatus*, and spotted gar. Hormone moiety and leucine- rich box in the C-terminal neurophysin are shaded and "GKR" (enzymatic processing signal) is boxed. The cysteine residues have been star marked. The *C. batrachus* sequences are partial at the N-terminal without the signal peptide and hormone moiety.

central conserved neurophysin having 14 cysteine residues. The poorly conserved C- terminal regions have leucine-rich boxes, "LLLRILH" in the VT precursor and "LLKLLHL" in the IT precursor (**Figure 1**).

In silico translation of the clones, recognized as the neurohypophyseal hormone precursors from the EST database of *I. punctatus* (Ip) by BLAST reveals that they indeed code for VT and IT precursors. The sequence read of the putative VT precursor clone (acc. no. BM495247) starts from 5′ UTR region and ends in the C-terminal part of the neurophysin. On the other hand, the putative IT precursor clone (acc. no. BE213165) sequence extends from the signal peptide region to the neurophysin (Supplementary Figures 1E,F and **Figure 1**).

The 3′ UTR region of the *H. fossilis* VT gene has a long stretch of 19 CA repeats. The *C. batrachus* VT gene has only 4 CA repeats in the 3′ UTR at approximately the same position as the *H. fossilis* VT gene (Supplementary Figures 1A,C).

Analysis of Spotted Gar Neurohypophyseal Nonapeptides

BLAST search revealed that the spotted gar has three neurohypophyseal nonapeptides, VT as the basic nonapeptide (XM 006626529.2) and two nonapeptides in the neutral family, IT (XM 006626499.1) and a novel peptide (XM 006626523.1, 1–366 nt) with a unique hormone "CFISNCPLG" is present. While the spotted gar IT has an extended C-terminal with a leucine- rich core, the novel nonapeptide has a short C-terminal like all other neutral nonapeptide precursors of vertebrates (**Figure 1**).

Tissue and Seasonal Expression of VT and IT Precursor Genes

The nonapeptide genes expressed only in the brain and ovary of the catfish (**Figure 2**). In the ovary, the expression was confined to the follicular envelope and not in oocytes. There was no expression in the gill, liver, kidney, testis and muscle. The VT and IT mRNA expressions were significantly higher in the brain than the ovary (**Figure 2**).

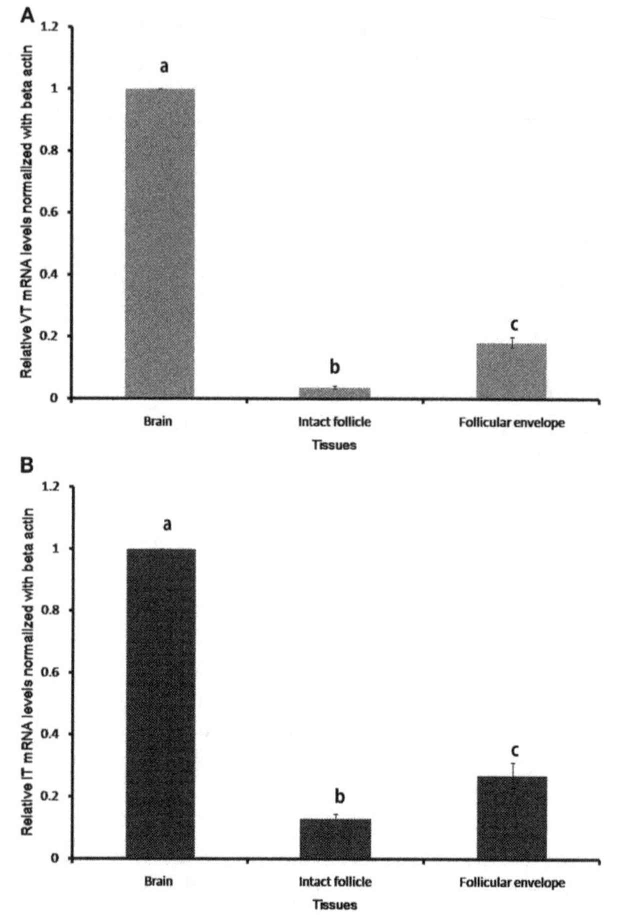

FIGURE 2 | Relative tissue expression levels of VT precursor (A) and IT precursor (B). Graphs were plotted with the mean RQ values ($2^{-\Delta\Delta CT}$) of expression in brain, intact follicle and follicular envelope. The RQ values (mean $\pm$ SEM; $n = 5$ fish each) were calculated with the resting phase brain cDNA as the calibrator. Groups with different alphabets show significant variations in the expression levels.

The sequence reads of the semi-nested 3′ RACE amplicons of VT and IT in the ovary were partial but good enough to indicate the presence of functional transcripts of the genes in ovarian follicles (not shown). Also, the sequences were similar to the brain transcripts, pointing to the same gene responsible for synthesis of the nonapeptides in both brain and ovary.

VT and IT expressions showed significant seasonal changes both in the brain and ovary (**Figure 3**). In the brain, the VT expression was low in the resting phase and increased in the preparatory, pre-spawning and spawning phases. The expression remained high in the post-spawning phase similar to the preparatory and pre-spawning phases. The expression of IT precursor was similar to that of the VT precursor but it decreased sharply in the post-spawning phase as in the resting phase.

The highest expression was observed in the spawning phase for both the genes (**Figures 3A,B**). In ovary too, the expression of both VT and IT increased in the reproductive phases compared to the resting phase (**Figures 3C,D**). However, while in the spawning phase the expression of the VT precursor was higher as compared to the preparatory and pre-spawning phases (**Figure 3C**), the IT precursor expression remained equally high in all the reproductive phases (**Figure 3D**).

Evolutionary History of Teleost NH Peptide Precursor Genes

Phylogenetic Analysis

The phylogenetic inference on vertebrate NH peptide precursors was drawn from both tree constructions as well as from the evolutionary distance calculation in between groups. Both the NJ and ML trees are similar and only the ML tree is shown in **Figure 4**. The NH sequences of salmonids and catastomids (teleosts) were included in the initial analysis but were removed from the tree as they did not make a definite cluster probably due to polyploidization that led to two copies of VT and IT genes, and gene conversions (Hyodo et al., 1991; Suzuki et al., 1992). Both the phylogenetic tree and evolutionary distance calculation in between the groups (**Figure 5**) show that the NH precursor paralogs of cartilaginous fish, coelacanth and mammals

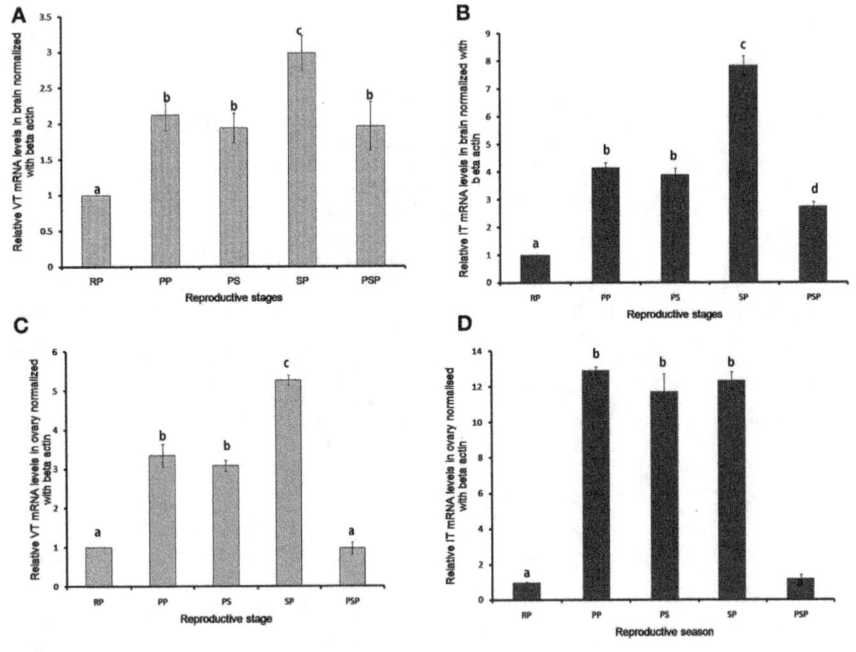

FIGURE 3 | Seasonal expression levels of VT and IT precursors in brain (A,B) and ovary (C,D). The RQ values ($2^{-\Delta\Delta CT}$) were calculated with the resting phase brain or ovary as the calibrator samples (mean ± SEM; 5 fish each). Groups with different alphabets show significant variations in the expression levels. RP, resting phase; PP, prepratory phase; PS, pre-spawning phase; SP, spawning phase; PSP, post-spawning phase.

are phylogenetically closer than their homologs in other groups. The cartilaginous fish VT and neutral hormone precursors share a distance of 0.350, coelacanth VT and MT precursor share a distance of 0.132, and the mammalian VP and OT precursors share a distance of 0.219. The evolutionary distances of the NH precursors of these groups with that of other vertebrate groups are larger (**Figure 5**). Amongst the cartilaginous fish, elephant shark VT and OT precursors share a closer phylogenetic relation, as shown by the ML tree.

The phylogenetic tree with the VT precursor of Agnatha as the outgroup also shows that the teleost VT and IT precursors form a cluster with those of the spotted gar (Holostei) while other gnathostome NH precursors form another cluster, which includes the cartilaginous fish VT and neutral hormone precursors, and coelacanth and lungfish VT and MT precursors. However, the bootstrap support for the node separating the teleost NH precursors and the other gnathostome NH precursors is low.

The catfish NH precursors expectedly segregated into their respective clusters, i.e., the HfVT, CbVT, IpVT and HfIT, CbIT, IpIT, making two distinct clusters. Within these clusters, the CbVT, HfVT and CbIT, HfIT are closer to each other than to IpVT and IpIT, respectively. The spotted gar NH precursors made a common cluster; the two neutral NH peptide precursors (IT precursor and the novel peptide precursor) are evolutionarily closer than the VT precursor. The Acanthoperygii VT and IT precursors are phylogenetically closer than their orthologs in the Ostariophysi. The evolutionary distance in between the groups confirms this. The evolutionary distance between the Acanthopterygii VT and IT precursors is only 0.269 while that between Acanthopterygii VT and Ostariophysi VT precursors is 0.426, and the Acanthopterygii IT and Ostariophysi IT precursors is 0.452. The ostariophysian VT precursor form a cluster having the catfish VT precursors and one of the two VT precursors of cavefish (*Astyanax mexicanus*), while zebrafish (*Danio rerio*) VT precursor does not form part of this cluster. The ostariophysian IT precursors make a cluster that includes the catfish and zebrafish IT precursors, and one of the IT precursors of the cavefish. The other cavefish VT and IT precursors, which do not form a part of the ostariophysian clusters, make a separate cluster and share a close phylogenetic relation with each other. Unlike the Acanthopterygii VT and IT precursors, the Ostariophysi VT and IT precursors are phylogenetically distant and share an evolutionary distance of 0.422 (**Figure 5**).

Linkage and Synteny Analysis of VT and IT in Teleosts and Spotted Gar

Details of the chromosome blocks and linkage groups used in the analysis are summarized in Supplementary Table 2. A schematic representation of conserved synteny in the spotted gar and teleosts is presented in **Figure 6**. In the spotted gar, VT, IT and the novel peptide precursors are present in the same linkage group. But, the VT precursor gene (*avp*-like) and IT precursor genes (*oxt*-like) are not arranged in tandem, unlike in human and *Xenopus* where the nonapeptide genes are present in tandem. However, the *oxt*-like gene and the novel peptide precursor gene (both in the neutral family) are arranged in tandem. Similarly, in acanthopterygian teleosts (fugu, tilapia, medaka, sticleback), the *avp*- like (VP- like) and *oxt*- like genes are in the same linkage group but are not present in tandem.

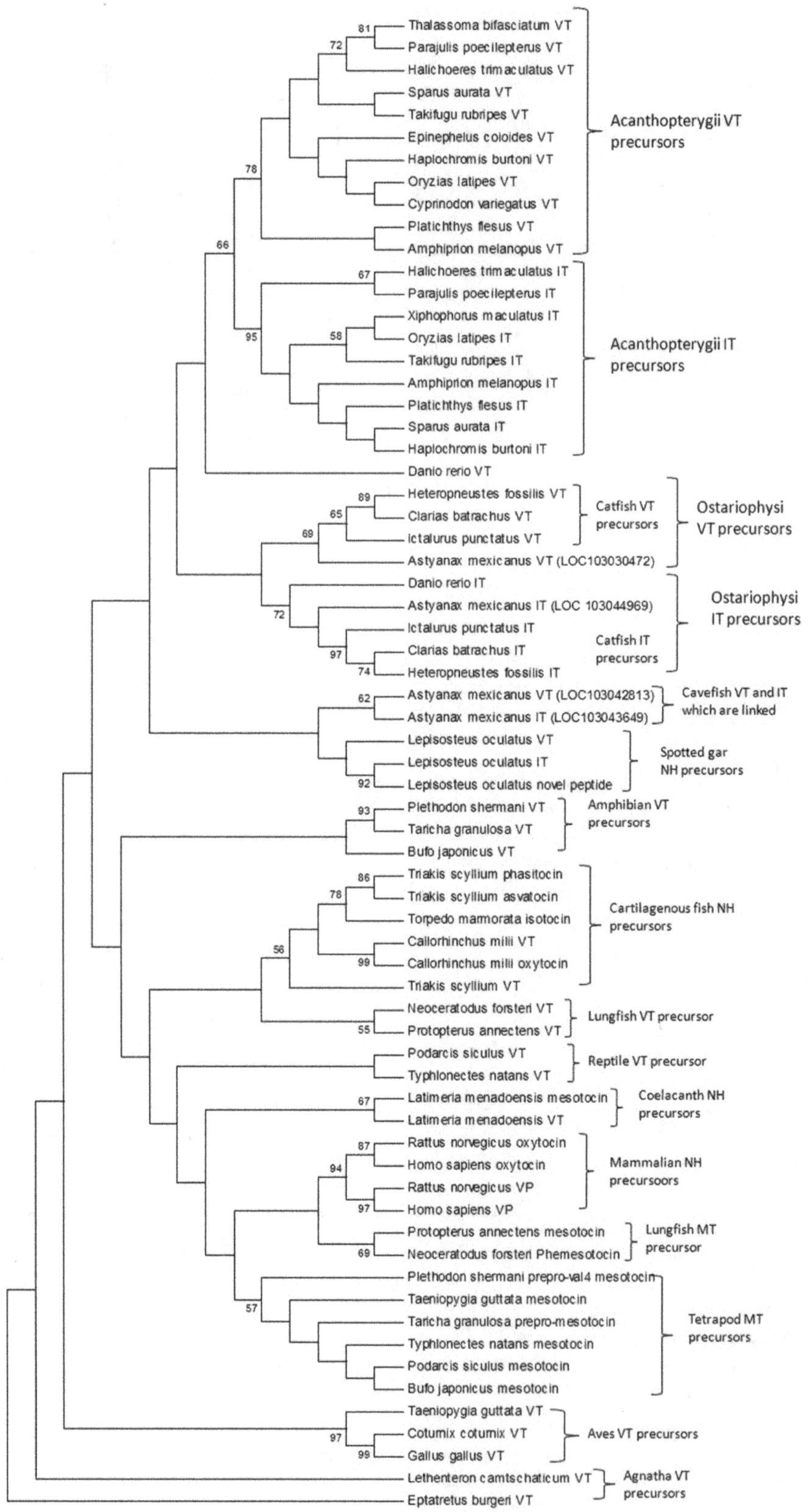

FIGURE 4 | The phylogenetic tree of vertebrate neurohypophyseal nonapeptides constructed by the Maximum-Likelihood method. The bootstrap consensus tree inferred from 500 replicates is taken to represent the evolutionary history of the taxa analyzed. The analysis involved 67 amino acid sequences. All positions with less than 95% site coverage were eliminated. There were a total of 97 positions in the final dataset. Evolutionary analyses were conducted in MEGA6. References to the sequence and species name are given in Supplementary Table 1.

	1	2	3	4	5	6	7	8	9	10	11	12	13	14	15	16	17	18	19	20	21
1. Ostariophysi IT		0.055	0.060	0.071	0.061	0.064	0.054	0.067	0.064	0.066	0.076	0.065	0.075	0.065	0.060	0.060	0.061	0.068	0.069	0.081	0.050
2. Acanthopterygii IT	0.395		0.045	0.070	0.070	0.068	0.060	0.076	0.069	0.077	0.084	0.071	0.076	0.068	0.075	0.066	0.072	0.079	0.080	0.090	0.058
3. Acanthopterygii VT	0.452	0.269		0.075	0.069	0.070	0.054	0.072	0.066	0.071	0.073	0.062	0.070	0.062	0.070	0.061	0.069	0.074	0.072	0.084	0.056
4. Cartilagenous fish neutral hormone	0.561	0.511	0.530		0.062	0.066	0.078	0.051	0.059	0.068	0.081	0.069	0.068	0.071	0.071	0.061	0.060	0.077	0.080	0.093	0.067
5. Coelacanth MT	0.424	0.416	0.461	0.429		0.049	0.064	0.060	0.047	0.039	0.078	0.056	0.055	0.063	0.060	0.043	0.043	0.070	0.073	0.082	0.055
6. Lungfish MT	0.463	0.440	0.482	0.485	0.258		0.067	0.064	0.061	0.060	0.071	0.070	0.059	0.062	0.061	0.049	0.047	0.058	0.062	0.088	0.064
7. Ostariophysi VT	0.422	0.426	0.384	0.593	0.437	0.476		0.070	0.064	0.065	0.074	0.064	0.071	0.066	0.070	0.059	0.068	0.067	0.068	0.078	0.058
8. Cartilagenous fish VT	0.517	0.530	0.489	0.350	0.386	0.440	0.524		0.054	0.067	0.077	0.071	0.070	0.061	0.072	0.051	0.060	0.076	0.078	0.093	0.065
9. Lungfish VT	0.476	0.440	0.410	0.409	0.257	0.398	0.469	0.343		0.052	0.075	0.052	0.062	0.058	0.064	0.043	0.055	0.072	0.072	0.083	0.055
10. Coelacanth VT	0.455	0.500	0.458	0.466	0.132	0.349	0.440	0.417	0.277		0.078	0.058	0.072	0.063	0.071	0.048	0.057	0.070	0.073	0.081	0.063
11. Agnatha VT	0.608	0.628	0.564	0.656	0.580	0.546	0.581	0.595	0.589	0.571		0.079	0.086	0.073	0.075	0.072	0.081	0.084	0.081	0.096	0.073
12. Reptile VT	0.453	0.445	0.399	0.481	0.244	0.408	0.434	0.457	0.264	0.257	0.590		0.063	0.066	0.070	0.047	0.058	0.070	0.069	0.084	0.061
13. Reptile MT	0.559	0.486	0.478	0.516	0.298	0.363	0.520	0.490	0.408	0.416	0.668	0.341		0.072	0.060	0.054	0.042	0.069	0.075	0.109	0.066
14. Avain VT	0.471	0.447	0.403	0.522	0.386	0.400	0.465	0.440	0.371	0.385	0.565	0.401	0.487		0.072	0.057	0.066	0.066	0.066	0.091	0.063
15. Avian MT	0.438	0.481	0.459	0.520	0.326	0.341	0.501	0.483	0.401	0.416	0.571	0.432	0.298	0.475		0.056	0.045	0.058	0.069	0.097	0.059
16. Amphibian VT	0.469	0.463	0.458	0.468	0.271	0.347	0.450	0.372	0.292	0.299	0.573	0.304	0.369	0.403	0.377		0.045	0.060	0.064	0.076	0.054
17. Amphibian MT	0.475	0.467	0.495	0.436	0.235	0.296	0.507	0.422	0.360	0.331	0.625	0.351	0.224	0.467	0.249	0.322		0.058	0.064	0.092	0.060
18. Mammalian OT	0.478	0.513	0.499	0.558	0.419	0.328	0.485	0.527	0.476	0.411	0.624	0.427	0.411	0.411	0.307	0.424	0.368		0.046	0.096	0.070
19. Mammalian VP	0.480	0.513	0.473	0.561	0.440	0.345	0.477	0.523	0.428	0.440	0.616	0.370	0.472	0.390	0.400	0.438	0.414	0.219		0.089	0.074
20. Spotted gar VT	0.560	0.549	0.549	0.667	0.503	0.594	0.534	0.615	0.513	0.484	0.730	0.503	0.741	0.563	0.626	0.532	0.604	0.620	0.543		0.075
21. Spotted gar neutral peptide precursor	0.341	0.333	0.354	0.480	0.334	0.416	0.412	0.444	0.342	0.395	0.567	0.357	0.436	0.395	0.373	0.394	0.411	0.434	0.451	0.415	

FIGURE 5 | Shows the number of amino acid substitutions per site from averaging overall sequence pairs between groups. Standard error estimate(s) shown above the diagonal were obtained by a bootstrap procedure (500 replicates). Analyses were conducted using the Poisson correction model (Zuckerkandl and Pauling, 1965). The analysis involved 67 amino acid sequences. All positions with less than 95% site coverage were eliminated. That is, fewer than 5% alignment gaps, missing data, and ambiguous bases were allowed at any position. There were a total of 97 positions in the final dataset. Evolutionary analyses were conducted in MEGA6 (Tamura et al., 2013).

In the ostariophysian teleosts, two contrasting situations exist. In zebrafish, *avp*- like and *oxt*- like are present on two different chromosomes. In contrast, in the cavefish where there are two genes each for VT and IT, one pair is present in the same linkage group like in the acanthopterygian fish. The other *avp*-like and *oxt*-like genes are present on different linkage groups so that in the cavefish, there are three linkage groups harboring the nonapeptide genes. The chromosome block in which the two genes are linked shares a conserved synteny with the acathopterygian NH loci and zebrafish *avp*-like containing linkage group. The other *oxt*-like gene is present in the paralogon of this block and shares a conserved synteny with the zebrafish *oxt*-like containing block and the Acanthopterygii paralogon of the NH loci. The genomic context of the other *avp*-like gene is considerably different from that of the teleost and spotted gar nonapeptide-harboring chromosome blocks or their paralogons. But, on a closer examination it seems to share a conserved synteny with the tetrapod nonapeptide loci as it is present in the same linkage group as the genes *fast kd 5* and *ddrgk* (genes linked with NH genes in tetrapods) but separated from them by 13 genes.

Discussion

Catfish VT and IT Precursor Genes and Proteins

In the present study, we cloned a full length cDNA of 618 bp from *H. fossilis* that coded for a VT precursor of 155 aa. There is no difference in the sequence of the brain and ovarian transcripts and hence the same gene expresses in both the tissues. We could also clone *C. batrachus* partial VT precursor gene from the N-terminal neurophysin coding region to the 3′ UTR. The catfish VT precursor gene does not show any major departure from the other known teleost sequences. However, a repeat of CA dinucleotide at the 3′ UTR is unique and the number of repeats is varied in different catfishes. In *H. fossilis,* there are 19 repeats, while in *C. batrachus*, there are only 4 repeats. The putative *Ictalurus* VT precursor gene from the database do not show any CA repeat. The available sequence read ended with the coding region of the neurophysin and did not extend to the 3′ UTR region so that no CA repeat was observed. It may be inferred that the clone has CA repeats in the 3′ UTR, as it belongs to the microsatellite enriched library. It is very likely that the CA repeats may be a conserved feature of the VT precursor genes of catfishes and may have a regulatory role.

The deduced amino acid sequence of the VT precursors shows that, like all other members of neurohypophyseal nonapeptide precursor superfamily, it has a multi- domain structure, each having a separate function. Apart from the signal peptide, the vasopressin family peptides have a three domain structure. The nine amino acid hormone forms the smallest domain, the most biologically active region, and is released with a C-terminal amidation after a three-step enzymatic process. The second domain called neurophysin is joined to the hormone moiety with a GKR, which is the site of the three-step enzymatic process of cleavage of the hormone and amidation. The N-terminal 9 amino acid of the neurophysin is poorly conserved, while the rest is conserved. The third domain is copeptin which is poorly conserved except for the presence of a leucine-rich core (de Bree and Burbach, 1998). The catfish VT precursors like the vasopressin family peptides have the three domain structure. Only in mammals, a second cleavage apart from the hormone-neurophysin cleavage has been reported, which separates the copeptin from the neurophysin. The copeptin domain possesses N- linked glycosylation sites in mammals, amphibians and lungfish (Hyodo et al., 1997) but unlike in teleosts. The catfish VT copeptin domain does not have a N-linked glycosylation site nor is cleaved. The isolated IT precursor has a multi-domain structure too and, like VT/VP precursors, has an extended C-terminal with a leucine-rich core, while no other vertebrate pre-prohormone in the neutral line has got an extended C-terminal.

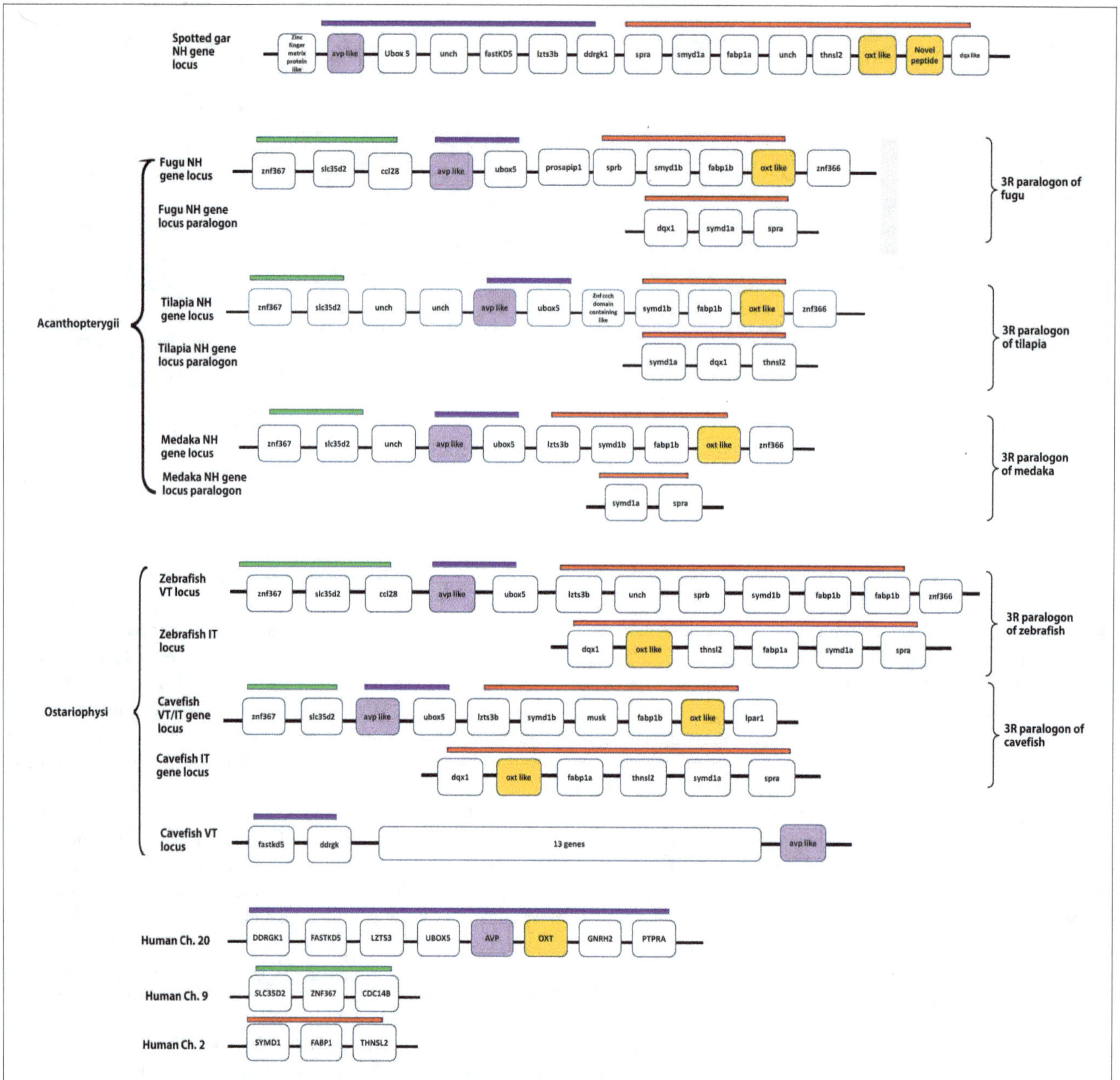

FIGURE 6 | A schematic representation of the genomic loci of spotted gar and teleost NH precursor genes and their paralogons. Human assembly is represented as a reference of tetrapod genomic context of the respective loci. The figure shows the linked situation of the genes in spotted gar (Holostei), acanthopterygian teleosts and one of the loci in cavefish, and unlinked situation in teleosts belonging to Ostariophysi. Conserved syntenic blocks have bars with the same colors. Details of genes and proteins encoded are: *ubox5*, ring finger protein 37; *fast KD5*, fast kinase domain containing protein5; *lzts3b*, leucine zipper, putative tumor suppressor family 3b; *DDRGK1*, DDRGK domain containing protein1; *spra*, sepiapterin reductase; *smyd1*, SET and MYND domain containing protein; *fabp1*, fatty acid binding protein1; *thnsl2*, threonine synthase like; *avp*, arginine vasopressin; *oxt*, oxytocin; *znf367*, zinc finger domain protein 367; *slc35d2*, UDP- N- acetylglucosamine transporter; *ccl28*, c-c motif chemokine 28; *prosapip1*, prosap interacting protein 1; *dqx*, DEAQ box RNA dependent ATPase; *znf366*, zinc finger protein 366; *ptpra*, protein phosphatase receptor type A, *GnRH2*, gonadotropin releasing hormone 2; *cdc14b*, cell divison cycle 14b; unch, uncharacterized gene.

Tissue Expression Profile of Nonapeptides and Functional Implications

In *H. fossilis*, VT and IT genes are expressed only in the brain and ovary. In a previous study, the distribution of VT has been reported in the preoptico-hypophyseal neurosecretory system of the catfish (Singh and Joy, 2008). Brain VT showed seasonal variation associated with the annual reproductive cycle of the catfish with an increase during the recrudescent phase and a decrease after spawning. The expression of the VT and IT genes shows differences in tissue and seasonal transcript levels. The transcript levels are high in the brain than ovary. In the ovary, the expression was confined to the follicular layer since the denuded oocytes did not show any signal. In the seasonal study, the VT and IT precursor transcripts in the brain and ovary show significant variations with higher levels during the reproductive phase, suggesting a prominent influence of the reproductive factors on the transcriptional activity of the genes. The expression of both VT and IT precursor genes in the ovary points to local synthesis of the peptides for a paracrine role in ovarian activity. This confirms the earlier findings from our laboratory showing HPLC characterization of both VT and IT, and immunocytochemical localization of VT in the follicular layer (Singh and Joy, 2008). The ovarian VT levels vary with the annual ovarian cycle closely associated with recrudescence and spawning (Singh and Joy, 2008). Moreover, steroid hormones estradiol-17β and 17, 20 β- dihydroxypregnen-3-one, the maturation- inducing steroid, modulate VT secretion as in the brain (Singh and Joy, 2009a, 2011). *In vitro* studies with ovarian follicles have showed that VT stimulated steroidogenesis, oocyte final maturation, oocyte hydration, ovulation and prostaglandin secretion (Singh and Joy, 2010, 2011; Joy and Singh, 2013). Gwee et al. (2009) have shown VT expression in the ovary of elephant shark. Bobe et al. (2006) have reported VT and IT mRNAs in the preovulatory ovaries of rainbow trout, while the transcripts were not detected in the ovary during the other stages of reproduction. In mammals, there are several reports of the presence of VP and OT in nonneuronal peripheral sites, where they have a paracrine role (Wathes et al., 1983; Clements and Funder, 1986; Sernia et al., 1994; Mechaly et al., 1999). Similarly, in other classes of vertebrates like aves, presence of VT has been reported in the reproductive tissues (Saito and Grossmann, 1999). The peripheral expression of VT and its homolog signifies a phylogenetic pattern and the phenomenon seems to be conserved in all major groups of vertebrates.

Evolutionary History of Teleost NH Precursors from Phylogenetic Analysis, Genomic Locations and Synteny Analysis

Phylogenetic inference from the present study shows that the precursor paralogs in some vertebrate groups (cartilaginous fish, coelacanth, mammals) are closer than their homologs in other groups. Similarly, studies in salmons (Hyodo et al., 1991; Suzuki et al., 1992) and flounder (Warne et al., 2000) showed that the VT and IT precursors share high sequence identity. Gwee et al. (2008, 2009) also showed that the sequence identity between the respective precursor paralogs is very high in coelacanth and elephant shark. The studies also reported that the high sequence similarity was mostly in the central portion of the neurophysin. Events of gene conversion between the paralogous genes may be responsible for diluting the distance created by the long evolutionary history and make them seem more closely related than what they actually are, typifying "concerted evolution." Concerted evolution is common in duplicated genes, for example, as reported in rRNA genes, the highly conserved histone and ubiquitin gene families, and the heat shock protein gene family (Nei and Rooney, 2005). For the NH precursors, gene conversions seem to encompass the central neurophysin region and, therefore, the high sequence similarity in the central portion. Further evidence in favor of frequent events of gene conversion in between the nonapeptide paralogs is given for the bovine VP and OT precursor mRNA and avian NH precursors, having their central neurophysin not merely similar but identical pointing to a recent event of gene conversion (Ruppert et al., 1984; Levy et al., 1987). Gwee et al. (2008) found a low GC3 content in all the three exons of coelacanth VT and MT precursors as compared to bovine and human VP and OT genes, and attributed the sequence similarity in coelacanth to purifying selection rather than due to gene conversion. In mammals and yeast, gene conversion events are known to be GC-biased so that the GC content increases after gene conversion (Galtier, 2003; Marais, 2003; Noonan et al., 2004; Duret and Galtier, 2009). However, a recent study showed that gene conversions might not always be GC-biased (Assis and Kondrashov, 2012) and in such a scenario one of the evidence in favor of gene conversion can be incompatibility between phylogenetic tree and known duplication history (Mansai and Innan, 2010), as is the case in the present study. The neurophysin is only concerned with precursor processing and axonal transport which is common to all nonapeptides in contrast to the hormone moieties that evolved under the constraints of stringent and differential ligand-receptor selectivity in the two families. Hence, gene conversion events encompassing only the neurophysin might have occurred during evolution. This might also be facilitated by the 3-exon structure of the nonapeptide genes where the central neurophysin is encoded by a separate exon, i.e., the 2nd exon.

Based on the gene structures of salmon VT and IT, Urano and Ando (2011) had proposed a distinct and independent origin of the teleost IT as compared to the neutral hormone precursors of other vertebrates. Evidence in support of it is the presence of an extended C-terminal in IT precursors with a leucine-rich core, like in VT/VP. However, the authors have added that the molecular divergence of VT and IT in teleosts is complicated because of the 3R. The recent addition of the spotted gar sequences in the database and the analysis in the present study has prompted a re-apprisal. The presence of IT with the extended C-terminal in the spotted gar suggests an origin of IT in the actinopterygian lineage before the 3R. The spotted gar has an additional neutral peptide with a short C-terminal, which may be related directly to the evolutionary line of other vertebrate neutral hormone precursors that has originated at the base of the gnathostome lineage. In no teleost studied till date, a neutral peptide with a short C-terminal has been reported. Therefore, it may be hypothesized that the neutral hormone precursor gene with the short C-terminal might have originated very early in vertebrates, as documented in the cartilaginous fish (Hyodo et al., 2004; Gwee et al., 2009) and this early neutral hormone precursor might be the evolutionary forerunner of MT and OT. In teleosts, this neutral hormone precursor gene might have been secondarily lost or needs to be traced in the teleost lineage.

An interesting result that surfaced due to the addition of the catfish nonapeptide precursor sequences in the phylogenetic study is about the differences in the evolutionary distance shared by the precursor paralogs of different groups within teleosts. While the Acanthopterygii VT and IT precursors share a very small evolutionary distance (0.269) between them, the Ostariophysi VT and IT precursors are phylogenetically distant (0.422). The distance between the VT precursors and IT precursors of Acanthopterygii and Ostariophysi is also high (0.426 and 0.452, respectively). Phylogenetic clustering of the teleost NH precursors further supports these results. In the phylogenetic tree, the Acanthopterygii VT and IT precursors clustered together and seemed to have diverged from a common lineage. While the Ostariophysi IT precursors formed a definite cluster that included the catfish IT precursors, one of the IT precursors of the cavefish and the zebrafish IT precursor. The VT precursors of the catfish and one of the cavefish make a cluster which does not include the zebrafish VT precursor. The results from the distance calculation between the groups and the phylogenetic tree suggest that underlying the apparent homogeneity in all teleosts having VT and IT, there might be a difference in the origin of VT and IT precursors in different groups, i.e., these may be lineage-specific paralogs.

The analysis of the genomic loci of the NH hormone genes and the synteny analysis of the loci in different groups of teleosts further support the above assumption. Gwee et al. (2008, 2009) showed that in coelacanth, lamprey, and elephant shark (cartilaginous fish), the NH gene loci has a conserved synteny with the tetrapod NH loci. In fugu, there is a rearrangement. In the present study, the NH gene loci were studied in the spotted gar and teleosts belonging to different groups, which are known to have suffered independent gene losses during the process of diploidization (Garcia de la serrana et al., 2014). Our study indicates that, indeed, the loci and 3R paralogons show the footprints of rearrangements and differential losses of the NH gene paralogs in the different teleost lineages. On examination of the different genes linked with the nonapeptide genes in the spotted gar chromosome segment and the human linkage groups (as a tetrapod reference), it may be inferred that a rearrangement in the position of the genes in the nonapeptide loci of the spotted gar occurred by the fusion of the two blocks of chromosomes after the origin of IT in the actinopterygian lineage, disrupting the tandem arrangement of the genes, before the 3R. After the 3R, in teleosts the two paralogous blocks (3R paralogons) harboring the nonapeptide genes suffered further rearrangement and differential gene losses during the process of diploidization. The rearrangement was common judging from the conserved synteny in both the NH gene loci and its paralogon in all teleosts. However, the gene losses in these loci were differential in the two teleost superorders Acanthopterygii and Ostariophysi. This led to the linked and nonlinked *avp*-like and *oxt-like* genes in these different groups. In the acanthopterygian lineage, both the genes might have been lost from the same paralogon maintaining the linked situation of the two genes similar to the spotted gar, i.e., the pre 3R genome. In the zebrafish, *avp* like and *oxt*-like genes were lost one each from two paralogons so that a single copy of the NH hormone genes was maintained and they remained unlinked. It is difficult to reconstruct the sequence of events that can explain the present picture of synteny in the NH loci and also the inconsistent phylogenetic relation between the VT and IT precursors in the different groups of teleosts. However, it may be inferred that in the base lineage of acanthopterygians, after one pair of VT and IT precursor genes was lost from one of the 3R paralogon, an event of gene conversion might have occurred between the remaining pair. This might have occurred in the time period between the 3R and the explosive adaptive radiation and could explain the phylogentic relation of the Acanthopterygii VT and IT precursors. The Acanthopterygii VT precursors and Acanthopterygii IT precursors make two distinct clusters but share a very close phylogenetic relation. In the Ostariophysi, the loss of the NH precursor paralog was differential as compared to the Acanthopterygii with VT and IT precursor genes being lost one each from the two 3R paralogons. Rapid speciation event might have occurred after this. Gene conversion might not have occurred in the ostariophysian lineage. This explains the unlinked state of the NH paralogs in the zebrafish and also the distant relation shared by the VT and IT precursors of the Ostariophysi. The situation in the cavefish is difficult to explain. It is likely that the VT precursor gene was lost from one of the 3R paralogons while in the other both genes were retained so that a pair of linked genes remained. An independent event of gene conversion might also have occurred in between the two linked genes explaining the close phylogenetic relation between the two. The evolutionary history of the VT precursor gene of the cavefish which is unlinked can be easily traced phylogenetically as it clusters with the catfish VT precursors. However, the synteny analysis shows that it is present in a unique genomic context which shares a conserved synteny with neither the tetrapod nor the teleost NH loci, making it impossible to arrive at a possible origin of this gene. Genomic information of the NH loci from more teleost species belonging to the Ostariophysi may be helpful in explaining this. Our future direction of work would involve isolating the NH gene loci in the catfish so that the evolutionary history of the VT and IT genes in the Ostariophysi may be inferred more clearly. With the available information from the phylogeny and synteny analysis, it is clear that in the different groups of teleosts the VT and IT precursors are lineage-specific paralogs arising from differential loss of the 3R paralogs in the different superorders. The independent yet consistent retention of VT and IT in the different groups despite the catastrophes of genome duplications, diploidizations and gene conversions might have been directed by stringent ligand- receptor selectivity, established early during the vertebrate evolution.

Conclusion

The complete VT and IT precursors were cloned from *H. fossilis*, and partially from *C. batrachus*. The deduced precursor proteins have the characteristics of the NH precursors. The precursors express in the brain and follicular envelope of the ovary. The expression in both brain and ovary shows seasonal variation with higher expression in the reproductive phases. The phylogenetic analysis of the vertebrate NH precursors and the synteny analysis of the NH gene loci show that the VT and IT precursors are lineage-specific paralogs in the superorders of Teleostei (Acanthopterygii and Ostariophysi).

Acknowledgments

This study was supported by a Department of Science and Technology, New Delhi Research Grant (No.

SA/SO/AS-43/2009) to KPJ and RC. PB is grateful to the Council of Scientific and Industrial Research, New Delhi for Junior and Senior Research Fellowships. We thank the Coordinator of DBT- BHU Interdisciplinary School of life Sciences for providing the qPCR facility.

References

Acher, R. (1996). Molecular evolution of fish neurohypophysial hormone: neutral and selective evolutionary mechanism. *Gen. Comp. Endocrinol.* 102, 157–172. doi: 10.1006/gcen.1996.0057

Assis, R., and Kondrashov, A. S. (2012). Non-allelic gene conversion is not GC-biased in *Drosophila* or Primates. *Mol. Biol. Evol.* 29, 1291–1295. doi: 10.1093/molbev/msr304

Bobe, J., Montfort, J., Nguyen, T., and Fosteir, A. (2006). Identification of new participants in the rainbow trout (*Onchorhynchus mykiss*) oocyte maturation and ovulation process using cDNA microarrays. *Reprod. Biol. Endocrinol.* 4, 39–54. doi: 10.1186/1477-7827-4-39

Chauvet, J., Hurpet, D., Colne, T., Michel, G., Chauvet, M. T., and Acher, R. (1985). Neurohypophyseal hormones as evolutionary tracers: identification of oxytocin, lysine vasopressin, and arginine vasopressin in two South American opossums (*Didelphis marsupialis* and *Philander opossum*). *Gen. Comp. Endocrinol.* 57, 320–328. doi: 10.1016/0016-6480(85)90277-1

Chauvet, J., Hurpet, D., Michel, G., Chauvet, M. T., and Acher, R. (1984). Two multigene families for marsupial neurohypophyseal hormones? Identification of oxytocin, mesotocin, lysipressin and arginine vasopressin in the North American opossum *Didelphis virginiana*. *Biochem. Biophys. Res. Commun.* 123, 306–311. doi: 10.1016/0006-291X(84)90413-3

Chauvet, M. T., Colne, T., Hurpet, D., Chauvet, J., and Acher, R. (1983). A multigene family for the vasopressin-like hormones? Identification of mesotocin, lysipressin and phenypressin in Australian macropods. *Biochem. Biophys. Res. Commun.* 116, 258–263. doi: 10.1016/0006-291X(83)90409-6

Chomczynski, P., and Sacchi, N. (1987). Single step method of RNA isolation by acid guanidinium thiocyanate- phenol- chloroform extraction. 1987. *Anal. Biochem.* 162, 156–159. doi: 10.1006/abio.1987.9999

Christoffels, A., Koh, E. G. L., Chia, J. M., Brenner, S., Aparicio, S., and Venkatesh, B. (2004). Fugu genome analysis provides evidence for a whole-genome duplication early during the evolution of ray-finned fishes. *Mol. Biol. Evol.* 21, 1146–1151. doi: 10.1093/molbev/msh114

Clements, J. A., and Funder, J. W. (1986). Arginine vasopressin (AVP) and AVP like immunoreactivity in peripheral tissues. *Endocr. Rev.* 7, 449–460. doi: 10.1210/edrv-7-4-449

Cruz, L. J., Santos, V. D., Zafaralla, G. C., Ramilo, C. A., Zeikus, R., Gray, W. R., et al. (1987). Characterization of peptides from *Conus geographus* and *Conus striatus* venoms. *J. Biol. Chem.* 262, 15821–15824.

de Bree, F. M., and Burbach, J. P. H. (1998). Structure-function relationship of the vasopressin prohormone domains. *Cell. Mol. Neurobiol.* 18, 173–191. doi: 10.1023/A:1022564803093

de Bree, F. M., Knight, D., Howell, L., and Murphy, D. (2000). Sorting of the vasopressin prohormone into the regulated secretory pathway. *FEBS Lett.* 475, 175–180. doi: 10.1016/S0014-5793(00)01623-9

Duret, L., and, Galtier, N. (2009). Biased gene conversion and the evolution of mammalian genomic landscapes. *Annu. Rev. Genomics Hum. Genet.* 10, 285–311. doi: 10.1146/annurev-genom-082908-150001

Galtier, N. (2003). Gene conversion drives GC content evolution in mammalian histones. *Trends Genet.* 19, 65–68. doi: 10.1016/S0168-9525(02) 00002-1

Garcia de la serrana, D., Marceo, E. A., and Johnston, I. A. (2014). Systematic variation in the pattern of gene paralog retention between teleost superorders Ostariophysi and Acanthopterygii. *Genome Biol. Evol.* 6, 981–987. doi: 10.1093/gbe/evu074

Grimmelikhuijzen, C. J. P., Dierickx, K., and Boer, G. J. (1982). Oxytocin/vasopressin-like immunoreactivity is present in the nervous system of *Hydra*. *Neuroscience* 7, 3191–3199. doi: 10.1016/0306-4522(82)90241-X

Grimmelikhuijzen, C. J. P., Williamson, M., and Hansen, G. N. (2002). Neuropeptides in cnidarians. *Can. J. Zool.* 80, 1690–1702. doi: 10.1139/z02-137

Gwee, P. C., Amemiya, C. T., Brenner, S., and Venkatesh, B. (2008). Sequence and organization of coelacanth neurohypophysial hormone genes: evolutionary history of the vertebrate neurohypophysial hormone gene locus. *BMC Evol. Biol.* 8:93. doi: 10.1186/1471-2148-8-93

Gwee, P. C., Tay, B. H., Brenner, S., and Venkatesh, B. (2009). Characterization of the neurohypophyseal gene loci in elephant shark and the Japnese lamprey. *BMC Evol. Biol.* 9:47. doi: 10.1186/1471-2148-9-47

Hamann, D., Hunt, N., and Ivell, R. (1992). The chicken vasotocin gene. *J. Neuroendocrinol.* 4, 505–513. doi: 10.1111/j.1365-2826.1992.tb00198.x

Heierhorst, J., Marley, S. D., Figueroa, J., Krentler, C., Lederis, K., and Richter, D. (1989). Vasotocin and isotocin precursor from the white sucker, *Catastomus commersoni*: cloning and sequence analysis of cDNA. *Proc. Natl. Acad. Sci. U.S.A.* 86, 5242–5246. doi: 10.1073/pnas.86.14.5242

Hyodo, S., Ishii, S., and Joss, J. M. P. (1997). Australian lungfish neurohypophyseal hormone genes encode vasotocin and (Phe2) mesotocin precursors homologous to tetrapod- type precursors. *Proc. Natl. Acad. Sci. U.S.A.* 94, 13339–13344. doi: 10.1073/pnas.94.24.13339

Hyodo, S., Kato, Y., Ono, M., and Urano, A. (1991). Cloning and sequence analysis of cDNAs encoding vasotocin and isotocin precursors of chum salmon, *Oncorhynchus keta:* evolutionary relationships of neurohypophysial hormone precursors. *J. Comp. Physiol. B.* 160, 601–608. doi: 10.1007/BF00571256

Hyodo, S., Tsukada, T., and Takei, Y. (2004). Neurohypophyseal hormones of dogfish *Triakis scyllium*: structure and salinity dependent secretion. *Gen. Comp. Endocrinol.* 138, 97–104. doi: 10.1016/j.ygcen.2004.05.009

Jaillon, O., Aury, J. M., Brunet, F., Petit, J. L., Stange-Thomann, N., Mauceli, E., et al. (2004). Genome duplication in the teleost fish *Tetraodon nigroviridis* reveals the early vertebrate proto-karyotype. *Nature* 431, 946–957. doi: 10.1038/nature03025

Jansen, S., Devaere, S., Weekers, P. H. H., and Adriaens, A. (2006). Phylogenetic relationship and divergence time estimate of African anguilliformes catfish (Siluriformes:claridae) inferred from ribososmal gene and spacer sequence. *Mol. Phylogenet. Evol.* 38, 65–78. doi: 10.1016/j.ympev.2005.09.011

Joy, K. P., and Singh, V. (2013). Functional interactions between vasotocin and prostaglandins during final oocyte maturation and ovulation in the catfish *Heteropneustes fossilis*. *Gen. Comp. Endocrinol.* 186, 126–135. doi: 10.1016/j.ygcen.2013.02.043

Kawada, T., Sekiguchi, T., Itoh, Y., and Ogasawara, M. (2008). Characterization of a novel vasopressin/oxytocin superfamily peptide and its receptor from an ascidian, *Ciona intestinalis*. *Peptides* 26, 1672–1678. doi: 10.1016/j.peptides.2008.05.030

Lagman, D., Daza, D. O., Widmark, J., Abalo, X. M., Sundstrom, G., and Larhammar, D. (2013). The vertebrate ancestral repertoire of visual opsins, transducin alpha subunits and oxytocin/ vasopressin receptors was established by duplication of their shared genomic region in the two rounds of early vertebrate genome duplications. *BMC Evol. Biol.* 13:238. doi: 10.1186/1471-2148-13-238

Lane, T. F., Sower, S. A., and Kawauchi, H. (1988). Arginine vasotocin from the pituitary gland of the lamprey *Petromyzon marinus*: isolation and amino acid sequence. *Gen. Comp. Endocrinol.* 70, 152–157. doi: 10.1016/0016-6480(88)90104-9

Larhammar, D., Sundstrom, G., Dreborg, S., Daza, D. O., and Larsson, T. A. (2009). Major genomic events and their consequences for vertebrate evolution and endocrinology. Trends in comparative endocrinology and neurobiology. *Ann. N.Y. Acad. Sci.* 1163, 201–208. doi: 10.1111/j.1749-6632.2008.03659.x

Levy, B., Michel, G., Chauvet, J., Chauvet, M. T., and Acher, R. (1987). Gene conversion in avian mesotocin and vasotocin genes: a recurrent mechanism linking two neurohypophyseal precursor lineages. *Biosci. Rep.* 8, 631–636. doi: 10.1007/BF01127675

Livak, K. J., and Schmittgen, T. D. (2001). Analysis of relative gene expression data using real-time quantitative PCR and the 2–ΔΔCT method. *Methods* 25, 402–408. doi: 10.1006/meth.2001.1262

Lu, J., Peatman, E., Yang, Q., Wang, S., Hu, Z., Reecy, J., et al. (2010). The catfish genome database cBARBEL: an informatics platform for genome biology of ictalurid catfish. *Nucl. Acids Res.* 39, 815–821. doi: 10.1093/nar/gkq765

Mansai, S. P., and Innan, H. (2010). The power of the methods for detecting interlocus gene conversion. *Genetics* 184, 517–527. doi: 10.1534/genetics.109.111161

Marais, G. (2003). Biased gene conversion: implications for genome and sex evolution. *Trends Genet.* 19, 330–338. doi: 10.1016/S0168-9525(03)00116-1

Mechaly, I., Macari, F., Lautier, C., Serrano, J. J., Cros, G., and Grigorescu, F. (1999). Identification by RT-PCR and immunolocalization of arginine vasopressin in rat pancreas. *Diabetes Metab.* 25, 498–501.

Meyer, A., and Schartl, M. (1999). Gene and genome duplications in vertebrates: the one-to-four (-to-eight in fish) rule and the evolution of novel gene functions. *Curr. Opin. Cell Biol.* 11, 699–704. doi: 10.1016/S0955-0674(99)00039-3

Mishra, A., and Joy, K. P. (2006). Effects of gonadotropin *in vivo* and 2-hydroxyestradiol- 17β *in vitro* on follicular steroid hormone profile associated with oocyte maturation in the catfish *Heteropneustes fossilis*. *J. Endocrinol.* 189, 341–353. doi: 10.1677/joe.1.06686

Montefiano, D. I., Spiess, R., Romano, A., Limatola, M., and Ivell, R. (2001). "Cloning of mesotocin (MT) and vasotocin (AVT) cDNA from the oviparous reptile *Podarcis sicula*," in *Perspectives in Comparative Endocrinology: Unity and Diversity*, eds H. Goos, R. Rastogi, and H. Vaudry (Bologna: Monduzzi Editore), 547–554.

Morley, S. D., Schonrock, C., Heierhorst, J., Figueroa, J., Lederis, K., and Richter, D. (1990). Vasotocin genes of the teleost fish *Catostomus commersoni:* gene structure, exon-intron boundary, and hormone precursor organization. *Biochemistry* 29, 2506–2511. doi: 10.1021/bi00462a011

Nei, M., and Rooney, A. P. (2005). Concerted and birth and death evolution of multigene families. *Annu. Rev. Genet.* 39, 121–152. doi: 10.1146/annurev.genet.39.073003.112240

Nojiri, H., Ishida, I., Miyashita, E., Sato, M., Urano, A., and Deguchi, T. (1987). Cloning and sequence analysis of cDNAs for neurohypophyseal hormones vasotocin and mesotocin from the hypothalamus of toad, *Bufo japonicus*. *Proc. Natl. Acad. Sci. U.S.A.* 84, 3043–3046. doi: 10.1073/pnas.84.9.3043

Noonan, J. P., Grimwood, J., Schmutz, J., Dickson, M., and Myers, R. M. (2004). Gene conversion and the evolution of protocadherin gene cluster diversity. *Genome Res.* 14, 354–366. doi: 10.1101/gr.2133704

Ocampo Daza, D., Lewicka, M., and Larhammar, D. (2012). The oxytocin/vasopressin receptor family has at least five members in the gnathostome lineage, including two distinct V2 type receptors subtypes. *Gen. Com. Endocrinol.* 175, 135–143. doi: 10.1016/j.ygcen.2011.10.011

Parry, L. J., Bathgate, R. A. D., and Ivell, R. (2000). Mammalian mesotocin: cDNA sequence and expression of an oxytocin- like gene in a macropodid marsupial. the tammar wallaby. *Gen. Comp. Endocrinol.* 118, 187–199. doi: 10.1006/gcen.2000.7464

Proux, J. P., Miller, C. A., Li, J. P., and Corney, R. L. (1987). Identification of an arginine vasopressin-like diuretic hormone from *Locusta migratoria*. *Biochem. Biophys. Res. Commun.* 149, 180–186. doi: 10.1016/0006-291X(87)91621-4

Rawat, A., Chaube, R., and Joy, K. P. (2015). Molecular cloning, sequencing and phylogeny of vasotocin receptor genes in the air-breathing catfish *Heteropneustes fossilis* with sex dimorphic and seasonal variations in tissue expression. *Fish Physiol. Biochem.* 41, 509–532. doi: 10.1007/s10695-015-0026-0

Rouille, Y., Chauvet, M.-T., Chauvet, J., and Acher, R. (1988). Dual duplication of neurohypophysial hormones in an Australian marsupial: mesotocin, oxytocin, lysine vasopressin and arginine vasopressin in a single gland of the northern bandicoot (*Isoodon macrourus*). *Biochem. Biophys. Res. Commun.* 154, 346–350. doi: 10.1016/0006-291X(88)90691-2

Rouille, Y., Michel, G., Chauvet, M. T., Chauvet, J., and Acher, R. (1989). Hydrins, new hydroosmotic neurohypophyseal peptides: osmoregulatory adaptation in amphibians through vasotocin precursor processing. *Proc. Natl. Acad. Sci. U.S.A.* 88, 5272–5275. doi: 10.1073/pnas.86.14.5272

Ruppert, S., Scherer, G., and Schutz, G. (1984). Recent gene conversion involving bovine vasopressin and oxytocin genes as suggested by nucleotide sequence. *Nature* 308, 554–557. doi: 10.1038/308554a0

Saito, N., and Grossmann, R. (1999). Gene expression of arginine vasotocin in ovarian and uterine tissue of chicken. *Asian Aus. J. Anim. Sci.* 12, 695–701. doi: 10.5713/ajas.1999.695

Santini, F., Harmon, L. J., Carnevale, G., and Alfaro, M. E. (2009). Did genome duplication drive the origin of teleosts? A comparative study of diversification in ray finned fishes. *BMC Evol. Biol.* 9:194. doi: 10.1186/1471-2148-9-194

Satake, H., Takawa, K., Minakata, H., and Matsushima, O. (1999). Evidence for conservation of the vasopressin/oxytocin superfamily in Annelida. *J. Biol. Chem.* 274, 5605–5611. doi: 10.1074/jbc.274.9.5605

Searcy, B. T., Walthers, E. A., Heppner, B. L., Thompson, R. R., and Moore, F. L. (2009). Identification of mesotocin and vasotocin nucleotide sequences in two species of urodele amphibian. *Gen. Comp. Endocrinol.* 160, 111–116. doi: 10.1016/j.ygcen.2008.11.013

Sernia, C., Bathgate, R. A. D., and Gemmell, R. T. (1994). Mesotocin and arginine-vasopressin in the corpus luteum of an Australian marsupial, the brushtail possum (*Trichosurus vulpecula*). *Gen. Comp. Endocrinol.* 93, 197–204. doi: 10.1006/gcen.1994.1023

Singh, V., and Joy, K. P. (2008). Immunocytochemical localization, HPLC characterization and seasonal dynamics of vasotocin in the brain, blood plasma and gonads of the catfish *Heteropneustes fossilis*. *Gen. Comp. Endocrinol.* 159, 214–225. doi: 10.1016/j.ygcen.2008.09.003

Singh, V., and Joy, K. P. (2009a). Effects of hCG and ovarian steroid hormones on vasotocin levels in the female catfish *Heteropneustes fossilis*. *Gen. Comp. Endocrinol.* 162, 172–178. doi: 10.1016/j.ygcen.2009.03.016

Singh, V., and Joy, K. P. (2009b). Relative *in vitro* seasonal effects of vasotocin and isotocin on ovarian steroid hormone levels in the catfish *Heteropneustes fossilis*. *Gen. Comp. Endocrinol.* 162, 257–264. doi: 10.1016/j.ygcen.2009.03.024

Singh, V., and Joy, K. P. (2010). An involvement of vasotocin in oocyte hydration in the catfish *Heteropneustes fossilis*: a comparison with effects of isotocin and hCG. *Gen. Comp. Endocrinol.* 166, 504–512. doi: 10.1016/j.ygcen.2010.02.020

Singh, V., and Joy, K. P. (2011). Vasotocin induces final oocyte maturation and ovulation through the production of a maturation-inducing steroid in the catfish *Heteropneustes fossilis*. *Gen. Comp. Endocrinol.* 174, 15–21. doi: 10.1016/j.ygcen.2011.07.009

Stafflinger, E., Karina, K. H., Hauser, F., Schneider, M., Cazzamali, G., Williamson, M., et al. (2008). Cloning and identification of an oxytocin/vasopressin-like receptor and its ligand from insects. *Proc. Natl. Acad. Sci. U.S.A.* 105, 3262–3267. doi: 10.1073/pnas.0710897105

Suzuki, M., Hyodo, S., and Urano, A. (1992). Cloning and sequence analyses of vasotocin and isotocin precursor cDNAs in the masu salmon, *Oncorhynchus masou:* evolution of neurohypophysial hormone precursors. *Zool. Sci.* 9, 157–167.

Suzuki, M., Kubokawa, K., Nagasawa, H., and Urano, A. (1995). Sequence analysis of vasopressin cDNAs of the lamprey, *Lampetra japonica,* and the hagfish, *Eptatretus burgeri:* evolution of cyclostome vasotocin precursors. *J. Mol. Endocrinol.* 14, 67–77. doi: 10.1677/jme.0.0140067

Takuwa-Kwodo, K., Iwakoshi-Ukena, E., Kanda, A., and Minakata, H. (2003). Octopus, which owns the most advanced brain in invertebrates, has two members of vasopressin/oxytocin superfamily as in vertebrates. *Regul. Pept.* 115, 139–149. doi: 10.1016/S0167-0115(03)00151-4

Tamura, K., Stecher, G., Peterson, D., Filipski, A., and Kumar, S. (2013). MEGA6: molecular evolutionary genetics analysis version 6.0. *Mol. Biol. Evol.* 30, 2725–2729. doi: 10.1093/molbev/mst197

Urano, A., and Ando, H. (2011). Diversity of the hypothalamo- neurohypophyseal system and its hormonal genes. *Gen. Comp. Endocrinol.* 170, 41–56. doi: 10.1016/j.ygcen.2010.09.016

Venkatesh, B., and Brenner, S. (1995). Structure and organization of the isotocin and vasotocin genes from teleosts. *Adv. Exp. Med. Biol.* 395, 629–638.

Warne, J. M., Hyodo, S., Harding, K., and Balment, R. J. (2000). Cloning of pro-vasotocin and pro-isotocin cDNAs from the flounder *Platichthys flesus*; levels of hypothalamic mRNA following acute osmotic challenge. *Gen. Comp. Endocrinol.* 119, 77–84. doi: 10.1006/gcen.2000.7495

Wathes, D. C., Swann, R. W., Birkett, S. D., Porter, D. G., and Pickering, B. T. (1983). Characterization of oxytocin, vasopressin and neurophysin from bovine corpus luteum. *Endocrinology* 113, 693–698. doi: 10.1210/endo-113-2-693

Yagamuchi, Y., Kaiya, H., Konno, N., Iwata, E., Miyazato, M., Uchiyama, M., et al. (2012). The fifth neurohypophyseal hormone receptor is structurally related to V2-type receptor but functionally similar to V1 type receptor. *Gen. Comp. Endocrinol.* 178, 519–528. doi: 10.1016/j.ygcen.2012.07.008

Zuckerkandl, E., and Pauling, L. (1965). Molecules as documents of evolutionary history. *J. Theor. Biol.* 8, 357–366. doi: 10.1016/0022-5193(65)90083-4

15

Melanocortin receptor accessory proteins in adrenal disease and obesity

David S. Jackson, Shwetha Ramachandrappa, Adrian J. Clark and Li F. Chan *

Centre for Endocrinology, William Harvey Research Institute, Barts and the London School of Medicine and Dentistry, Queen Mary University of London, London, UK

Edited by:
Olivier Kah,
Centre National de la Recherche Scientifique UMR 6026, France

Reviewed by:
Rafael Vazquez-Martinez,
University of Cordoba, Spain
Andreas Stengel,
Charité Universitätsmedizin Berlin, Germany

***Correspondence:**
Li F. Chan,
Centre for Endocrinology, William Harvey Research Institute, Barts and the London School of Medicine and Dentistry, Queen Mary University of London, Charterhouse Square, London EC1M 6BQ, UK
l.chan@qmul.ac.uk

Melanocortin receptor accessory proteins (MRAPs) are regulators of the melanocortin receptor family. MRAP is an essential accessory factor for the functional expression of the MC2R/ACTH receptor. The importance of MRAP in adrenal gland physiology is demonstrated by the clinical condition familial glucocorticoid deficiency type 2. The role of its paralog melanocortin-2-receptor accessory protein 2 (MRAP2), which is predominantly expressed in the hypothalamus including the paraventricular nucleus, has recently been linked to mammalian obesity. Whole body deletion and targeted brain specific deletion of the Mrap2 gene result in severe obesity in mice. Interestingly, Mrap2 complete knockout (KO) mice have increased body weight without detectable changes to food intake or energy expenditure. Rare heterozygous variants of MRAP2 have been found in humans with severe, early-onset obesity. *In vitro* data have shown that Mrap2 interaction with the melanocortin-4-receptor (Mc4r) affects receptor signaling. However, the mechanism by which Mrap2 regulates body weight *in vivo* is not fully understood and differences between the phenotypes of Mrap2 and Mc4r KO mice may point toward Mc4r independent mechanisms.

Keywords: melanocortin receptors, accessory proteins, adrenal function, obesity, knockout mouse model

The Melanocortin Receptor Family

Melanocortin receptors (MCRs) comprise a family of five, class A, G protein-coupled receptors designated MC1R-MC5R with diverse physiological roles. MCRs are found in chordates and are regarded as having evolved from a single ancestral receptor, possibly corresponding most closely to MC4R (Dores, 2013). Signaling by MCRs has primarily been observed as occurring through the stimulatory α unit Gs which activates adenylyl cyclase to produce cAMP, although other pathways have been implicated (Yang, 2011). Receptor properties such as biased agonism (MC4R) and constitutive activity (MC3R and MC4R) have also been reported (Nijenhuis et al., 2001; Breit et al., 2011).

The melanocortin agonist ligands for MCRs, adrenocorticotropic hormone (ACTH) and the melanocyte stimulating hormones αMSH, βMSH, and γMSH, are neuropeptides derived by enzymatic cleavage from proopiomelanocortin (Pritchard et al., 2002). Their relative potencies are set out together with the natural antagonists in **Table 1**. The natural peptide antagonists comprise agouti and agouti related protein (AgRP) (Cone, 2006). Agouti was first discovered as a high affinity MC1R antagonist, following studies on genetic determinants of yellow coat color and obese phenotype observed in agouti mouse strains (Lu et al., 1994). Agouti-related

TABLE 1 | Natural ligands of the melanocortin receptor family (Kiefer et al., 1997; MacNeil et al., 2002; Cone, 2006).

Receptor	Relative potency of agonists	Antagonists	Main site of expression	Primary Function
MC1R	αMSH = βMSH = ACTH > γMSH	Agouti	Melanocytes	Pigmentation, inflammation
MC2R	ACTH only		Adrenal cortex	Adrenal steroidogenesis
MC3R	αMSH = βMSH = ACTH ≈ γMSH	Agouti; AgRP	CNS, GI tract, Kidney	Energy homoestasis, inflammation, Entrainment to meal intake
MC4R	αMSH = βMSH = ACTH >> γMSH	Agouti; AgRP	CNS	Energy homeostasis, thermogenesis, appetite regulation, erectile function
MC5R	αMSH > βMSH = ACTH >> γMSH		Exocrine cells	Exocrine function, regulation of sebaceous glands

protein (AgRP) was later identified as a MC3R and MC4R antagonistic peptide almost identical in size and genomic structure to Agouti (Ollmann et al., 1997; Shutter et al., 1997). Since then it has been shown that both Agouti and AgRP can act as inverse agonists in cAMP assays inhibiting MC1R and MC4R constitutive activity respectively (Vage et al., 1997; Chai et al., 2003). However, such inverse agonists to the MC4R can act as agonists through intracellular ERK1/2 signaling (Breit et al., 2011; Mo and Tao, 2013). A number of additional molecules have been shown to alter MCR function in a variety of ways including β-defensin 3 (Beaumont et al., 2012; Swope et al., 2012), attractin (also known as mahogany), and mahogunin (He et al., 2001).

MC1R

Pigmentation and the control of the inflammatory functions of the immune system are dependent on MC1R. Stimulation of MC1R in skin and hair follicle cells by αMSH results in melanogenesis producing dark skin or hair in many species, including humans (Beaumont et al., 2011). Variants in MC1R in humans are associated with red hair, pale skin, and increased risk to skin cancer. This action of αMSH is antagonized *in vivo* by agouti (Lu et al., 1994). MC1R is present on human leukocytes, and on murine macrophages, and has been implicated in the anti-inflammatory properties of αMSH (Star et al., 1995; Catania et al., 2004).

MC2R

MC2R is unique as it is the only MCR that binds to a specific ligand ACTH. The receptor is predominantly expressed in the adrenal gland. In humans, the inability of ACTH to activate MC2R leads to failure of the adrenal gland to generate cortisol, resulting in the potentially lethal condition of familial glucocorticoid deficiency (FGD) (Clark et al., 1993). Mutation in MC2R leads to FGD type 1. The FGD phenotype was reproduced in the MC2R knockout mouse, although the mice also had evidence of mineralocorticoid deficiency (Chida et al., 2007). MC2R is also found in human and mouse bone where it is thought to be involved in osteoblast proliferation (Zhong et al., 2005). Interestingly, patients with FGD type 1 have tall stature (Elias et al., 2000). MC2R has also been detected in human subcutaneous fat (Smith et al., 2003) and the developing testis (O'Shaughnessy et al., 2007). In mouse adipose tissue, MC2R may be implicated in the release of non-esterified fatty acids from adipocytes (Moller et al., 2011).

MC3R

MC3R is primarily expressed in the central nervous system in the arcuate nucleus of the hypothalamus and limbic areas, where it affects food utilization/partitioning and food anticipatory behavior (Sutton et al., 2008, 2010; Begriche et al., 2011). Although loss-of-function mutations in MC3R have been identified in humans with obesity, there is still uncertainty if these variants are truly causative (Lee et al., 2007; Mencarelli et al., 2011). In mice, MC3R is essential for the maintenance of a circadian rhythm of activity related to feeding behavior (Begriche et al., 2012). Both central and peripheral MC3R are involved in energy utilization (Begriche et al., 2011). MC3R has also been implicated in the anti-inflammatory processes in murine macrophages (Getting et al., 2006; Leoni et al., 2008; Montero-Melendez et al., 2014).

MC4R

MC4R is thought to bind principally to αMSH in the paraventricular nucleus (PVN) of the hypothalamus (CNS), a region crucial in the control of food intake. Global homozygous deletion of MC4R in mice results in hyperphagia, increased fat and lean mass, increased body length, reduced activity, and reduced metabolic rate (Huszar et al., 1997; Balthasar et al., 2005). Inactivating mutations in MC4R are the single most common form of monogenic obesity in humans (Farooqi et al., 2003). Common variants near the MC4R locus are associated with adiposity, body weight, risk of obesity and insulin resistance at a population level (Chambers et al., 2008; Loos et al., 2008). The function of MC4R has also expanded over recent years and involvement in autonomic regulation of thermogenesis and glycaemia (Berglund et al., 2014), regulation of sympathetic and parasympathetic control of blood pressure (Sohn et al., 2013) and anhedonia (Lim et al., 2012) have all been described. A role in erectile function and sexual behavior have also been reported (van der Ploeg et al., 2002). Most recently, MC4R expression has been demonstrated in enteroendocrine L cells and regulates the release of peptide YY (PYY) and glucagon-like peptide 1 (GLP-1) (Panaro et al., 2014).

MC5R

The need for MC5R activity in the secretory function of exocrine glands is well-known (Chen et al., 1997; van der Kraan et al., 1998). MC5R is widely expressed and mice deficient of Mc5r have impaired water repulsion and thermoregulation (Chen et al., 1997). There are some suggestions that MC5R expression in the zona glomerulosa of the adrenal gland may be involved in melanocortin stimulated aldosterone secretion (Vinson et al., 1980; Griffon et al., 1994; van der Kraan et al., 1998), although this is not in keeping with the lack of an adrenal phenotype in Mc5r knockout mice (Chen et al., 1997). Stimulation of MC5R in 3T3-L1 adipocytes with αMSH has been shown to result in lipolysis, through cAMP production, and impairment of re-esterification of fatty acids, through the ERK1/2 pathway (Rodrigues et al., 2013).

The Melanocortin Receptor Accessory Proteins, MRAP, and MRAP2

Discovery of MRAP and MRAP2

The discovery of MRAP (sometimes referred to as MRAP1) in 2005 by Metherell et al. has provided insight into a novel aspect of MCR regulation, previously unknown (Metherell et al., 2005). By studying the clinical condition FGD it was noted that only approximately 25% of FGD cases were attributable to mutations of MC2R (Chan et al., 2009). Failure of MC2R to traffick to the cell surface in cells other than those derived from an adrenal lineage suggested the presence of an adrenal specific accessory protein (Noon et al., 2002). Using whole genome SNP array genotyping on informative families, mutations in the gene encoding a protein derived from open reading frame 61 of human chromosome 21 (C21orf61), corresponding to a murine adipocyte transmembrane protein (Xu et al., 2002), was identified to cause FGD type 2 (Metherell et al., 2005). This gene was subsequently named melanocortin-2-receptor accessory protein (MRAP). The human MRAP gene contains six exons, exons 5 and 6 are alternatively spliced to give rise to two MRAP isoforms, MRAPα (exon1–5), and MRAPβ (exon 1–4 and 6). Exons 1 and 2 are not translated in the human isoforms whilst rodents do not have the corresponding exons 1 and 2 and produce only one form of the protein (Webb and Clark, 2010). The translated small single pass transmembrane domain protein differs from other known GPCR accessory proteins (Webb and Clark, 2010) and has been shown to adopt a unique anti-parrallel homodimer conformation at the cell surface (Sebag and Hinkle, 2007; Cooray et al., 2008). Both isoforms are present with MC2R in human adrenal tissue (Metherell et al., 2005). The presence of either MRAPα or MRAPβ is essential for MC2R cell surface expression and signaling (Metherell et al., 2005; Roy et al., 2007; Cooray et al., 2008; Hinkle and Sebag, 2009), but the response of MC2R to ACTH may differ between the two isoforms, with MRAPα increasing potency but MRAPβ increasing maximal response (Roy et al., 2007).

Human C6orf117 was identified as a possible paralog to MRAP (Metherell et al., 2005). This gene was subsequently designated MRAP2. The human MRAP2 gene has four exons, exons 2–4 code for a 205 amino acid residue protein (Chan et al., 2009). MRAP2 is thought to adopt a similar dual topology at the cell surface (Chan et al., 2009). Mouse Mrap2 gene differs in having two small untranslated exons 1 and 1a (Asai et al., 2013). Zebra fish has a single Mrap and two forms of Mrap2, designated mrap2a and mrap2b (Agulleiro et al., 2010). Mrap2a and mrap2b appear to have different actions and appear at differing time points in zebrafish development (Sebag et al., 2013). Study of the conservation between the Mraps of lampreys, cartilaginous fish, teleosts, and tetrapods has indicated that MRAP2 is the ancestral gene (Webb and Clark, 2010; Dores, 2013).

Tissue Expression of MRAPs

Both MRAPα mRNA and MRAPβ mRNA are found in human adrenal tissue, testis, breast tissue, ovary, fat, skin, and jejunum, MRAPα mRNA alone being more widely distributed in digestive tract tissues, the immune system, and in thyroid and pituitary, and MRAPβ mRNA alone appearing in brain (Metherell et al., 2005). Evidence for human MRAP mRNA has been detected in the hippocampus, prefrontal cortex, cerebellum, and spinal cord, among other tissues (Gardiner et al., 2002). MRAP expression clearly extends beyond MC2R expression, where expression of MC2R has been reported in the adrenal, bone, adipose tissue, ovaries, testes, skin, and the pituitary (Metherell et al., 2005). MRAP2 mRNA was detected in human adrenal and brain tissue (Chan et al., 2009). In mice Mrap2 mRNA was detected by RT-PCR in a wider number of tissues including hypothalamus, pons, brainstem, cerebellum, eye, thymus, pituitary, adrenal, gonads, skin, and fat (Asai et al., 2013). A recent report demonstrated that MRAP2 expression in human endometrium was significantly down regulated during endometrial transition from its pre-receptive state to the receptive state (Hu et al., 2014), although the physiological significance of this change is unknown.

MRAPs and Melanocortin Receptors *In vitro*

Several groups have studied the effects of MRAPs on MCR cell surface expression and function in a number of heterologous systems. The absolute requirement of MRAP for the MC2R trafficking and function is clear and recapitulated by many groups (Metherell et al., 2005; Roy et al., 2007; Sebag and Hinkle, 2007). Transient transfection of MRAPα and MRAP2 with MCRs into CHO cells confirmed that MRAP is necessary for surface expression of MC2R and showed that MRAP2 also can enable surface expression of MC2R (Chan et al., 2009). One study using HEK293 cells reported MC2R surface expression in the absence of MRAP (Roy et al., 2007), although this may well have been due to endogenous MRAP2 in some HEK293 cell-lines (Roy et al., 2010). In addition to surface expression, there are suggestions that MRAPs could influence the post-translational glycosylation of MC2R and MC4R (Kay et al., 2013a). MRAP is essential for MC2R to respond to ACTH and although the presence of MRAP2 can enable MC2R to respond to ACTH this is unlikely to be of physiological significance (Gorrigan et al., 2011). The interplay between MRAP and MRAP2 on MC2R function is less clear. Some suggest that MRAP and MRAP2 act in an antagonistic manner whilst others show no effect or an additive effect on MC2R function in the presence of both MRAPs (Chan et al., 2009; Agulleiro et al., 2010; Sebag and Hinkle, 2010).

The reported results on other MCRs vary, which in part may be due to differences in ligands, cell-lines, ratio of MRAP to MCR expressed or be dependent on the ortholog studied. MRAPs have no effect on the trafficking of MC1R and MC3R but reduce surface expression of MC4R and MC5R (Chan et al., 2009; Sebag and Hinkle, 2009, 2010). In the case of MC5R, MRAP appeared to disrupt MC5R dimerization (Sebag and Hinkle, 2009). Reduced cAMP generation in response to NDP-MSH was demonstrated for human MC1-5R (Chan et al., 2009). Other groups have also shown a significant reduction in MC5R signaling in the presence of MRAPs (Sebag and Hinkle, 2010; Kay et al., 2013b). These studies however found no change in MC4R potency (Sebag and Hinkle, 2010) or an increase in MC4R function (Asai et al., 2013; Sebag et al., 2013). MC4R constitutive activity does appear to be affected in the presence of MRAP/MRAP2 (Asai et al., 2013; Kay et al., 2013b; Sebag et al., 2013). The two isoforms of Mrap2 in zebrafish appears to have differing effects on Mc4r function. Mrap2a inhibits activation of Mc4r whilst Mrap2b suppressed the constitutive activity of the receptor but greatly increased the potency of αMSH (Sebag et al., 2013).

MRAP2

In vitro, MRAP2 has been shown to enable MC2R trafficking to the cell surface and subsequent signaling. N-linked glycosylation appears critical in this process (Chan et al., 2009). The dose of ACTH required to activate the receptor is however 1000 times higher than that compared to MRAP (Sebag and Hinkle, 2010; Gorrigan et al., 2011), which would explain the inability of MRAP2 to rescue MC2R function in patients with MRAP mutations. Furthermore, significantly lower levels of Mrap2 expression compared with Mrap expression are found in adult rat adrenal gland. Unlike Mrap, which is highly expressed in the zona fasciculata, Mrap2 appears sparsely expressed throughout the adult adrenal cortex (Gorrigan et al., 2011). Although, Mrap2 appears highly expressed in the developing adrenal gland, to date no adrenal phenotype have been described in the Mrap2 KO mice (Gorrigan et al., 2011; Asai et al., 2013).

MRAPs and Adrenal Disease

MRAP

Loss-of-function mutations in MRAP give rise to FGD type 2 (Metherell et al., 2005). Patients with FGD type 2 present with symptoms and signs resulting from isolated glucocorticoid deficiency and excess plasma ACTH (Chung et al., 2010). FGD type 2 patients present significantly earlier than those with FGD type 1 individuals harboring MC2R mutations, with the exception of those patients with missense MRAP mutations who present later and with a milder phenotype (Hughes et al., 2010).

In keeping with the importance of MRAP's role in glucocorticoid production, with both MRAP and MC2R are highly expressed in the zona fasciculata. However, the highest levels of expression are found in the undifferentiated zone, believed to contain adrenal stem cells, suggesting that MC2R and MRAP maybe important in adrenal development and/or maintenance (Gorrigan et al., 2011). The adrenal histology from deceased FGD patients would support this notion revealing glomerulosa cell disorganization and loss of fasciculata and reticularis cells (Clark and Weber, 1998).

MRAP is a critical component of the hypothalamic-pituitary-adrenal axis, involved in adrenal responsiveness to ACTH and possibly other adrenal disease processes. In rats, the transcription of Mrap RNA closely tracks the normal ultradian pulses of ACTH and, together with similar patterns of transcription and related protein processing of other components of adrenal steroidogenesis, suggests that Mrap protein availability is closely tied to need for signaling in response to ACTH (Liu et al., 2003).

One study assessed MC2R, MRAP, and MRAP2 expression in human adrenal tissue derived from normal and hyperplastic adrenal gland, and from adrenocortical adenomas and carcinomas (Hofland et al., 2012). Their data suggested that the effect of ACTH stimulation on the expression of the ACTH receptor complex comprising MC2R, MRAP and MRAP2 assists in the production of a functioning complex, although the level of MRAP2 being insufficient to reduce its sensitivity to ACTH.

MRAPs and Obesity

MRAP2

MRAP2 was shown to interact with all MCRs and the expression in the hypothalamus and PVN pointed to a role in central melanocortin regulation of metabolism and appetite (Chan et al., 2009). A recent publication describing obesity in rodents and humans with MRAP2 deficiency has demonstrated that this is indeed the case (Asai et al., 2013). Furthermore, zebrafish deficient of MRAP2 isoforms was shown to have disrupted growth and development supporting the role of MRAP2 in metabolism homeostasis (Sebag et al., 2013).

Phenotypically, global Mrap2 KO mice on an sv129 genetic background fed a chow *ad libitum* diet develop severe obesity at a young age and were found to be significantly heavier than their wild type counterparts at approximately 6 weeks of age. Mrap2$^{-/-}$ mice have increased body length and fat deposits, whilst percentage lean mass was reduced. Heterozygous Mrap2$^{+/-}$ mice have an intermediate phenotype (Asai et al., 2013).

Serum leptin was elevated in Mrap2 null mice, which normalized following weight loss through food restriction. No differences in fasting serum insulin concentration, response to glucose load or serum T3 and T4 levels were detectable between null and wild-type animals, whilst Mrap2$^{-/-}$ males have lower 24 h urine epinephrine and norepinephrine. AgRP mRNA levels in the hypothalamus are increased in Mrap2 null animals without changes in POMC mRNA. Although brown fat deposit was enlarged in obese mice, response to cold challenge normal and Ucp1 mRNA levels in brown fat increased appropriately when mice were subjected to 4°C for 18 h (Asai et al., 2013).

Interestingly, no increase in food intake was detected and despite paired feeding, Mrap2$^{-/-}$ mice became significantly heavier in weight compared with Mrap$^{+/+}$ littermates. Food restriction in Mrap2$^{-/-}$ mice (90% (females) or 87% (males) of wild type intake) was required to normalize their weight gain to that of wild-type Mrap2$^{+/+}$ mice. Faecal energy content was also indistinguishable between Mrap2$^{-/-}$ and Mrap2$^{+/+}$ mice (Asai et al., 2013).

Analysis of young mice prior the divergence of weight between null and wild-type mice demonstrated indistinguishable 24 h energy expenditure and respiratory exchange ratio (RER) when measured by indirect calorimetry. There was no difference in locomotor activity during the day or night and body temperature even when challenged by cold was not different (Asai et al., 2013).

Asai et al. demonstrated that Mrap2 was expressed in several sites of the mouse brain and in the PVN co-localized with Mc4r expressing neurons (Asai et al., 2013), suggestive of an MC4R dependent mechanisms. Mrap2$^{-/-}$ mice share some phenotypic similarities with Mc4r KO mice, which are heavier with increased length and adiposity. Heterozygous Mc4r$^{+/-}$ mice have an intermediate weight phenotype (Huszar et al., 1997). In support of an MC4R mechanism, mice with conditional deletion of Mrap2 in Sim1 neurons that express Mc4r were equally obese and phenotypically similar to global Mrap2$^{-/-}$ mice (Asai et al., 2013). However, differences exist between Mrap2$^{-/-}$ and Mc4r$^{-/-}$ mice. In Mc4r$^{-/-}$ mice, obesity is attributable to hyperphagia and reduced energy expenditure. The Mc4r null mice also have increased lean mass (Balthasar et al., 2005; Sutton et al., 2006).

In humans, disabling mutations of MC4R are the most common cause of monogenic obesity and found in up to 6% of severely obese patients (Vaisse et al., 1998; Yeo et al., 1998). In comparison, genetic screening of two large obese pediatric cohorts identified only four rare heterozygous MRAP2 variants (N88Y, L115V, R125C, E24X) in patients with severe early onset obesity (Asai et al., 2013). The individual carrying the most damaging variant, E24X variant, was the most severely affected with a reported BMI of 63 kg/m2 (BMI SDS 4.7) at the age of 19 years.

Data from zebrafish supports the notion that MRAP2 is an MC4R accessory protein capable of regulating the function of MC4R (Asai et al., 2013; Sebag et al., 2013). However, several lines of evidence from the Mrap2$^{-/-}$ mice data would suggest the possibility of Mc4r independent mechanisms. Firstly, Mrap2$^{-/-}$ mice remain responsive to treatment with MTII, a Mc3r and Mc4r agonist, whilst anorexic response to MTII is abolished in Mc4r$^{-/-}$ mice. Secondly, Mrap2$^{-/-}$ and Mc4r$^{-/-}$ double KOs are less obese compared with Mc4r$^{-/-}$ mice alone and finally the Mrap2$^{-/-}$ does not completely replicate Mc4r$^{-/-}$ mice phenotype.

The phenotype of the Mc3r homozygous knockout mice is of interest. Mc3r$^{-/-}$ animals are not obviously hyperphagic but eventually become heavier than wild type mice on a standard chow diet, and have more adipose tissue and smaller bones, but no significant difference in energy expenditure (Chen et al., 2000; Begriche et al., 2011). Heterozygous Mc3r knockout mice are similar to wild type mice (Chen et al., 2000). More recently it has been shown that MRAP2, but not MRAP, localizes at the apical plasma membrane in the presence of MC3R in a polarized cell, MC3R also localizing at the apical membrane (Park et al., 2014). Receptors and other structures in neurons have precisely determined locations and are associated with dedicated trafficking mechanisms in which MRAPs may have a role.

There is no suggestion that Mrap2 plays a role in MC1R or MC2R function as Mrap2$^{-/-}$ mice have normal coat color and corticosterone production (at baseline and when stressed) (Asai et al., 2013).

MRAP

It is not yet known if MRAP is associated with mammalian obesity. There is a single case report describing a family with a splice site mutation of MRAP. Family members homozygous and heterozygous for the mutation were obese compared with normal weighted unaffected members (Rumie et al., 2007). As yet the knockout mouse has not been reported. In murine 3T3-L1 cells,

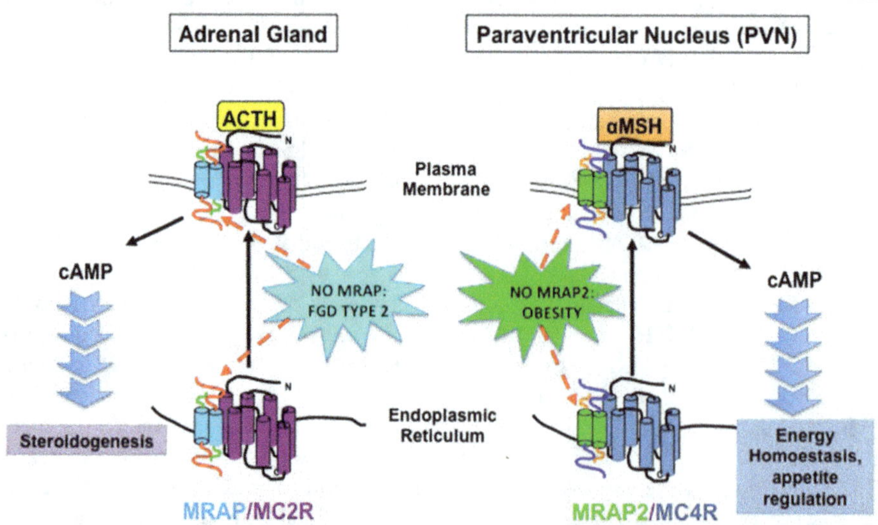

FIGURE 1 | Schematic Diagram illustrating MRAP and MRAP2 action on MC2R and MC4R, respectively and physiological consequence of MRAP and MRAP2 deficiency on adrenal steroidogenesis and energy homeostasis.

ACTH triggers lipolysis and knockdown of Mrap in these cells substantially inhibits lipolysis (Kim et al., 2013). Furthermore, the promoter of Mrap was found to include a region binding the transcription factor PPARγ that regulates adipogenesis in fibroblasts (Tontonoz et al., 1994; Kim et al., 2013).

Future of MRAPs

The discovery of MRAP and MRAP2 has initiated a paradigm shift in our understanding of MCR and GPCR signaling (**Figure 1**). For MRAP, the ability to functionally express MC2R in non-adrenal cell lines has opened up many opportunities including screening for MC2R peptide antagonists (Bouw et al., 2014). Moreover, the finding that MRAP2 is associated with mammalian obesity is exciting and could provide a novel therapeutic target at a time when obesity is at epidemic levels. There are many scientific questions yet to be answered. For example, the precise mechanism of how MRAP2 causes obesity is not fully understood. It is intriguing that no difference in food intake or energy expenditure was detected in $Mrap2^{-/-}$ compared to wild-type littermates. This may represent the lack of sensitivity of the systems in place to detect the relatively small changes in food intake and energy expenditure. If so this demonstrates the fine balance in energy homeostasis, where small changes could tip the scale leading to significant weight gain. However, in light of the differences between $Mc4r^{-/-}$ and $Mrap2^{-/-}$ mice, it is likely that MC4R independent mechanisms as well as MCR independent pathways are at play. The complexity of these proteins and how they regulate MCR and GPCR function is only just beginning to be explored.

Acknowledgments

Research on MRAPs is supported by an MRC/Academy of Medical Sciences Clinician Scientist Fellowship to LFC (grant number G0802796).

References

Agulleiro, M. J., Roy, S., Sanchez, E., Puchol, S., Gallo-Payet, N., and Cerda-Reverter, J. M. (2010). Role of melanocortin receptor accessory proteins in the function of zebrafish melanocortin receptor type 2. *Mol. Cell Endocrinol.* 320, 145–152. doi: 10.1016/j.mce.2010.01.032

Asai, M., Ramachandrappa, S., Joachim, M., Shen, Y., Zhang, R., Nuthalapati, N., et al. (2013). Loss of function of the melanocortin 2 receptor accessory protein 2 is associated with mammalian obesity. *Science* 341, 275–278. doi: 10.1126/science.1233000

Balthasar, N., Dalgaard, L. T., Lee, C. E., Yu, J., Funahashi, H., Williams, T., et al. (2005). Divergence of melanocortin pathways in the control of food intake and energy expenditure. *Cell* 123, 493–505. doi: 10.1016/j.cell.2005.08.035

Beaumont, K. A., Smit, D. J., Liu, Y. Y., Chai, E., Patel, M. P., Millhauser, G. L., et al. (2012). Melanocortin-1 receptor-mediated signalling pathways activated by NDP-MSH and HBD3 ligands. *Pigment Cell Melanoma Res.* 25, 370–374. doi: 10.1111/j.1755-148X.2012.00990.x

Beaumont, K. A., Wong, S. S., Ainger, S. A., Liu, Y. Y., Patel, M. P., Millhauser, G. L., et al. (2011). Melanocortin MC(1) receptor in human genetics and model systems. *Eur. J. Pharmacol.* 660, 103–110. doi: 10.1016/j.ejphar.2010.11.040

Begriche, K., Levasseur, P. R., Zhang, J., Rossi, J., Skorupa, D., Solt, L. A., et al. (2011). Genetic dissection of the functions of the melanocortin-3 receptor, a seven-transmembrane G-protein-coupled receptor, suggests roles for central and peripheral receptors in energy homeostasis. *J. Biol. Chem.* 286, 40771–40781. doi: 10.1074/jbc.M111.278374

Begriche, K., Marston, O. J., Rossi, J., Burke, L. K., McDonald, P., Heisler, L. K., et al. (2012). Melanocortin-3 receptors are involved in adaptation to restricted feeding. *Genes Brain Behav.* 11, 291–302. doi: 10.1111/j.1601-183X.2012.00766.x

Berglund, E. D., Liu, T., Kong, X., Sohn, J. W., Vong, L., Deng, Z., et al. (2014). Melanocortin 4 receptors in autonomic neurons regulate thermogenesis and glycemia. *Nat. Neurosci.* 17, 911–913. doi: 10.1038/nn.3737

Bouw, E., Huisman, M., Neggers, S. J., Themmen, A. P., van der Lely, A. J., and Delhanty, P. J. (2014). Development of potent selective competitive-antagonists of the melanocortin type 2 receptor. *Mol. Cell Endocrinol.* 394, 99–104. doi: 10.1016/j.mce.2014.07.003

Breit, A., Buch, T. R., Boekhoff, I., Solinski, H. J., Damm, E., and Gudermann, T. (2011). Alternative G protein coupling and biased agonism: new insights into melanocortin-4 receptor signalling. *Mol. Cell Endocrinol.* 331, 232–240. doi: 10.1016/j.mce.2010.07.007

Catania, A., Gatti, S., Colombo, G., and Lipton, J. M. (2004). Targeting melanocortin receptors as a novel strategy to control inflammation. *Pharmacol. Rev.* 56, 1–29. doi: 10.1124/pr.56.1.1

Chai, B. X., Neubig, R. R., Millhauser, G. L., Thompson, D. A., Jackson, P. J., Barsh, G. S., et al. (2003). Inverse agonist activity of agouti and agouti-related protein. *Peptides* 24, 603–609. doi: 10.1016/S0196-9781(03)00104-9

Chambers, J. C., Elliott, P., Zabaneh, D., Zhang, W., Li, Y., Froguel, P., et al. (2008). Common genetic variation near MC4R is associated with waist circumference and insulin resistance. *Nat. Genet.* 40, 716–718. doi: 10.1038/ng.156

Chan, L. F., Webb, T. R., Chung, T. T., Meimaridou, E., Cooray, S. N., Guasti, L., et al. (2009). MRAP and MRAP2 are bidirectional regulators of the melanocortin receptor family. *Proc. Natl. Acad. Sci. U.S.A.* 106, 6146–6151. doi: 10.1073/pnas.0809918106

Chen, A. S., Marsh, D. J., Trumbauer, M. E., Frazier, E. G., Guan, X. M., Yu, H., et al. (2000). Inactivation of the mouse melanocortin-3 receptor results in increased fat mass and reduced lean body mass. *Nat. Genet.* 26, 97–102. doi: 10.1038/79254

Chen, W., Kelly, M. A., Opitz-Araya, X., Thomas, R. E., Low, M. J., and Cone, R. D. (1997). Exocrine gland dysfunction in MC5-R-deficient mice: evidence for coordinated regulation of exocrine gland function by melanocortin peptides. *Cell* 91, 789–798. doi: 10.1016/S0092-8674(00)80467-5

Chida, D., Nakagawa, S., Nagai, S., Sagara, H., Katsumata, H., Imaki, T., et al. (2007). Melanocortin 2 receptor is required for adrenal gland development, steroidogenesis, and neonatal gluconeogenesis. *Proc. Natl. Acad. Sci. U.S.A.* 104, 18205–18210. doi: 10.1073/pnas.0706953104

Chung, T. T., Chan, L. F., Metherell, L. A., and Clark, A. J. (2010). Phenotypic characteristics of familial glucocorticoid deficiency (FGD) type 1 and 2. *Clin. Endocrinol. (Oxf.)* 72, 589–594. doi: 10.1111/j.1365-2265.2009.03663.x

Clark, A. J., and Weber, A. (1998). Adrenocorticotropin insensitivity syndromes. *Endocr. Rev.* 19, 828–843. doi: 10.1210/edrv.19.6.0351

Clark, A. J., McLoughlin, L., and Grossman, A. (1993). Familial glucocorticoid deficiency associated with point mutation in the adrenocorticotropin receptor. *Lancet* 341, 461–462. doi: 10.1016/0140-6736(93)90208-X

Cone, R. D. (2006). Studies on the physiological functions of the melanocortin system. *Endocr. Rev.* 27, 736–749. doi: 10.1210/er.2006-0034

Cooray, S. N., Almiro Do Vale, I., Leung, K. Y., Webb, T. R., Chapple, J. P., Egertova, M., et al. (2008). The melanocortin 2 receptor accessory protein exists as a homodimer and is essential for the function of the melanocortin 2 receptor in the mouse y1 cell line. *Endocrinology* 149, 1935–1941. doi: 10.1210/en.2007-1463

Dores, R. M. (2013). Observations on the evolution of the melanocortin receptor gene family: distinctive features of the melanocortin-2 receptor. *Front. Neurosci.* 7:28. doi: 10.3389/fnins.2013.00028

Elias, L. L., Huebner, A., Metherell, L. A., Canas, A., Warne, G. L., Bitti, M. L., et al. (2000). Tall stature in familial glucocorticoid deficiency. *Clin. Endocrinol. (Oxf.)* 53, 423–430. doi: 10.1046/j.1365-2265.2000.01122.x

Farooqi, I. S., Keogh, J. M., Yeo, G. S., Lank, E. J., Cheetham, T., and O'Rahilly, S. (2003). Clinical spectrum of obesity and mutations in the melanocortin 4 receptor gene. *N.Engl. J. Med.* 348, 1085–1095. doi: 10.1056/nejmoa022050

Gardiner, K., Slavov, D., Bechtel, L., and Davisson, M. (2002). Annotation of human chromosome 21 for relevance to Down syndrome: gene structure and expression analysis. *Genomics* 79, 833–843. doi: 10.1006/geno.2002.6782

Getting, S. J., Lam, C. W., Leoni, G., Gavins, F. N., Grieco, P., and Perretti, M. (2006). [D-Trp8]-gamma-melanocyte-stimulating hormone exhibits anti-inflammatory efficacy in mice bearing a nonfunctional MC1R (recessive yellow e/e mouse). *Mol. Pharmacol.* 70, 1850–1855. doi: 10.1124/mol.106.028878

Gorrigan, R. J., Guasti, L., King, P., Clark, A. J., and Chan, L. F. (2011). Localisation of the melanocortin-2-receptor and its accessory proteins in the developing and adult adrenal gland. *J. Mol. Endocrinol.* 46, 227–232. doi: 10.1530/JME-11-0011

Griffon, N., Mignon, V., Facchinetti, P., Diaz, J., Schwartz, J. C., and Sokoloff, P. (1994). Molecular cloning and characterization of the rat fifth melanocortin receptor. *Biochem. Biophys. Res. Commun.* 200, 1007–1014. doi: 10.1006/bbrc.1994.1550

He, L., Gunn, T. M., Bouley, D. M., Lu, X. Y., Watson, S. J., Schlossman, S. F., et al. (2001). A biochemical function for attractin in agouti-induced pigmentation and obesity. *Nat. Genet.* 27, 40–47. doi: 10.1038/89022

Hinkle, P. M., and Sebag, J. A. (2009). Structure and function of the melanocortin2 receptor accessory protein (MRAP). *Mol. Cell Endocrinol.* 300, 25–31. doi: 10.1016/j.mce.2008.10.041

Hofland, J., Delhanty, P. J., Steenbergen, J., Hofland, L. J., van Koetsveld, P. M., van Nederveen, F. H., et al. (2012). Melanocortin 2 receptor-associated protein (MRAP) and MRAP2 in human adrenocortical tissues: regulation of expression and association with ACTH responsiveness. *J. Clin. Endocrinol. Metab.* 97, E747–E754. doi: 10.1210/jc.2011-2328

Hu, S., Yao, G., Wang, Y., Xu, H., Ji, X., He, Y., et al. (2014). Transcriptomic changes during the pre-receptive to receptive transition in human endometrium detected by RNA-Seq. *J. Clin. Endocrinol. Metab.* 99, E2744–E2753. doi: 10.1210/jc.2014-2155

Hughes, C. R., Chung, T. T., Habeb, A. M., Kelestimur, F., Clark, A. J., and Metherell, L. A. (2010). Missense mutations in the melanocortin 2 receptor accessory protein that lead to late onset familial glucocorticoid deficiency type 2. *J. Clin. Endocrinol. Metab.* 95, 3497–3501. doi: 10.1210/jc.2009-2731

Huszar, D., Lynch, C. A., Fairchild-Huntress, V., Dunmore, J. H., Fang, Q., Berkemeier, L. R., et al. (1997). Targeted disruption of the melanocortin-4 receptor results in obesity in mice. *Cell* 88, 131–141. doi: 10.1016/S0092-8674(00)81865-6

Kay, E. I., Botha, R., Montgomery, J. M., and Mountjoy, K. G. (2013a). hMRAPa specifically alters hMC4R molecular mass and N-linked complex glycosylation in HEK293 cells. *J. Mol. Endocrinol.* 50, 217–227. doi: 10.1530/JME-12-0220

Kay, E. I., Botha, R., Montgomery, J. M., and Mountjoy, K. G. (2013b). hMRAPa increases alphaMSH-induced hMC1R and hMC3R functional coupling and hMC4R constitutive activity. *J. Mol. Endocrinol.* 50, 203–215. doi: 10.1530/JME-12-0221

Kiefer, L. L., Ittoop, O. R., Bunce, K., Truesdale, A. T., Willard, D. H., Nichols, J. S., et al. (1997). Mutations in the carboxyl terminus of the agouti protein decrease agouti inhibition of ligand binding to the melanocortin receptors. *Biochemistry* 36, 2084–2090. doi: 10.1021/bi962647v

Kim, N. S., Kim, Y. J., Cho, S. Y., Lee, T. R., and Kim, S. H. (2013). Transcriptional activation of melanocortin 2 receptor accessory protein by PPARgamma in adipocytes. *Biochem. Biophys. Res. Commun.* 439, 401–406. doi: 10.1016/j.bbrc.2013.08.061

Lee, Y. S., Poh, L. K., Kek, B. L., and Loke, K. Y. (2007). The role of melanocortin 3 receptor gene in childhood obesity. *Diabetes* 56, 2622–2630. doi: 10.2337/db07-0225

Leoni, G., Patel, H. B., Sampaio, A. L., Gavins, F. N., Murray, J. F., Grieco, P., et al. (2008). Inflamed phenotype of the mesenteric microcirculation of melanocortin type 3 receptor-null mice after ischemia-reperfusion. *FASEB J.* 22, 4228–4238. doi: 10.1096/fj.08-113886

Lim, B. K., Huang, K. W., Grueter, B. A., Rothwell, P. E., and Malenka, R. C. (2012). Anhedonia requires MC4R-mediated synaptic adaptations in nucleus accumbens. *Nature* 487, 183–189. doi: 10.1038/nature11160

Liu, H., Kishi, T., Roseberry, A. G., Cai, X., Lee, C. E., Montez, J. M., et al. (2003). Transgenic mice expressing green fluorescent protein under the control of the melanocortin-4 receptor promoter. *J. Neurosci.* 23, 7143–7154.

Loos, R. J., Lindgren, C. M., Li, S., Wheeler, E., Zhao, J. H., Prokopenko, I., et al. (2008). Common variants near MC4R are associated with fat mass, weight and risk of obesity. *Nat. Genet.* 40, 768–775. doi: 10.1038/ng.140

Lu, D., Willard, D., Patel, I. R., Kadwell, S., Overton, L., Kost, T., et al. (1994). Agouti protein is an antagonist of the melanocyte-stimulating-hormone receptor. *Nature* 371, 799–802. doi: 10.1038/371799a0

MacNeil, D. J., Howard, A. D., Guan, X., Fong, T. M., Nargund, R. P., Bednarek, M. A., et al. (2002). The role of melanocortins in body weight regulation: opportunities for the treatment of obesity. *Eur. J. Pharmacol.* 450, 93–109. doi: 10.1016/S0014-2999(02)01989-1

Mencarelli, M., Dubern, B., Alili, R., Maestrini, S., Benajiba, L., Tagliaferri, M., et al. (2011). Rare melanocortin-3 receptor mutations with *in vitro* functional consequences are associated with human obesity. *Hum. Mol. Genet.* 20, 392–399. doi: 10.1093/hmg/ddq472

Metherell, L. A., Chapple, J. P., Cooray, S., David, A., Becker, C., Ruschendorf, F., et al. (2005). Mutations in MRAP, encoding a new interacting partner of the ACTH receptor, cause familial glucocorticoid deficiency type 2. *Nat. Genet.* 37, 166–170. doi: 10.1038/ng1501

Mo, X. L., and Tao, Y. X. (2013). Activation of MAPK by inverse agonists in six naturally occurring constitutively active mutant human melanocortin-4 receptors. *Biochim. Biophys. Acta* 1832, 1939–1948. doi: 10.1016/j.bbadis.2013.06.006

Moller, C. L., Raun, K., Jacobsen, M. L., Pedersen, T. A., Holst, B., Conde-Frieboes, K. W., et al. (2011). Characterization of murine melanocortin receptors mediating adipocyte lipolysis and examination of signalling pathways involved. *Mol. Cell Endocrinol.* 341, 9–17. doi: 10.1016/j.mce.2011.03.010

Montero-Melendez, T., Madeira, M. F., Norling, L. V., Alsam, A., Curtis, M. A., da Silva, T. A., et al. (2014). Association between periodontal disease and inflammatory arthritis reveals modulatory functions by melanocortin receptor type 3. *Am. J. Pathol.* 184, 2333–2341. doi: 10.1016/j.ajpath.2014.04.009

Nijenhuis, W. A., Oosterom, J., and Adan, R. A. (2001). AgRP(83-132) acts as an inverse agonist on the human-melanocortin-4 receptor. *Mol. Endocrinol.* 15, 164–171. doi: 10.1210/mend.15.1.0578

Noon, L. A., Franklin, J. M., King, P. J., Goulding, N. J., Hunyady, L., and Clark, A. J. (2002). Failed export of the adrenocorticotrophin receptor from the endoplasmic reticulum in non-adrenal cells: evidence in support of a requirement for a specific adrenal accessory factor. *J. Endocrinol.* 174, 17–25. doi: 10.1677/joe.0.1740017

O'Shaughnessy, P. J., Baker, P. J., Monteiro, A., Cassie, S., Bhattacharya, S., and Fowler, P. A. (2007). Developmental changes in human fetal testicular cell numbers and messenger ribonucleic acid levels during the second trimester. *J. Clin. Endocrinol. Metab.* 92, 4792–4801. doi: 10.1210/jc.2007-1690

Ollmann, M. M., Wilson, B. D., Yang, Y. K., Kerns, J. A., Chen, Y., Gantz, I., et al. (1997). Antagonism of central melanocortin receptors *in vitro* and *in vivo* by agouti-related protein. *Science* 278, 135–138. doi: 10.1126/science.278.5335.135

Panaro, B. L., Tough, I. R., Engelstoft, M. S., Matthews, R. T., Digby, G. J., Moller, C. L., et al. (2014). The Melanocortin-4 receptor is expressed in enteroendocrine L cells and regulates the release of peptide YY and Glucagon-like peptide 1 *in vivo*. *Cell Metab.* 20, 1018–1029. doi: 10.1016/j.cmet.2014.10.004

Park, J., Sharma, N., and Cutting, G. R. (2014). Melanocortin 3 receptor has a 5' exon that directs translation of apically localized protein from the second in-frame ATG. *Mol. Endocrinol.* 28, 1547–1557. doi: 10.1210/me.2014-1105

Pritchard, L. E., Turnbull, A. V., and White, A. (2002). Pro-opiomelanocortin processing in the hypothalamus: impact on melanocortin signalling and obesity. *J. Endocrinol.* 172, 411–421. doi: 10.1677/joe.0.1720411

Rodrigues, A. R., Almeida, H., and Gouveia, A. M. (2013). Alpha-MSH signalling via melanocortin 5 receptor promotes lipolysis and impairs re-esterification in adipocytes. *Biochim. Biophys. Acta* 1831, 1267–1275. doi: 10.1016/j.bbalip.2013.04.008

Roy, S., Perron, B., and Gallo-Payet, N. (2010). Role of asparagine-linked glycosylation in cell surface expression and function of the human adrenocorticotropin receptor (melanocortin 2 receptor) in 293/FRT cells. *Endocrinology* 151, 660–670. doi: 10.1210/en.2009-0826

Roy, S., Rached, M., and Gallo-Payet, N. (2007). Differential regulation of the human adrenocorticotropin receptor [melanocortin-2 receptor (MC2R)] by human MC2R accessory protein isoforms alpha and beta in isogenic human embryonic kidney 293 cells. *Mol. Endocrinol.* 21, 1656–1669. doi: 10.1210/me.2007-0041

Rumie, H., Metherell, L. A., Clark, A. J., Beauloye, V., and Maes, M. (2007). Clinical and biological phenotype of a patient with familial glucocorticoid deficiency type 2 caused by a mutation of melanocortin 2 receptor accessory protein. *Eur. J. Endocrinol.* 157, 539–542. doi: 10.1530/EJE-07-0242

Sebag, J. A., and Hinkle, P. M. (2007). Melanocortin-2 receptor accessory protein MRAP forms antiparallel homodimers. *Proc. Natl. Acad. Sci. U.S.A.* 104, 20244–20249. doi: 10.1073/pnas.0708916105

Sebag, J. A., and Hinkle, P. M. (2009). Opposite effects of the melanocortin-2 (MC2) receptor accessory protein MRAP on MC2 and MC5 receptor dimerization and trafficking. *J. Biol. Chem.* 284, 22641–22648. doi: 10.1074/jbc.m109.022400

Sebag, J. A., and Hinkle, P. M. (2010). Regulation of G protein-coupled receptor signaling: specific dominant-negative effects of melanocortin 2 receptor accessory protein 2. *Sci. Signal.* 3:ra28. doi: 10.1126/scisignal.2000593

Sebag, J. A., Zhang, C., Hinkle, P. M., Bradshaw, A. M., and Cone, R. D. (2013). Developmental control of the melanocortin-4 receptor by MRAP2 proteins in zebrafish. *Science* 341, 278–281. doi: 10.1126/science.1232995

Shutter, J. R., Graham, M., Kinsey, A. C., Scully, S., Luthy, R., and Stark, K. L. (1997). Hypothalamic expression of ART, a novel gene related to agouti, is up-regulated in obese and diabetic mutant mice. *Genes Dev.* 11, 593–602. doi: 10.1101/gad.11.5.593

Smith, S. R., Gawronska-Kozak, B., Janderova, L., Nguyen, T., Murrell, A., Stephens, J. M., et al. (2003). Agouti expression in human adipose tissue: functional consequences and increased expression in type 2 diabetes. *Diabetes* 52, 2914–2922. doi: 10.2337/diabetes.52.12.2914

Sohn, J. W., Harris, L. E., Berglund, E. D., Liu, T., Vong, L., Lowell, B. B., et al. (2013). Melanocortin 4 receptors reciprocally regulate sympathetic and parasympathetic preganglionic neurons. *Cell* 152, 612–619. doi: 10.1016/j.cell.2012.12.022

Star, R. A., Rajora, N., Huang, J., Stock, R. C., Catania, A., and Lipton, J. M. (1995). Evidence of autocrine modulation of macrophage nitric oxide synthase by alpha-melanocyte-stimulating hormone. *Proc. Natl. Acad. Sci. U.S.A.* 92, 8016–8020. doi: 10.1073/pnas.92.17.8016

Sutton, G. M., Begriche, K., Kumar, K. G., Gimble, J. M., Perez-Tilve, D., Nogueiras, R., et al. (2010). Central nervous system melanocortin-3 receptors are required for synchronizing metabolism during entrainment to restricted feeding during the light cycle. *FASEB J.* 24, 862–872. doi: 10.1096/fj.09-142000

Sutton, G. M., Perez-Tilve, D., Nogueiras, R., Fang, J., Kim, J. K., Cone, R. D., et al. (2008). The melanocortin-3 receptor is required for entrainment to meal intake. *J. Neurosci.* 28, 12946–12955. doi: 10.1523/JNEUROSCI.3615-08.2008

Sutton, G. M., Trevaskis, J. L., Hulver, M. W., McMillan, R. P., Markward, N. J., Babin, M. J., et al. (2006). Diet-genotype interactions in the development of the obese, insulin-resistant phenotype of C57BL/6J mice lacking melanocortin-3 or -4 receptors. *Endocrinology* 147, 2183–2196. doi: 10.1210/en.2005-1209

Swope, V. B., Jameson, J. A., McFarland, K. L., Supp, D. M., Miller, W. E., McGraw, D. W., et al. (2012). Defining MC1R regulation in human melanocytes by its agonist alpha-melanocortin and antagonists agouti signaling protein and beta-defensin 3. *J. Invest. Dermatol.* 132, 2255–2262. doi: 10.1038/jid.2012.135

Tontonoz, P., Hu, E., and Spiegelman, B. M. (1994). Stimulation of adipogenesis in fibroblasts by PPAR gamma 2, a lipid-activated transcription factor. *Cell* 79, 1147–1156. doi: 10.1016/0092-8674(94)90006-X

Vage, D. I., Lu, D., Klungland, H., Lien, S., Adalsteinsson, S., and Cone, R. D. (1997). A non-epistatic interaction of agouti and extension in the fox, Vulpes vulpes. *Nat. Genet.* 15, 311–315. doi: 10.1038/ng0397-311

Vaisse, C., Clement, K., Guy-Grand, B., and Froguel, P. (1998). A frameshift mutation in human MC4R is associated with a dominant form of obesity. *Nat. Genet.* 20, 113–114. doi: 10.1038/2407

van der Kraan, M., Adan, R. A., Entwistle, M. L., Gispen, W. H., Burbach, J. P., and Tatro, J. B. (1998). Expression of melanocortin-5 receptor in secretory epithelia supports a functional role in exocrine and endocrine glands. *Endocrinology* 139, 2348–2355. doi: 10.1210/en.139.5.2348

van der Ploeg, L. H., Martin, W. J., Howard, A. D., Nargund, R. P., Austin, C. P., Guan, X., et al. (2002). A role for the melanocortin 4 receptor in sexual function. *Proc. Natl. Acad. Sci. U.S.A.* 99, 11381–11386. doi: 10.1073/pnas.172378699

Vinson, G. P., Whitehouse, B. J., Dell, A., Etienne, T., and Morris, H. R. (1980). Characterisation of an adrenal zona glomerulosa-stimulating component of posterior pituitary extracts as alpha-MSH. *Nature* 284, 464–467. doi: 10.1038/284464a0

Webb, T. R., and Clark, A. J. (2010). Minireview: the melanocortin 2 receptor accessory proteins. *Mol. Endocrinol.* 24, 475–484. doi: 10.1210/me.2009-0283

Xu, A., Choi, K. L., Wang, Y., Permana, P. A., Xu, L. Y., Bogardus, C., et al. (2002). Identification of novel putative membrane proteins selectively expressed during adipose conversion of 3T3-L1 cells. *Biochem. Biophys. Res. Commun.* 293, 1161–1167. doi: 10.1016/S0006-291X(02)00354-6

Yang, Y. (2011). Structure, function and regulation of the melanocortin receptors. *Eur. J. Pharmacol.* 660, 125–130. doi: 10.1016/j.ejphar.2010.12.020

Yeo, G. S., Farooqi, I. S., Aminian, S., Halsall, D. J., Stanhope, R. G., and O'Rahilly, S. (1998). A frameshift mutation in MC4R associated with dominantly inherited human obesity. *Nat. Genet.* 20, 111–112.

Zhong, Q., Sridhar, S., Ruan, L., Ding, K. H., Xie, D., Insogna, K., et al. (2005). Multiple melanocortin receptors are expressed in bone cells. *Bone* 36, 820–831. doi: 10.1016/j.bone.2005.01.020

Pineal melatonin is a circadian time-giver for leptin rhythm in *Syrian hamsters*

Ibtissam Chakir[1,2], Stéphanie Dumont[2], Paul Pévet[2], Ali Ouarour[1], Etienne Challet[2] and Patrick Vuillez[2]**

[1] Laboratory of Biology and Health, Faculty of Science, Abdelmalek Essaâdi University, Tetouan, Morocco, [2] Regulation of Circadian Clocks Team, Institute for Cellular and Integrative Neurosciences, UPR3212, Centre National de la Recherche Scientifique and University of Strasbourg, Strasbourg, France

Edited by:
Hubert Vaudry, University of Rouen, France

Reviewed by:
Andries Kalsbeek, University of Amsterdam, Netherlands
Jonathan Johnston, University of Surrey, UK

***Correspondence:**
Etienne Challet and Patrick Vuillez, Institute for Cellular and Integrative Neurosciences, UPR3212, Centre National de la Recherche Scientifique and University of Strasbourg, 5 rue Blaise Pascal, 67000 Strasbourg, France
challet@ inci-cnrs.unistra.fr; vuillez@inci-cnrs.unistra.fr

Nocturnal secretion of melatonin from the pineal gland may affect central and peripheral timing, in addition to its well-known involvement in the control of seasonal physiology. The Syrian hamster is a photoperiodic species, which displays gonadal atrophy and increased adiposity when adapted to short (winter-like) photoperiods. Here we investigated whether pineal melatonin secreted at night can impact daily rhythmicity of metabolic hormones and glucose in that seasonal species. For that purpose, daily variations of plasma leptin, cortisol, insulin and glucose were analyzed in pinealectomized hamsters, as compared to sham-operated controls kept under very long (16 h light/08 h dark) or short photoperiods (08 h light/16 h dark). Daily rhythms of leptin under both long and short photoperiods were blunted by pinealectomy. Furthermore, the phase of cortisol rhythm under a short photoperiod was advanced by 5.6 h after pinealectomy. Neither plasma insulin, nor blood glucose displays robust daily rhythmicity, even in sham-operated hamsters. Pinealectomy, however, totally reversed the decreased levels of insulin under short days and the photoperiodic variations in mean levels of blood glucose (i.e., reduction and increase in long and short days, respectively). Together, these findings in *Syrian hamsters* show that circulating melatonin at night drives the daily rhythmicity of plasma leptin, participates in the phase control of cortisol rhythm and modulates glucose homeostasis according to photoperiod-dependent metabolic state.

Keywords: golden hamster, pinealectomy, photoperiod, cortisol rhythm, plasma glucose

Introduction

Photoperiodic animals, such as *Syrian hamsters*, are species whose physiology is specifically and reversibly regulated on a seasonal basis. Notably, they display seasonal changes in gonadal activity. When *Syrian hamsters* are exposed to long, summer-like photoperiods, gonadal function is active and their adiposity is decreased. Conversely, after transfer to short, winter-like photoperiods, these hamsters become sexually quiescent, while their adiposity increases (Bartness and Wade, 1985).

In mammals, melatonin can be synthesized by several organs, including the pineal gland, retina and gastrointestinal tract (Pevet, 2003; Hardeland et al., 2011; Tosini et al., 2012). The pineal gland, however, is the main source of the nocturnal peak of circulating melatonin, as evidenced by the lack of detectable levels in the blood after pinealectomy. The daily fluctuations of melatonin synthesis and release by the pineal are tightly controlled by the master clock in the suprachiasmatic nuclei of the hypothalamus (SCN). The daily duration of nocturnal melatonin transduces photoperiodic cues into neuroendocrine changes that modulate seasonal physiology, thus highlighting the pivotal role of pineal melatonin in the integration of seasonal changes in day length (Malpaux et al., 2001; Pevet, 2003).

Besides, the nocturnal peak of melatonin may also play a role as an internal time-giver on a daily basis (Pevet and Challet, 2011). Among others, circadian rhythmicity of the pups during gestation and weaning can be synchronized by maternal melatonin via placenta and milk (Torres-Farfan et al., 2008, 2011). In adults, nocturnal melatonin can control the rhythmic activity of brain and peripheral regions, including striatum, pars tuberalis of the hypophysis and spleen, as shown by the disappearance of clock gene oscillations in these structures after pinealectomy (Messager et al., 2001; Uz et al., 2003; Prendergast et al., 2013). Melatoninergic cues may even feed-back on the master clock in the SCN where they affect clock gene expression (Agez et al., 2007) and firing rate (Rusak and Yu, 1993).

The aim of the present study was to investigate whether rhythmic melatonin can also affect the daily timing of other hormones, such as leptin and glucocorticoids. Plasma leptin is secreted by adipocytes in proportion with adiposity (Ahima and Flier, 2000). Accordingly, levels of plasma leptin are higher in *Syrian hamsters* adapted to short photoperiod compared to animals exposed to long photoperiod (Horton et al., 2000). In addition, leptin is rhythmically secreted, with peak phases depending on the species. Adrenal glucorticoids are other hormones rhythmically secreted, with endogenous peaks occurring around activity onsets (Dickmeis, 2009). The main glucocorticoid is cortisol in humans and hamsters, and corticosterone in rats and mice. To test whether nocturnal melatonin can have chronomodulatory effects on leptin, cortisol and insulin rhythms, we investigated the impact of pinealectomy on these rhythms in *Syrian hamsters* kept under long or short photoperiods.

Material and Methods

Animals

Ninety-seven male *Syrian hamsters (Mesocricetus auratus)* bred in-house (Chronobiotron platform, UMS3415, CNRS and University of Strasbourg) were 6-month-old at the end of the experiment. From birth, they were maintained in a Long Photoperiod (LP) consisting of 16-h light and 8-h dark (around 150 lux within the cages during the light period), with lights on at 05:00 AM, defining Zeitgeber time (ZT) 0. Animals were housed 3–5 per cage and kept at 22 ± 1°C with *ad libitum* access to water and food. All experiments were conducted in accordance with the French National Law (License 67–88) implementing the European Union Directive 2010/63/EU. All efforts were made to minimize the number of animals used and their suffering, and the study met the ethical standards.

Experimental Design

All hamsters were initially kept under LP. Around half of the animals were sham-operated ($n = 48$), while the others were pinealectomized ($n = 49$).

Hamsters (weighing approximately 140 g) were anesthetized during the light phase with i.p. injections of a mixture of Zoletil 20 (Virbac, Carros, France) and Rompun (Bayer Pharma, Puteaux, France). After being placed into a stereotaxic instrument (Kopf), a midline circular incision of the skull was gently performed to expose the pineal gland. The pineal was removed with a pair of fine forceps, the skull cap replaced and the incision closed. After surgery, hamsters were housed individually for 1–2 days until complete recovery. Thereafter, hamsters were either kept in LP ($n = 21$) or transferred to a Short Photoperiod (SP; $n = 28$) consisting of 8 h light and 16 h dark, with lights on at 09:00 AM, defining ZT0 under SP. This photoperiodic condition triggers in that species an inhibition of the reproductive axis, including gonadal atrophy.

Ten weeks later, all animals under LP and SP were killed every 4 h ($n = 1$ of the same cage per ZT) throughout the 24 h, from ZT3, 7, 11, 15, 19 to 23.

Blood samples were collected in heparinized tubes and centrifuged for 10 min at 4600 g at 4°C.

Hormonal Assays

Plasma concentrations of leptin were determined by a multi-species leptin RIA kit (XL-85K, Millipore, Molsheim, France). The limit of sensitivity of the assay was 2 ng·mL^{-1} and the inter- and intra-assay coefficients of variance were <9 and <4%, respectively.

Plasma concentrations of cortisol were determined by a Cortisol Express EIA Kit (AYN830, Cayman Chemical, Ann Arbor, MI, USA). The limit of sensitivity of the assay was 0.1 ng·mL^{-1}, while the coefficients of variance for a dose of 5 ng were equal, respectively, to 11 and 6% for inter- and intra-assays. Plasma levels of insulin were assayed with Ultra Rat Insulin ELISA Kit (# 90060, Crystal Chem, Downers Grove, IL, USA) using hamster insulin standard (# 90330, Crystal Chem) following the instructions of the manufacturer. The limit of sensitivity of the assay was 0.1 ng·mL^{-1} and the coefficients of variance were <10% for both inter- and intra-assays.

Glucose Assay

Blood glucose was determined with GOD-PAP Kit (LP80009, Biolabo, Maizy, France).

Statistical Analysis

Data are presented as means ± S.E.M. Three-Way analyses of variance (ANOVA) followed by *post-hoc* comparisons with the Fisher's least significant difference Test were used to compare the effects of Zeitgeber time × photoperiod × treatment. Level of significance was set at $P < 0.05$. For each blood parameter in either photoperiod, One-Way ANOVAs, or ANOVAs on ranks when normality test (Shapiro–Wilk) failed, were performed to determine if the effect of Zeitgeber time was significant (i.e., if the blood parameters display time-dependent variations). For assessing daily rhythmicity, we used a cosinor analysis to determine mean level, amplitude and acrophase of the considered parameter with SigmaPlot software (Systat software Inc., San Jose, CA, USA). Individual data of each experimental group (Long or short photoperiod, sham-operated or pinealectomized) were fitted to the following regression: $[y = a+b\cdot\cos(2\cdot\pi\cdot(x-c)/24)]$ where a is the mean level, b the amplitude, and c the acrophase of the rhythm. For a given parameter, we used the Mean, Size, standard Error (MSE) format of SigmaPlot to compare the acrophases of significant regressions with *t*-tests or One-Way ANOVA followed by Fisher's *post-hoc* test for two or more groups, respectively.

Results

Body mass at the end of the experiment was not significantly modified by pinealectomy, either in LP or SP (**Table 1**). Pinealectomy is routinely used in this and other labs to suppress the nocturnal rise of circulating melatonin. Indeed, after visual extirpation of the pineal gland in hamsters, levels of plasma melatonin at night become systematically undetectable (i.e., less than 1 pg/tube according to the limit of sensitivity of our RIA melatonin assay) (Schuster et al., 2001). In this study, we attribute the differences in pinealectomized hamsters compared to sham-operated controls, as due to impaired melatonin secretion. Based on the present protocol without hormonal replacement in pinealectomized animals, we cannot fully exclude the possibility of melatonin-independent effects of pinealectomy.

Cortisol Rhythm

Levels of plasma cortisol were significantly affected by Zeitgeber time (Three-Way ANOVA; $P = 0.01$). Independently of photoperiod and treatment, higher values were found at ZT11 (i.e., 11 h after lights on) compared to ZT3 (early morning) and ZT23 (late night; **Figure 1**). There was also a significant effect of photoperiod (Three-Way ANOVA; $P = 0.003$) on plasma cortisol, mean values being larger under short days compared to long days. By contrast, plasma cortisol was not modified by Treatment (Three-Way ANOVA; sham-operated vs. pinealectomized; $P = 0.09$). In addition, the triple interaction [Zeitgeber time × photoperiod × treatment] was significant (Three-Way ANOVA; $P = 0.004$), but only for sham-operated animals, indicating that in these animals the daily pattern differs between photoperiods. Cosinor analysis detected a significant daily rhythm for both sham-operated and pinealectomized hamsters under short photoperiod (**Table 2**). Of note, the cortisol acrophase was phase-advanced by almost 6 h in pinealectomized hamsters compared to intact animals (from ZT14.3 to ZT8.7; $P < 0.05$; One-Way ANOVA; **Figure 1**; **Table 2**). By contrast, under long photoperiod, a significant daily rhythm was found only in pinealectomized hamsters (delayed by more than 5 h as compared to pinealectomized hamsters under short days; $P < 0.05$; One-Way ANOVA; **Table 2**). The lack of significant daily rhythmicity in intact animals under long days is probably due to the bimodal pattern characterized by daytime and nocturnal peaks (**Figure 1**).

TABLE 1 | Body mass of hamsters.

	LP Sham ($n = 23$)	LP PinX ($n = 21$)	SP Sham ($n = 25$)	SP PinX ($n = 28$)
Mean (g)	129.7	127.6	136.5	131.9
±SEM	±2.9	±2.6	±2.7	±2.1

Mean body mass of hamsters, either sham-operated (Sham) or pinealectomized (PinX) under long (LP) or short photoperiods (SP).

Leptin Rhythm

Levels of plasma leptin were changed according to Zeitgeber times (Three-Way ANOVA; $P = 0.002$), the values at ZT15 being larger than those at both ZT11 and ZT23 (**Figure 2**). Moreover, the levels of leptin were modified by photoperiod (Three-Way ANOVA; $P = 0.004$), with increased values in short days. Levels of plasma leptin were not affected by pinealectomy (Three-Way ANOVA; $P = 0.9$). However, the triple interaction [Zeitgeber time × photoperiod × treatment] was significant (Three-Way ANOVA; $P = 0.003$), but only after pinealectomy, indicating that the daily patterns of leptin in these animals differ in both photoperiods, as compared to respective controls (**Figure 2**). Accordingly, a significant rhythm was detected only in sham-operated animals, demonstrating a role of time-giver of circulating melatonin upon leptin rhythm (**Figure 2; Table 2**). Furthermore, the leptin acrophase under long photoperiod was delayed by 8 h as compared to short photoperiod (from ZT13.2 to ZT21.3; $P < 0.05$; *t*-test; **Table 2**).

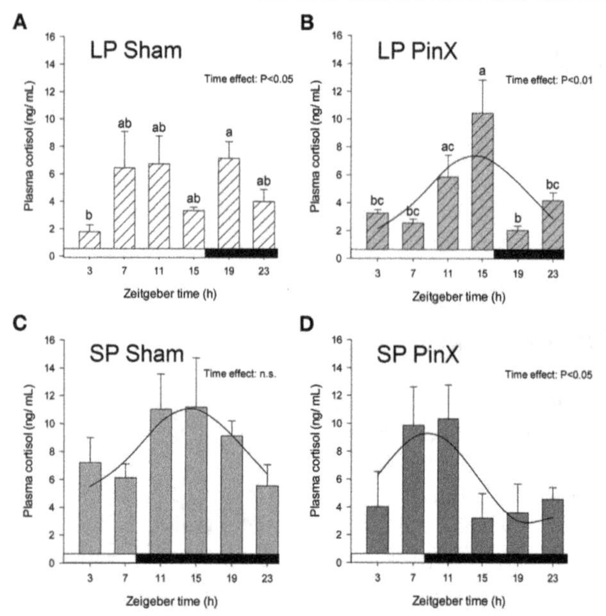

FIGURE 1 | Effects of photoperiod and pinealectomy on daily variations of plasma cortisol in the *Syrian hamster*. Light and dark bars represent photoperiod and scotoperiod, respectively. LP, long photoperiod (16 h light/08 h dark) **(A,B)**; SP, short photoperiod (08 h light/16 h dark) **(C,D)**; Sham, sham-operated hamsters **(A,C)**; PinX, pinealectomized hamsters **(B,D)**. Fitted curves represent significant cosinor analyses (for details, see Materials and Methods and **Table 2**). The absence of a curve in the LP Sham panel indicates that the daily variations of cortisol are not significant in these conditions. The inset for each graph indicates the effect of Zeitgeber time, evaluated by One-Way ANOVAs or ANOVAs on ranks when normality test (Shapiro-Wilk) failed; n.s., non-significant. For a given panel, histograms lacking common letters are significantly different ($P < 0.05$).

TABLE 2 | Parameters of cosinor regressions.

		Plasma leptin			Plasma cortisol			Plasma insulin			Plasma glucose		
		Mean	SEM	*P*	Mean	SEM	*P*	Mean	SEM	*P*	Mean	SEM	*P*
LP Sham (*n* = 23)	a	7.06	0.49	<0.001	5.03	0.71	<0.001	1.79	0.22	<0.001	1.02	0.05	<0.001
	b	2.18	0. 70	0.006	1.46	1.02	0.17	0.21	0.32	0.53	0.04	0.08	0.62
	c	21.34*	1.22	<0.001	13.43	2.60	<0.001	6.68	5.36	0.27	14.60	7.20	<0.001
LP PinX (*n* = 21)	a	6.95	0.67	<0.001	4.72	0.65	<0.001	1.78	0.10	<0.001	1.24	0.03	<0.001
	b	0.75	0.95	0.43	2.66	0.92	0.009	0.38	0.15	0.017	0.05	0.04	0.19
	c	6.75	4.80	0.17	14.08*	1.32	<0.001	4.84*	1.48	0.004	13.84	2.81	<0.001
SP Sham (*n* = 25)	a	8.48	0.61	<0.001	8.27	0.74	<0.001	1.32	0.09	<0.001	1.12	0.05	<0.001
	b	2.45	0.85	0.01	2.82	1.09	0.015	0.12	0.13	0.37	0.11	0.06	0.09
	c	13.22#	1.34	<0.001	14.26*	1.36	<0.001	18.92	4.22	0.11	18.80	2.36	<0.001
SP PinX (*n* = 28)	a	8.70	0.05	<0.001	6.01	0.88	<0.001	1.81	0.20	<0.001	1.00	0.035	<0.001
	b	0.11	0.06	0.91	3.30	1.21	0.011	0.61	0.28	0.037	0.10	0.05	0.041
	c	8.81	2.36	0.81	8.67#	1.45	<0.001	20.18#	1.79	<0.001	12.96	1.81	<0.001

The table shows the three parameters of cosinor regression, including a the mean level, b the amplitude, and c the acrophase of the rhythm (see Material and Methods for details). For the acrophase, the reference time is Zeitgeber 0 (i.e., lights on) for both photoperiods. LP, long photoperiod; SP, short photoperiod; Sham, sham-operated; PinX, pinealectomized. Italicized parameters are not statistically significant (P > 0.05). For a given hormone (column), mean acrophases lacking common superscripts (or #) are significantly different (t-test or One-Way ANOVA for 2 or more groups, respectively). No superscript is included in case the overall regression was not significant due to non-significant acrophase (c) and/or amplitude (b), or when there was only one significant regression precluding statistical comparison with the other groups (as in the case of plasma glucose).*

Insulin Rhythm

The mains effects of Zeitgeber time, photoperiod and treatment were not significant for insulin levels (Three-Way ANOVA; $P = 0.14$, $P = 0.17$, and $P = 0.11$, respectively). However, the double interactions [Zeitgeber time × photoperiod] and [Zeitgeber time × treatment] were significant (Three-Way ANOVA; $P = 0.01$ for both), indicating that the daily profiles of insulin differ according to photoperiodic conditions. In particular, the mean levels of plasma insulin were lower in hamsters exposed to short photoperiod as compared to long photoperiod, but only for sham-operated animals (Fisher's *post-hoc* test; $P = 0.02$). Finally, the double interaction [photoperiod × treatment] was also significant (Three-Way ANOVA; $P = 0.04$), revealing that insulin levels were increased by pinealectomy under short photoperiod (Fisher's *post-hoc* test; $P < 0.01$), but they were unaffected by this treatment under long photoperiod (**Figure 3**; **Table 2**). Cosinor analysis detected a significant daily rhythm of plasma insulin only in pineactomized hamsters, with different acrophases between short and long photoperiods (**Figure 3**; **Table 2**).

Glucose Rhythm

Levels of blood glucose were hardly affected by Zeitgeber time (Three-Way ANOVA; $P = 0.056$), and unchanged by photoperiod (Three-Way ANOVA; $P = 0.4$) or treatment (Three-Way ANOVA; $P = 0.6$). The lack of daily rhythmicity in blood glucose might be due to the 4-h sampling. Nonetheless, the double interaction [Zeitgeber time × treatment] was highly significant (Three-Way ANOVA; $P < 0.001$). In particular, mean blood glucose in pinealectomized hamsters was significantly increased under long photoperiod, while it was decreased in short photoperiod (Fisher's *post-hoc* test; $P < 0.001$, **Figure 4**; **Table 2**). Moreover, mean glycemia in sham-operated hamsters was increased in short vs. long photoperiods (Fisher's *post-hoc* test; $P = 0.007$), while the values in pinealectomized animals was decreased in short vs. long photoperiods (Fisher's *post-hoc* test; $P < 0.001$). Cosinor analysis detected a significant daily rhythm of blood glucose only in pineactomized hamsters under short days (**Figure 4**; **Table 2**), precluding any comparison with the other studied groups. Nevertheless, these results indicate that circulating melatonin differentially affects overall glucose regulation according the photoperiod-induced metabolic changes.

Discussion

The main findings of this study are that pineal melatonin not only acts as a time-giver for hormonal rhythms, but also affects glucose homeostasis in a photoperiod-dependent way.

The first conclusion is supported by the fact that pinealectomy in *Syrian hamsters* suppresses the daily rhythmicity of plasma leptin and can lead to shifts of the daily rhythm of plasma cortisol. The second conclusion relies on the differential impact of pinealectomy on glycemia and plasma insulin according to the photoperiod (**Figure 5**).

Pinealectomy Affects Glucose and Insulin Levels According to Photoperiods

This study is mainly based on cosinor analysis with a relatively small number of observations per time point ($n = 4$–6) and 4-h sampling (6 time-points over 24 h). In contrast to what is found in other rodents (La Fleur et al., 1999; Kalsbeek et al., 2001; Cuesta et al., 2009), no significant daily rhythm in blood glucose is found in control (sham-operated) *Syrian hamsters* housed under long

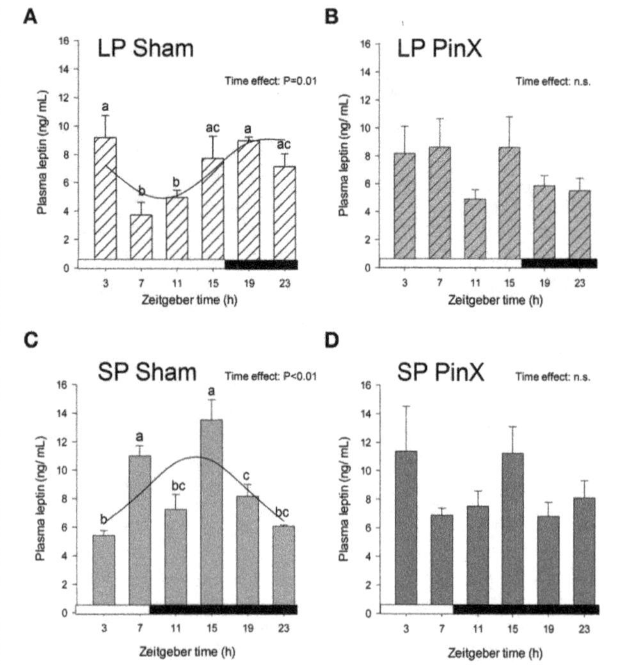

FIGURE 2 | Effects of photoperiod and pinealectomy on daily variations of plasma leptin in the *Syrian hamster*. Light and dark bars represent photoperiod and scotoperiod, respectively. LP, long photoperiod (16 h light/08 h dark) **(A,B)**; SP, short photoperiod (08 h light/16 h dark) **(C,D)**; Sham, sham-operated hamsters **(A,C)**; PinX, pinealectomized hamsters **(B,D)**. Fitted curves represent significant cosinor analyses (for details, see Materials and Methods and **Table 2**). The absence of a curve in LP PinX and SP PinX **(B,D)** indicates that the daily rhythmicity of leptin is not significant after pinealectomy. The inset for each graph indicates the effect of Zeitgeber time, evaluated by One-Way ANOVAs or ANOVAs on ranks when normality test (Shapiro-Wilk) failed; n.s., non-significant. For a given panel, histograms lacking common letters are significantly different ($P < 0.05$).

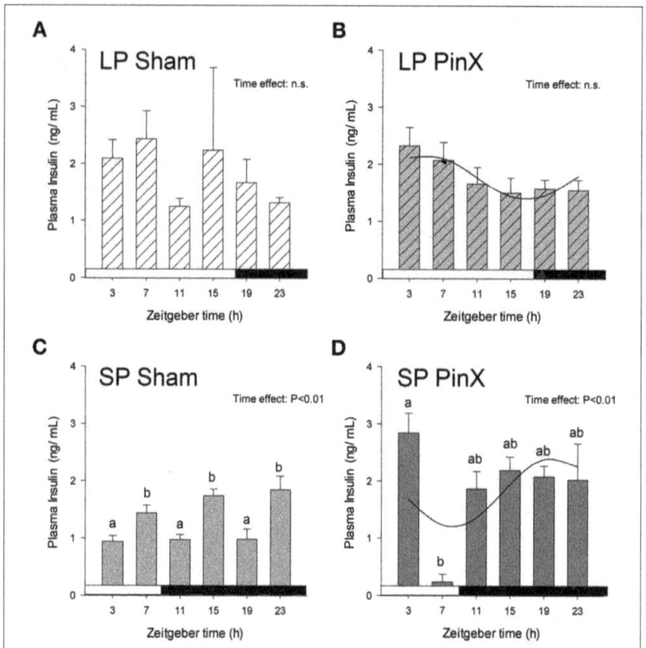

FIGURE 3 | Effects of photoperiod and pinealectomy on daily variations of plasma insulin in the *Syrian hamster*. Light and dark bars represent photoperiod and scotoperiod, respectively. LP, long photoperiod (16 h light/08 h dark) **(A,B)**; SP, short photoperiod (08 h light/16 h dark) **(C,D)**; Sham, sham-operated hamsters **(A,C)**; PinX, pinealectomized hamsters **(B,D)**. Fitted curves represent significant cosinor analyses (for details, see Materials and Methods and **Table 2**). The absence of a curve in LP Sham and SP Sham **(A,C)** indicates that the daily rhythmicity of insulin is not significantly rhythmic in sham-operated hamsters. The inset for each graph indicates the effect of Zeitgeber time, evaluated by One-Way ANOVAs or ANOVAs on ranks when normality test (Shapiro-Wilk) failed; n.s., non-significant. For a given panel, histograms lacking common letters are significantly different ($P < 0.05$).

or short photoperiods. This prevented us to assess the possible time-giving property of melatonin on that parameter. Based on a study in pinealectomized rats, the endogenous rhythm of pineal melatonin may enhance the amplitude of the daily rhythm of plasma glucose (la Fleur et al., 2001). In any case, the lack of rhythmic glycemia in *Syrian hamsters* has been already reported (Rowland, 1984). This specific feature is actually concomitant with a lack of marked day-night difference in feeding behavior (Rowland, 1984). Because hamsters in the present study were not fasted before blood sampling, meal-induced rise in plasma glucose may have blunted any small endogenous rhythm.

Contrary to mice fed *ad libitum* (Ahren, 2000), no daily variations of plasma insulin were found in intact *Syrian hamsters* exposed to either long or short photoperiods. Nonetheless, a significant rhythm of plasma insulin with low amplitude was only detected in pinealectomized hamsters. As noted for glucose levels, possible interactions with meal-induced secretion of insulin may have interfered with the endogenous rhythmicity of insulin. Alternativly, the fed state of the hamsters studied here avoided fasting-induced bias in hormonal/glucose levels due to variable mobilization of body stores according to photoperiods, times of day and associated differences in fasting duration.

Nevertheless, the present study provides novel information on how melatonin can modulate glucose homeostasis. We found that the effects of pinealectomy on plasma glucose and insulin depend on the metabolic state (i.e., short-day, fattier phenotype with more plasma glucose and leptin, and less insulin vs. long-day, leaner phenotype with less plasma glucose and leptin, and more insulin). In relatively lean hamsters (exposed to long photoperiod), pinealectomy leads to mild hyperglycemia. This finding is in accordance with the fact that pineal ablation in non-photoperiodic lean rats also increases nighttime glucose levels (la Fleur et al., 2001). This relative hyperglycemia at night in rats without pineal gland is not due to a reduced insulin secretion to meal cues because in hamsters exposed to long photoperiod, mean insulin levels were not significantly affected by pinealectomy. Accordingly, another work in pinealectomized rats did not detect changes in plasma insulin levels and provides experimental arguments for a decreased sensitivity of cells to circulating insulin (Alonso-Vale et al., 2004). Therefore, the mild hyperglycemia in pinealectomized hamsters in long days may be, as observed in rats, due to a reduced responsiveness of the target cells to insulin.

In sharp contrast, pinealectomy in relatively fatty hamsters (exposed to short photoperiod) reduces the mild hyperglycemia

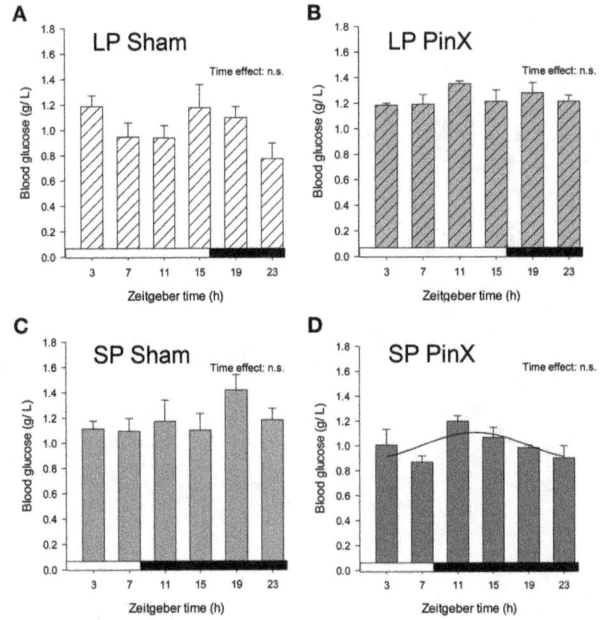

FIGURE 4 | Effects of photoperiod and pinealectomy on daily variations of plasma glucose in the *Syrian hamster*. Light and dark bars represent photoperiod and scotoperiod, respectively. LP, long photoperiod (16 h light/08 h dark) **(A,B)**; SP, short photoperiod (08 h light/16 h dark) **(C,D)**; Sham, sham-operated hamsters **(A,C)**; PinX, pinealectomized hamsters **(B,D)**. The absence of curves indicates that the daily variations of plasma glucose are not significant, except for SP PinX animals in which cosinor analysis detected a significant daily rhythm (for details, see Materials and Methods and **Table 2**). The inset for each graph indicates the effect of Zeitgeber time, evaluated by one-way ANOVAs or ANOVAs on ranks when normality test (Shapiro-Wilk) failed; n.s., non-significant. For a given panel, histograms lacking common letters are significantly different ($P < 0.05$).

observed in sham-operated hamsters. Thus, pinealectomy in that case normalizes glycemia to levels close to those in long-day control hamsters. High-fat feeding triggers obesity in non-photoperiodic rats. Pineal ablation, however, does not modulate their concentration of blood glucose, at least in the morning (Prunet-Marcassus et al., 2003). In the present work, we also found that concentrations of plasma insulin were increased by pinealectomy in hamsters exposed to short photoperiod. Therefore, considering that insulin sensitivity is improved under short days compared to long days, the increased concentrations of circulating insulin can explain the lower levels of blood glucose. Meanwhile, our results reveal that the lack of circulating melatonin in hamsters markedly modifies glucose homeostasis, with opposite effects according to their seasonal metabolic state.

Pinealectomy Shifts the Daily Rhythm of Cortisol

In sham-operated hamsters, the daily pattern of plasma cortisol was found to be unimodal and bimodal in short and long photoperiods, respectively. Furthermore, plasma levels of cortisol are larger in short compared to long photoperiods. This contrasts with previous results in the Syrian hamster that found unchanged levels in males (de Souza and Meier, 1987) or decreased levels of cortisol in short days (Ottenweller et al., 1987; Nexon et al., 2011). These discrepancies are puzzling, and may be related to the more extreme photoperiods used in the present study and the fact the hamsters here were all operated upon. Furthermore, the reported quiescent hypothalamo-hypophyso-adrenal axis in *Syrian hamsters* under short photoperiods can be profoundly modulated by social interactions (Morgan, 2012). It is therefore possible that the present housing conditions (3–5 animals per cage) may have led to social instability and/or inter-individual differences in social status, thus keeping an activated hypothalamo-hypophyso-adrenal axis in *Syrian hamsters* under short photoperiods. Regarding the effects of melatonin on glucorticoids, pinealectomy in *Syrian hamsters* does not affect the mean levels of cortisol, whatever the photoperiod. This confirms what is found by several studies in rats for corticoterone levels (Szafarczyk et al., 1983; Kaplanski and Ronen, 1986), albeit other investigations report increased levels of plasma corticosterone in pinealectomized rats (Oxenkrug et al., 1984; Alonso-Vale et al., 2004).

In terms of daily timing, a clear phase-advance is induced by pinealectomy in hamsters exposed to short days. Previous studies in adult rats found no effect of pinealectomy on the phase of corticosterone profile (Szafarczyk et al., 1983; Kaplanski and Ronen, 1986), while adrenal glands of rat fetus is entrained by maternal melatonin (Torres-Farfan et al., 2011). Furthermore, melatonin modulates *in vitro* molecular oscillations in the adrenal gland of adult monkeys (Valenzuela et al., 2008). Together, these findings suggest that circulating melatonin can participate in the control of adrenal rhythmicity.

Pinealectomy Flattens the Daily Rhythm of Leptin

In accordance with the increased adiposity in hamsters exposed to short photoperiods (Bartness and Wade, 1985), mean levels of plasma leptin are higher in hamsters exposed to short photoperiods in comparison with animals in long photoperiods, as found by others (Horton et al., 2000). Furthermore, whatever the photoperiod, pinealectomy in hamsters does not affect mean leptin levels, in keeping with results in the non-photoperiodic laboratory rat (Alonso-Vale et al., 2004).

In the present study, the peak of plasma leptin in hamsters exposed to long or short photoperiods takes place at night, as in other nocturnal rodents like rats and mice (Ahren, 2000; Kalsbeek et al., 2001; Cuesta et al., 2009). Other reports in *Syrian hamsters*, however, found either hardly rhythmic profile (Horton et al., 2000) or rhythmic leptin peaking during daytime (Karakas and Gunduz, 2006). The daily rhythm of leptin is thought to be controlled both by the master clock in the SCN and by the adipose clock (Kalsbeek et al., 2001; Karakas and Gunduz, 2006; Otway et al., 2009). In addition, in cultured adipocytes, rhythmic treatment with melatonin has been shown to synchronize their metabolic and hormonal function, including leptin secretion (Alonso-Vale et al., 2008). This result perfectly fits with our *in vivo* demonstration that in hamsters without circulating melatonin at night, the daily rhythm of leptin is blunted. These findings highlight that rhythmic melatonin is a time-giver for rhythmic secretion of leptin. To firmly demonstrate that interpretation, further experiments in pinealectomized hamsters treated with melatonin are needed. It is expected that in contrast to continuous melatonin replacement, only restoration

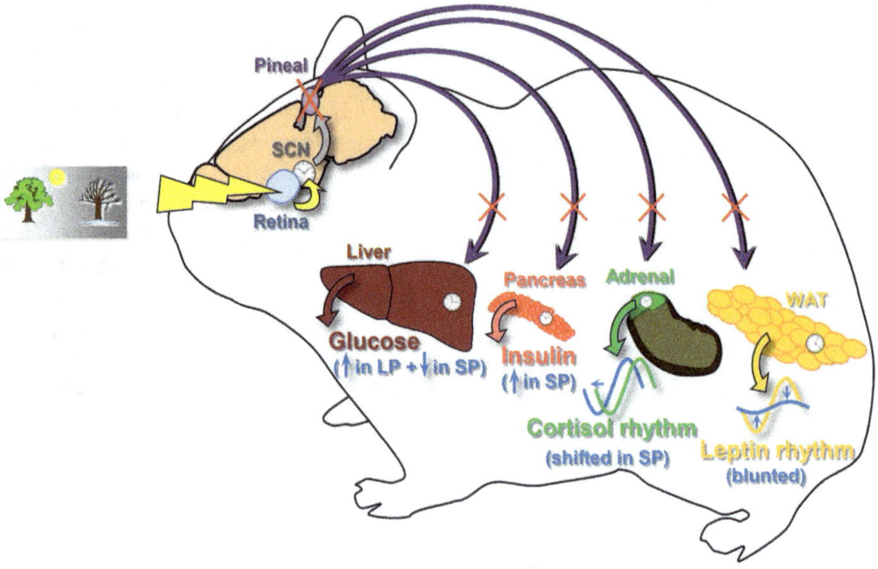

FIGURE 5 | Schematic view summarizing the effects of pinealectomy on metabolic physiology in the *Syrian hamster*. For each parameter, changes after pinealectomy are drawn in blue. Pinealectomy in *Syrian hamsters* suppresses the daily rhythmicity of plasma leptin synthesized by the white adipose tissue (WAT), whatever the photoperiod. Pinealectomy leads to shifts of the daily rhythm of plasma cortisol in hamsters adapted to a short photoperiod. Furthemore, pinealectomy leads to increased levels of insulin in hamsters exposed to a short photoperiod (SP). Finally, pinealectomy increases plasma glucose in leaner hamsters exposed to a long photoperiod (LP), and decreases glycemia in fattier animals adapted to a short photoperiod (SP). SCN, suprachiasmatic nuclei, site of the master clock.

of a melatonin rhythm will reinstate daily variations of plasma leptin.

Organ-Specific Sensitivity to Rhythmic Melatonin or Glucocorticoids

Because of the presence of melatonin receptors in a multitude of central and peripheral organs, the daily rhythm of plasma melatonin is thought to distribute temporal cues generated by the master clock throughout the body, thus playing a role of coupling between the central and secondary clocks (Pevet and Challet, 2011). In the present study, we noticed that pinealectomy affects daily rhythms of plasma leptin, cortisol, and insulin in different ways depending on the rhythm considered (**Figure 5**). We suggest that these differential effects of melatonin (or its absence) *in vivo* are indicative of direct effects on targeted peripheral tissues, rather than indirect effects on upstream structures (e.g., in the central nervous system). Previous studies on organs (white adipose tissue, adrenal gland or pancreas) isolated *in vitro* are in accordance with this hypothesis (Peschke and Peschke, 1998; Alonso-Vale et al., 2008; Valenzuela et al., 2008).

It is worth reminding that rhythmic glucocorticoids, such as cortisol and corticosterone, are also considered themselves as internal time-givers. The prevalent view is that most, if not all, peripheral organs that express glucocorticoid receptors are sensitive to the synchronizing effects of applications of glucocorticoid agonist (dexamethasone) (Balsalobre et al., 2000). Therefore, a given structure expressing the *ad hoc* receptors could theoretically be sensitive to the two hormonal synchronizers. Accordingly, in the white adipose tissue, both glucocorticoids and melatonin can modulate timing of daily profiles of metabolic gene expression (Alonso-Vale et al., 2008; Su et al., 2015), or hormonal output (i.e., leptin; Alonso-Vale et al., 2008; this study). In fact, this dual sensitivity may not be so widespread.

Some tissues, indeed, appear to be more specifically sensitive to the synchronizing effects of either melatonin or glucocorticoids. In the mouse liver for instance, glucocorticoids play a strong synchronizing effect, as shown by arrhythmicity in metabolic gene expression after adrenalectomy (Oishi et al., 2005), while melatonin cues do not markedly affect hepatic timing (Houdek et al., 2015). In the brain of mice, the daily variations of dopamine in the striatum are controlled by rhythmic melatonin, as evidenced by disappearance of rhythmicity after pineal ablation and restoration with daily injections of melatonin, while adrenalectomy does not impair the timing of the dopaminergic variations (Khaldy et al., 2002). Conversely, daily variations of serotonin in the rodent brain, known to be controlled by rhythmic glucocorticoids (Segall et al., 2006; Malek et al., 2007), are not affected by pinealectomy or daily injections of melatonin (Khaldy et al., 2002). Finally, circadian timing in the pars tuberalis of the hypophysis appears to be driven by circulating melatonin (Dardente, 2007).

These data, together with our differential findings on plasma cortisol and leptin after pinealectomy, favor the hypothesis that rhythmic melatonin acts as an internal synchronizer on targeted structures. The functional implication of these specific temporal regulations for physiology and health remains to be investigated. The seasonal species that display annual and reversible changes in metabolic physiology, like *Syrian hamsters* studied here, provide promising models in that respect.

Acknowledgments

We are indebted to Christiane Calgari-Tavernier for the RIA assay. This work was supported by the Comité Mixte Inter-Universitaire Franco-Marocain, PHC Volubilis MA/07/177, the Centre National de la Recherche Scientifique, and University of Strasbourg. Ibtissam Chakir was supported by scholarships from the GDRI Neurosciences Fondamentales et Cliniques (CNRS/INSERM, France and CNRST, Morocco) and N€uromed project (European FP7).

References

Agez, L., Laurent, V., Pevet, P., Masson-Pevet, M., and Gauer, F. (2007). Melatonin affects nuclear orphan receptors mRNA in the rat suprachiasmatic nuclei. *Neuroscience* 144, 522–530. doi: 10.1016/j.neuroscience.2006.09.030

Ahima, R. S., and Flier, J. S. (2000). Leptin. *Annu. Rev. Physiol.* 62, 413–437. doi: 10.1146/annurev.physiol.62.1.413

Ahren, B. (2000). Diurnal variation in circulating leptin is dependent on gender, food intake and circulating insulin in mice. *Acta Physiol. Scand.* 169, 325–331. doi: 10.1046/j.1365-201x.2000.00746.x

Alonso-Vale, M. I., Andreotti, S., Mukai, P. Y., Borges-Silva, C., Peres, S. B., Cipolla-Neto, J., et al. (2008). Melatonin and the circadian entrainment of metabolic and hormonal activities in primary isolated adipocytes. *J. Pineal Res.* 45, 422–429. doi: 10.1111/j.1600-079X.2008.00610.x

Alonso-Vale, M. I., Borges-Silva, C. N., Anhe, G. F., Andreotti, S., Machado, M. A., Cipolla-Neto, J., et al. (2004). Light/dark cycle-dependent metabolic changes in adipose tissue of pinealectomized rats. *Horm. Metab. Res.* 36, 474–479. doi: 10.1055/s-2004-825723

Balsalobre, A., Brown, S. A., Marcacci, L., Tronche, F., Kellendonk, C., Reichardt, H. M., et al. (2000). Resetting of circadian time in peripheral tissues by glucocorticoid signaling. *Science* 289, 2344–2347. doi: 10.1126/science.289.5488.2344

Bartness, T. J., and Wade, G. N. (1985). Photoperiodic control of seasonal body weight cycles in hamsters. *Neurosci. Biobehav. Rev.* 9, 599–612. doi: 10.1016/0149-7634(85)90006-5

Cuesta, M., Clesse, D., Pevet, P., and Challet, E. (2009). From daily behavior to hormonal and neurotransmitters rhythms: comparison between diurnal and nocturnal rat species. *Horm. Behav.* 55, 338–347. doi: 10.1016/j.yhbeh.2008.10.015

Dardente, H. (2007). Does a melatonin-dependent circadian oscillator in the pars tuberalis drive prolactin seasonal rhythmicity? *J. Neuroendocrinol.* 19, 657–666. doi: 10.1111/j.1365-2826.2007.01564.x

de Souza, C. J., and Meier, A. H. (1987). Circadian and seasonal variations of plasma insulin and cortisol concentrations in the *Syrian hamster, Mesocricetus auratus. Chronobiol. Int.* 4, 141–151. doi: 10.3109/07420528709078520

Dickmeis, T. (2009). Glucocorticoids and the circadian clock. *J. Endocrinol.* 200, 3–22. doi: 10.1677/JOE-08-0415

Hardeland, R., Cardinali, D. P., Srinivasan, V., Spence, D. W., Brown, G. M., and Pandi-Perumal, S. R. (2011). Melatonin–a pleiotropic, orchestrating regulator molecule. *Prog Neurobiol.* 93, 350–384. doi: 10.1016/j.pneurobio.2010.12.004

Horton, T. H., Buxton, O. M., Losee-Olson, S., and Turek, F. W. (2000). Twenty-four-hour profiles of serum leptin in siberian and golden hamsters: photoperiodic and diurnal variations. *Horm. Behav.* 37, 388–398. doi: 10.1006/hbeh.2000.1592

Houdek, P., Polidarova, L., Novakova, M., Mateju, K., Kubik, S., and Sumova, A. (2015). Melatonin administered during the fetal stage affects circadian clock in the suprachiasmatic nucleus but not in the liver. *Dev. Neurobiol.* 75, 131–144. doi: 10.1002/dneu.22213

Kalsbeek, A., Fliers, E., Romijn, J. A., La Fleur, S. E., Wortel, J., Bakker, O., et al. (2001). The suprachiasmatic nucleus generates the diurnal changes in plasma leptin levels. *Endocrinology* 142, 2677–2685. doi: 10.1210/endo.142.6.8197

Kaplanski, J., and Ronen, J. (1986). Effect of neonatal pinealectomy on circadian periodicity of adrenocortical activity. *J. Neural Transm.* 66, 59–67. doi: 10.1007/BF01262958

Karakas, A., and Gunduz, B. (2006). Suprachiasmatic nuclei may regulate the rhythm of leptin hormone release in *Syrian hamsters* (*Mesocricetus auratus*). *Chronobiol. Int.* 23, 225–236. doi: 10.1080/07420520500545821

Khaldy, H., Leon, J., Escames, G., Bikjdaouene, L., Garcia, J. J., and Acuna-Castroviejo, D. (2002). Circadian rhythms of dopamine and dihydroxyphenyl acetic acid in the mouse striatum: effects of pinealectomy and of melatonin treatment. *Neuroendocrinology* 75, 201–208. doi: 10.1159/000048238

La Fleur, S. E., Kalsbeek, A., Wortel, J., and Buijs, R. M. (1999). A suprachiasmatic nucleus generated rhythm in basal glucose concentrations. *J. Neuroendocrinol.* 11, 643–652. doi: 10.1046/j.1365-2826.1999.00373.x

la Fleur, S. E., Kalsbeek, A., Wortel, J., van der Vliet, J., and Buijs, R. M. (2001). Role for the pineal and melatonin in glucose homeostasis: pinealectomy increases night-time glucose concentrations. *J. Neuroendocrinol.* 13, 1025–1032. doi: 10.1046/j.1365-2826.2001.00717.x

Malek, Z. S., Sage, D., Pevet, P., and Raison, S. (2007). Daily rhythm of tryptophan hydroxylase-2 messenger ribonucleic acid within raphe neurons is induced by corticoid daily surge and modulated by enhanced locomotor activity. *Endocrinology* 148, 5165–5172. doi: 10.1210/en.2007-0526

Malpaux, B., Migaud, M., Tricoire, H., and Chemineau, P. (2001). Biology of mammalian photoperiodism and the critical role of the pineal gland and melatonin. *J. Biol. Rhythms.* 16, 336–347. doi: 10.1177/0748730011290 02051

Messager, S., Garabette, M. L., Hastings, M. H., and Hazlerigg, D. G. (2001). Tissue-specific abolition of Per1 expression in the pars tuberalis by pinealectomy in the *Syrian hamster. Neuroreport* 12, 579–582. doi: 10.1097/00001756-200103050-00029

Morgan, C. (2012). Plasticity in photoperiodic regulation of adrenal, but not testicular, function in *Syrian hamsters. Gen. Comp. Endocrinol.* 178, 441–449. doi: 10.1016/j.ygcen.2012.06.023

Nexon, L., Sage, D., Pevet, P., and Raison, S. (2011). Glucocorticoid-mediated nycthemeral and photoperiodic regulation of tph2 expression. *Eur. J. Neurosci.* 33, 1308–1317. doi: 10.1111/j.1460-9568.2010.07586.x

Oishi, K., Amagai, N., Shirai, H., Kadota, K., Ohkura, N., and Ishida, N. (2005). Genome-wide expression analysis reveals 100 adrenal gland-dependent circadian genes in the mouse liver. *DNA Res.* 12, 191–202. doi: 10.1093/dnares/dsi003

Ottenweller, J. E., Tapp, W. N., Pitman, D. L., and Natelson, B. H. (1987). Adrenal, thyroid, and testicular hormone rhythms in male golden hamsters on long and short days. *Am. J. Physiol.* 253, R321–R328.

Otway, D. T., Frost, G., and Johnston, J. D. (2009). Circadian rhythmicity in murine pre-adipocyte and adipocyte cells. *Chronobiol. Int.* 26, 1340–1354. doi: 10.3109/07420520903412368

Oxenkrug, G. F., McIntyre, I. M., and Gershon, S. (1984). Effects of pinealectomy and aging on the serum corticosterone circadian rhythm in rats. *J. Pineal Res.* 1, 181–185. doi: 10.1111/j.1600-079X.1984.tb00209.x

Peschke, E., and Peschke, D. (1998). Evidence for a circadian rhythm of insulin release from perifused rat pancreatic islets. *Diabetologia* 41, 1085–1092. doi: 10.1007/s001250051034

Pevet, P. (2003). Melatonin: from seasonal to circadian signal. *J. Neuroendocrinol.* 15, 422–426. doi: 10.1046/j.1365-2826.2003.01017.x

Pevet, P., and Challet, E. (2011). Melatonin: both master clock output and internal time-giver in the circadian clocks network. *J. Physiol. Paris* 105, 170–182. doi: 10.1016/j.jphysparis.2011.07.001

Prendergast, B. J., Cable, E. J., Patel, P. N., Pyter, L. M., Onishi, K. G., Stevenson, T. J., et al. (2013). Impaired leukocyte trafficking and skin inflammatory responses in hamsters lacking a functional circadian system. *Brain Behav. Immun.* 32, 94–104. doi: 10.1016/j.bbi.2013.02.007

Prunet-Marcassus, B., Desbazeille, M., Bros, A., Louche, K., Delagrange, P., Renard, P., et al. (2003). Melatonin reduces body weight gain in sprague dawley rats with diet-induced obesity. *Endocrinology* 144, 5347–5352. doi: 10.1210/en.2003-0693

Rowland, N. (1984). Metabolic fuel homeostasis in *Syrian hamsters*: nycthemeral and exercise variables. *Physiol. Behav.* 33, 243–252. doi: 10.1016/0031-9384(84)90106-9

Rusak, B., and Yu, G. D. (1993). Regulation of melatonin-sensitivity and firing-rate rhythms of hamster suprachiasmatic nucleus neurons: pinealectomy effects. *Brain Res.* 602, 200–204. doi: 10.1016/0006-8993(93)90683-E

Schuster, C., Gauer, F., Malan, A., Recio, J., Pevet, P., and Masson-Pevet, M. (2001). The circadian clock, light/dark cycle and melatonin are differentially involved in the expression of daily and photoperiodic variations in mt(1) melatonin receptors in the Siberian and *Syrian hamsters. Neuroendocrinology* 74, 55–68. doi: 10.1159/000054670

Segall, L. A., Perrin, J. S., Walker, C. D., Stewart, J., and Amir, S. (2006). Glucocorticoid rhythms control the rhythm of expression of the clock protein, Period2, in oval nucleus of the bed nucleus of the stria terminalis and central nucleus of the amygdala in rats. *Neuroscience* 140, 753–757. doi: 10.1016/j.neuroscience.2006.03.037

Su, Y., van der Spek, R., Foppen, E., Kwakkel, J., Fliers, E., and Kalsbeek, A. (2015). Effects of adrenalectomy on daily gene expression rhythms in the rat suprachiasmatic and paraventricular hypothalamic nuclei and in white adipose tissue. *Chronobiol. Int.* 32, 211–224. doi: 10.3109/07420528.2014.963198

Szafarczyk, A., Pelzer, E., Ixart, G., Malaval, F., Nouguier-Soule, J., and Assenmacher, I. (1983). [Persistence of circadian rhythms of plasma ACTH and corticosterone after pinealectomy in sighted or blind rats]. *C. R. Seances Acad. Sci. III* 297, 471–476.

Torres-Farfan, C., Mendez, N., Abarzua-Catalan, L., Vilches, N., Valenzuela, G. J., and Seron-Ferre, M. (2011). A circadian clock entrained by melatonin is ticking in the rat fetal adrenal. *Endocrinology* 152, 1891–1900. doi: 10.1210/en.2010-1260

Torres-Farfan, C., Valenzuela, F. J., Mondaca, M., Valenzuela, G. J., Krause, B., Herrera, E. A., et al. (2008). Evidence of a role for melatonin in fetal sheep physiology: direct actions of melatonin on fetal cerebral artery, brown adipose tissue and adrenal gland. *J. Physiol.* 586, 4017–4027. doi: 10.1113/jphysiol.2008.154351

Tosini, G., Baba, K., Hwang, C. K., and Iuvone, P. M. (2012). Melatonin: an underappreciated player in retinal physiology and pathophysiology. *Exp. Eye Res.* 103, 82–89. doi: 10.1016/j.exer.2012.08.009

Uz, T., Akhisaroglu, M., Ahmed, R., and Manev, H. (2003). The pineal gland is critical for circadian Period1 expression in the striatum and for circadian cocaine sensitization in mice. *Neuropsychopharmacology* 28, 2117–2123. doi: 10.1038/sj.npp.1300254

Valenzuela, F. J., Torres-Farfan, C., Richter, H. G., Mendez, N., Campino, C., Torrealba, F., et al. (2008). Clock gene expression in adult primate suprachiasmatic nuclei and adrenal: is the adrenal a peripheral clock responsive to melatonin? *Endocrinology* 149, 1454–1461. doi: 10.1210/en.2007-1518

17

DeepGP: An integrated deep learning method for endocrine disease gene prediction using omics data

*Ningyi Zhang[1], Haoyan Wang[1], Chen Xu[2], Liyuan Zhang[1] and Tianyi Zang[1]**

[1] School of Computer Science and Technology, Harbin Institute of Technology, Harbin, China, [2] Center for Bioinformatics, Harbin Institute of Technology, Harbin, China

Edited by:
Lei Deng,
Central South University, China

Reviewed by:
Tao Huang,
Shanghai Institute of Nutrition and Health, Chinese Academy of Sciences, China
Xiaofang Zhao,
Institute of Computing Technology, Chinese Academy of Sciences (CAS), China

***Correspondence:**
Tianyi Zang
tianyi.zang@hit.edu.cn

Endocrinology is the study focusing on hormones and their actions. Hormones are known as chemical messengers, released into the blood, that exert functions through receptors to make an influence in the target cell. The capacity of the mammalian organism to perform as a whole unit is made possible based on two principal control mechanisms, the nervous system and the endocrine system. The endocrine system is essential in regulating growth and development, tissue function, metabolism, and reproductive processes. Endocrine diseases such as diabetes mellitus, Grave's disease, polycystic ovary syndrome, and insulin-like growth factor I deficiency (IGFI deficiency) are classical endocrine diseases. Endocrine dysfunction is also an increasing factor of morbidity in cancer and other dangerous diseases in humans. Thus, it is essential to understand the diseases from their genetic level in order to recognize more pathogenic genes and make a great effort in understanding the pathologies of endocrine diseases. In this study, we proposed a deep learning method named DeepGP based on graph convolutional network and convolutional neural network for prioritizing susceptible genes of five endocrine diseases. To test the performance of our method, we performed 10-cross-validations on an integrated reported dataset; DeepGP obtained a performance of the area under the curve of ~83% and area under the precision-recall curve of ~65%. We found that type 1 diabetes mellitus (T1DM) and type 2 diabetes mellitus (T2DM) share most of their associated genes; therefore, we should pay more attention to the rest of the genes related to T1DM and T2DM, respectively, which could help in understanding the pathogenesis and pathologies of these diseases.

Keywords: endocrine disease, Graves' disease, T2DM, PCOS, T1DM, IGF-I, deep learning methods

INTRODUCTION

Endocrine diseases fall into broad categories of hormone over- or underproduction, modulate tissue response to hormones, or tumors caused by endocrine tissue (Belfiore and LeRoith, 2018). Hormones synthesized and released by the endocrine glands exert their functions by regulating the biological process of cells. There are several examples of common endocrine diseases: type I/II diabetes mellitus, Graves' disease (GD), polycystic ovary syndrome (PCOS), and insulin-like growth factor I (IGFI) deficiency, etc. To date, genome-wide association studies (GWAS) have reported numerous gene regions associated with different endocrine diseases. The aim of GWAS analysis is to determine how the combined allele frequency of multiple susceptibility genes can affect autoimmunity and/or disease risk.

Graves' disease is an organ-specific autoimmune thyroid disease, resulting from excessive secretion of thyroid hormones by thyroid tissue (Dvornikova et al., 2020). The pathogenesis of GD is mediated by the production of antibodies to TSH receptors, which provide increased secretion of thyroid hormones and a rapid growth of the thyroid after stimulation (Smith et al., 2018; Soh and Aw, 2019). Since, GD is a hereditary and polygenic transmission disease (Perricone and Shoenfeld, 2019). It has been identified that associations between CTLA-4, FOXP3, TLR class polymorphism, and a number of pathological conditions develop in GD (Xiao et al., 2015; Fathima et al., 2019).

Diabetes mellitus, such as type 1 diabetes mellitus (TIDM) and type 2 diabetes mellitus (T2DM) are also a typical group of endocrine diseases. But basic pathogenic differences exist in these two types of diabetes mellitus. T1DM is immune mediated while T2DM is mediated by metabolic mechanisms (Eizirik et al., 2020). Glucagon secretion is observed to be reduced in patients with T1DM, with an increasing risk of insulin-induced hypoglycemia, but it is enhanced in T2DM, exacerbating the effects of reduced insulin release and action on glucose of blood levels (Gromada et al., 2018). Recent studies have detected several novel and promising TDM-susceptible genes, such as GCKR, SLC30A8, TLR4, and FTO (Ehrmann et al., 1999; Rotterdam ESHRE/ASRM-Sponsored PCOS Consensus Workshop Group, 2004; Day et al., 2015).

Polycystic ovary syndrome is a common endocrinopathy among women, with symptoms including irregular menstrual cycles, hyperandrogenism and polycystic ovarian morphology (Rotterdam ESHRE/ASRM-Sponsored PCOS Consensus Workshop Group, 2004). It is also accompanied with obesity and insulin resistance, increasing the risk of diabetes, metabolic syndrome, and other cardiovascular diseases (Ehrmann et al., 1999). There are several published causal variants from GWAS studies associated with PCOS (Day et al., 2015; Hayes et al., 2015). Despite the detrimental impact of the disorder on women's health, the etiology remains poorly understood.

Insulin-like growth factor I production is mainly mediated by growth hormones (GH); both GH and IGF-I have an anabolic effect on skeletal muscle and bone. Despite the effects on growing process in childhood, GH also plays an important role in the regulation of metabolism, body composition, and mood, which persist into adult life (Gazzaruso et al., 2014). However, low serum levels of IGF-I have been detected in patients suffering from chronic liver disease and malnutrition despite normal or elevated GH secretion (Cuneo et al., 1995).

Though there have been numerous susceptible loci identified by GWAS that are associated with endocrine diseases, etiology and pathology is still unclear. Analogous to other complex traits, common susceptibility loci identified by GWAS account for only a small proportion of the genetic heritability of the traits. As GWAS were designed to detect the common allelic variants with a minor allele frequencies of 2 to 5%, the variants occurred less frequently but with greater effect sizes being ignored which may account for the observed deficit in heritability (Manolio et al., 2009). Since SNPs detected by GWAS may not be the real causative regions, the SNPs related to them may be the real causative genes of complex diseases due to the theory of linkage disequilibrium (LD). Therefore, we take the expression level of genes regulated by SNPs into account to reduce the impact of LD. eQTL research plays an important role in prioritizing SNP loci in GWAS susceptible regions (Barral et al., 2012). Previous studies usually investigate susceptible genes of complex diseases based on the regulation function of SNPs on gene expression. MR analysis, for example, is proposed to explain the causative effect on a phenotype of gene expression based on the regulation of genetic variants (Freeman et al., 2013). However, it is rarely available in practice to obtain such a large sample size of different types of data, such as phenotype, genome-wide SNP genotype, and gene expression data, to perform a MR analysis. To overcome this, a SMR method was proposed which integrates summary-level data from independent GWAS with eQTL data to identify disease susceptible genes (Zhu et al., 2016).

Machine learning methods have been widely used in prediction problems, such as support vector machine (SVM), network embedding algorithms (such as node2vec), network diffusion algorithms (such as Laplacian heat diffusion, random walk with restart), etc. Combined with multiple biomolecular features, novel biomarkers, genes, and proteins can be predicted (Chen et al., 2018, 2019; Zhang et al., 2020). Nowadays, deep learning methods have also been utilized in bioinformatics. Liu et al. (2017) applied convolutional neural network (CNN) model to identify cell cycle-regulated genes. Graph convolutional network (GCN) was utilized to predict disease-related metabolites in the study by Zhao et al. (2020). Most machine learning and deep learning methods focused on feature extraction and selection. However, no computational method has been developed to predict the susceptible genes of endocrine diseases based on integrated omics data to eliminate the LD disequilibrium bias.

In this study, we developed "DeepGP," a method to prioritize susceptible genes of endocrine diseases based on deep learning approaches. First, we obtained curated disease-gene associations of five endocrine diseases from disGeNET database; susceptible regions and expression level data were downloaded from GWAS catalog and GTEx database, respectively. After mapping the genes to susceptible loci based on position information of genes, the feature vector of each gene was composed of two types of features, a phenotype-based feature derived from GWAS dataset and a transcriptome-based feature derived from eQTL data. Disease similarity network can be obtained from our previous work, which can represent disease features. GCN was then utilized to decipher the integrated feature representations of the gene. Finally, the classification of candidate genes was performed by CNN.

MATERIALS AND METHODS

Work Frame

DeepGP contains three main parts, data preprocessing (feature extraction), feature reconstruction based on GCN, and endocrine disease-related gene prediction based on CNN. In the feature extraction process, we obtained endocrine disease-related gene information from DisGeNET (Bauer-Mehren et al., 2010), GWAS Catalog (Buniello et al., 2019), and GTEx Portal databases (Carithers and Moore, 2015). After extracting the features of genes and diseases, we built a heterogeneous network composed of genes and diseases. We then utilized the GCN method to reconstruct the integrated gene features to obtain a more precise feature representation of each gene. In the disease gene prediction part, CNN is used to prioritize the causative genes related to endocrine diseases based on a comprehensive feature representation of disease-gene pairs. The workflow of DeepGP is shown in **Figure 1**.

Data Collection and Preprocessing

Genome-wide association studies have identified thousands of genetic variants that are associated with diseases and traits of medical importance in humans. However, the genes detected from the SNPs identified by GWAS which are pathogenic on diseases remain largely unknown due to the complicated LD between SNPs. Intuitively, genes closest to the top associated variants in position are the most likely causative genes. However, there have been studies reporting that causal genes are distinct from the nearest genes (Zhu et al., 2016). Studies have verified that gene expression may be influenced by different genetic variants among genes with different genotypes of the genetic variants, which means the phenotypes can be influenced by genetic variants through regulating the expression of their target genes. Therefore, we used a GCN network embedding method based on two types of omics data to obtain the comprehensive feature vector of each gene.

We first collected endocrine diseases from the "Endocrine diseases" chapter according to the International Classification of Diseases 11th Revision released by the World Health Organization. The major glands of the endocrine system include the pineal gland, pituitary gland, pancreas, ovaries, testes, thyroid gland, parathyroid gland, hypothalamus, and adrenal glands. Considering that some of the endocrine diseases have not been previously widely investigated, we chose five of the endocrine diseases, GD (which is mainly related to thyroid gland), T1DM/T2DM (which is mainly related to pancreas), PCOS (which is mainly related to ovaries), and IGFI deficiency (which is mainly related to pituitary gland). We then collected curated disease genes from the DisGeNET database (Piñero et al., 2016), causative loci from the GWAS database (Buniello et al., 2019), and expression level data from the GTEx database (Carithers and Moore, 2015). In addition, gene–gene interaction network was downloaded from HumanNet v2.0, where the correlation scores between a pair of genes were calculated. We then utilized an R package named biomaRt to obtain detailed information, such as gene location, chromosome number, and start and end position of each gene. BiomaRt can also be used to transform different gene IDs, such as gene symbol, Ensembl ID, and entrez ID, from different databases. After mapping the genes to the susceptible loci identified by GWAS and eQTL, genes with at least one susceptible SNP were kept. Finally, we obtained 7,406 genes, including 4,212 known causal genes and 3,194 candidate genes obtained from HumanNet v2.0.

Therefore, each gene has a feature of 2 × 25D based on GWAS and eQTL summary data according to five diseases. For the phenotype-based feature of each gene, we used the p-value of top 5 related SNPs of each disease to indicate the gene feature vector, for genes with less than five related SNPs, the feature vector is filled with 1. Thus, the phenotype-based feature of each gene could be denoted as:

$$G_S^i = [P_S^1 P_S^2, \cdots, P_S^{25}] \quad (1)$$

where P_S^i denotes the p-value of SNPs mapped by gene locations. Transcriptome-based feature of each gene can be extracted by the same method:

$$G_S^T = [P_T^1, P_T^2, \cdots, P_T^{25}] \quad (2)$$

where P_T^i denotes the p-value of susceptible loci consistent with that from the phenotype-based feature vector of each gene obtained from eQTL data. Thus, an initial integrated 2 × 25D feature vector of each gene is constructed.

Feature Reconstruction by GCN

In this section, we introduced a network-embedding algorithm based on GCN in order to present a new representation of gene features. GCN is a graph deep learning method based on node features and network architecture to classify the nodes

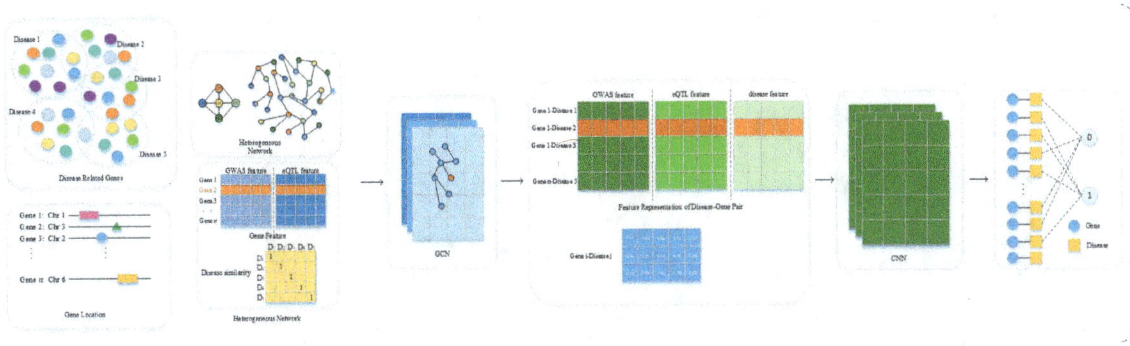

FIGURE 1 | Workflow of DeepGP.

of a network. Although GCNs have been successfully applied in other domains, to our knowledge, this is the first time that GCN was utilized to represent latent gene features from several omics datasets and network properties, while also being capable of disentangling the underlying molecular mechanisms driving the etiology of endocrine diseases.

Considering a graph $G = (V, E, W)$, where V denotes the nodes of the network, E denotes the edges of the network, and W the weight matrix encoding the interacting weight between nodes, which is obtained from HumanNet v2.0 as the gene interactions between gene pairs, the feature matrix of the nodes can be denoted as $X \in R^{N\times F}$. Thus, the eigenvectors of the graph Laplacian L can be denoted as:

$$\mathrm{L} = D^{-\frac{1}{2}}\tilde{A}D^{-\frac{1}{2}} \tag{3}$$

where the adjacency matrix $\tilde{A} = A + I$ has added self-connections since gene nodes should contain both gene interaction and gene itself information and D is the degree matrix.

Finally, we can define a propagation rule for each layer:

$$H^{l+1} = (LH^{l}XW^{l}) \tag{4}$$

$$\mathrm{ReLU}\,(x) = \begin{cases} x, & x>0 \\ 0, & x\leq 0 \end{cases} \tag{5}$$

where σ denotes a nonlinearity, such as the Rectified Linear Unit activation function. The input of the first layer is X, which includes the gene expression feature and gene variation feature of five interested traits, so $H^0=X$. Therefore, the feature of the gene network could be extracted by formula (4). Since we combined two omics types of data, each gene feature could be represented as a 2 × 25D vector. Thus, we have a feature representation of each gene; the feature can be denoted as: $g_i = \begin{bmatrix} P^1_{i,s}, P^2_{i,s}, P^3_{i,s}, \cdots, P^{25}_{i,s} \\ P^1_{i,T}, P^2_{i,T}, P^3_{i,T}, \cdots, P^{25}_{i,T} \end{bmatrix}$.

Causal Gene Prediction With CNN

After obtaining the best combination of initial feature representation by GCN, we constructed disease features based on disease similarity matrix calculated by the method ImpAESim. Each disease feature can be denoted as a 1 × 5D vector:

$$D_i = \{S_{i,j}\},\ \mathrm{j} = 1, 2, 3, 4, 5 \tag{6}$$

$S_{i,j}$ denotes the similarity between D_i and D_j, $S_{i,j}$ is 1 if $i = j$. We then combined the gene feature and disease feature as a 3 × 5D feature of disease–gene pair.

We then trained a CNN model to predict causal genes based on the gene features derived from GCN. Analogous to other machine learning methods, CNN consists of a training step where the estimation of network parameters from a given training dataset is learned, and the testing step utilized the well-trained network to predict outputs of new testing dataset (Min et al., 2017). Since our feature format of each gene–disease pair is 3 × 5D, which can be regarded as an image with three channels, in this work, the structure of the CNN section is shown in **Figure 2**. The CNN section includes four parts as follows: convolution layer, max-pooling layer, fully connected layer, and an output layer. Convolution layer is responsible for extracting the subspace features of the input. Max-pooling layer is used for dimension reduction to discard the redundant information. The final fully connected layer connects all the nodes and the output layer applying sigmoid as the activation function to solve the binary classification problem.

The tanh function is the activation function in each convolutional layer.

$$\tanh\,(x) = \frac{\sinh x}{\cosh x} = \frac{e^x - e^{-x}}{e^x + e^{-x}} \tag{7}$$

The sigmoid function is used as the activation function in the output layer.

$$\delta\,(x) = 1/(1 + e^{-x}) \tag{8}$$

Since our disease gene prediction can be treated as a binary classification problem, we chose the binary cross-entropy function as the loss function to assess the probability of the output.

$$\mathrm{loss} = -\sum_{i\ 1}^{n} y_i' \log\left(y_i\right) + (1 - y_i')\log(1 - y_i') \tag{9}$$

$$\frac{\partial \mathrm{loss}}{\partial y} = -\sum_{i=1}^{n} \frac{y_i'}{y_i} - \frac{1 - y_i'}{1 - y_i'} \tag{10}$$

According to formulas (7, 8), loss is 0 as long as y_i' is equal to y_i.

As a result, each disease–gene pair was assigned a correlation score with a range of [0, 1], where 1 denotes the pair having the strongest association and 0 means no association.

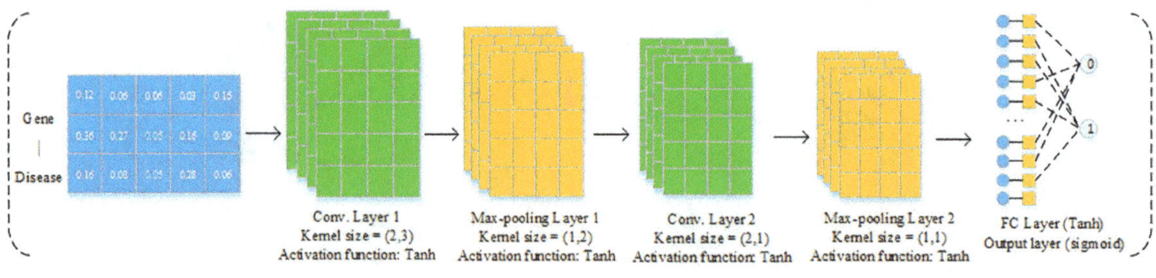

FIGURE 2 | Structure of CNN model.

Training Steps

According to the 4,212 curated disease-related genes to five endocrine diseases, there are 6,258 positive disease–gene pairs derived from the curated disease–gene associations, and 14,802 (4,212 × 5–6,258) pairs are not reported to be associated; we randomly selected 6,258 pairs to construct the negative samples. However, the sample size of different diseases are extremely unbalanced, as shown in **Table 1**; the sample size ranges from 28 IGFI–gene pairs to 3,058 T2D–gene pairs due to the insufficiency of studies related to these diseases, which may have a serious negative impact on the classification performance. From the analysis for summary data derived from GWAS and eQTL, T1D, and T2D share as much as 950 genes in total, with 679/1,629 genes merely related to T1D and 2,108/3,058 genes merely related to T2D.

After obtaining the new dataset that consisted of 6,258 positive samples and 6,258 negative samples, we conducted a 10-cross-validation on this new dataset to test the performance. First, the dataset is randomly divided into 10 groups, then 10 times of iterations were performed based on nine of 10 groups as training set and one group as test set, which made sure that each group can be used as an independent test set.

RESULTS

Performance Evaluation on Predicting Disease–Gene Associations

The area under the curve (AUC) and the area under the precision-recall curve (AUPR) are used to assess DeepGP. The AUC and AUPR of each iteration in 10-cross-validation process are shown in **Table 2**. As a result, DeepGP achieved a mean AUC of 0.845 and a mean AUPR of 0.833, which have shown better and stable in disease–gene prediction.

TABLE 1 | Number of curated disease genes.

Disease	T2D	T1D	PCOS	GD	IGFI deficiency
No. of samples	3,058	1,629	974	568	28

TABLE 2 | AUC and AUPR of DeepGP in 10 times 10 cross-validation.

	1	2	3	4	5	6	7	8	9	10	Average
AUC	0.832	0.845	0.821	0.854	0.864	0.855	0.831	0.861	0.856	0.831	0.845
AUPR	0.827	0.837	0.816	0.845	0.838	0.825	0.816	0.858	0.842	0.826	0.833

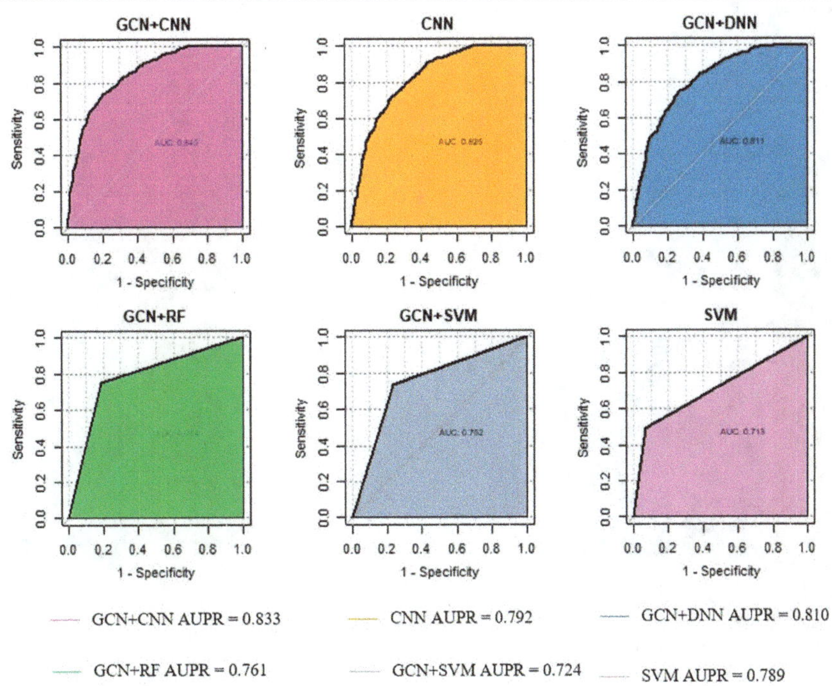

FIGURE 3 | Performance comparison among different methods.

Comparison Experiments With Classic Methods

We evaluated the performance of DeepGP and classic machine learning methods, such as SVM, random forest (RF), Naïve Bayes, and deep neural network (DNN) for predicting disease-gene associations. To validate the performance of extracting best combination of gene features by GCN, we alternatively only used CNN for feature extraction and prediction. Then, to assess the effect of convolution layers in CNN, we applied a typical deep learning method DNN and two classic machine learning methods SVM and RF. As a contrast, we also only used a SVM model for the classification task. Therefore, we compared the performance of five methods with DeepGP: CNN, GCN-DNN, GCN-SVM, GCN-RF, and SVM.

The method of training and testing was performed the same as DeepGP. As shown in **Figure 3**, comparing with other classic machine learning methods, DeepGP achieves the highest performance according to both AUC and AUPR. CNN and DNN achieved the second and third highest AUROC which infers deep learning methods are better than classic machine learning methods in this disease-gene prediction task; however, it can also be inferred that convolution layers are essential. In addition, the performance was improved after feature encoding by GCN.

It has been shown that the depth of CNN models can affect the classification performance. To assess the influence of the depth of CNN models, we compared DeepGP with a shallower CNN model, denoted as GCN+CNN (B), consisting of one set of one convolution layer and one max-pooling layer. Since the feature dimension of each disease-gene pair is 3 × 5, we also enlarged the kernel size to detect the effect of dimension reduction. The performance is shown in **Figure 4**. GCN+CNN (A) denotes the structure of DeepGP, GCN+CNN (B) denotes the shallower CNN model, and GCN+CNN (C) denotes the structure of CNN with enlarged kernel size. As a result, DeepGP achieved the best performance comparing with other methods even though the feature dimension of each sample is low. Hence, according to the above results, we conclude that our proposed DeepGP is competitive against other methods.

Validation of Prediction Results

After verifying the effectiveness of DeepGP based on the comparison experiments. We conducted the disease-gene prediction process among all the unknown disease-gene pairs. We set a threshold of 0.5 as default to screen the scores and identified 7,702 of 14,903 pairs to be true. Among the predicted associations, 971 novel genes were identified to be associated with GD, 3,142 novel genes associated with PCOS, and 2,437 and 1,154 novel genes associated with T1DM and T2DM, respectively. Due to deficiency of studies focused on IGFI deficiency, only 28 of 4,212 were reported as curated genes related to the trait. The highest score of IGFI gene pairs was 0.33, which is under the threshold, and was predicted to be have no

TABLE 3 | Top 5 related genes with four diseases.

GD	PCOS	T1D	T2D
CCL27	RBM14	ADM2 (+)	UPK3B (+)
CXCL16	miR-1307	Enho (+)	miR-592
BECN1	CMKLR1	FUT6 (+)	NELFCD (+)
PROX1	AKT3	FUT7	miR-589 (+)
PTX3	GCGR	ATRNL1 (+)	Linc00641 (+)

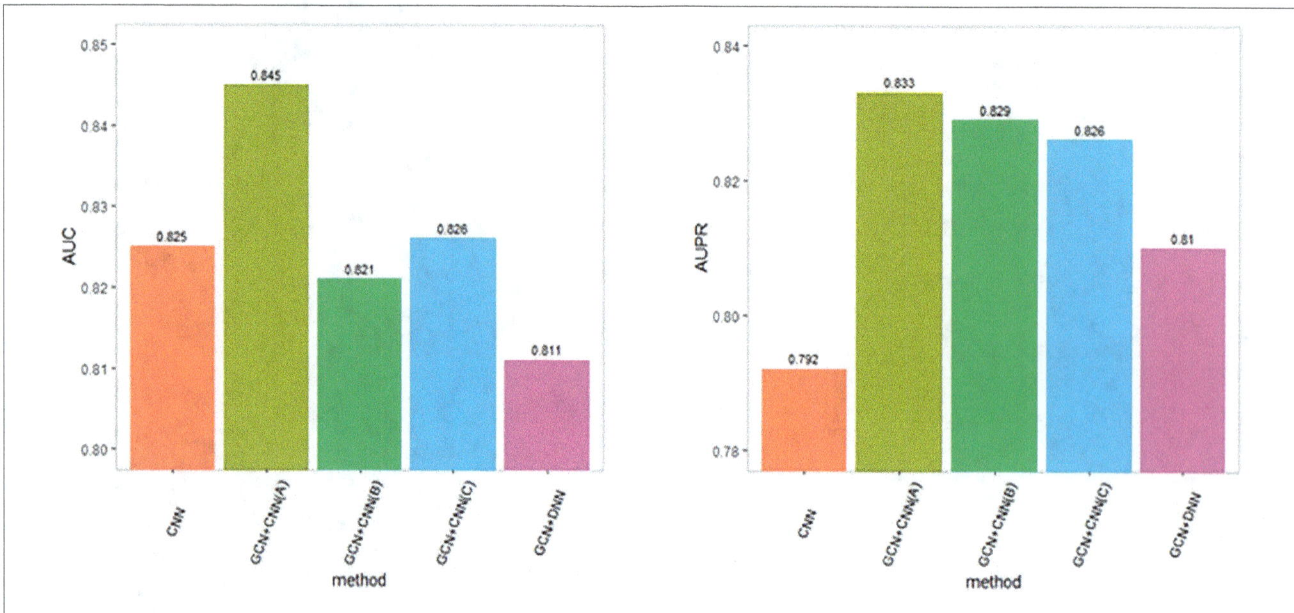

FIGURE 4 | Performance comparison with variational deep learning methods.

associations by DeepGP. For the rest of the diseases, 772 of 3,778 genes were shared.

Case Study

Graves' Disease

Graves' disease is mainly mediated by T cells which produce cytokines and chemokines in abnormal amounts. CCL27 is reported to be associated with serum chemokine concentrations detected in GD, which might be a good biomarker for GD (Hiratsuka et al., 2015). CXCL16 have been demonstrated to bind to the unique receptor CXCR6, which is expressed on a subset of multiple types of T cells, and it has been implicated in the pathogenesis of atherosclerosis and GD (Günther et al., 2012). It has been identified that loci at BECN1 can be denoted as a significant extract differentially methylated region for Graves' orbitopathy under the context of GD (Shi et al., 2019).

Polycystic Ovary Syndrome

RBM14 and miR-1307 have been reported to be up-regulated in PCOS patients in the study of Xu et al. (2015) and Che et al. (2020). Besides, CMKLR1, known as chemerin chemokine-like receptor 1, is the receptor of chemerin which is expressed at both mRNA and protein levels in human granulosa cells, and it has been reported to vary in women with PCOS (Bongrani et al., 2019).

Diabetes Mellitus

Due to the pathophysiological characteristics and many other potential etiopathogenesis factors T1DM and T2DM share, there are genes linked to both diseases such as *GLIS3* (Mahajan et al., 2014), *EIL2AK3* (also named as *PERK*; Delépine et al., 2000), etc. According to the result obtained from our method, we identified 2,582 genes related to T1D and 1,153 genes related to T2D, with a number of 474 shared genes. We then searched the top-ranked predicted genes related to T1D and T2D. According to the work of Ahmed et al., ADM2 is found to be preferentially up-regulated by bacteroides dorei (BD), which is a bacteria increased significantly at the time of onset of T1D. Enho is an energy homeostasis-associated gene that can produce a regulatory peptides named adropin, which has been identified to be strongly associated with type 1 diabetes in children (Polkowska et al., 2019). *FUT7* gene has been demonstrated to be linked with an antigen termed bile salt-dependent lipase which is reported to be associated with type 1 diabetes (Panicot et al., 1999). UPK3B is regarded as a mesothelial-like cell marker of a major adipocyte progenitor cell subpopulations which may induce adipocyte dysfunction in visceral adipose tissue in type 2 diabetes (Strieder-Barboza et al., 2020). miR-592 is reported to be associated with T2D due to its background of insulin resistance by Song et al. (2019). NELFCD has been identified to be matched with risk haplotypes across five FDM-risk haplotype, which is further identified in a common T2D gene, *ANK1*.

Therefore, we can illustrate that the predicted disease-gene pairs are reliable from the case studies mentioned above; top related genes with diseases are shown in **Table 3**. The "+" means the gene identified with T1D (T2D) is also related to T2D (T1D) according to the DisGeNET database.

DISCUSSION

In summary, we proposed a disease gene prediction method based on integrated deep learning models. We construct gene features considering both biological process and "linkage disequilibrium" theory. Identifying disease genes merely based on disease-susceptible loci identified by GWAS studies may be inaccurate due to LD. It has been indicated that genetic variants can affect the phenotype by regulating the gene expression level. In this study, eQTL data are also utilized to extract gene features. To fully use the underlying information contained in a gene interaction network, GCN was applied to extract comprehensive gene features based on the constructed gene network. Therefore, our method exploits the predictive power derived from complementary data types and the underlying network simultaneously. Disease features are derived based on disease similarity, which is calculated by the method named ImpAESim. Finally, we combined gene and disease features as a disease–gene pair feature. CNN was then used to classify the disease–gene pairs as a binary classification task.

As a result, DeepGP achieved an average AUC of 0.845 and an average AUPR of 0.833 after a 10 times 10-cross-validation based on the constructed training set, which is superior to other classic machine learning and deep learning methods. We then used the well-trained model to predict the novel disease-gene associations based on the disease–gene pairs which have not been reported to be associated before. We verified the prediction results based on a case study. Most of the top disease-related genes have reported evidences to illustrate that the genes may have associations with the diseases. In addition, we also identified 474 genes shared by T1DM and T2DM which may be helpful in designing therapeutic methods for diabetes mellitus patients. Therefore, the novel disease genes identified by DeepGP provide a strong support for the feasibility of extracting diagnostic markers for future validation and shed light on new strategies for the diagnosis and treatment of endocrine diseases.

DATA AVAILABILITY STATEMENT

The original contributions presented in the study are included in the article/supplementary material; further inquiries can be directed to the corresponding author/s.

AUTHOR CONTRIBUTIONS

NZ did most of the work and wrote the manuscript. HW, CX, and LZ assisted in completing the experiments. TZ proposed the idea of the manuscript. HW made a great contribution in modifying the manuscript. All authors contributed to the article and approved the submitted version.

REFERENCES

Barral, S., Bird, T., Goate, A., Farlow, M. R., Diaz-Arrastia, R., Bennett, D. A., et al. (2012). Genotype patterns at PICALM, CR1, BIN1, CLU, and APOE genes are associated with episodic memory. *Neurology* 78, 1464–1471. doi: 10.1212/wnl.0b013e3182553c48

Bauer-Mehren, A., Rautschka, M., Sanz, F., and Furlong, L. I. (2010). DisGeNET: a cytoscape plugin to visualize, integrate, search and analyze gene–disease networks. *Bioinformatics* 26, 2924–2926. doi: 10.1093/bioinformatics/btq538

Belfiore, A., and LeRoith, D. (2018). *Principles of Endocrinology and Hormone Action*. New York, NY: Springer.

Bongrani, A., Mellouk, N., Rame, C., Cornuau, M., Guérif, F., Froment, P., et al. (2019). Ovarian expression of adipokines in polycystic ovary syndrome: a role for chemerin, omentin, and apelin in follicular growth arrest and ovulatory dysfunction? *Int. J. Mol. Sci.* 20:3778. doi: 10.3390/ijms2015 3778

Buniello, A., MacArthur, J. A. L., Cerezo, M., Harris, L. W., Hayhurst, J., Malangone, C., et al. (2019). The NHGRI-EBI GWAS Catalog of published genome-wide association studies, targeted arrays and summary statistics. *Nucleic Acids Res.* 47, D1005–D1012.

Carithers, L. J., and Moore, H. M. (2015). *The Genotype-Tissue Expression (GTEx) Project*. New Rochelle, NY: Mary Ann Liebert, Inc.

Che, Q., Liu, M., Zhang, D., Lu, Y., Xu, J., Lu, X., et al. (2020). Long noncoding RNA HUPCOS promotes follicular fluid androgen excess in PCOS patients via aromatase inhibition. *J. Clin. Endocrinol. Metab.* 105, 1086–1097. doi: 10.1210/clinem/dgaa060

Chen, L., Zhang, Y.-H., Huang, G., Pan, X., Huang, T., and Cai, Y. D. (2019). Inferring novel genes related to oral cancer with a network embedding method and one-class learning algorithms. *Gene Ther.* 26, 465–478. doi: 10.1038/s41434-019-0099-y

Chen, L., Zhang, Y.-H., Zhang, Z., Huang, T., and Cai, Y. D. (2018). Inferring novel tumor suppressor genes with a protein-protein interaction network and network diffusion algorithms. *Mol. Ther. Methods Clin. Dev.* 10, 57–67. doi: 10.1016/j.omtm.2018.06.007

Cuneo, R. C., Hickman, P. E., Wallace, J. D., Teh, B. T., Ward, G., Veldhuis, J. D., et al. (1995). Altered endogenous growth hormone secretory kinetics and diurnal GH—binding protein profiles in adults with chronic liver disease. *Clin. Endocrinol.* 43, 265–275. doi: 10.1111/j.1365-2265.1995.tb02031.x

Day, F. R., Hinds, D. A., Tung, J. Y., Stolk, L., Styrkarsdottir, U., Saxena, R., et al. (2015). Causal mechanisms and balancing selection inferred from genetic associations with polycystic ovary syndrome. *Nat. Commun.* 6, 1–7.

Delépine, M., Nicolino, M., Barrett, T., Golamaully, M., Lathrop, G. M., and Julier, C. (2000). EIF2AK3, encoding translation initiation factor 2-α kinase 3, is mutated in patients with Wolcott-Rallison syndrome. *Nat. Genet.* 25, 406–409. doi: 10.1038/78085

Dvornikova, K. A., Bystrova, E. Y., Platonova, O. N., and Churilov, L. P. (2020). Polymorphism of toll-like receptor genes and autoimmune endocrine diseases. *Autoimmun. Rev.* 19:102496. doi: 10.1016/j.autrev.2020.102496

Ehrmann, D. A., Barnes, R. B., Rosenfield, R. L., Cavaghan, M. K., and Imperial, J. (1999). Prevalence of impaired glucose tolerance and diabetes in women with polycystic ovary syndrome. *Diabetes Care* 22, 141–146. doi: 10.2337/diacare.22.1.141

Eizirik, D. L., Pasquali, L., and Cnop, M. (2020). Pancreatic β-cells in type 1 and type 2 diabetes mellitus: different pathways to failure. *Nat. Rev. Endocrinol.* 16, 349–362. doi: 10.1038/s41574-020-0355-7

Fathima, N., Narne, P., and Ishaq, M. (2019). Association and gene–gene interaction analyses for polymorphic variants in CTLA-4 and FOXP3 genes: role in susceptibility to autoimmune thyroid disease. *Endocrine* 64, 591–604. doi: 10.1007/s12020-019-01859-3

Freeman, G., Cowling, B. J., and Schooling, C. M. (2013). Power and sample size calculations for Mendelian randomization studies using one genetic instrument. *Int. J. Epidemiol.* 42, 1157–1163. doi: 10.1093/ije/dyt110

Gazzaruso, C., Gola, M., Karamouzis, I., Giubbini, R., and Giustina, A. (2014). Cardiovascular risk in adult patients with growth hormone (GH) deficiency and following substitution with GH—an update. *J. Clin. Endocrinol. Metab.m* 99, 18–29. doi: 10.1210/jc.2013-2394

Gromada, J., Chabosseau, P., and Rutter, G. A. (2018). The α-cell in diabetes mellitus. *Nat. Rev. Endocrinol.* 14, 694–704.

Günther, C., Carballido-Perrig, N., Kaesler, S., Carballido, J. M., and Biedermann, T. (2012). CXCL16 and CXCR6 are upregulated in psoriasis and mediate cutaneous recruitment of human CD8+ T cells. *J. Invest. Dermatol.* 132, 626–634. doi: 10.1038/jid.2011.371

Hayes, M. G., Urbanek, M., Ehrmann, D. A., Armstrong, L. L., Lee, J. Y., Sisk, R., et al. (2015). Genome-wide association of polycystic ovary syndrome implicates alterations in gonadotropin secretion in European ancestry populations. *Nat. Commun.* 6, 1–13.

Hiratsuka, I., Itoh, M., Yamada, H., Yamamoto, K., Tomatsu, E., Makino, M., et al. (2015). Simultaneous measurement of serum chemokines in autoimmune thyroid diseases: possible role of IP-10 in the inflammatory response. *Endocr. J.* 62, EJ15–EJ0448.

Liu, C., Cui, P., and Huang, T. (2017). Identification of cell cycle-regulated genes by convolutional neural network. *Comb. Chem. High Throughput Screen.* 20, 603–611.

Mahajan, A., Go, M. J., Zhang, W., Below, J. E., Gaulton, K. J., Ferreira, T., et al. (2014). Genome-wide trans-ancestry meta-analysis provides insight into the genetic architecture of type 2 diabetes susceptibility. *Nat. Genet.* 46, 234–244. doi: 10.1038/ng.2897

Manolio, T. A., Collins, F. S., Cox, N. J., Goldstein, D. B., Hindorff, L. A., Hunter, D. J., et al. (2009). Finding the missing heritability of complex diseases. *Nature* 461, 747–753.

Min, S., Lee, B., and Yoon Deep, S. (2017). learning in bioinformatics. *Brief. Bioinformatics* 18, 851–869.

Panicot, L., Mas, E., Thivolet, C., and Lombardo, D. (1999). Circulating antibodies against an exocrine pancreatic enzyme in type 1 diabetes. *Diabetes* 48, 2316–2323. doi: 10.2337/diabetes.48.12.2316

Perricone, C., and Shoenfeld, Y. (2019). *Mosaic of Autoimmunity: the Novel Factors of Autoimmune Diseases*. Cambridge, MA: Academic Press.

Piñero, J., Bravo, À, Queralt-Rosinach, N., Gutiérrez-Sacristán, A., Deu-Pons, J., Centeno, E., et al. (2016). DisGeNET: a comprehensive platform integrating information on human disease-associated genes and variants. *Nucleic Acids Res.* 45:gkw943.

Polkowska, A., Pasierowska, I. E., Pasławska, M., Pawluczuk, E., and Bossowski, A. (2019). Assessment of serum concentrations of adropin, afamin, and neudesin in children with type 1 diabetes. *BioMed. Res. Int.* 2019:6128410.

Rotterdam ESHRE/ASRM-Sponsored PCOS Consensus Workshop Group (2004). Revised 2003 consensus on diagnostic criteria and long-term health risks related to polycystic ovary syndrome. *Fertil. Steril.* 81, 19–25. doi: 10.1016/j.fertnstert.2003.10.004

Soh, S-B, and Aw, T-C (2019). Laboratory testing in thyroid conditions-pitfalls and clinical utility. *Ann. Lab. Med.* 39:3. doi: 10.3343/alm.2019.39.1.3

Shi, T.-T., Hua, L., Xin, Z., Li, Y., Liu, W., and Yang, Y. L. (2019). Identifying and validating genes with DNA methylation data in the context of biological network for Chinese patients with Graves' orbitopathy. *Int. J. Endocrinol.* 2019:6212681.

Smith, M. J., Rihanek, M., Coleman, B. M., Gottlieb, P. A., Sarapura, V. D., and Cambier, J. C. (2018). Activation of thyroid antigen-reactive B cells in recent onset autoimmune thyroid disease patients. *J. Autoimmun.* 89, 82–89. doi: 10.1016/j.jaut.2017.12.001

Song, Y., Wu, L., Li, M., Xiong, X., Fang, Z., Zhou, J., et al. (2019). Down-regulation of MicroRNA-592 in obesity contributes to hyperglycemia and insulin resistance. *EBioMedicine* 42, 494–503. doi: 10.1016/j.ebiom.2019.03.041

Strieder-Barboza, C., Flesher, C. G., Geletka, L. M., Orourke, RW., and Lumeng, CN. (2020). 1973-P: single-Nuclei transcriptomics of human adipose tissue identify distinct adipocyte progenitor subpopulations in type 2 diabetes. *Am. Diabetes Assoc.* 69(Suppl. 1).

Xiao, W., Liu, Z., Lin, J., Li, J., Wu, K., Ma, Y., et al. (2015). Polymorphisms in TLR1, TLR6 and TLR10 genes and the risk of Graves' disease. *Autoimmunity* 48, 13–18.

Xu, B., Zhang, Y.-W., Tong, X.-H., and Liu, Y. S. (2015). Characterization of microRNA profile in human cumulus granulosa cells: identification of microRNAs that regulate Notch signaling and are associated with PCOS. *Mol. Cell. Endocrinol.* 404, 26–36. doi: 10.1016/j.mce.2015.01.030

Zhang, H., Wang, S., and Huang, T. (2020). Identification of chronic hypersensitivity pneumonitis biomarkers with machine learning and differential co-expression analysis. *Curr. Gene Ther.* 21.

Zhao, T., Hu, Y., and Cheng, L. (2020). Deep-DRM: a computational method for identifying disease-related metabolites based on graph deep learning approaches. *Brief. Bioinformatics* 20:bbaa212.

Zhu, Z., Zhang, F., Hu, H., Bakshi, A., Robinson, M. R., Powell, J. E., et al. (2016). Integration of summary data from GWAS and eQTL studies predicts complex trait gene targets. *Nat. Genet.* 48, 481–487. doi: 10.1038/ng.3538

18

Reporter cell lines to evaluate the selectivity of chemicals for human and zebrafish estrogen and peroxysome proliferator activated γ receptors

Marina Grimaldi[1,2,3,4], *Abdelhay Boulahtouf*[1,2,3,4], *Vanessa Delfosse*[5,6], *Erwan Thouennon*[1,2,3,4], *William Bourguet*[5,6] *and Patrick Balaguer*[1,2,3,4*]

[1] *Institut de Recherche en Cancérologie de Montpellier, Montpellier, France,* [2] *Institut National de la Santé et de la Recherche Médicale U1194, Montpellier, France,* [3] *Université Montpellier, Montpellier, France,* [4] *Institut Reigional du Cancer de Montpellier, Montpellier, France,* [5] *Institut National de la Santé et de la Recherche Médicale U1054, Montpellier, France,* [6] *Centre National de la Recherche Scientifique UMR5048, Centre de Biochimie Structurale, Université Montpellier, Montpellier, France*

Edited by:
Hubert Vaudry,
University of Rouen, France

Reviewed by:
Berta Levavi-Sivan,
The Hebrew University, Israel
Taisen Iguchi,
National Institute for Basic Biology, Japan

***Correspondence:**
Patrick Balaguer,
Institut de Recherche en Cancérologie de Montpellier, Institut National de la Santé et de la Recherche Médicale 1194, Institut Reigional du Cancer de Montpellier, Parc Euromédecine, 208 rue des Apothicaires, 34090 Montpellier, France
patrick.balaguer@inserm.fr

Zebrafish is increasingly used as an animal model to study the effects of environmental nuclear receptors (NRs) ligands. As most of these compounds have only been tested on human NRs, it is necessary to measure their effects on zebrafish NRs. Estrogen receptors (ER) α and β and peroxysome proliferator activated receptor (PPAR) γ are main targets of environmental disrupting compounds (EDCs). In humans there are two distinct nuclear ERs (hERα and hERβ), whereas the zebrafish genome encodes three ERs, zfERα, zfERβ1, and zfERβ2. Only one isoform of PPARγ is expressed in both humans and zebrafish. In this review, we described reporter cell lines that we established to study the interaction of EDCs with human and zebrafish ERs and PPARγ. Using these cell lines, we observed that zfERs are thermo-sensitive while zfPPARγ is not. We also showed significant differences in the ability of environmental and synthetic ligands to modulate activation of zfERs and zfPPARγ in comparison to hERs and hPPARγ. Some environmental estrogens (bisphenol A, mycoestrogens) which are hER panagonists displayed greater potency for zfERα as compared to zfERβs. hERβ selective agonists (8βVE2, DPN, phytoestrogens) also displayed zfERα selectivity. Among hERα selective synthetic agonists, 16α-LE2 was the most zfERα selective compound. Almost all zfPPARγ environmental ligands (halogenated bisphenol A derivatives, phthalates, perfluorinated compounds) displayed similar affinity for human and zebrafish PPARγ while pharmaceutical hPPARγ agonists like thiazolidones are not recognized by zfPPARγ. Altogether, our studies show that all hERs and hPPARγ ligands do not control in a similar manner the transcriptional activity of zfERs and zfPPARγ and point out that care has to be taken in transposing the results obtained using the zebrafish as a model for human physiopathology.

Keywords: estrogen receptor, peroxysome proliferator activated receptor γ, environmental disrupting compounds, reporter cell lines, human, zebrafish

Introduction

Human nuclear hormone receptors (NHRs) are a family of 48 transcription factors, many of which have been shown to be activated by ligands. NHRs regulate cognate gene networks involved in key physiological functions such as cell growth and differentiation, development, homeostasis, or metabolism (Gronemeyer et al., 2004; Germain et al., 2006). Consequently, inappropriate exposure to environmental pollutants often leads to proliferative, reproductive, and metabolic diseases, including hormonal cancers, infertility, obesity or diabetes. NHRs are modular proteins composed of several domains, most notably an N-terminal domain, which harbors a ligand-independent activation function (AF-1), a central DNA-binding domain (DBD), and a C-terminal ligand-binding domain (LBD) hosting a ligand-dependent transcriptional activation function (AF-2) (Gronemeyer et al., 2004). In the absence of the cognate ligand, some NHRs are located in the nucleus, bind to the DNA response elements of their target genes, and recruit corepressors, while others are located in the cytoplasm in an inactive complex with chaperones.

Ligand binding induces major structural alterations of the receptor LBDs, leading to (1) destabilization of corepressor or chaperone interfaces, (2) exposure of nuclear localization signals to allow nuclear translocation and DNA binding of cytoplasmic receptors, and (3) recruitment of coactivators triggering gene transcription through chromatin remodeling and activation of the general transcription machinery. The crystal structures of many NHR LBDs have been determined, revealing a conserved core of 12 α-helices (H1–H12) and a short two-stranded antiparallel β-sheet (S1 and S2) arranged into a three-layered sandwich fold. This arrangement generates a mostly hydrophobic cavity in the lower half of the domain, which can accommodate the cognate ligand. In all hormone-bound LBD structures, the ligand-binding pocket (LBP) is sealed by helix H12. This conformation is specifically induced by the binding of hormones or synthetic agonists and is referred to as the "active conformation" because it allows the dissociation of corepressors and favors the recruitment of transcriptional coactivators (Bourguet et al., 2000; Renaud and Moras, 2000; Pike, 2006).

In contrast to agonist binding, interaction with antagonists prevents the correct positioning of helix H12, thus avoiding association with the LxxLL motifs of coactivators. The LBD also contributes to the modulation of the N-terminal AF-1 through interdomain crosstalk so that both AF-1 and AF-2 domains can recruit a range of coregulatory proteins and act individually or in a synergistic manner (Benecke et al., 2000; Bommer et al., 2002; Wilson, 2011).

Among nuclear receptors, ERs and PPARγ are main targets of numerous synthetic substances released into the environment by human activities. These substances can act as endocrine-disrupting chemicals (EDCs) causing reproductive, developmental, metabolic, or neurological diseases as well as hormone-related cancers (Diamanti-Kandarakis et al., 2009). Many EDCs are man-made compounds, for example bisphenols, phthalates, parabens, dioxins, pesticides, alkylphenols, organotins, polychlorinated biphenyls, or perfluoroalkyl compounds. Some natural EDCs can also be found in plants and fungi. Standard methods to study interaction of EDCs with these nuclear receptors use stable cell reporter gene assays based on human ERs and PPARγ activation (Balaguer et al., 1999; Legler et al., 1999; Seimandi et al., 2005; Riu et al., 2011a). To address whether chemicals exert an effect at the organismal level, ER activity assays have been developed for zebrafish. In these animals, GFP reporter constructs are designed to act in certain tissues exclusively (such as liver or brain) (Kurauchi et al., 2005; Brion et al., 2012) or in all tissues of embryos and larvae (Gorelick and Halpern, 2011; Lee et al., 2012). Zebrafish has also been used as an *in vivo* model to study the effect of environmental compounds on PPARγ (Riu et al., 2014). Zebrafish stores neutral lipid triglycerides in visceral, intramuscular, and subcutaneous adipocyte depots (Tingaud-Sequeira et al., 2012). Studies of the zebrafish embryo, which is optically transparent thus facilitating the labeling and detection of lipid depots using lipid staining (Minchin and Rawls, 2011), have shown that white adipose tissue appearance is correlated with size rather than the age of the fish. By using zebrafish as a PPARγ ligand screening model, we have showed that halogenated-BPA analogs are potent inducers of lipid accumulation *in vivo* through PPARγ signaling (Riu et al., 2014).

In order to evaluate the effects of environmental and pharmaceutical compounds on the transcriptional activity of zfERs and zfPPARγ and to compare the data with their activity on hERs and hPPARγ, we established human and zebrafish ERs and PPARγ reporter cell lines in the same cellular context (Balaguer et al., 1999; Seimandi et al., 2005; Pinto et al., 2014; Riu et al., 2014). In HeLa cells stably expressing an ERE-driven luciferase reporter (HELN cells), we expressed the full-length hERα, hERβ, zfERα, zfERβ1, and zfERβ2, respectively. Similarly, in HeLa cells stably expressing a GAL4RE-driven luciferase reporter (HG5LN cells), we expressed a fusion protein consisting of the hPPARγ or zfPPARγ ligand binding domain (LBD) and the DNA binding domain (DBD) of the yeast transcription factor GAL4 (GAL4-PPARγ).

The resulting HELN-ERs and HG5LN PPARγ cell lines were used to evaluate the effects of environmental compounds on gene transactivation by the five ERs and the two PPARγ, and to compare these effects with results obtained on hER and PPARγ orthologs. Since zebrafish is used as a model for studying the effects of environmental compounds *in vivo*, determining the transcriptional profiles of these compounds on the zfERs and zfPPARγ is crucial to support the zebrafish model for ER- and PPARγ-related studies and their extrapolation to the mammalian system.

Estrogen Receptors

Estrogen signaling is mainly mediated by the two estrogen receptors ERα (also called NR3A1) and ERβ (also called NR3A2) (Jensen and Jordan, 2003; Dahlman-Wright et al., 2006) which play important roles in the growth and maintenance of various tissues such as the mammary gland, uterus, bones, or the cardiovascular system. Like most NRs, ERs bind as dimers to DNA response elements in the promoter region of target genes and respond to the naturally occurring sex hormone 17β-estradiol (E_2). Both hERs are widely distributed throughout the body, displaying distinct but overlapping expression patterns in a variety of tissues (Couse and Korach, 1999). hERα is primarily expressed in the uterus, liver, kidney, and heart, whereas hERβ is preferentially expressed in the ovary, prostate, lung, gastrointestinal tract, bladder, and hematopoietic and central nervous systems (Kuiper et al., 1997). However, hERα and hERβ are coexpressed in a number of tissues including the mammary gland, thyroid, adrenal, bones, and some regions of the brain. Although hERα and hERβ share similar mechanisms of action, several differences in the transcriptional abilities of each receptor and distinct phenotypes between gene-null animals have been identified, suggesting that these receptors may regulate distinct cellular pathways (Curtis et al., 1996; Couse and Korach, 1999). Interestingly, when hERs are coexpressed, hERβ exhibits an inhibitory action on ERα-mediated gene expression (Pettersson et al., 2000; Liu et al., 2002), so that hERβ has been shown to antagonize several hERα-mediated effects including fat reduction and cell proliferation in breast, uterus, or prostate (Ogawa et al., 1998; Weihua et al., 2000; Lindberg et al., 2003). Furthermore, in addition to controlling the normal development and function of the reproductive system and other tissues, estrogens are key regulators of primary breast and prostatic cancer growth (Jensen and Jordan, 2003). Roughly 40% of human cancers require steroid hormones for their growth and the first-line therapy for treatment of hormone-dependent cancers is based on androgen and estrogen antagonists interacting with AR or ERs and shutting down the corresponding hormone-responsive pathway. Interestingly, ERβ has been shown to antagonize ERα-mediated effects on cell proliferation in the breast, uterus, ovary, and prostate (Weihua et al., 2000; Lindberg et al., 2003; Ellem and Risbridger, 2009). In this regard, estrogens with selectivity for either ER subtypes may produce different biological outcomes, particularly on cancer cell proliferation. Given the widespread role of ERs in human physiology, it is not surprising that environmental compounds which bind to ERs, thus substituting for the natural hormone and deregulating the fine-tuned action of E_2, can lead to ER-related disorders including breast, endometrial, colorectal, or prostate cancers, as well as neurodegenerative, inflammatory, immune, cardiovascular, and metabolic diseases.

Small fish including zebrafish (*Danio rerio*) are increasingly being used as model species to study *in vivo* effects of EDCs (Segner, 2009; Vosges et al., 2010; Brion et al., 2012). In zebrafish, three zfER subtypes (zfERα, zfERβ1, and zfERβ2) are present (Menuet et al., 2002; Hawkins and Thomas, 2004). Zebrafish ERα (esr1) is orthologous to the human ERα, while ERβ1 (esr2b) and ERβ2 (esr2a) are orthologs of the human ERβ (Bardet et al., 2002). The overall amino-acid sequence identity between the zfER subtypes and their corresponding human ER orthologs is approximately 50% (Menuet et al., 2002). ZfERs are differently expressed and regulated in reproductive tissue like gonads, liver, as well as in brain. In adult liver, E2 induces zfERα expression while it has no effect on zfERβ2 and represses zfERβ1 expression (Menuet et al., 2002). Moreover, both zfERα and zfERβ2 upregulate zfERα expression after E2 exposure, whereas zfERβ1 has no effect on this expression (Menuet et al., 2004). These studies suggest that the different forms of zfERs have partially distinct and nonredundant functions. Hence, in the perspective of developing fish *in vitro* assays, it is essential to take into account all zfER subtypes in the assessment of chemical estrogenicity in zebrafish. Since these three zfERs are thought to mediate different biological effects, there is an increased interest in finding subtype-selective zfER ligands.

Estrogen Receptors Reporter Cell Lines

To understand and to evaluate impact of xenoestrogens on ER-signaling pathway, it is necessary to develop cell-based transcription assay systems that could reflect different cellular contexts and/or different model species. *In vitro* assays based on reporter gene driven by ERE have been proven to be useful and relevant screening tools to address the large number of chemicals yet needed to be tested for their estrogenic potential. We and other groups have developed stable reporter gene assays based on human ERα and ERβ activation in different cell contexts and successfully used them to characterize estrogenic potency of chemicals (Balaguer et al., 1999; Legler et al., 1999; Wilson et al., 2004; Sotoca et al., 2008; Docquier et al., 2013). In order to take into account the species of origin of studied receptor in hazard assessment of estrogenic chemicals in fish, we have developed *in vitro* stable reporter gene assays derived from fish species (Molina-Molina et al., 2008; Cosnefroy et al., 2012; Pinto et al., 2014). Among them, HELN-zfERα, -zfERβ1, and -zfERβ2 (Pinto et al., 2014) reporter cell lines were established in a similar way than HELN-hERα and -hERβ cell lines (Pinto et al., 2014). Briefly, HELN-ERs cell lines cells were obtained by transfection of HELN cells (HeLa cells stably transfected with the ERE-βGlobin-Luc-SVNeo plasmid) (Balaguer et al., 1999) by the corresponding pSG5-puro plasmids (pSG5-hERα-puro, -hERβ-puro -zfERα-puro, -zfERβ1-puro, and -zfERβ2-puro, respectively).

Selectivity of Chemicals for Human and Zebrafish Estrogen Receptors

Screening of endogenous, environmental and synthetic ligands in the HELN-zfER cell lines showed that known mammalian ER ligands are also able to induce transcriptional activity of zebrafish ER subtypes (Pinto et al., 2014). This screening allowed us to assess differences in the potency of the estrogenic compounds among the three zfER subtypes, and compare their selectivity toward hERs using a similar human cellular context. The HELN-zfERs cells were incubated at 28°C after addition of chemicals to the cells because it is a more physiologically relevant temperature for zebrafish, which increased the potency of estradiol approximately 10-fold compared to incubation at 37°C. Temperature sensitivity of fish ERs has already been reported using reporter gene assays (Matthews et al., 2002; Cosnefroy et al., 2009) and the reason seems to be thermo-dependence of estrogen binding (Tan et al., 1999; Matthews et al., 2002; Sumida et al., 2003).

We have shown that there are clear differences between the selectivity of various (anti)estrogens for zebrafish and human ER isoforms, establishing the fact that a direct translation of (anti)estrogenic effects (activities or potencies) from mammals to zebrafish is not possible. Although none of the tested compounds specifically activated either zebrafish or human ERs, transcriptional activities toward human and zebrafish ERs need to be studied.

Natural (E2) and pharmaceutical (EE2) estrogens display similar affinities for hERs and zfERs. Some environmental estrogens (α-zearalanol, bisphenol-A) with similar affinity for hERs preferentially activated zfERα rather than zfERβs. Other environmental estrogens (nonylphenol mixture, 4-tert-octylphenol) with similar affinity for hERs displayed slightly higher affinity for zfERα and zfERβ2 than for zfERβ1. Benzophenone 2 and phytoestrogens (genistein, liquiritigenin) which have higher affinity for hERβ than for hERα also displayed slightly higher affinity for zfERα and zfERβ2 than for zfERβ1. Finally, hERβ selective synthetic compounds (8β-vE2, DPN) preferentially activated zfERα compared to zfERβs. On the contrary and similar to hERs, the synthetic compound 16α-E2, which has 1000-fold more selectivity for hERα (Escande et al., 2006), also exhibited higher affinity for zfERα compared to the zfERβ subtypes and is the most selective compound for zfERα nowadays (**Figure 1**; **Table 1**).

To gain structural insights into the zfERα selectivity of 16α-LE2 in human and zebrafish ERs, we used the web-based server EDMon (Endocrine Disruptor Monitoring; http://atome2.cbs.cnrs.fr/AT2B/SERVER/EDMon.html) (Delfosse et al., 2012) to model zfERs in complex with this ligand. The structural basis of the hERα and hERβ selectivity toward certain ligands has been associated with two amino acid differences in their ligand-binding pockets. Indeed, L384 and M421 of hERα are replaced by M336 and I373 in hERβ, respectively (**Figure 2** and Manas et al., 2004). Superimposition of the 16α-LE2-bound zfERα model on the crystal structure of hERα in complex with E2 (PDB code 3UUD) showed that the phenol ring of 16α-LE2 occupies the same position as that of E2 and is engaged in a network of hydrogen bonds with E353 from helix 3 (H3) and R394 from H5 (**Figure 2A**). On the other side of the ligand-binding pocket (LBP), it appears that the hydrogen bond observed between the 17-hydroxyl group of E2 and H524 (H11) is conserved in 16α-LE2. The difference

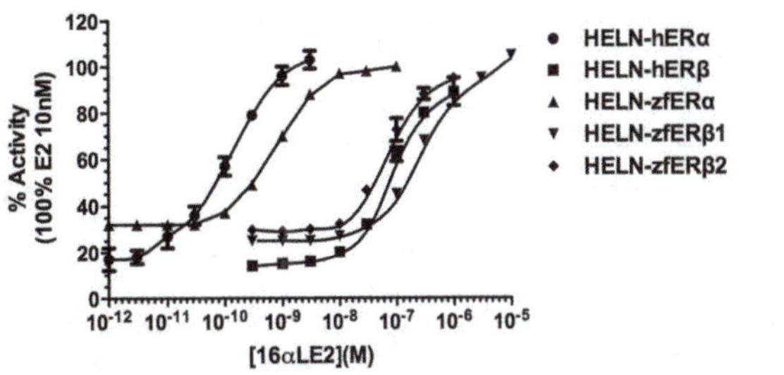

FIGURE 1 | Transcriptional activity of hERα, hERβ, zfERα, zfERβ1, and zfERβ2 in response to the synthetic pharmaceutical compound 16α-LE2. HELN-hERα (●), -hERβ1 (■), -zfERα (○), HELN-zfERβ1 (□), HELN-zfERβ2 (◇) cells were exposed to different concentrations of 16α-LE2. Results are expressed as % of 10 nM E2 treatment and are derived from Escande et al. (2006) and Pinto et al. (2014).

TABLE 1 | 16αLE2 ERs EC_{50} and maximal activities.

NR	EC_{50} (nM)	Maximal activity (%)
hERα	0.093 ± 0.025	100
hERβ	92.9 ± 1.4	100
zfERα	0.79 ± 0.43	100
zfERβ1	240 ± 30.2	100
zfERβ2	74.6 ± 7.08	100

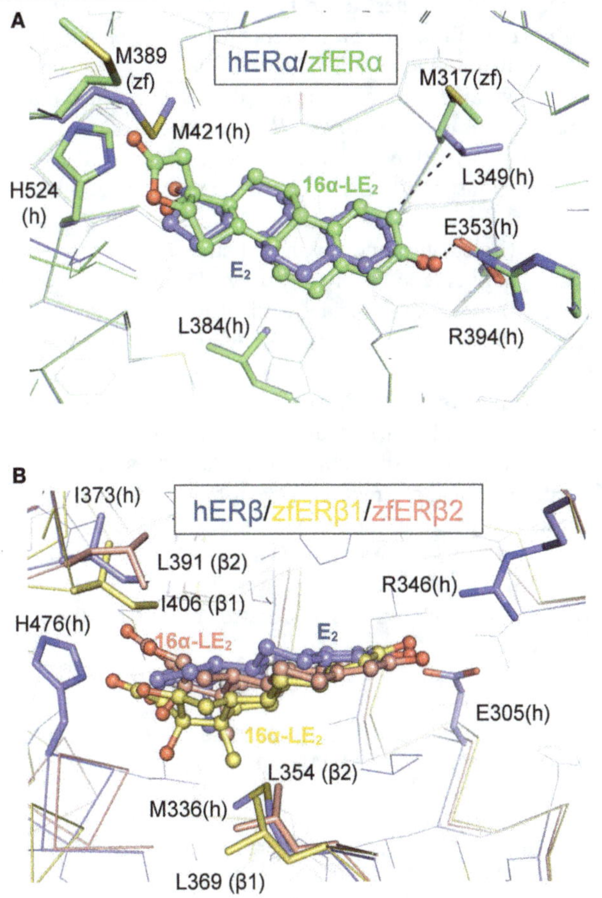

FIGURE 2 | Modeling of the interaction between 16α-LE2 and the human (h) and zebrafish (zf) estrogen receptors. Superposition of the structures of hERα **(A)** and hERβ **(B)** LBDs bound to E2 (blue) on to the molecular models of the 16α-LE2-bound zfERα **(A)** (green) and 16α-LE2-bound hERβ1 (red) and 16α-LE2-bound hERβ2 (yellow) **(B)** LBDs. In zfERα, the lactone ring of 16α-LE2 points toward M421 (H7) which undergoes a large conformational change (black arrow) to accommodate this additional group. In hERβ, the linear M421 present in ERα (M389 in zfERα) is replaced by branched residues (I373 in hERβ, I406 in zfERβ1 and L391 in zfERβ2), which are characterized by a much smaller intrinsic flexibility that maintains the synthetic ligand in a position where it interacts unfavorably with M336 in hERβ, L369 in zfERβ1 and L354 in zfERβ2. This figure is derived from Pinto et al. (2014).

between the two complexes resides in the lactone ring of 16α-LE2 which points toward M421 (H7) that must undergo a large conformational change to accommodate this additional group. In hERβ, the linear M421 is replaced by the branched residue Ileu 373 characterized by a much smaller intrinsic flexibility (**Figure 2B**). As a consequence, I373 maintains the synthetic ligand in a position where it interacts unfavorably with M336 (H3). Therefore, 16α-LE2 adopts different positions in hERα and hERβ, the more constrained environment provided by the latter accounting for the weaker affinity of the ligand for this receptor subtype. The affinity values measured with the zebrafish receptors reflect the variations in the space constraints provided by the different combinations of residues in the three receptor subtypes. With H3 and H7 residues identical to those of the human receptor, zfERα interacts with 16α-LE2 with the highest affinity. The slight difference in the binding affinity of 16α-LE2 for hERα and zfERα relies most likely on the replacement of L349 (H3) by a methionine residue (M317) (**Figure 2A**) and a possible loss of a favorable interaction provided by the branched but not by the linear residue (**Figure 2A**). With a conserved isoleucine in H7 (I406) and a leucine residue in H3 (L369) (**Figure 2B**), zfERβ1 displays the most constrained LBP reflecting the weakest binding affinity for 16α-LE2. This receptor combines two large residues with low (isoleucine) and medium (leucine) flexibilities. The replacement of I406 in H7 of zfERβ1 by a leucine residue (L391) (**Figure 2B**) in zfERβ2 provides a slight gain in LBP plasticity, in agreement with the slightly better affinity of 16α-LE2 for the latter.

The inability of hERβ-selective phytoestrogens (genistein and liquiritigenin) and pharmaceuticals (8bv-E2, DPN) to activate preferentially the zfERβ isoforms is explained by the mutation of a critical amino acid involved in genistein binding in hERβ. In all zfERs, the position homologous to hERβ M336 is occupied, as in hERα, by a leucine residue (**Figure 2**) (Sassi-Messai et al., 2009). This amino acid change most likely accounts for the lack of obvious selectivity of the phytoestrogens toward the zfERβ subtypes.

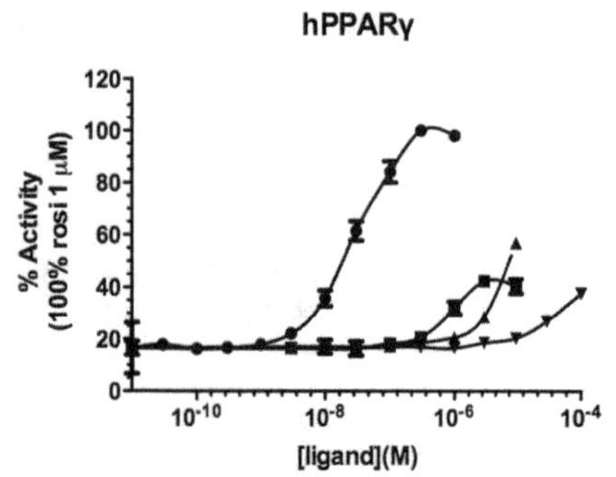

FIGURE 3 | Transcriptional activity of hPPARγ in response to the synthetic pharmaceutical compound rosiglitazone and the environmental compounds TBBPA, MEHP, and PFOA. HG5LN hPPARγ and zfPPARγ cells were exposed to different concentrations of rosiglitazone (●), TBBPA (□), MEHP (○), and PFOA (◊). Results are expressed as % of basal activity and are derived from Riu et al. (2011a).

Peroxysome Proliferator γ

PPARs are involved in the regulation of glucose, lipid, and cholesterol metabolism in response to fatty acids and their derivatives, eicosanoids, and drugs used in the treatment of hyperlipidemia and diabetes. The human PPAR subfamily contains three members known as hPPARα, hPPARβ, and hPPARγ. Each hPPAR subtype shows a distinct tissue distribution and ligand preference. hPPARγ is highly expressed in adipose tissue and is a central regulator of lipid storage and adipocyte gene expression and differentiation (Tontonoz et al., 1995) and is involved in various pathophysiological disorders, including metabolic disease, insulin resistance, and diabetes (Rosen and Spiegelman, 2001). hPPARγ is the target for antidiabetic agents of the thiazolidinedione class, which includes troglitazone, pioglitazone, and rosiglitazone. The LBD of hPPARγ is rather large and the diversity of ligands that can be accommodated within its pocket, mainly represented by lipid derivatives, may contribute to the large array of roles that have been assigned to hPPARγ. Given the physiological role of hPPARγ in adipose tissue development and maintenance, it has been proposed that disruption of regulation pathways under the control of hPPARγ may be involved in the onset of diabetes and obesity (Swedenborg et al., 2009). Indeed, activation of this receptor by certain xenobiotic compounds has been shown to stimulate adipogenesis *in vitro* and *in vivo* through induction

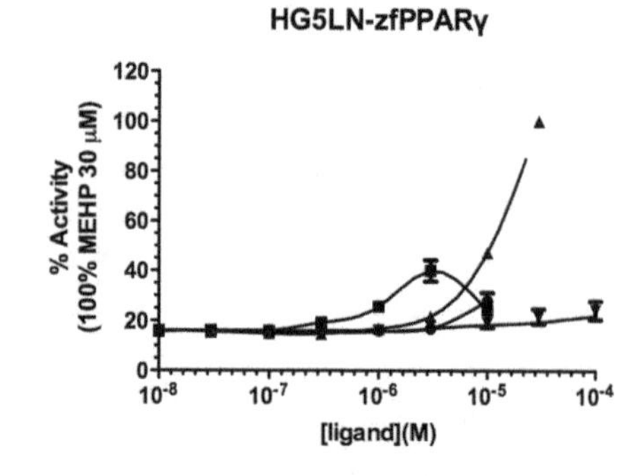

FIGURE 4 | Transcriptional activity of zfPPARγ in response to the synthetic pharmaceutical compound rosiglitazone and the environmental compounds TBBPA, MEHP, and PFOA. HG5LN hPPARγ and zfPPARγ cells were exposed to different concentrations of rosiglitazone (●), TBBPA (□), MEHP (○), and PFOA (◊). Results are expressed as % of basal activity and are derived from Riu et al. (2011a) and Riu et al. (2014).

TABLE 2 | EC_{50} and maximal activities of PPARγ ligands.

Ligand	hPPARγ EC_{50} (μM) (maximal activity %)	zfPPARγ E_{50} (μM) (maximal activity %)
Rosiglitazone	0.027 ± 0.003 (100)	ND (27.9)
TBBPA	0.762 ± 0.136 (42,4)	1.45 ± 0.33 (40)
MEHP	1050 ± 73 (57)	11.3 ± 1.29 (100)
PFOA	380 ± 71 (37.8)	ND (24.2)

ND, Not determined.

of the differentiation of preadipocytes of the fibroblastic lineage into mature adipocytes (Grun and Blumberg, 2009; le Maire et al., 2009; Janesick and Blumberg, 2011; Riu et al., 2011a). This has led to the "obesogen hypothesis," according to which, in addition to disruption of the balance between caloric intake and expenditure characterizing modern life-style, the rapidly growing obesity epidemic could also implicate environmental risk factors including an increased exposure to chemicals that interfere with any aspects of metabolism (Grun and Blumberg, 2009; Janesick and Blumberg, 2011, 2012). Accordingly, compounds that have the potential to disrupt any metabolic signaling pathways and lead to increased fat accumulation and obesity are referred to as "obesogens" (Grun and Blumberg, 2006).

Like for ERs, zebrafish begin to be used as model species to study *in vivo* effects of EDCs on PPARγ (Lyche et al., 2011; Riu et al., 2014). Similar to mammals, zebrafish store neutral lipid triglycerides in the visceral, intramuscular, and subcutaneous adipocyte depots. The first adipocytes, which can be observed from day 8 to 12, or at a minimal size of about 5 mm (Imrie and Sadler, 2010), appear in the pancreatic region, then in the viscera, and later on, in the subcutaneous and cranial regions (Flynn et al., 2009; Imrie and Sadler, 2010). Lipid staining can be detected before this stage; however, at this time point, the lipids are not stored in adipocytes, but rather in the yolk, hepatocytes, blood vessels, skeletal myocytes, jaw chondrocytes, and neuronal tissue in the brain (Imrie and Sadler, 2010).

Pparγ reporter cell lines

HG5LN-hPPARγ and -zfPPARγ reporter cell lines were established in a similar way (Seimandi et al., 2005; Riu et al., 2014). Briefly, HG5LN-PPARγ cell line was obtained by transfection of HG5LN cells (HeLa cells stably transfected with the GALRE5-βGlobin-Luc-SVNeo plasmid) (Seimandi et al., 2005) by the corresponding pSG5-puro plasmids [pSG5-GAL4(DBD)-hPPARγ(LBD)-puro and -zfPPARγ(LBD)-puro, respectively]. Interestingly, the thermodependence observed for zfERs is not shared by zfPPARγ (Riu et al., 2014).

Selectivity of chemicals for human and zebrafish PPARγ

Screening of environmental and pharmaceutical ligands in the HG5LN-zfPPARγ cell lines showed that known hPPARγ ligands are not always able to induce transcriptional activity of zebrafish

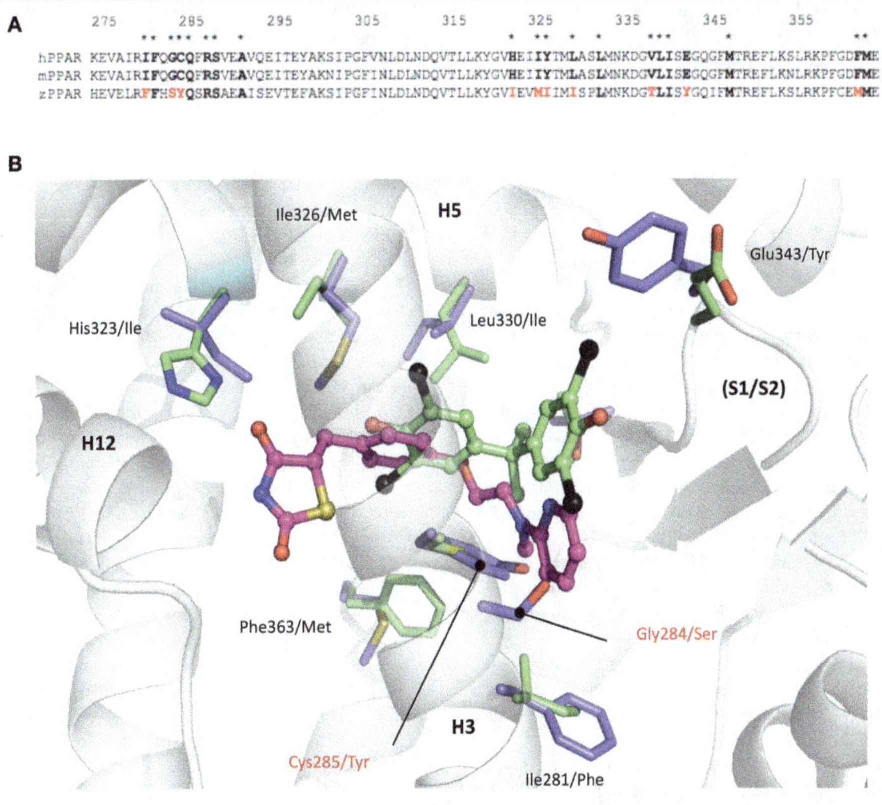

FIGURE 5 | (A) Sequence alignment of human, mouse, and zebrafish PPARγ ligand binding pocket residues. Asterisks denote residues in contact with TBBPA and/or rosiglitazone (PDB code 2PRG). Interacting residues that differ between sequences are highlighted in red. **(B)** TBBPA (carbon atoms colored in green) and rosiglitazone (magenta, PDB code 2PRG) as they are positioned in the human PPARγ. Residues that differ in the ligand binding pocket of human and zebrafish PPARγ are displayed as green and blue sticks, respectively. The human PPARγ Gly284 and Cys285 which are replaced by serine and tyrosine residues in zebrafish PPARγ are indicated in red. This figure is derived from Riu et al. (2011a).

PPARγ (Riu et al., 2011a). Pharmaceutical hPPARγ ligands like thiazolidones (rosiglitazone, troglitazone) do not or very weakly bind to zfPPARγ. On the contrary, environmental PPARγ compounds including phthalates (MEHP), perfluorinated compounds (PFOA, PFOS) and halogenated derivatives of BPA (TBBPA, TCBPA) are common activators of hPPARγ and zfPPARγ (**Figures 3, 4; Table 2**). We also provide evidence that activation of ERs and PPARγ depends on the halogenation degree of BPA analogs. The bulkier are brominated BPA analogs, the greater is their capability to activate PPARγ and the weaker is their estrogenic potential (Riu et al., 2011b).

Comparison of human and zebrafish PPARγ sequences reveals several residue differences which could explain the differential ligand specificity of the various species (**Figure 5A**). In particular, the replacement of human PPARγ Gly284 and Cys285 by serine and tyrosine residues in zebrafish PPARγ provides a rationale for the weak binding affinity of rosiglitazone for this receptor as compared to that observed for the human homolog (**Figure 4B**). In contrast, the different binding mode of halogenated compounds allows both hPPARγ and zfPPARγ to accommodate TBBPA and TCBPA (**Figure 5B**).

Structural and biophysical studies revealed that TBT binds to both hRXR and hPPARγ through formation of a covalent bond between the tin atom and the sulfur atom of cysteine residues located in the LBP of both receptors (le Maire et al., 2009; Delfosse et al., 2014). In RXR, this cysteine (Cys432) is located in helix H11 and is conserved in several species. In contrast, the cysteine residue of PPARγ (Cys285) resides in H3 and is not conserved in several species including zebrafish.

Conclusion

We have shown above that there are clear differences between the activity of various EDCs for zebrafish and human ERs and PPARs, demonstrating that a direct translation of effects from mammals to zebrafish is not possible. The differences revealed in this study, in terms of transcriptional activities toward human and zebrafish ERs and PPARs, highlight the need to take into account the species of origin when assessing the potency of chemicals. This is particularly important with regard to EDCs screening for hazard assessment since at the present time established test guidelines are only based on human cell lines expressing human nuclear receptors.

To this end, such *in vitro* cell lines expressing zebrafish nuclear receptors can serve as useful screening tools to address nuclear receptor potency of chemicals for fish models. Hence, an initial screening should be followed up with an NR-subtype specific analysis using both human and zebrafish NRs to elucidate the full spectrum of NR-mediated EDCs effects.

Acknowledgments

We would like to acknowledge the financial support from the Agence Nationale de la Recherche, project PROOFS and TOXSYN.

References

Balaguer, P., François, F., Comunale, F., Fenet, H., Boussioux, A. M., Pons, M. et al. (1999). Reporter cell lines to study the estrogenic effects of xenoestrogens. *Sci. Total Environ.* 233, 47–56. doi: 10.1016/S0048-9697(99)00178-3

Bardet, P. L., Horard, B., Robinson-Rechavi, M., Laudet, V., and Vanacker, J. M. (2002). Characterization of oestrogen receptors in zebrafish (Danio rerio). *J. Mol. Endocrinol.* 28, 153–163. doi: 10.1677/jme.0.0280153

Benecke, A., Chambon, P., and Gronemeyer, H. (2000). Synergy between estrogen receptor alpha activation functions AF1 and AF2 mediated by transcription intermediary factor TIF2. *EMBO Rep.* 1, 151–157. doi: 10.1093/embo-reports/kvd028

Bommer, M., Benecke, A., Gronemeyer, H., and Rochette-Egly, C. (2002). TIF2 mediates the synergy between RARalpha 1 activation functions AF-1 and AF-2. *J. Biol. Chem.* 277, 37961–37966. doi: 10.1074/jbc.M206001200

Bourguet, W., Germain, P., and Gronemeyer, H. (2000). Nuclear receptor ligand-binding domains: three-dimensional structures, molecular interactions and pharmacological implications. *Trends Pharmacol. Sci.* 21, 381–388. doi: 10.1016/S0165-6147(00)01548-0

Brion, F., Le Page, Y., Piccini, B., Cardoso, O., Tong, S. K., Chung, B. C., et al. (2012). Screening estrogenic activities of chemicals or mixtures *in vivo* using transgenic (*cyp19a1b*-GFP) zebrafish embryos. *PLoS ONE* 7:e36069. doi: 10.1371/journal.pone.0036069

Cosnefroy, A., Brion, F, Guillet, B, Laville, N, Porcher, J. M., Balaguer, P., et al. (2009). A stable fish reporter cell line to study estrogen receptor transactivation by environmental (xeno)estrogens. *Toxicol. In Vitro* 23, 1450–1454. doi: 10.1016/j.tiv.2009.07.003

Cosnefroy, A., Brion, F., Maillot-Maréchal, E., Porcher, J. M., Pakdel, F., Balaguer, P., et al. (2012). Selective activation of zebrafish estrogen receptor subtypes by chemicals by using stable reporter gene assay developed in a zebrafish liver cell line. *Toxicol. Sci.* 125, 439–449. doi: 10.1093/toxsci/kfr297

Couse, J. F., and Korach, K. S. (1999). Estrogen receptor null mice: what have we learned and where will they lead us? *Endocr. Rev.* 20, 358–417. doi: 10.1210/edrv.20.3.0370

Curtis, S. W., Washburn, T., Sewall, C., DiAugustine, R., Lindzey, J., and Couse, J. F., et al. (1996). Physiological coupling of growth factor and steroid receptor signaling pathways: estrogen receptor knockout mice lack estrogen-like response to epidermal growth factor. *Proc. Natl. Acad. Sci. U.S.A.* 93, 12626–12630 doi: 10.1073/pnas.93.22.12626

Dahlman-Wright, K., Cavailles, V., Fuqua, S. A., Jordan, V. C., Katzenellenbogen, J. A., Korach, K. S., et al. (2006). International union of pharmacology. LXIV. Estrogen receptors. *Pharmacol. Rev.* 58, 773–781. doi: 10.1124/pr.58.4.8

Delfosse, V., Grimaldi, M., Cavaillès, V., Balaguer, P., and Bourguet, W. (2014). Structural and functional profiling of environmental ligands for estrogen receptors. *Environ. Health Perspect.* 122, 1306–1313. doi: 10.1289/ehp.1408453

Delfosse, V., Grimaldi, M., Pons, J. L., Boulahtouf, A., le Maire, A., Cavailles, V., et al. (2012). Structural and mechanistic insights into bisphenols action provide guidelines for risk assessment and discovery of bisphenol A substitutes. *Proc. Natl. Acad. Sci. U.S.A.* 109, 14930–14935. doi: 10.1073/pnas.1203574109

Diamanti-Kandarakis, E., Bourguignon, J. P., Giudice, L. C., Hauser, R., Prins, G. S., Soto, A. M., et al. (2009). Endocrine-disrupting chemicals: an endocrine society scientific statement. *Endocr. Rev.* 30, 293–342. doi: 10.1210/er.2009-0002

Docquier, A., Garcia, A., Savatier, J., Boulahtouf, A., Bonnet, S., Bellet, V., et al. (2013). Negative regulation of estrogen signaling by ERβ and RIP140 in ovarian cancer cells. *Mol. Endocrinol.* 27, 1429–1441. doi: 10.1210/me.2012-1351

Ellem, S. J., and Risbridger, G. P. (2009). The dual, opposing roles of estrogen in the prostate. *Ann. N.Y. Acad. Sci.* 1155, 174–186. doi: 10.1111/j.1749-6632.2009.04360.x

Escande, A., Pillon, A., Servant, N., Cravedi, J. P., Larrea, F., and Muhn, P., et al. (2006). Evaluation of ligand selectivity using reporter cell lines stably expressing estrogen receptor alpha or beta. *Biochem. Pharmacol.* 71, 1459–1469. doi: 10.1016/j.bcp.2006.02.002

Flynn, E. J. III., Trent, C. M., and Rawls, J. F. (2009). Ontogeny and nutritional control of adipogenesis in zebrafish (Danio rerio). *J. Lipid. Res.* 50, 1641–1652. doi: 10.1194/jlr.M800590-JLR200

Germain, P., Staels, B., Dacquet, C., Spedding, M., and Laudet, V. (2006). Overview of nomenclature of nuclear receptors. *Pharmacol. Rev.* 58, 685–704. doi: 10.1124/pr.58.4.2

Gorelick, D. A. and Halpern, M. E. (2011). Visualization of estrogen receptor transcriptional activation in zebrafish. *Endocrinology* 152, 2690–2703. doi: 10.1210/en.2010-1257

Gronemeyer, H., Gustafsson, J. A., and Laudet, V. (2004). Principles for modulation of the nuclear receptor superfamily. *Nat. Rev. Drug Discov.* 3, 950–964. doi: 10.1038/nrd1551

Grun, F., and Blumberg, B. (2006). Environmental obesogens: organotins and endocrine disruption via nuclear receptor signaling. *Endocrinology* 147, S50–S55 doi: 10.1210/en.2005-1129

Grun, F., and Blumberg, B. (2009). Endocrine disrupters as obesogens. *Mol. Cell. Endocrinol.* 304, 19–29. doi: 10.1016/j.mce.2009.02.018

Hawkins, M. B., and Thomas, P. (2004). 17alpha-ethinylestradiol disrupts the ontogeny of the forebrain GnRH system and the expression of brain aromatase during early development of zebrafish. *Endocrinology* 145, 2968–2977. doi: 10.1210/en.2003-0806

Imrie, D., Sadler, K. C. (2010). White adipose tissue development in zebrafish is regulated by both developmental time and fish size. *Dev. Dyn.* 239, 3013–3023. doi: 10.1002/dvdy.22443

Janesick, A., and Blumberg, B. (2011). Minireview: PPARγ as the target of obesogens. *J. Steroid Biochem. Mol. Biol.* 127, 4–8. doi: 10.1016/j.jsbmb.2011.01.005

Janesick, A., and Blumberg, B. (2012). stem cells and the developmental programming of obesity. *Int. J. Androl.* 35, 437–448. doi: 10.1111/j.1365-2605.2012.01247.x

Jensen, E. V., and Jordan, V. C. (2003). The estrogen receptor: a model for molecular medicine. *Clin. Cancer Res.* 9, 1980–1989.

Kuiper, G. G., Carlsson, B., Grandien, K., Enmark, E., Häggblad, J., Nilsson, S., et al. (1997). Comparison of the ligand binding specificity and transcript tissue distribution of estrogen receptors alpha and beta. *Endocrinology* 138, 863–870.

Kurauchi, K., Nakaguchi, Y., Tsutsumi, M., Hori, H., Kurihara, R., Hashimoto, S., et al. (2005). *In vivo* visual reporter system for detection of estrogen-like substances by transgenic medaka. *Environ. Sci. Technol.* 39, 2762–2768. doi: 10.1021/es0486465

Lee, O., Tyler, C. R., and Kudoh, T. (2012). Development of a transient expression assay for detecting environmental oestrogens in zebrafish and medaka embryos. *BMC Biotechnol.* 12:32. doi: 10.1186/1472-6750-12-32

Legler, J., van den Brink, C. E., Brouwer, A., Murk, A. J., van der Saag, P. T., Vethaak, A. D., et al. (1999). Development of a stably transfected estrogen receptor-mediated luciferase reporter gene assay in the human T47D breast cancer cell line. *Toxicol. Sci.* 48, 55–66. doi: 10.1093/toxsci/48.1.55

le Maire, A., Grimaldi, M., Roecklin, D., Dagnino, S., Vivat-Hannah, V., Balaguer, P., et al. (2009). Activation of RXR-PPAR heterodimers by organotin environmental endocrine disruptors. *EMBO Rep.* 10, 367–373. doi: 10.1038/embor.2009.8

Lindberg, M. K., Moverare, S., Skrtic, S., Gao, H., Dahlman-Wright, K., Gustafsson, J. A., et al. (2003). Estrogen receptor (ER)-beta reduces ERalpha-regulated gene transcription, supporting a "ying yang" relationship between ERalpha and ERbeta in mice. *Mol. Endocrinol.* 17, 203–208. doi: 10.1210/me.2002-0206

Liu, M. M., Albanese, C., Anderson, C. M., Hilty, K., Webb, P., Uht, R. M., et al. (2002). Opposing action of estrogen receptors alpha and beta on cyclin D1 gene expression. *J. Biol. Chem.* 277, 24353–24360. doi: 10.1074/jbc.M201829200

Lyche, J. L., Nourizadeh-Lillabadi, R, Karlsson, C, Stavik, B, Berg, V, Skåre, J. U., et al. (2011). Natural mixtures of POPs affected body weight gain and induced transcription of genes involved in weight regulation and insulin signaling. *Aquat. Toxicol.* 102, 197–204. doi: 10.1016/j.aquatox.2011.01.017

Manas, E. S., Xu, Z. B., Unwalla, R. J., and Somers, W. S. (2004). Understanding the selectivity of genistein for human estrogen receptor-beta using X-ray crystallography and computational methods. *Structure* 12, 2197–2207. doi: 10.1016/j.str.2004.09.015

Matthews, J. B., Fertuck, K. C., Celius, T., Huang, Y. W., Fong, C. J., and Zacharewski, T. R. (2002). Ability of structurally diverse natural products and synthetic chemicals to induce gene expression mediated by estrogen receptors from various species. *J. Steroid Biochem. Mol. Biol.* 82, 181–194. doi: 10.1016/S0960-0760(02)00159-0

Menuet, A., Le Page, Y., Torres, O., Kern, L., Kah, O., and Pakdel, F. (2004). Analysis of the estrogen regulation of the zebrafish estrogen receptor (ER) reveals distinct effects of ERalpha, ERbetal and ERbeta2. *J. Mol. Endocrinol.* 32, 975–986. doi: 10.1677/jme.0.0320975

Menuet, A., Pellegrini, E, Anglade, I, Blaise, O, Laudet, V, Kah, O., et al. (2002). Molecular characterization of three estrogen receptor forms in zebrafish: binding characteristics, transactivation properties, and tissue distributions. *Biol. Reprod.* 66, 1881–1892. doi: 10.1095/biolreprod66.6.1881

Minchin, J. E., and Rawls, J. F. (2011). *In vivo* analysis of white adipose tissue in zebrafish. *Methods Cell Biol.* 105, 63–86. doi: 10.1016/b978-0-12-381320-6.00003-5

Molina-Molina, J. M., Escande, A., Pillon, A., Gomez, E., Pakdel, F., Cavaillès, V., et al. (2008). Profiling of benzophenone derivatives using fish and human estrogen receptor-specific *in vitro* bioassays. *Toxicol. Appl. Pharmacol.* 232, 384–395. doi: 10.1016/j.taap.2008.07.017

Ogawa, S., Eng, V., Taylor, J., Lubahn, D. B., Korach, K. S., and Pfaff, D. W. (1998). Roles of estrogen receptor alpha gene expression in reproduction-related behaviors in female mice. *Endocrinology* 139:5070–5081.

Pettersson, K., Delaunay, F., and Gustafsson, J. A. (2000). Estrogen receptor beta acts as a dominant regulator of estrogen signaling *Oncogene* 19, 4970–4978 doi: 10.1038/sj.onc.1203828

Pike, A. C. (2006). Lessons learnt from structural studies of the oestrogen receptor. *Best Pract. Res. Clin. Endocrinol. Metab.* 20, 1–14. doi: 10.1016/j.beem.2005.09.002

Pinto, C., Grimaldi, M., Boulahtouf, A., Pakdel, F., Brion, F., Aït-Aïssa, S., et al. (2014). Selectivity of natural, synthetic and environmental estrogens for zebrafish estrogen receptors. *Toxicol. Appl. Pharmacol.* 280, 60–69. doi: 10.1016/j.taap.2014.07.020

Renaud, J. P., and Moras, D. (2000). Structural studies on nuclear receptors. *Cell. Mol. Life Sci.* 57, 1748–1769. doi: 10.1007/PL00000656

Riu, A., Grimaldi, M., le Maire, A., Bey, G., Phillips, K., Boulahtouf, A., et al. (2011a). Peroxisome proliferator-activated receptor γ is a target for halogenated analogs of bisphenol A. *Environ. Health Perspect.* 119, 1227–1232. doi: 10.1289/ehp.1003328

Riu, A., le Maire, A., Grimaldi, M., Audebert, M., Hillenweck, A., Bourguet, W., et al. (2011b). Characterization of novel ligands of ERα, ERβ, and PPARγ: the case of halogenated bisphenol A and their conjugated metabolites. *Toxicol. Sci.* 122, 372–382. doi: 10.1093/toxsci/kfr132

Riu, A., McCollum, C. W., Pinto, C. L., Grimaldi, M., Hillenweck, A., Perdu, E., et al. (2014). Halogenated bisphenol-A analogs act as obesogens in zebrafish larvae (Danio rerio). *Toxicol. Sci.* 139, 48–58. doi: 10.1093/toxsci/kfu036

Rosen, E. D., and Spiegelman, B. M. (2001). PPARγ: a nuclear regulator of metabolism, differentiation, and cell growth. *J. Biol. Chem.* 276, 37731–37734. doi: 10.1074/jbc.R100034200

Sassi-Messai, S., Gibert, Y., Bernard, L., Nishio, S., Ferri Lagneau, K. F., Molina, J., et al. (2009). The phytoestrogen genistein affects zebrafish development through two different pathways. *PLoS ONE* 4:e4935. doi: 10.1371/journal.pone.0004935

Segner, H. (2009). Zebrafish (Danio rerio) as a model organism for investigating endocrine disruption. *Comp. Biochem. Physiol. C Toxicol. Pharmacol.* 149, 187–195. doi: 10.1016/j.cbpc.2008.10.099

Seimandi, M., Lemaire, G., Pillon, A., Perrin, A., Carlavan, I., Voegel, J. J., et al. (2005). Differential responses of PPARα, PPARδ, and PPARγ reporter cell lines to selective PPAR synthetic ligands. *Anal. Biochem.* 344, 8–15. doi: 10.1016/j.ab.2005.06.010

Sotoca, A. M., Ratman, D., van der Saag, P., Ström, A., Gustafsson, J. A., Vervoort, J., et al. (2008). Phytoestrogen-mediated inhibition of proliferation of the human T47D breast cancer cells depends on the ERalpha/ERbeta ratio. *J. Steroid Biochem. Mol. Biol.* 112, 171–178. doi: 10.1016/j.jsbmb.2008.10.002

Sumida, K., Ooe, N, Saito, K, and Kaneko, H. (2003). Limited species differences in estrogen receptor alpha-medicated reporter gene transactivation by xenoestrogens. *J. Steroid. Biochem. Mol. Biol.* 84, 33–40. doi: 10.1016/S0960-0760(03)00003-7

Swedenborg, E., Ruegg, J., Makela, S., and Pongratz, I. (2009). Endocrine disruptive chemicals: mechanisms of action and involvement in metabolic disorders. *J. Mol. Endocrinol.* 43, 1–10. doi: 10.1677/JME-08-0132

Tan, N. S., Frecer, V., Lam, T. J., and Ding, J. L. (1999). Temperature dependence of estrogen binding: importance of a subzone in the ligand binding domain of a novel piscine estrogen receptor. *Biochim. Biophys. Acta* 1452, 103–120. doi: 10.1016/S0167-4889(99)00128-7

Tingaud-Sequeira, A., Knoll-Gellida, A., André M., and Babin, P. J. (2012). Vitellogenin expression in white adipose tissue in female teleost fish. *Biol. Reprod.* 86, 38. doi: 10.1095/biolreprod.111.093757

Tontonoz, P., Hu, E., and Spiegelman, B. M. (1995). Regulation of adipocyte gene expression and differentiation by peroxisome proliferator activated receptor gamma. *Curr. Opin. Genet. Dev.* 5, 571–576. doi: 10.1016/0959-437X(95)80025-5

Vosges, M., Le Page, Y., Chung, B. C., Combarnous, Y., Porcher, J. M., Kah, O., et al. (2010). 17alpha-ethinylestradiol disrupts the ontogeny of the forebrain GnRH system and the expression of brain aromatase during early development of zebrafish. *Aquat Toxicol.* 99, 479–491. doi: 10.1016/j.aquatox.2010.06.009

Weihua, Z., Saji, S., Makinen, S., Cheng, G., Jensen, E. V., Warner, M., et al. (2000). Estrogen receptor (ER) beta, a modulator of ERalpha in the uterus. *Proc. Natl. Acad. Sci. U.S.A.* 97, 5936–5941. doi: 10.1073/pnas.97.11.5936

Wilson, E. M. (2011). Analysis of interdomain interactions of the androgen receptor. *Methods Mol. Biol.* 776, 113–129. doi: 10.1007/978-1-61779-243-4_8

Wilson, V. S., Bobseine, K., and Gray, L. E. Jr. (2004). Development and characterization of a cell line that stably expresses an estrogen-responsive luciferase reporter for the detection of estrogen receptor agonist and antagonists. *Toxicol. Sci.* 81, 69–77. doi: 10.1093/toxsci/kfh180

19

Local modulation of steroid action: Rapid control of enzymatic activity

Thierry D. Charlier[1,2], Charlotte A. Cornil[3], Christine Patte-Mensah[4], Laurence Meyer[4], A. Guy Mensah-Nyagan[4] and Jacques Balthazart[3]*

[1] Institut de Recherche en Santé, Environnement et Travail, University of Rennes 1, Rennes, France, [2] Department of Biological Sciences, Ohio University, Athens, OH, USA, [3] GIGA Neuroscience, University of Liège, Liege, Belgium, [4] INSERM1119, University of Strasbourg, Strasbourg, France

Edited by:
Olivier Kah,
CNRS UMR 6026, France

Reviewed by:
Barney A. Schlinger,
University of California, Los Angeles, USA
Nobuhiro Harada,
Fujita Health University School of Medicine, Japan

***Correspondence:**
Thierry D. Charlier,
IRSET-INSERM U1085, University of Rennes 1, Campus Beaulieu, Bat 13, Room 135/2, 35042 Rennes, France
thierry.charlier@univ-rennes1.fr

Estrogens can induce rapid, short-lived physiological and behavioral responses, in addition to their slow, but long-term, effects at the transcriptional level. To be functionally relevant, these effects should be associated with rapid modulations of estrogens concentrations. 17β-estradiol is synthesized by the enzyme aromatase, using testosterone as a substrate, but can also be degraded into catechol-estrogens via hydroxylation by the same enzyme, leading to an increase or decrease in estrogens concentration, respectively. The first evidence that aromatase activity (AA) can be rapidly modulated came from experiments performed in Japanese quail hypothalamus homogenates. This rapid modulation is triggered by calcium-dependent phosphorylations and was confirmed in other tissues and species. The mechanisms controlling the phosphorylation status, the targeted amino acid residues and the reversibility seem to vary depending of the tissues and is discussed in this review. We currently do not know whether the phosphorylation of the same amino acid affects both aromatase and/or hydroxylase activities or whether these residues are different. These processes provide a new general mechanism by which local estrogen concentration can be rapidly altered in the brain and other tissues.

Keywords: aromatase, hypothalamus, 17β-estradiol, catechol-estrogens, phosphorylation, neurosteroidogenesis

Introduction

The local conversion of androgens into estrogens in specific areas of the central nervous system is an essential step in the activation of numerous testosterone-dependent physiological and behavioral processes, including sexual differentiation of the brain, negative feedback on the secretion of gonadotrophin releasing hormone and the activation of male sexual and aggressive behaviors (Beyer et al., 1976; MacLusky and Naftolin, 1981; Bagatell et al., 1994; Fisher et al., 1998; Honda et al., 1998; Toda et al., 2001; Rochira et al., 2006; Trainor et al., 2006). This transformation is catalyzed by the enzyme aromatase, also known as CYP 19 or estrogen synthase. In most vertebrates, central aromatase expression is restricted to specific neuronal populations mainly located in the hypothalamic/preoptic areas including the medial preoptic nucleus and in the limbic system (Roselli et al., 1985; Foidart et al., 1995a,b; Wagner and Morrell, 1997; Trainor et al., 2007; Metzdorf et al., 1999; Roselli and Resko, 2001). It should be noted that songbirds have an additional population of aromatase expressing neurons in the caudomedial nidopallium, in the telencephalon (NCM; Shen et al., 1995; Saldanha et al., 2000). Aromatase is also abundantly expressed in the whole brain of teleost fishes but only in glial cells

(Forlano et al., 2001, 2006; Diotel et al., 2010). The presence of aromatase in defined brain areas allows for local increase in estrogens (17β-estradiol or E2) without affecting the periphery or surrounding brain regions. The estrogens resulting from local aromatization bind to estrogen receptors alpha or beta, trigger a conformational change and dimerization of the receptor, and lead the receptor to translocate to the nucleus. The receptor dimer then binds to a specific response element on the DNA, usually but not only, upstream of the target gene, recruits a set of transcriptional coregulators and enhances or reduces gene transcription. This modulation of transcription affects the physiology of the cell and ultimately the functioning of the organ and the entire organism. The actions of estrogens at this genomic level develop relatively slowly (several minutes but usually several hours to several days) and have long lasting effects on the physiology, from several days to a life time. However, numerous laboratories have now described estrogen-dependent physiological changes that occur much more rapidly and independently of mRNA transcription and protein synthesis. For example, an acute estrogenic treatment *in vitro* triggers the activation of numerous intracellular signaling pathways including phosphorylation of the mitogen-activated protein kinase (MAPK) and cAMP response element binding protein (CREB) and changes in intracellular calcium concentrations (Mermelstein et al., 1996; Moss et al., 1997; Kenealy et al., 2011; Roepke et al., 2005). In the brain, these modifications lead to modulations of neuronal activity (Joels, 1997; Moss et al., 1997; Rønnekleiv and Kelly, 2002; Abraham et al., 2003, 2004; Boulware et al., 2005) and can in some instance rapidly affect behavior in numerous species (Hayden-Hixson and Ferris, 1991; Remage-Healey and Bass, 2004; Dewing et al., 2007; Micevych and Mermelstein, 2008; Lord et al., 2009; Seredynski et al., 2013; see Cornil et al., 2012a for review). These observations led to the hypothesis that estrogens are not only slow acting signaling molecules, or hormones, but can also function more rapidly like classical neurotransmitters, such as glutamate or dopamine (Balthazart and Ball, 2006; Saldanha et al., 2011).

While these rapid, non-genomic, effects of estrogens are currently the focus of intense research, they raise the question of how rapid increases of estrogens can occur. Indeed, estrogens, like other steroids, cannot be stored in synaptic vesicles before rapid release due to their lipophilic nature. We therefore suggested that the fast effects of estrogens require a rapid change of local steroid concentration via rapid changes in their synthesis rate by androgen conversion (Balthazart and Ball, 2006; Cornil et al., 2006), therefore implicating changes in aromatase activity (AA). Changes in AA often reflect changes in aromatase protein concentration resulting from relatively slow transcriptional control. For example, aromatase expression in the hypothalamus in most vertebrates is controlled by sex steroids: weak aromatase expression is detected in castrated males, while testosterone replacement markedly increases aromatase transcript, protein and activity (Roselli and Resko, 1984, 1989; Schumacher and Balthazart, 1986; Fusani et al., 2001). These changes in AA generally occur after several hours or days of treatment. However, the rapid effects of E2 introduced above require mechanisms affecting the synthesis of the steroid more rapidly, suggesting posttranslational change(s) of the protein activity.

Rapid Modulation of Aromatase Activity

The first evidence that AA is rapidly modulated was obtained in preoptic area/hypothalamus explants from Japanese quail. A rise in extracellular K^+ concentration or an increase of intracellular calcium concentration rapidly (5 min) and transiently reduced AA (Balthazart et al., 2001b). These results suggested that the K^+-induced transient depolarization resulted in an increase of Ca^{++} from intracellular stores and led to a rapid reduction of AA. In agreement with this hypothesis, the inhibition of enzymatic activity was significantly hindered when the K^+-induced depolarization was performed in a Ca^{++}-free medium (Balthazart et al., 2001b). In a different model, the zebra finch telencephalon, Remage-Healey and colleagues showed that a K^+-induced depolarization and the increase of intracellular calcium concentrations were also able to significantly reduce AA, as suggested by the rapid reduction of E2 concentrations measured by ELISA on NCM microdialysates (Remage-Healey et al., 2011). However, the increase in calcium concentrations in this model resulted from the activation of voltage-gated calcium channels, and not from a release from intracellular stores. Indeed, the use of ω-conotoxin, a specific inhibitor of N-type Ca^{++} channel, blocked the K^+-induced decrease in E2 concentration (Remage-Healey et al., 2011).

Glutamate

Our group investigated physiologically relevant signaling molecules that could affect the local concentrations of calcium in the brain and investigated whether the activation of glutamate receptors could lead to a rapid modulation of AA in male quail preoptic/hypothalamic explants. We found that the glutamate agonists AMPA [2-amino-3-(5-methyl-3-oxo-1,2- oxazol-4-yl) propanoic acid], kainate and, to a some extent, NMDA (N-methyl-D-aspartate) rapidly and reversibly down-regulated AA from quail hypothalamic explants. Addition of the glutamate receptor antagonist NBQX blocked the effect of kainate on AA, confirming the specificity of the treatments (Balthazart et al., 2006). Interestingly, intracellular recording combined with biocytin labeling of aromatase-positive neurons confirm that these neurons are sensitive to glutamate, a finding consistent with the idea that glutamatergic inputs on aromatase cells acutely regulate AA (Cornil et al., 2000, 2004). In parallel, *in vivo* retrodialysis of glutamate in the zebra finch telencephalon induced a significant reduction of local E2 concentration, while NMDA had no apparent effect (Remage-Healey et al., 2008).

Dopamine

It should be noted that dopaminergic signaling could also be involved in the rapid modulation of AA. Double immunocytochemistry highlighted a close interaction between dopaminergic fibers (tyrosine hydroxylase-positive structures) and aromatase-positive cells in the hypothalamus of Japanese quail (Balthazart et al., 1998). More importantly, several dopaminergic drugs rapidly inhibited AA in homogenates and *in vitro* explants obtained from the preoptic area hypothalamus of male Japanese quail (Baillien and Balthazart, 1997; Balthazart et al., 2002).This inhibition was fully reversible in explant when the compounds were removed from the incubation medium (Absil et al., 2001). Surprisingly, agonists as well as antagonists of dopamine, specific for the D1 or D2 receptors, depressed AA in explants incubated *in vitro*, raising questions about the exact mechanism underlying the potential implication of D1 or D2 receptors. In addition, the observation that the dopamine reuptake inhibitor nomifensine had no effect in homogenates but strongly inhibits AA in explants suggests that the accumulation of dopamine within the synaptic cleft is the cause of AA inhibition.

GABA

Another neurotransmitter, the inhibitory amino acid GABA, did not affect the enzymatic activity in quail preoptic hypothalamus explants nor *in vivo* in zebra finch telencephalon (Balthazart et al., 2001b; Remage-Healey et al., 2008). It is therefore obvious that the direct links between the activation of the membrane receptor, calcium release and the exact intracellular pathway(s) involved in the rapid modulation of AA require further investigation.

Post-translational Modifications of Aromatase Activity by Phosphorylation

Post-translational modifications are a common mechanism involved in the control of protein activity and is a widely used regulatory mechanism in the brain to control for example NMDA receptor activity in hippocampal neurons (Chen and Roche, 2007) and tyrosine hydroxylase activity, the rate-limiting enzyme in catecholamine synthesis (Albert et al., 1984; Daubner et al., 1992). These phosphorylations are catalyzed by specific kinases that critically depend on the intracellular concentration of Ca^{++} and Mg^{++}. Interestingly, previous studies have implicated divalent cations in the control of AA (Ca^{++}: Onagbesan and Peddie, 1989; Mg^{++}: Steimer and Hutchison, 1991). We therefore wondered whether Ca^{++} and Mg^{++}, in addition of adenosine triphosphate ATP as a phosphate donor, during phosphorylation process could also potentially affect AA. We showed that exposure to ATP (2–8 mM), Ca^{++} (0.5–2 mM), and Mg^{++} (2–10 mM) rapidly and significantly inhibited AA in male Japanese quail preoptic area/hypothalamus homogenate (Balthazart et al., 2001b), strongly suggesting that phosphorylations rapidly inhibit this enzymatic activity. To test whether ATP/Mg/Ca conditions induce kinase-dependent protein phosphorylations or whether these conditions result in a non-specific inactivation of AA, we tested effects of the second messengers cAMP and cGMP, respectively activators of protein kinase A, PKA and protein kinase G, PKG. These kinase activators did not modify AA in the absence or presence of ATP/Mg/Ca (Balthazart et al., 2003). We also tested the effects of numerous kinase inhibitors on the AA of preoptic area/hypothalamic homogenates in the presence or absence of ATP/Mg/Ca (Balthazart et al., 2003). Several of these inhibitors significantly blocked the inhibition of AA induced by the addition of ATP/Mg/Ca while others had no effect. The general serine/threonine (Ser/Thr) kinase inhibitor Staurosporine (STAU), and the general tyrosine (Tyr) kinase inhibitor genistein (GEN) significantly blocked the inhibition produced by ATP/Mg/Ca while they had no effect on basal AA. Similar effects (blockade of inhibition) were also observed in presence of the PKC inhibitor bisindolylmaleimide, the myosin light chain kinase inhibitor ML7, the inhibitor of PKA and PKC H7, the specific inhibitor of PKA/PKG H9, the PKA inhibitor H89 and the calmodulin antagonist trifluoperazin. Altogether, these data indicate that rapid modulation of AA results from the phosphorylation of both Tyr and Ser/Thr residues (Balthazart et al., 2001a, 2003). It should be noted that the potential quantitative role of each kinase family in the rapid modulation of AA in homogenates seems to vary according to the sex: While the addition of protein kinase inhibitors blocked the ATP/Mg/Ca-dependent inhibition AA in both sexes, the magnitude of these effects were sexually differentiated and usually more pronounced in females compared to males (Konkle and Balthazart, 2011). Moreover, phosphorylating conditions affected AA differentially in 2 subcellular compartments isolated via differential ultracentrifugation from zebra finch telencephalon. The reduction of AA by phosphorylating conditions was significantly more pronounced in the fraction containing synaptosomes (P2), as compared to microsomes (endoplasmic reticulum, P3 fractions, Cornil et al., 2012b).

We further investigated whether the rapid inhibition of AA by ATP/Mg/Ca-dependent phosphorylation processes is specific to the neuronal environment or can be observed in other aromatase-rich tissues. Effects of phosphorylating conditions were quantified in ovary and ovarian follicles homogenates from Japanese quail and demonstrated a drastic decrease in enzymatic activity within 15 min (Charlier et al., 2011). We also transiently and stably expressed human aromatase in HEK293 cells. Similarly to what was observed in the preoptic area/hypothalamus of Japanese quail and telencephalon of zebra finch, a K^+-induced depolarization triggered a pronounced but transient inhibition of AA expressed by transfected HEK293 cells. In addition, we also showed that phosphorylating conditions did not affect the enzyme affinity for the substrate but only changed the maximum velocity of reaction. Interestingly, the rapid enzymatic inhibition induced by depolarization also involved the activity of protein kinases as the addition of staurosporine (Ser/Thr kinase inhibitor) or Genistein (Tyr kinase inhibitor) blocked the effect of K^+-induced depolarizations on AA (Charlier et al., 2011). These observations are contrasting to what is observed in the breast cancer cell line MCF-7. Indeed, Catalano et al. (2009) showed that E2 rapidly modulates c-Src kinase action on aromatase tyrosine residues to enhance AA. It should however be noted that these effects were observed after 5 h of incubation and might be underlying different physiological processes.

In both cases however, the rapid change in AA is reversible, suggesting (1) that phosphorylation does not involve protein degradation when AA is reduced (Charlier et al., 2011) and (2) phosphatase is required to restore the un-phosphorylated stage. Interestingly, the general inhibitor of protein phosphatases (PPase), vanadate, did not significantly increase AA but reduced it in male quail preoptic area/hypothalamic homogenates. In addition, alkaline PPase inhibited AA in a dose-dependent manner in the presence, as well as in the absence, of ATP/Mg/Ca (Balthazart et al., 2005). In contrast, preincubation with acid

PPase completely blocked the inhibitory effects of ATP/Mg/Ca on AA although the addition of the PPase was unable to restore AA after the enzymatic activity had been inhibited by the phosphorylating conditions. Moreover, high concentrations of acid PPase also moderately inhibited AA in the absence of ATP/Mg/Ca (Balthazart et al., 2005). It should be noted that recent work on human placental choriocarcinoma cell line JEG-3 demonstrated that microsomal aromatase was rapidly inactivated with calcium, magnesium, and ATP, similarly to what is observed in quail preoptic area/hypothalamus homogenate and transfected cell lines, but the protein was then subsequently degraded in these conditions (Hayashi and Harada, 2014). More specifically, aromatase was protected from protein degradation by treatment with alkaline phosphatase, whereas degradation was enhanced by treatment with the phosphatase (calcineurin) inhibitors FK506 and cyclosporin A. Furthermore, aromatase was protected from degradation by treatment with kinase inhibitors, especially the calcium/calmodulin kinase inhibitors KN62 and KN93 (Hayashi and Harada, 2014).

It is therefore possible aromatase can first be rapidly inactivated by phosphorylation, then follow 2 different paths: either (1) its activity is restituted by dephosphorylation following interaction with phosphatase, or (2) the absence of dephosphorylation leads to subsequent degradation, i.e., a permanent inactivity of the enzyme. However, the specific enzymes involved in the phosphorylation-dephosphorylation mechanisms associated to the rapid and reversible control of AA are not fully defined and are currently under further investigation. It should also be noted that tyrosine phosphatase PTP1B was shown to reduce AA in MCF-7 and ZR75 breast cancer cells (Barone et al., 2012). Altogether, this suggests that some level of phosphorylation is required for a fully functional activity but future work should define in more detail the intricate role of phosphatases and kinases in the control of AA in different cell types.

Evidence for the Direct Phosphorylation of the Aromatase Protein

Our next question was to define whether phosphorylations controlling enzymatic activity directly affect the aromatase itself or modulate the activity of a cofactor that could secondarily regulate AA. We purified by immunoprecipitation the aromatase protein from quail preoptic area/hypothalamic homogenates and the presence of phosphorylated residues on the purified protein was investigated by Western blotting using anti-phosphoserine, anti-phosphothreonine or anti-phosphotyrosine antibodies. Confirming the pharmacological finding described above, phosphorylated Ser, Thr, or Tyr were identified by the specific antibodies at the level of the electrophoresis band corresponding to aromatase and the intensity of the phosphorylation signal was denser when homogenates were pre-incubated with ATP/Mg/Ca as compared to homogenates incubated in control conditions (Balthazart et al., 2003).

Similar experiments were performed on engineered human aromatase containing a c-myc tag that allows its specific immunoprecipitation. HEK293 cells transfected with this construct were incubated with [γ-^{32}P]-ATP in phosphorylating or non-phosphorylating (control) conditions. The radioactive aromatase c-myc in phosphorylating conditions was clearly observed at the expected molecular weight while only a low-intensity band was present in control conditions (Charlier et al., 2011). In additional experiments, the immunoprecipitated aromatase obtained after a 5 min-incubation of the cell lysate in phosphorylating conditions was clearly visible at the expected size on immunoblot when visualized with anti-phosphoserine antibody, while that band was not present in different control conditions (Charlier et al., 2011). This set of experiments clearly supports the hypothesis that the aromatase protein itself is rapidly phosphorylated in the presence of ATP/Mg/Ca, leading to a reduction of its enzymatic activity. Similarly, immunoprecipitation of His6-tagged aromatase in MCF-7 cells and investigation of phosphorylated amino acid by immunoblotting revealed that aromatase tyrosine residue is directly targeted by the kinase c-Src (Catalano et al., 2009, 2014).

Identification of Aromatase Residues Involved in the Rapid Control of Activity

This set of pharmacological experiments on quail hypothalamus explants and homogenates and the manipulations performed with immunoprecipitated human aromatase indicated that the inhibition of AA by phosphorylation is likely to be catalyzed by the activity of two Ser/Thr kinases, protein kinase A (PKA) and C (PKC), although the implication of tyrosine kinase and other Ser/Thr kinases cannot be completely ruled out (Balthazart et al., 2003; Charlier et al., 2011). The quail and human aromatase protein sequence were analyzed using bioinformatic tools to identify the potential phosphorylation sites, highly conserved amongst several avian and mammalian species. Fifteen and nineteen putative phosphorylation sites were identified for quail and human sequences respectively using the open access NETPHOS 2.0 program. These sites included 10 of the 27 serines, 5 of the 24 threonines, and 4 of the 17 tyrosines residues on the human sequence and we paralleled these findings with the results obtained using NETPHOSK, highlighting consensus sequences corresponding to PKC and PKA, protein kinases shown to affect quail and human AA during the pharmacological experiments (Balthazart et al., 2003; Charlier et al., 2011). The output pointed to 6 different residues, five serines (S118, S167, S247, S267, S497), and one threonine (T143) on the human sequence. It should be pointed out that other kinases might also be involved, as consensus binding sequence were observed on both quail and human aromatase. These were however not investigated. From this analysis, we decided to focus our attention on 6 different residues: S247, S267, and S497 that had high scores in both the predictive phosphorylation sites and PKA or PKC recognition consensus sequence; T462 and T493 that correspond to positions S455 and S486 in quail aromatase, two 2 residues that were predicted to be involved in the phosphorylation of aromatase (Balthazart et al., 2003). In addition, *in vitro* studies of the mouse aromatase performed by 2 different groups suggested that 2 other amino acid residues, namely serine S118 (Miller et al., 2008) or tyrosine

Y361 (Catalano et al., 2009) can be phosphorylated. Indeed, the phosphorylation of Y361 triggered by the tyrosine-kinase c-Src seems involved in the E2-dependent upregulation of AA in breast cancer cell lines (Catalano et al., 2009) while phosphorylation of S188 by AGC-like kinases, including PKC and PKA, seems important for the stabilization of the protein, and therefore for the expression of AA (Miller et al., 2008). It should be noted that the effects of the phosphorylation status of these 2 residues on the rapid change of AA was not investigated and we explored the potential implication of S188 phosphorylation (not Y361) in the rapid control of AA.

Altogether, we investigated the consequence of mutating 6 S/T residues into alanine (A) using the human aromatase as template. All mutants expressed normal baseline AA and pre-incubation with ATP/Ca/Mg for 15 min markedly reduced this enzymatic activity in the 6 different mutants alone (S118A, S247A, S267A, T462A, T493A, S497A) or in combination (S267A-S247A, T493A-T462A-S267A, T493A-T462A-S267A-S247A, S497A-T493A-T462A-S267A-S247A) roughly to the same extent as in wild type enzyme, clearly showing that these single or combined mutations did not block the rapid inhibition of aromatase by phosphorylating conditions. The absence of effect, against all expectations, was thoroughly discussed in the original article (Charlier et al., 2011). In summary, it is likely that a combination of several phosphorylated residues that was not tested here is required to control AA. The control by multiple kinases reinforces the idea that several amino acids must concomitantly be phosphorylated to modify AA. It is possible that other consensus sites for phosphorylations and for other types of kinases that were also predicted on the quail and human aromatase sequences might be involved. Alternatively, it is possible that the control of AA by phosphorylations depends on the modulation of certain factors interacting with aromatase, in addition to the enzyme itself. Aromatase requires the presence of an active NADPH-cytochrome P450 reductase for electron transfer (Thompson and Siiteri, 1974; Miller, 2005; Hong et al., 2009). The phosphorylation of the reductase could be a control mechanism affecting the electron transfer and this idea should be further investigated.

Behavior and Rapid Modulation of Aromatase Activity

It is important to note that the change in enzymatic activity resulting from the phosphorylation of aromatase is physiologically and behaviorally relevant. Indeed, rapid changes in AA were demonstrated to occur *in vivo* in response to social interactions in a few species investigated to date, including birds and fish. For example, expression of appetitive or consummatory sexual behavior rapidly reduces AA in specific brain regions in the preoptic-hypothalamic area of quail after 5–30 min of sexual interaction with a receptive female (Cornil et al., 2005a; de Bournonville et al., 2013) while exposure to acute restraint stress, or stress-related hormones such as AVT and corticosterone lead to an increase in AA in both male and female quail (Dickens et al., 2011, 2013). Male removal from a socially stable group of the

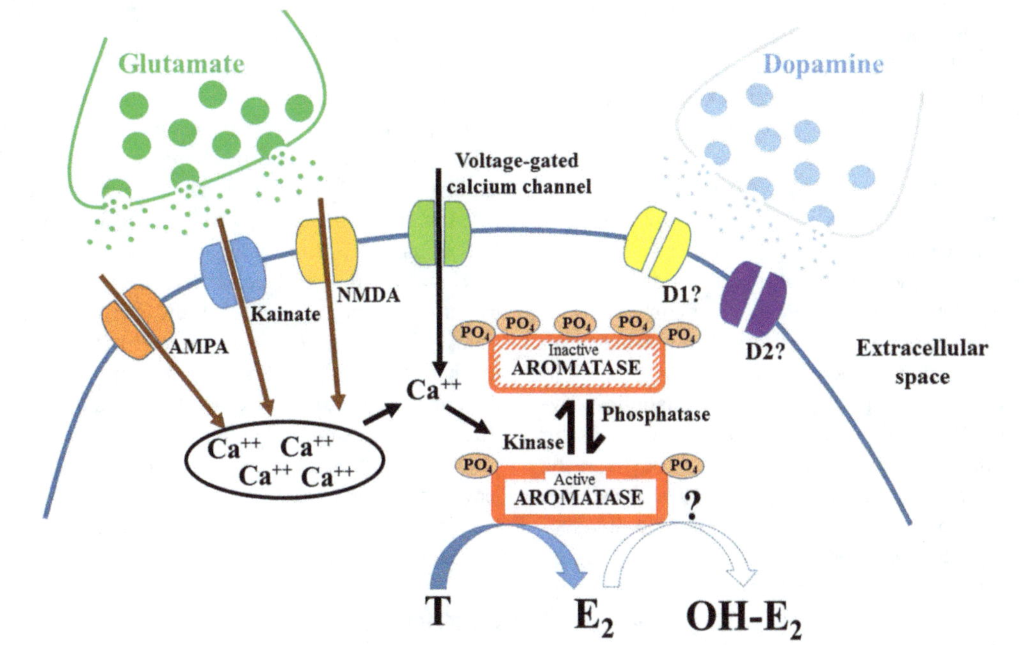

FIGURE 1 | Schematic diagram representing the mechanisms involved in the rapid control of aromatase activity.
Phosphorylations (PO_4) rapidly modulate aromatase activity, inhibiting the transformation of testosterone (T) into 17β-estradiol (E2). It is likely that these modifications are induced by calcium-voltage channels, by glutamatergic receptors and/or by dopaminergic receptors. The increase of intracellular calcium (Ca^{++}), either from intracellular storage or from the activation of voltage-gated channel is in most cases a prerequisite for the inhibition of aromatase activity. Change in phosphorylation level could also affect the hydroxylase activity of aromatase.

sex-changing fish *Lythrypnus dalli* resulted in rapid increases in aggression associated with a rapid reduction in brain AA in the dominant female (Black et al., 2005, 2011). Conversely in zebra finches, a brief exposure to song (30 min) resulted in an increase of AA in NCM within the telencephalon (Remage-Healey et al., 2009). While behavior can affect AA, the reverse is also true and recent studies showed that rapid changes in AA modulate behavior and sensory processing. Indeed, an acute systemic or central administration of aromatase inhibitors such as Vorozole or Androstatrienedione significantly and rapidly reduced male sexual behavior in quail and mice (Cornil et al., 2005b; Taziaux et al., 2007; Seredynski et al., 2013), approach behavior toward females in male goldfish (Lord et al., 2009), aggressive behavior in Beach and California mice (Trainor et al., 2007, 2008) and vocalizations in midshipman fish (Remage-Healey and Bass, 2004). Fadrozole, another aromatase inhibitor, rapidly suppressed the preference for a bird's own song in male zebra finches (Remage-Healey et al., 2010) and reduced song-elicited neuronal firing rate in zebra finches and prevented the expression of hearing-driven gene expression in NCM, a brain regions involved in song discrimination in songbirds (Tremere et al., 2009). Altogether, this clearly confirms that the rapid modulation of AA, likely by phosphorylation, is of physiological importance. This also shows that the rapid inhibition of AA rapidly influences the physiology and behavior.

Catabolism of Estrogens

Therefore, there must exist some mechanisms that are able to rapidly clear locally-produced estrogens to terminate their effects. The half-life of E2 in the brain is not known, although calculations derived from pharmacokinetic data estimated that its half-life in the blood is below 30 min (Johnson and van Tienhoven, 1981; Tsang and Grunder, 1984). The liver is known to express several enzymes involved in the clearance of circulating estrogens, notably CYP1A1, CYP1A2, CYP1B1, and CYP3A (Whirl-Carrillo et al., 2012). These enzymes catalyze the conversion of estrogen into inactive (or less active) water-soluble metabolites by oxidative metabolism and allow for further sulfation by sulfotransferases, glucuronidation by glucoronyltransferases, or methylation by catecholmethyltransferases. The elimination of plasma estrogens from the organism is ensured through excretion following their conjugation. Although this type of degradation of estrogens occurs mainly in the liver, some catabolic activity is also observed in the brain, albeit to a much lower extent. We hypothesized that the rapid elimination of estrogens in the brain involves the enzyme aromatase itself. Indeed, a few studies suggest that, in addition to its estrogen synthase activity, aromatase also catalyzes estrogen hydroxylation. A previous study in Japanese quail showed that 2-hydroxylase enzymatic activity is present in all brain regions that are known to contain a high level of AA, including the median preoptic nucleus and the ventromedial nucleus of the hypothalamus (Balthazart et al., 1994), suggesting that the same protein is involved in both the production and the conversion of estrogens. However, no sex difference in 2-hydroxylase activity was identified here, while AA is higher in males than in females in almost every brain region.

The first evidence that aromatase protein also had estrogen hydroxylase activity came from Osawa et al. (1993). They demonstrated that purified aromatase obtained from placental microsomes demonstrates an estrogen-2-hydroxylase activity in certain conditions. Both aromatase and estradiol 2-hydroxylase activities were observed after purification of human placental microsomal cytochrome P-450 by monoclonal antibody-based immunoaffinity chromatography and gradient elution. Moreover, they confirmed the concomitant existence of estradiol hydroxylase activity with AA by expressing human aromatase in CHO cells. Not only did the purified aromatase exhibit the hydroxylase activity but testosterone and androstenedione competitively inhibited estradiol 2-hydroxylation, and conversely, estrone and estradiol competitively inhibited aromatization of both testosterone and androstenedione. Similarly, equine aromatase expressed *in vitro* has a clear hydroxylase activity (Almadhidi et al., 1996). A specific antiserum raised against purified testicular equine P450arom and known to inhibit AA was also found to inhibit the estrogen hydroxylase activity of equine placental microsomes. Furthermore, the estrogen hydroxylase activity was inhibited in a dose-dependent manner by different aromatase inhibitors, including fadrozole and 4-hydroxyandrostenedione (Almadhidi et al., 1996). It remains to be determined whether the phosphorylation of the same residue(s) leads to the rapid reduction of both estrogen synthase and estrogen hydroxylase activity.

Conclusions

Altogether, a few laboratories have accumulated strong evidence showing that AA can be rapidly modulated via post-translational modifications, most notably via phosphorylation (see **Figure 1** for general model). The rapid modulation of AA by phosphorylating conditions is a widespread mechanism present in different tissues affecting aromatase from various species, including humans. The mechanisms leading to these modifications remain poorly understood, but it is increasingly clear that the enzymatic changes must result in a local rapid modulation of estrogens availability and consequently in a modification of cellular estrogen-dependent events that are not mediated by the genomic actions of these steroids. The phosphorylation/dephosphorylation processes provide a new widespread mechanism by which estrogens concentration could be rapidly altered in the brain and other tissues, albeit likely in different directions. It would be interesting to test whether precise phosphorylation patterns affect one type of enzymatic activity while leaving the other untouched or whether phosphorylation is a general shut-down switch for all enzymatic activity displayed by the aromatase protein.

Acknowledgments

Some of these data were obtained thanks to the Fonds Leon Frederic (ULg, Belgium) and FNRS-FRS to TDC and grant from NIH/NIMH (R01MH50388) to GF Ball and JB. TDC was a F.R.S.-FNRS Post-doctoral Researcher. CAC is a F.R.S.-FNRS Research Associate.

References

Abraham, I. M., Todman, M. G., Korach, K. S., and Herbison, A. E. (2004). Critical *in vivo* roles for classical estrogen receptors in rapid estrogen actions on intracellular signaling in mouse brain. *Endocrinology* 145, 3055–3061. doi: 10.1210/en.2003-1676

Abraham, I. M., Han, S.-K., Todman, M. G., Korach, K. S., and Herbison, A. E. (2003). Estrogen receptor Beta mediates rapid estrogen actions on gonadotropin-releasing hormone neurons *in vivo*. *J. Neurosci.* 23, 5771–5777.

Absil, P., Baillien, M., Ball, G. F., Panzica, G. C., and Balthazart, J. (2001). The control of preoptic aromatase activity by afferent inputs in Japanese quail. *Brain Res. Brain Res. Rev.* 37, 38–58. doi: 10.1016/S0165-0173(01)00122-9

Albert, K. A., Helmer-Matyjek, E., Nairn, A. A., Müller, T. H., Haycock, J. W., Greene, L. A., et al. (1984). Calcium/phospholipid-dependent protein kinase (protein kinase C) phosphorylates and activates tyrosine hydroxylase. *Proc. Natl. Acad. Sci. U.S.A.* 81, 7713–7717. doi: 10.1073/pnas.81.24.7713

Almadhidi, J., Moslemi, S., Drosdowsky, M. A., and Seralini, G. E. (1996). Equine cytochrome P450 aromatase exhibits an estrogen 2-hydroxylase activity *in vitro*. *J. Steroid Biochem. Mol. Biol.* 59, 55–61. doi: 10.1016/S0960-0760(96)00085-4

Bagatell, C. J., Dahl, K. D., and Bremner, W. J. (1994). The direct pituitary effect of testosterone to inhibit gonadotropin secretion in men is partially mediated by aromatization to estradiol. *J. Androl.* 15, 15–21.

Baillien, M., and Balthazart, J. (1997). A direct dopaminergic control of aromatase activity in the quail preoptic area. *J. Steroid Biochem. Mol. Biol.* 63, 99–113. doi: 10.1016/S0960-0760(97)00080-0

Balthazart, J., Baillien, M., and Ball, G. F. (2001a). Phosphorylation processes mediate rapid changes of brain aromatase activity. *J. Steroid Biochem. Mol. Biol.* 79, 261–277. doi: 10.1016/S0960-0760(01)00143-1

Balthazart, J., Baillien, M., and Ball, G. F. (2002). Interactions between aromatase (estrogen synthase) and dopamine in the control of male sexual behavior in quail. *Comp. Biochem. Physiol. B Biochem. Mol. Biol.* 132, 37–55. doi: 10.1016/S1096-4959(01)00531-0

Balthazart, J., Baillien, M., and Ball, G. F. (2005). Interactions between kinases and phosphatases in the rapid control of brain aromatase. *J. Neuroendocrinol.* 17, 553–559. doi: 10.1111/j.1365-2826.2005.01344.x

Balthazart, J., Baillien, M., and Ball, G. F. (2006). Rapid control of brain aromatase activity by glutamatergic inputs. *Endocrinology* 147, 359–366. doi: 10.1210/en.2005-0845

Balthazart, J., Baillien, M., and Ball, G. F. (2001b). Rapid and reversible inhibition of brain aromatase activity. *J. Neuroendocrinol.* 13, 61–71. doi: 10.1046/j.1365-2826.2001.00598.x

Balthazart, J., Baillien, M., Charlier, T. D., and Ball, G. F. (2003). Calcium-dependent phosphorylation processes control brain aromatase in quail. *Eur. J. Neurosci.* 17, 1591–1606. doi: 10.1046/j.1460-9568.2003.02598.x

Balthazart, J., and Ball, G. F. (2006). Is brain estradiol a hormone or a neurotransmitter. *Trends Neurosci.* 29, 241–249. doi: 10.1016/j.tins.2006.03.004

Balthazart, J., Foidart, A., Baillien, M., Harada, N., and Ball, G. F. (1998). Anatomical relationships between aromatase and tyrosine hydroxylase in the quail brain: double-label immunocytochemical studies. *J. Comp. Neurol.* 391, 214–226.

Balthazart, J., Stoop, R., Foidart, A., Granneman, J. C., and Lambert, J. G. (1994). Distribution and regulation of estrogen-2-hydroxylase in the quail brain. *Brain Res. Bull.* 35, 339–345. doi: 10.1016/0361-9230(94)90111-2

Barone, I., Giordano, C., Malivindi, R., Lanzino, M., Rizza, P., Casaburi, I., et al. (2012). Estrogens and PTP1B function in a novel pathway to regulate aromatase enzymatic activity in breast cancer cells. *Endocrinology* 153, 5157–5166 doi: 10.1210/en.2012-1561

Beyer, C., Morali, G., Naftolin, F., Larsson, K., and Perez-Palacios, G. (1976). Effect of some antiestrogens and aromatase inhibitors on androgen induced sexual behavior in castrated male rats. *Horm. Behav.* 7, 353–363. doi: 10.1016/0018-506X(76)90040-4

Black, M. P., Balthazart, J., Baillien, M., and Grober, M. S. (2005). Socially induced and rapid increases in aggression are inversely related to brain aromatase activity in a sex-changing fish, *Lythrypnus dalli*. *Proc. Biol. Sci.* 272, 2435–2440. doi: 10.1098/rspb.2005.3210

Black, M. P., Balthazart, J., Baillien, M., and Grober, M. S. (2011). Rapid increase in aggressive behavior precedes the decrease in brain aromatase activity during socially mediated sex change in *Lythrypnus dalli*. *Gen. Comp. Endocrinol.* 170, 119–124. doi: 10.1016/j.ygcen.2010.09.019

Boulware, M. I., Weick, J. P., Becklund, B. R., Kuo, S. P., Groth, R. D., and Mermelstein, P. G. (2005). Estradiol activates group I and II metabotropic glutamate receptor signaling, leading to opposing influences on cAMP response element-binding protein. *J. Neurosci.* 25, 5066–5078. doi: 10.1523/JNEUROSCI.1427-05.2005

Catalano, S., Barone, I., Giordano, C., Rizza, P., Qi, H., Gu, G., et al. (2009). Rapid estradiol/ERalpha signaling enhances aromatase enzymatic activity in breast cancer cells. *Mol. Endocrinol.* 23, 1634–1645. doi: 10.1210/me.2009-0039

Catalano, S., Barone, I., and Andò, S. (2014). Rapid estrogen effects on aromatase phosphorylation in breast cancer cells. *Methods Mol. Biol.* 1204, 155–163. doi: 10.1007/978-1-4939-1346-6_14

Charlier, T. D., Harada, N., Balthazart, J., and Cornil, C. A. (2011). Human and quail aromatase activity is rapidly and reversibly inhibited by phosphorylating conditions. *Endocrinology* 152, 4199–4210 doi: 10.1210/en.2011-0119

Chen, B. S., and Roche, K. W. (2007). Regulation of NMDA receptors by phosphorylation. *Neuropharmacology* 53, 362–368. doi: 10.1016/j.neuropharm.2007.05.018

Cornil, C. A., Ball, G. F., and Balthazart, J. (2006). Functional significance of the rapid regulation of brain estrogen action: where do the estrogens come from? *Brain Res.* 1126, 2–26. doi: 10.1016/j.brainres.2006.07.098

Cornil, C. A., Ball, G. F., and Balthazart, J. (2012a). Rapid control of male typical behaviors by brain-derived estrogens. *Front. Neuroendocrinol.* 33, 425–446. doi: 10.1016/j.yfrne.2012.08.003

Cornil, C. A., Dalla, C., Papadopoulou-Daifoti, Z., Baillien, M., Dejace, C., Ball, G. F., et al. (2005a). Rapid decreases in preoptic aromatase activity and brain monoamine concentrations after engaging in male sexual behavior. *Endocrinology* 1416, 2809–2820. doi: 10.1210/en.2005-0441

Cornil, C. A., Leung, C. H., Pletcher, E. R., Naranjo, K. C., Blauman, S. J., and Saldanha, C. J. (2012b). Acute and specific modulation of presynaptic aromatization in the vertebrate brain. *Endocrinology* 153, 2562–2567. doi: 10.1210/en.2011-2159

Cornil, C. A., Seutin, V., Motte, P., and Balthazart, J. (2004). Electrophysiological and neurochemical characterization of neurons of the medial preoptic area in Japanese quail (*Coturnix japonica*). *Brain Res.* 1029, 224–240. doi: 10.1016/j.brainres.2004.09.047

Cornil, C. A., Taziaux, M., Baillien, M., Ball, G. F., and Balthazart, J. (2005b). Rapid effects of aromatase inhibition on male reproductive behaviors in Japanese quail. *Horm. Behav.* 49, 45–67. doi: 10.1016/j.yhbeh.2005.05.003

Cornil, C. A., Foidart, A., Minet, A., and Balthazart, J. (2000). Immunocytochemical localization of ionotropic glutamate receptors subunits in the adult quail forebrain. *J. Comp. Neurol.* 428, 577–608. doi: 10.1002/1096-9861(20001225)428:43.3.CO;2-B

Daubner, S. C., Lauriano, C., Haycock, J. W., and Fitzpatrick, P. F. (1992). Site-directed mutagenesis of serine 40 of rat tyrosine hydroxylase. Effects of dopamine and cAMP-dependent phosphorylation on enzyme activity. *J. Biol. Chem.* 267, 12639–12646.

de Bournonville, C., Dickens, M. J., Ball, G. F., Balthazart, J., and Cornil, C. A. (2013). Dynamic changes in brain aromatase activity following sexual interactions in males: where, when and why? *Psychoneuroendocrinology* 38, 789–799. doi: 10.1016/j.psyneuen.2012.09.001

Dewing, P., Boulware, M. I., Sinchak, K., Christensen, A., Mermelstein, P. G., and Micevych, P. (2007). Membrane estrogen receptor-alpha interactions with metabotropic glutamate receptor 1a modulate female sexual receptivity in rats. *J. Neurosci.* 27, 9294–9300. doi: 10.1523/JNEUROSCI.0592-07.2007

Dickens, M. J., Cornil, C. A., and Balthazart, J. (2011). Acute stress differentially affects aromatase activity in specific brain nuclei of adult male and female quail. *Endocrinology* 152, 4242–4251. doi: 10.1210/en.2011-1341

Dickens, M. J., Cornil, C. A., and Balthazart, J. (2013). Neurochemical control of rapid stress-induced changes in brain aromatase activity. *J. Neuroendocrinol.* 25, 329–339. doi: 10.1111/jne.12012

Diotel, N., Le Page, Y., Mouriec, K., Tong, S. K., Pellegrini, E., Vaillant, C., et al. (2010). Aromatase in the brain of teleost fish: expression, regulation and putative functions. *Front. Neuroendocrinol.* 31, 172–192 doi: 10.1016/j.yfrne.2010.01.003

Fisher, C. R., Graves, K. H., Parlow, A. F., and Simpson, E. V. (1998). Characterization of mice deficient in aromatase (ArKO) because of targeted disruption of *cyp19* gene. *Proc. Natl. Acad. Sci. U.S.A.* 95, 6965–6970. doi: 10.1073/pnas.95.12.6965

Foidart, A., Harada, N., and Balthazart, J. (1995a). Aromatase-immunoreactive cells are present in mouse brain areas that are known to express high levels of aromatase activity. *Cell Tissue Res.* 280, 561–574. doi: 10.1007/BF00318360

Foidart, A., Reid, J., Absil, P., Yoshimura, N., Harada, N., and Balthazart, J. (1995b). Critical re-examination of the distribution of aromatase-immunoreactive cells in the quail forebrain using antibodies raised against human placental aromatase and against the recombinant quail, mouse or human enzyme. *J. Chem. Neuroanat.* 8, 267–282. doi: 10.1016/0891-0618(95)00054-B

Forlano, P. M., Schlinger, B. A., and Bass, A. H. (2006). Brain aromatase: new lessons from non-mammalian model systems. *Front. Neuroendocrinol.* 27, 247–274. doi: 10.1016/j.yfrne.2006.05.002

Forlano, P. M., Deitcher, D. L., Myers, D. A., and Bass, A. H. (2001). Anatomical distribution and cellular basis for high levels of aromatase activity in the brain of teleost fish: aromatase enzyme and mRNA expression identify glia as a source. *J. Neurosci.* 21, 8943–8955.

Fusani, L., Hutchison, J. B., and Gahr, M. (2001). Testosterone regulates the activity and expression of aromatase in the canary neostriatum. *J. Neurobiol.* 49, 1–8. doi: 10.1002/neu.1061

Hayashi, T., and Harada, N. (2014). Post-translational dual regulation of cytochrome P450 aromatase at the catalytic and protein levels by phosphorylation/dephosphorylation. *FEBS J.* 281, 4830–4840. doi: 10.1111/febs.13021

Hayden-Hixson, D. M., and Ferris, C. F. (1991). Steroid-specific regulation of agonistic responding in the anterior hypothalamus of male hamsters. *Physiol. Behav.* 50, 793–799. doi: 10.1016/0031-9384(91)90020-O

Honda, S., Harada, N., Ito, S., Takagi, Y., and Maeda, S. (1998). Disruption of sexual behavior in male aromatase-deficient mice lacking exons 1 and 2 of the *cyp 19* gene. *Biochem. Biophys. Res. Commun.* 252, 445–449. doi: 10.1006/bbrc.1998.9672

Hong, Y., Li, H., Yuan, Y. C., and Chen, S. (2009). Sequence-function correlation of aromatase and its interaction with reductase. *J. Steroid Biochem. Mol. Biol.* 118, 203–206 doi: 10.1016/j.jsbmb.2009.11.010

Joels, M. (1997). Steroid hormones and excitability in the mammalian brain. *Front. Neuroendocrinol.* 18, 2–48. doi: 10.1006/frne.1996.0144

Johnson, A. L., and van Tienhoven, A. (1981). Pharmacokinetics of estradiol-17 beta in the laying hen. *J. Endocrinol.* 60, 2720–2723.

Kenealy, B. P., Keen, K. L., Ronnekleiv, O. K., and Terasawa, E. (2011). STX, a novel nonsteroidal estrogenic compound, induces rapid action in primate GnRH neuronal calcium dynamics and peptide release. *Endocrinology* 152, 3182–3191. doi: 10.1210/en.2011-0097

Konkle, A. T., and Balthazart, J. (2011). Sex differences in the rapid control of aromatase activity in the quail preoptic area. *J. Neuroendocrinol.* 23, 424–434. doi: 10.1111/j.1365-2826.2011.02121.x

Lord, L. D., Bond, J., and Thompson, R. R. (2009). Rapid steroid influences on visually guided sexual behavior in mal goldfish. *Horm. Behav.* 56, 519–526. doi: 10.1016/j.yhbeh.2009.09.002

MacLusky, N. J., and Naftolin, F. (1981). Sexual differentiation of the central nervous system. *Science* 211, 1294–1303. doi: 10.1126/science.6163211

Mermelstein, P. G., Becker, J. B., and Surmeier, D. J. (1996). Estradiol reduces calcium currents in rat neostriatal neurons via a membrane receptor. *J. Neurosci.* 16, 595–604.

Metzdorf, R., Gahr, M., and Fusani, L. (1999). Distribution of aromatase, estrogen receptor, and androgen receptor mRNA in the forebrain of songbirds and nonsongbirds. *J. Comp. Neurol.* 407, 115–129.

Micevych, P. E., and Mermelstein, P. G. (2008). Membrane estrogen receptors acting through metabotropic glutamate receptors: an emerging mechanism of estrogen action in the brain. *Mol. Neurobiol.* 38, 66–77. doi: 10.1007/s12035-008-8034-z

Miller, T. W., Shin, I., Kagawa, N., Evans, D. B., Waterman, M. R., and Arteaga, C. L. (2008). Aromatase is phosphorylated in situ at serine-118. *J. Steroid Biochem. Mol. Biol.* 112, 95–101 doi: 10.1016/j.jsbmb.2008.09.001

Miller, W. L. (2005). Minireview: regulation of steroidogenesis by electron transfer. *Endocrinology* 146, 2544–2550. doi: 10.1210/en.2005-0096

Moss, R. L., Gu, Q., and Wong, M. (1997). Estrogen: nontranscriptional signaling pathway. *Recent Prog. Horm. Res.* 52, 33–68. discussion: 68–69.

Onagbesan, O. M., and Peddie, M. J. (1989). Calcium-dependent stimulation of estrogen secretion by FSH from theca cells of the domestic hen (*Gallus domesticus*). *Gen. Comp. Endocrinol.* 75, 177–186. doi: 10.1016/0016-6480(89)90069-5

Osawa, Y., Higashiyama, T., Shimizu, Y., and Yarborough, C. (1993). Multiple functions of aromatase and the active site structure; aromatase is the placental estrogen 2-hydroxylase. *J. Steroid Biochem. Mol. Biol.* 44, 469–480. doi: 10.1016/0960-0760(93)90252-R

Remage-Healey, L., and Bass, A. H. (2004). Rapid, hierarchical modulation of vocal patterning by steroid hormones. *J. Neurosci.* 24, 5892–5900. doi: 10.1523/JNEUROSCI.1220-04.2004

Remage-Healey, L., Coleman, M. J., Oyama, R. K., and Schlinger, B. A. (2010). Brain estrogens rapidly strengthen auditory encoding and guide song preference in a songbird. *Proc. Natl. Acad. Sci. U.S.A.* 107, 3852–3857. doi: 10.1073/pnas.0906572107

Remage-Healey, L., Dong, S., Maidment, N. T., and Schlinger, B. A. (2011). Presynaptic control of rapid estrogen fluctuations in the songbird auditory forebrain. *J. Neurosci.* 31, 10034–10038. doi: 10.1523/JNEUROSCI.0566-11.2011

Remage-Healey, L., Maidment, N. T., and Schlinger, B. A. (2008). Forebrain steroid levels fluctuate rapidly during social interactions. *Nat. Neurosci.* 11, 1327–1334. doi: 10.1038/nn.2200

Remage-Healey, L., Oyama, R. K., and Schlinger, B. A. (2009). Elevated aromatase activity in forebrain synaptic terminals during song. *J. Neuroendocrinol.* 21, 191–199. doi: 10.1111/j.1365-2826.2009.01820.x

Rochira, V., Zirilli, L., Genazzani, A. D., Balestrieri, A., Aranda, C., Fabre, B., et al. (2006). Hypothalamic-pituitary-gonadal axis in two men with aromatase deficiency: evidence that circulating estrogens are required at the hypothalamic level for the integrity of gonadotropin negative feedback. *Eur. J. Endocrinol.* 155, 513–522. doi: 10.1530/eje.1.02254

Roepke, T. A., Ronnekleiv, O. K., and Kelly, M. J. (2005). Physiological consequences of membrane-initiated estrogen signaling in the brain. *Front. Biosci.* 16, 1560–1573. doi: 10.2741/3805

Rønnekleiv, O. K., and Kelly, M. J. (2002). "Rapid membrane effects of estrogen in the central nervous system," in *Hormones, Brain and Behavior*, eds D. W. Pfaff, A. P. Arnold, A. M. Etgen, S. E. Fahrbach, and R. T. Rubin (San Diego, CA: Elsevier Science), 361–380.

Roselli, C. E., Horton, L. E., and Resko, J. A. (1985). Distribution and regulation of aromatase activity in the rat hypothalamus and limbic system. *Endocrinology* 117, 2471–2477. doi: 10.1210/endo-117-6-2471

Roselli, C. E., and Resko, J. A. (1984). Androgens regulate brain aromatase activity in adult male through a receptor mechanism. *Endocrinology* 114, 2183–2189. doi: 10.1210/endo-114-6-2183

Roselli, C. E., and Resko, J. A. (1989). Testosterone regulates aromatase activity in discrete brain areas of male rhesus macaques. *Biol. Reprod.* 40, 929–934. doi: 10.1095/biolreprod40.5.929

Roselli, C. E., and Resko, J. A. (2001). Cytochrome P450 aromatase (CYP19) in the non-human primate brain: distribution, regulation, and functional significance. *J. Steroid Biochem. Mol. Biol.* 79, 247–253. doi: 10.1016/S0960-0760(01)00141-8

Saldanha, C. J., Remage-Healey, L., and Schlinger, B. A. (2011). Synaptocrine signaling: steroid synthesis and action at the synapse. *Endocr Rev.* 32, 532–549. doi: 10.1210/er.2011-0004

Saldanha, C. J., Tuerk, M. J., Kim, Y. H., Fernandes, A. O., Arnold, A. P., and Schlinger, B. A. (2000). Distribution and regulation of telencephalic aromatase expression in the zebra finch revealed with a specific antibody. *J. Comp. Neurol.* 423, 619–630. doi: 10.1002/1096-9861(20000807)423:4<619::AID-CNE7>3.0.CO;2-U

Schumacher, M., and Balthazart, J. (1986). Testosterone-induced brain aromatase is sexually dimorphic. *Brain Res.* 370, 285–293. doi: 10.1016/0006-8993(86)90483-X

Seredynski, A. L., Balthazart, J., Christophe, V. J., Ball, G. F., and Cornil, C. A. (2013). Neuroestrogens rapidly regulate sexual motivation but not performance. *J. Neurosci.* 33, 164–174. doi: 10.1523/JNEUROSCI.2557-12.2013

Shen, P., Schlinger, B. A., Campagnoni, A. T., and Arnold, A. P. (1995). An atlas of aromatase mRNA expression in the zebra finch brain. *J. Comp. Neurol.* 360, 172–184. doi: 10.1002/cne.903600113

Steimer, T., and Hutchison, J. B. (1991). "Micromethods for the *in vitro* study of steroid metabolism in the brain using radiolabelled tracers," in *Neuroendocrine Research Methods*, Vol. 2, ed B. Greenstein (Chur: Harwood Academic Publishers), 875–919.

Taziaux, M., Keller, M., Bakker, J., and Balthazart, J. (2007). Sexual behavior activity tracks rapid changes in brain estrogen concentrations. *J. Neurosci.* 27, 6563–6572. doi: 10.1523/JNEUROSCI.1797-07.2007

Thompson, E. A. Jr., and Siiteri, P. K. (1974). Utilization of oxygen and reduced nicotinamide adenine dinucleotide phosphate by human placental microsomes during aromatization of androstenedione. *J. Biol. Chem.* 249, 5364–5372.

Toda, K., Saibara, T., Okada, T., Onishi, S., and Shizuta, Y. (2001). A loss of aggressive behaviour and its reinstatement by oestrogen in mice lacking the aromatase gene (Cyp19). *J. Endocrinol.* 168, 217–220. doi: 10.1677/joe.0.1680217

Trainor, B. C., Finy, M. S., and Nelson, R. J. (2008). Rapid effects of estradiol on male aggression depend on photoperiod in reproductively non-responsive mice. *Horm. Behav.* 53, 192–199. doi: 10.1016/j.yhbeh.2007.09.016

Trainor, B. C., Lin, S., Finy, M. S., Rowland, M. R., and Nelson, R. J. (2007). Photoperiod reverses the effects of estrogens on male aggression via genomic and nongenomic pathways. *Proc. Natl. Acad. Sci. U.S.A.* 104, 9840–9845. doi: 10.1073/pnas.0701819104

Trainor, B. C., Kyomen, H. H., and Marler, C. A. (2006). Estrogenic encounters: how interaction between aromatase and the environment modulate agression. *Front. Neuroendocrinol.* 27, 170–179. doi: 10.1016/j.yfrne.2005.11.001

Tremere, L. A., Jeong, J. K., and Pinaud, R. (2009). Estradiol shapes auditory processing in the adult brain by regulating inhibitory transmission and plasticity-associated gene expression. *J. Neurosci.* 29, 5949–5963. doi: 10.1523/JNEUROSCI.0774-09.2009

Tsang, C. P., and Grunder, A. A. (1984). Production, clearance rates and metabolic fate of estradiol-17 beta in the plasma of the laying hen. *Steroids* 43, 71–84. doi: 10.1016/0039-128X(84)90059-X

Wagner, C. K., and Morrell, J. I. (1997). Neuroanatomical distribution of aromatase mRNA in the rat brain: indications of regional regulation. *J. Steroid Biochem. Mol. Biol.* 61, 307–314. doi: 10.1016/S0960-0760(97)80028-3

Whirl-Carrillo, M., McDonagh, E. M., Hebert, J. M., Gong, L., Sangkuhl, K., Thorn, C. F., et al. (2012). Pharmacogenomics knowledge for personalized medicine. *Clin. Pharmacol. Ther.* 92, 414–417. doi: 10.1038/clpt.2012.96

20

AMPK: A master energy regulator for gonadal function

Michael J. Bertoldo [1], *Melanie Faure* [2], *Joëlle Dupont* [2] *and Pascal Froment* [2*]

[1] *Discipline of Obstetrics and Gynaecology, School of Women's and Children's Health, University of New South Wales, Sydney, NSW, Australia,* [2] *Unité de Physiologie de la Reproduction et des Comportements, Institut National de la Recherche Agronomique, UMR85, Nouzilly, France*

Edited by:
Hubert Vaudry,
University of Rouen, France

Reviewed by:
Luis J. Garcia-Marin,
University of Extremadura, Spain
Maria Fernanda Riera,
Centro de Investigaciones Endocrinologicas-CONICET-GCBA, Argentina

***Correspondence:**
Pascal Froment,
Unité de Physiologie de la Reproduction et des Comportements, Institut National de la Recherche Agronomique, UMR85, 37380 Nouzilly, France
pascal.froment@tours.inra.fr

From *C. elegans* to mammals (including humans), nutrition and energy metabolism significantly influence reproduction. At the cellular level, some detectors of energy status indicate whether energy reserves are abundant (obesity), or poor (diet restriction). One of these detectors is AMPK (5′ AMP-activated protein kinase), a protein kinase activated by ATP deficiency but also by several natural substances such as polyphenols or synthetic molecules like metformin, used in the treatment of insulin resistance. AMPK is expressed in muscle and liver, but also in the ovary and testis. This review focuses on the main effects of AMPK identified in gonadal cells. We describe the role of AMPK in gonadal steroidogenesis, in proliferation and survival of somatic gonadal cells and in the maturation of oocytes or spermatozoa. We discuss also the role of AMPK in germ and somatic cell interactions within the cumulus-oocyte complex and in the blood testis barrier. Finally, the interface in the gonad between AMPK and modification of metabolism is reported and discussion about the role of AMPK on fertility, in regards to the treatment of infertility associated with insulin resistance (male obesity, polycystic ovary syndrome).

Keywords: AMPK, testis, ovary, germ cells, fertility

Introduction

The 5′ AMP-activated protein kinase (AMPK) is a serine/threonine heterotrimeric kinase composed of one catalytic α-subunit bound with β- and γ-regulatory subunits. The genes encoding the three subunits of AMPK are highly conserved in eukaryotic species including vertebrates, invertebrates, plants, fungi, and protozoa (Hardie et al., 2003; Ghillebert et al., 2011). Activation of AMPK occurs with the phosphorylation of the α-subunit at Threonine 172. AMPK is sensitive to the AMP to ATP ratio and is activated by an increasing AMP concentration and by the upstream kinases including liver kinase B1 (LKB1) and calcium/calmodulin (CaM) kinase (CaMKK) (Woods et al., 2003; Hawley et al., 2005). It can also be dephosphorylated by phosphatases [Protein kinase phosphatase-1 and -2A (PP2A and PP2C)] (Lu et al., 2010; Joseph et al., 2015). AMPK is activated in pathophysiological situations (exercise, stress), by metabolic hormones (leptin, adiponectin, ghrelin) or pharmacological agents [5-aminoimidazole-4-carboxamide-1-β-D-riboside (AICAR), metformin and thiazolidinediones (TZD)] (Hardie, 2015). It regulates energy homeostasis by maintaining constant intracellular ATP concentrations by stimulation of catabolic pathways and inhibition of anabolic pathways (Hardie, 2015). Several studies have also shown that AMPK is expressed in gonads (Tosca et al., 2005; Dupont et al., 2012; Tartarin et al., 2012a) and could play a key role in the reproductive function in linking the gonadal axis with energy balance. More precisely, AMPK is present in ovarian (granulosa and theca cells, oocytes and corpora lutea) and testicular (Sertoli, leydig and germinal cells) cells in different species [oyster (Guévelou et al., 2013),

C. elegans (Lee et al., 2008), bird (Tosca et al., 2006a; Nguyen et al., 2014), mammals: cow (Tosca et al., 2007a), pig (Mayes et al., 2007), rodents (Tosca et al., 2005; Downs et al., 2010; Tartarin et al., 2012a) and human (Pellatt et al., 2011)]. This kinase controls gonad steroidogenesis and germinal cell maturation but also cell proliferation and survival, polarity, formation, and maintenance of cellular junctional complexes, and cytoskeletal dynamics. In this review we report briefly some of the known functions of AMPK in the female and male gonad, and then we describe the potential role of this kinase in the interactions between metabolism and gonadal function. Most of the studies and conclusions are based on animal studies. However, we reported human studies (about granulosa and thecal cells or human embryonic testis) when it was possible.

Gonadal Steroidogenesis

In female mammals and birds, the role of AMPK has been studied in detail in granulosa cell cultures by using pharmacological agents and adenovirus-mediated expression of dominant negative forms of AMPK (Tosca et al., 2005). AMPK activators inhibit the secretion of progesterone and/or estradiol by granulosa cells in mammals (Tosca et al., 2005, 2007a). In rat and bovine species, this inhibition is associated with a decrease in 3beta-hydroxysteroid dehydrogenase (3β-HSD) mRNA and protein levels and a decrease in MAP kinase (MAPK) extracellular signal-regulated kinases (ERK) 1/2 phosphorylation (Tosca et al., 2005, 2007a, 2010). In rats, AMPK activation induced by metformin does not reduce aromatase expression and estradiol production. However, it decreases progesterone synthesis and the expression of different proteins involved in steroidogenesis [3β-HSD, cytochrome P450 (CYP11A1), steroidogenic acute regulatory protein (StAR)] (Tosca et al., 2006b). Metformin reduces follicle-stimulating hormone (FSH) but not forskolin-stimulated aromatase expression and activity in an AMP-activated protein kinase-independent manner in a human granulosa cell line (Rice et al., 2013). Also in human granulosa cells, metformin decreases androgen synthesis, by directly inhibiting cytochrome P450 17alpha-hydroxylase (Cyp17) activity (La Marca et al., 2000). In contrast, it has been shown that AMPK could improve androgen production by adrenal cells (Hirsch et al., 2012). Even if no studies have shown a role of AMPK in ovarian steroidogenesis *in vivo*, this has been largely demonstrated *in vitro*.

A total α1AMPK knock out mouse model has been developed (Tartarin et al., 2012a). The male $\alpha 1AMPK^{-/-}$ have high levels of testosterone that are not due to adrenal disorders or to glucorticoid resistance but to hyperactive Leydig cells (Tartarin et al., 2012a). Indeed, the Leydig cells of these animals have an increased volume, an altered endoplasmic reticulum area, a high intratesticular cholesterol concentration and a greater expression of proteins involved in steroid production (Tartarin et al., 2012a). These data accord with those described previously *in vitro* in granulosa cells but also in Leydig cells in response to a modulation of AMPK activity either pharmacologically or genetically. Certainly in MA-10 and MLTC-1 Leydig cells, AMPK activation inhibits cAMP-induced steroidogenesis by repressing the expression of key regulators of steroidogenesis, including the cholesterol carrier, StAR and the nuclear receptor Nr4a1 (Abdou et al., 2014). In the latter study, the authors suggest that some AMPK-sensitive element(s) containing sites for nuclear receptors of NR4A1 are located in the StAR promoter and are required for elevated cAMP dependent activation (Abdou et al., 2014). This suggests that activation of AMPK reduce the activity of NR4A1 and StAR expression. Furthermore, in primary rat Leydig cells, resveratrol, an AMPK agonist impairs human chorionic gonadotropin (hCG)-mediated testosterone production by repressing StAR expression (Svechnikov et al., 2009). In humans, the association of increased steroid production and the inhibition of AMPK could be associated to the Peutz-Jeghers Syndrome (PJS) (Ham et al., 2013). Peutz-Jeghers syndrome is an autosomal-dominant disorder that arises as a consequence of mutations in the serine/threonine kinase 11 (STK11) gene that encodes LKB1. In these PJS patients, excess estrogen and an increase in testicular aromatase expression is associated with a decrease in AMPK phosphorylation in the testis (Ham et al., 2013). Thus, AMPK could be a molecular modulator that inhibits gonadal steroidogenesis to preserve cellular energy homeostasis and prevent excess steroid production.

An important study for human health found that when human and mouse fetal testes were cultured in the presence of metformin, there was a reduction in testosterone secretion and mRNA of key factors which are involved in steroidogenesis (Tartarin et al., 2012b). This was also associated with an increase in lactate production. Furthermore, *in vivo* administration of metformin during pregnancy reduced the testicular size of fetal and neonatal testes. Although the number of germ cells was not altered by metformin treatment, the number of Sertoli cells was reduced in both fetal and neonatal testes. Interestingly the androgen producing Leydig cell population was only reduced in the fetal period at 16 days post-coitum (Tartarin et al., 2012b). This study presented a potentially harmful effect of metformin treatment on the development of fetal testes (Tartarin et al., 2012b). These effects were likely to result from a metformin-stimulated AMPK-mediated reduction in cellular proliferation (Kayampilly and Menon, 2012), indicating that the reduction in steroidogenesis occurred as a result of reduced testicular growth.

Proliferation and Survival of Somatic Gonadal Cells

Gonadal somatic cells comprise the granulosa, cumulus and theca cells of the ovary, and the Sertoli and Leydig cells of the testis. Proliferation and survival of somatic cells are indispensable for fertility. Indeed, it is well known that proliferating granulosa cells support the progression of follicular growth and oocyte maturation. In males, testis size and sperm production are directly correlated to the total number of adult Sertoli cells. Regulation of proliferation and survival processes involves different hormones including FSH. As AMPK has previously been described as inhibiting proliferation of somatic cells (Tosca et al., 2010; Hardie, 2011; Kayampilly and Menon, 2012; Riera et al., 2012), we will examine the proliferative role of AMPK for these critical cell types.

In *C. elegans*, AMPK promotes survival and arrests germline development during nutrient stress (Fukuyama et al., 2012). More precisely, AMPKα1 and AMPKα2 (aak-1 and aak-2), the two catalytic α subunits of AMP-activated protein kinase, regulate germline quiescence by suppressing activity of target of rapamycin complex 1 (TORC1) that is involved in cell growth, cell proliferation, cell motility, cell survival, protein synthesis, and transcription. Similarly in rat Sertoli cells, Riera et al. (2012) observed that activation of AMPK induces a decrease in FSH-stimulated Sertoli cell proliferation through a phosphatidylinositol 3-kinase (PI3K)/protein kinase B (Akt)/mTORC1 mechanisms but also an increase in cyclin dependent kinase inhibitor (CDKI, p19INK4d, p21Cip1, and p27Kip1) expression (Riera et al., 2012). In agreement with these data, Tosca et al. (2010) observed that metformin-induced AMPK activation reduces cell growth, protein synthesis and MAPK ERK1/2 and ribosomal protein S6 kinase (p90rsk) phosphorylation in response to insulin-like growth factor 1 (IGF1) in cultured bovine granulosa cells. Furthermore, Kayampilly and Menon observed that exposure of rat granulosa cells with a pharmacological activator of AMPK increased p27kip expression, an inhibitor of the cell cycle (Kayampilly and Menon, 2009). These latter authors have also observed that activation of AMPK induced by dihydrotestosterone (DHT) treatment decreases granulosa cell mitogenesis and consequently could contribute to ovulatory dysfunction observed in hyperandrogenic states (Kayampilly and Menon, 2012).

Maturation of Germ Cells

The Oocyte

The role of AMPK in mammalian oocyte maturation is strikingly species specific. AMPK improves resumption of oocyte meiosis in mice (Chen et al., 2006; Downs and Chen, 2006; Larosa and Downs, 2007; Chen and Downs, 2008) but not in rats (Downs, 2011) and pharmacological activation of AMPK blocks nuclear oocyte maturation in pigs and cattle (Mayes et al., 2007; Tosca et al., 2007b; Santiquet et al., 2014). The oocyte is reliant on the metabolism of lactate and pyruvate from the tricarboxylic acid cycle (TCA cycle) and oxidative phosphorylation for most of its energy stores (Biggers et al., 1967; Leese and Barton, 1984; Roberts et al., 2002). In human granulosa cells, AMPK could be also involved in lactate production which is important for follicular development (Richardson et al., 2009). The cumulus-oocyte complex (COC) also metabolizes glucose via numerous important pathways such as the pentose phosphate pathway and glycolysis. These metabolic pathways are critical for successful oocyte maturation and resumption of meiosis (Downs and Mastropolo, 1994; Downs et al., 1996; Sutton et al., 2003a,b). Cyclic adenosine monophosphate (cAMP), synthesized by adenylate cyclase downstream of the pentose phosphate pathway, is an important negative regulator of meiotic maturation. It is well known that degradation of cAMP by phosphodiestrases triggers resumption of meiosis. The depletion of cAMP results in an increase in the AMP/ATP ratio. As AMP levels rise, AMPK is triggered and activates a number of enzymes involved in energy producing pathways and inhibiting energy consuming pathways (Downs et al., 2002). This makes AMPK critically important for oocyte developmental competence.

In mouse oocytes, the α1AMPK subunit is more abundant than α2AMPK. Immunolocalization of the α1 catalytic subunit of AMPK showed an association with condensed chromatin and the meiotic spindle but not in the spindle poles or midbody. In the absence of α1AMPK specifically in the oocyte, a decrease in mdm2 protein level, a strong negative regulator of p53, leads to an increase in the p53 content and probably induces cell cycle arrest as shown by the few number of oocyte fertilized in IVF or by the lower litter size in comparison to control mice (Bertoldo et al., 2014b, 2015). AMPK activation increases the rate of germinal vesicle breakdown (GVBD), spindle formation and polar body (PB) extrusion whereas the kinase has no effect on peripheral movement of the spindle. The meiosis-inducing actions and localization of AMPK are regulated by microtubule spindle integrity during mouse oocyte maturation (Ya and Downs, 2014). Interestingly, in mice, fatty acid oxidation is required for AMPK-induced maturation *in vitro* (Vasangkar and Downs, 2013).

The AMPK activator, AICAR, is a potent stimulator of maturation in mouse cumulus cell-enclosed oocytes (CEO) and denuded oocytes (DO), but only marginally stimulatory in rat CEO and ineffective in rat DO (Downs, 2011). AICAR and compound C produced contrasting results on polar body formation in cultured CEO in rat and mouse. Active AMPK was colocalized with chromatin after GVBD in rat and mouse oocytes, but did not appear at the spindle poles in rat oocytes as it did in mouse oocytes. These data highlight significant differences in meiotic regulation between the two species (Downs, 2011).

Contrary to results obtained with mouse oocytes, bovine and porcine oocyte meiosis is inhibited by activators of AMPK which is activated by AMP, the degradation product of cAMP (Bilodeau-Goeseels et al., 2007; Mayes et al., 2007; Bilodeau-Goeseels, 2011). During oocyte *in vitro* maturation (IVM), Santiquet et al. (2014) cultured porcine oocytes in the presence of AICAR and assessed the oocytes response in reference to oocyte nuclear maturation and cumulus cell expansion. Nuclear maturation was inhibited, however, this effect was only observed in cumulus enclosed oocytes, suggesting that cumulus cells are essential for AICAR's effect on oocyte maturation. In addition, AICAR inhibited cumulus expansion, which normally occurs in response to FSH and/or epidermal growth factor (EGF) during IVM (Harper and Brackett, 1993; Lonergan et al., 1996; Ritter et al., 2015). The results in porcine are supported by those in bovine where supplementation of metformin during embryo *in vitro* production resulted in AMPK mediated activation of TSC2 (Pikiou et al., 2015) and probably a reduction in TOR complex signaling and protein synthesis inhibition. In bovine COCs, metformin blocks meiotic progression at the germinal vesicle stage, activates AMPK, and inhibits MAPK3/1 phosphorylation in both the oocytes and cumulus cells during *in vitro* maturation. Moreover, cumulus cells were essential for the effects of metformin on bovine oocyte maturation, whereas MAPK ERK1/2 phosphorylation was not (Tosca et al., 2007b). While the precise targets of AMPK in the COCs are not entirely known, AMPK has been shown to modulate protein synthesis in various cell types (Hormon et al., 2002; Proud, 2004) and proteins involved in communication with somatic cells (see next section).

As observed in the large animal species, AMPK signaling keeps nemertean oocytes from maturing (Stricker et al., 2013). Unlike in mice, where the onset of oocyte maturation (germinal vesicle breakdown, GVBD) is blocked by cAMP and triggered by AMPK, oocytes of the marine nemertean worm Cerebratulus undergo GVBD in response to cAMP elevations and AMPK deactivation (Stricker, 2011). In addition these effects are observed only in the absence of the surrounding somatic cells (Stricker et al., 2010). These results also provide evidence for a novel GVBD-regulating mechanism involving AMPK deactivation by cAMP-mediated S485/491 phosphorylation and further highlight the highly species specific effects of AMPK in regard to oocyte maturation.

Male Germ Cells

αAMPK is present in male germ cells of oyster (Guévelou et al., 2013), chicken (Nguyen et al., 2014) and mammals (Hurtado de Llera et al., 2012a; Tartarin et al., 2012a; Cordova et al., 2014). In oyster, it is more highly expressed in male gonad than in female and its expression is more important during the first stage of gametogenesis when germ cells proliferate (Guévelou et al., 2013).

To traverse the female reproductive tract, it is essential that mammalian spermatozoa acquire the functional competence to achieve this objective in order to successfully fertilize the oocyte. These functional markers include motility, capacitation, hyperactivation and the acrosome reaction (Hurtado de Llera et al., 2015). It was recently demonstrated that AMPK protein is highly expressed in ejaculated boar and chicken spermatozoa (Hurtado de Llera et al., 2012a; Nguyen et al., 2014), and in mouse epididymal sperm (Tartarin et al., 2012a; Bertoldo et al., 2014a) and that it localizes in the head of the spermatozoon and in the midpiece of the flagellum (Hurtado de Llera et al., 2013). In the boar, pharmacological inhibition of AMPK lead to a reduction in motility (Hurtado de Llera et al., 2012a) while concomitantly causing changes in mitochondrial membrane potential, sperm plasma membrane fluidity and organization and acrosome integrity (Hurtado de Llera et al., 2013; Martin-Hidago et al., 2013). Similar results have been described in the chicken. These studies highlight the conservation of the AMPK function in sperm activity.

Interestingly, Hurtado de Llera *et al.* noted that the majority of studies to date that had studied sperm physiology as a function of AMPK had only done so under conditions where AMPK was inhibited (Hurtado de Llera et al., 2012b, 2015) or was genetically silenced (Tartarin et al., 2012a). Consequently they conducted a study to assess sperm physiology while activating AMPK indirectly. They observed under extended periods (24 h) of AMPK activation, boar spermatozoa had reduced motility, acrosome membrane integrity and organization and fluidity of the plasma membrane which was associated with an increase in lipid disorganization (Hurtado de Llera et al., 2015). As these processes are critical under the different environmental conditions experienced by spermatozoa when transiting through the female reproductive tract to accomplish fertilization, it becomes obvious from studies carried out so far that an optimal level of AMPK activation is essential for regulating spermatozoa function (Hurtado de Llera et al., 2015).

Nakada *et al.* demonstrated that spermatogenesis is intimately linked to mitochondrial respiration (Nakada et al., 2006), and recently Pellicione et al. associated asthenozoospermia with abnormal mitochondrial ultrastructure (Pelliccione et al., 2011). Therefore, it is likely that the motility disturbances observed in our α1AMPK KO model and in the LKB1 KO model that presented with abnormalities in spermatozoa functionality and morphology (motility and head morphology) (Towler et al., 2008; Tartarin et al., 2012a), was directly linked to mitochondrial dysgenesis. Similarly, incubation of sperm from boar with an AMPK inhibitor, compound C, lead to a reduction in motility (Martin-Hidago et al., 2013). Surprisingly, a mouse model inactivated for an oxidative stress sensor protein like glutathione peroxydase 4 (Liang et al., 2009; Schneider et al., 2009) is described with structural abnormalities in spermatozoa analogous to those observed in α1AMPK KO, suggesting that mitochondria dysfunction could affect oxidative stress oxidative status.

Diabetic and infertile men present with a decrease in anti-oxidant concentrations and an increase in ROS generation in their semen, even before cryopreservation, demonstrating that the sperm from this group are at increased risk of oxidative damage (Lewis et al., 1995; Garcez et al., 2010). Several studies have demonstrated that metformin can reduce the levels of oxidative DNA damage and afford anti-oxidant protection (Attia et al., 2009; Onken and Driscoll, 2010; Martin-Montalvo et al., 2013). Metformin has been shown to guard against diabetes-induced genomic instability in sperm cells and the bone marrow of diabetic rats (Attia et al., 2009), so we can hypothesize that the use of metformin in diabetic patients would have no negative effect in the integrity of spermatozoa. However, we cannot exclude consequences on the paternal genome for oocyte fertilization. For example, treatment of murine sperm with high concentration of metformin increased histone deacetylase activity (Bertoldo et al., 2014a). Curiously, treatment of sperm with known natural activators of AMPK such as resveratrol or a synthetic activator like metformin, present positive effects such as reduction in DNA damage and lipid peroxidation (Bertoldo et al., 2014a). A study in the wood frog (*Rana sylvatica*), a species with a high freeze tolerance, has revealed that AMPK was more activated in liver and muscle tissue, thus presenting AMPK as a molecule with cryoprotective properties (Rider et al., 2006). Subsequently modification of AMPK has been exploited in the freezing protocols of mammalian semen (Bertoldo et al., 2014a; Cordova et al., 2014). Metformin was used in mouse semen extender (Bertoldo et al., 2014a) and following thawing, spermatozoa showed an improvement in fertilization capability *in vitro*. This was associated with a reduction in the number of abnormal zygotes following IVF when mouse spermatozoa was frozen in the presence of metformin compared to controls (Bertoldo et al., 2014a). AMPK was also modulated in stallion semen extender where there was an improvement in sperm quality post-thaw (Cordova et al., 2014). As the reports of AMPK presence in spermatozoa are growing in number, we believe it is reasonable to assume that AMPK activity is likely required for optimal mammalian spermatozoa physiology.

Germinal and Somatic Cells Interactions

Cumulus-oocyte Complex

Gap junction communication between cumulus cells and oocytes is crucial for oocyte meiotic maturation and to acquire full developmental competence (Gilchrist et al., 2004; Gilchrist, 2011; Li and Albertini, 2013). Such that maintenance of gap junction communication and delayed meiotic resumption have been shown to increase oocyte developmental competence (Thomas et al., 2004; Gharibi et al., 2013). Gap junction communication between the oocyte and the surrounding cumulus cells is established by the formation of bidirectional channels. The connexins family, which compose gap junctions is involved in oocyte/cumulus cell communication and allows passage of ions and small organic molecules. Loss of connexin 37 and connexin 43 in mouse oocytes or cumulus cells impaired fertility through inhibiting oocyte growth and folliculogenesis (Winterhager and Kidder, 2015). Electron microscopic analysis has shown that junctions between granulosa cells and oocytes are altered or absent as in connexin $37^{-/-}$ mice (Simon et al., 1997). In the mouse, deletion of α1AMPK specifically in the oocyte lead to a reduction in connexin 37 between the oocyte and cumulus cells at the Metaphase II stage which was associated with reduced fertility following IVF, and suggests a reduction in gap junction communication (Bertoldo et al., 2015). Reductions in connexin 26 and connexin 37 expression were also described in a diabetic mouse model, where oocyte quality is poor (Ratchford et al., 2008). In an non-mammalian example, Alesutan et al., demonstrated that active AMPK decreased connexin 26 abundance in the cell membrane in xenopus oocytes (Alesutan et al., 2011), suggesting disparate regulation of gap junction communication by AMPK between species.

Deletion of α1AMPK in oocytes leads to reductions in other proteins associated with intercellular communication within the cumulus oocyte complexes (Bertoldo et al., 2015). These include N-cadeherin and β-catenin (markers for adherens junctions) and occludin (a marker for tight junctions) (Bertoldo et al., 2015). The cumulus-oocyte complex interacts with granulosa cells through adhesion junctions composed of proteins such as E-cadherin and N-cadherin (Rufas et al., 2000; Machell and Farookhi, 2003). Expression of N-cadherin for example, increases throughout maturation, fertilization and early embryogenesis (Ziv et al., 2002), and N-cadherin mediated cell contact is associated with the maintenance of meiotic arrest (Peluso, 2006). Deregulation of these proteins impacts oocyte maturation, fertilization and early embryogenesis (Ziv et al., 2002; Peluso, 2006).

Furthermore in the bovine, it was recently demonstrated that the transzonal processes (TZP) that traverse the zona pellucida transfer RNA molecules from cumulus cells to the oocyte (Macaulay et al., 2014). It was proposed that these TZPs are held in place by adherens like junctions (Macaulay et al., 2014) and are critical for oocyte developmental competence. During repair of lung capillary endothelium α1AMPK promotes the development of intercellular adherens junctions by binding with N-cadherin and contributes to repair (Creighton et al., 2011). This supports the notion that AMPK may have a critical role in oocyte developmental competence by maintaining open oocyte-somatic cell communication channels through at least gap, adherens and tight junctions. Taken together the literature supports the concept that AMPK plays a crucial role in maintaining metabolic and molecular intercellular coupling between the oocyte and its somatic cells and breakdown of this coupling results in reduced oocyte developmental competence.

Blood Testis Barrier

As in the cumulus oocyte complex, male germ cells are closely linked their support cells; the Sertoli cells during their maturation. Sertoli cells have an important role in the shaping of the spermatid head for example (Kierszenbaum and Tres, 2004). Different transgenic mouse models show that AMPK plays a role in intra-testicular communication. Absence of the upstream AMPK kinase, LKB1 reduced mature spermatozoa production associated with abnormal acrosome morphology and a defect in Sertoli cell polarity and testicular junctional complexes (Towler et al., 2008). Patients with Peutz-Jeghers syndrome present a similar phenotype with alteration of sperm production associated with modifications of tight junctions in the blood-testis-barrier (Ulbright et al., 2007; Chen et al., 2012; Tanwar et al., 2012). The disruption of the *α1AMPK* gene in the whole murine testis induced altered sperm morphology without presenting abnormalities in Sertoli cell nucleus polarization (Tartarin et al., 2012a). Nonetheless, transmission electron microscopy analyses have shown the presence of some disrupted Sertoli cell/elongated spermatid germ cell junctions (Tartarin et al., 2012a). Interestingly, a similar phenotype in sperm head or midpiece morphology has been already described in mice deleted for adhesion molecules like nectin-2 (Mueller et al., 2003) or Tslc1 (Surace et al., 2006). The fact that absence of the *α1AMPK* gene lead to a mild phenotype in contrast to LKB1 could be explained by the activation of LKB1 through several other AMPK-related kinases present in the testis such as microtubule-associated protein/microtubule affinity-regulating kinases (MARK2) (Bessone et al., 1999) or SNRK (Jaleel et al., 2005) as a compensatory mechanism. This hypothesis is supported by the decrease in phosphorylation of MARK in testis in LKB1-KO mice (Kojima et al., 2007; Tanwar et al., 2012). The reduction and/or incorrect relocalization of markers of adherens junctions (β-catenin and N-Cadherin) (Kopera et al., 2010) and tight junctions (occludin and ZO-1) (Kopera et al., 2010) in Sertoli cells from LKB1-KO mice suggests a loss of contact with germ cells leading probably to alteration in germ cell shape (Kleymenova et al., 2005). Notably, altered β-catenin expression has previously been described to compromise Sertoli cell function and the maturation of germ cells and lead to infertility (Lee et al., 2005; Tanwar et al., 2010; Kerr et al., 2013).

The use of the AMPK activator (AICAR) can also influence junction complex integrity in rat Sertoli cells as has been described by Galardo et al. (2010). Rat Sertoli cells incubated with AICAR stabilized ZO-1 protein as observed by immunofluorescence (Galardo et al., 2010). The use of EGTA to limit the free calcium concentration in culture medium induced a redistribution of ZO-1 between Sertoli cells. Addition of AICAR or adenosine, in the presence of EGTA permitted the rescue of ZO-1 distribution to normal conditions at the cell membranes (Galardo et al., 2010). As in oocytes, the cAMP/PKA pathway is modified in the absence of α1AMPK in Sertoli cells, raising the question about the interaction between AMPK/cAMP signaling and the functionality of the blood-testis barrier permeability. Indeed, the cAMP signal has been described to be involved for the formation and maturation of male germ cells (Scobey et al., 2001), and can perturb junctions in rat Sertoli cells (Lui and Lee, 2005).

Interface between AMPK and Modification of Metabolism

Diet restriction is well known to promote longevity and reduce fertility in several species like *C. elegans*, *drosophila melanogaster*, birds and mammals. Diet restriction induces a negative energy balance which activates some energy sensors such as AMPK and the sirtuins which promote respiration and energy production by mitochondria. In mice, a deficiency in LKB1 or AMPK in mature Sertoli cells negatively impacts mitochondrial function, and has been associated with loss of quiescence and an activation of cell proliferation (Bertoldo et al., 2013). The association between nutrient availability, mitochondrial function and fertility has been already observed in invertebrates. In *C. elegans* the germinal stem cells regulate longevity through the TOR pathway (Arrantes-Oliveira et al., 2002), and similarly in drosophila TOR signaling is involved in the regulation of female germinal stem cell proliferation as a function of the availability of nutrients (Drummond-Barbosa and Spradling, 2001; Lafever and Drummond-Barbosa, 2005; Lafever et al., 2010; Shyh-Chang et al., 2013). These results are also observed in Sertoli cells where stimulation with an AMPK activator such as metformin or AICAR has consequences on lactate production and the increase in glucose transport (Galardo et al., 2007). One hypothesis of the action of metformin, is an indirect effect: an inhibition of the respiratory chain in mitochondria leading to an increase in lactate production, and in the AMP: ATP ratio inducing the activation of AMPK. On the other hand, the inactivation of α1AMPK in Sertoli cells, reduces the expression of mitochondrial markers (cytochrome c and PGC1a) and the ATP content, and increases the lactate production (Bertoldo et al., 2013). The increase in lactate, in this case, could be due to a switch in the cell between energy production by respiration to the aerobic glycolysis. Thus, α1AMPK deficiency enhances the Warburg Effect which can be associated with increased cell proliferation *in vitro* (Faubert et al., 2013). In addition, glycolysis could increase the allocation of glucose carbon into lipids and explain the increase in lipid vesicles. We cannot exclude that a modification in lipid metabolism in Sertoli cells has a consequence on germ cells. Indeed, some studies have described lipid transport from the Sertoli cells to the germ cells (Saether et al., 2003). Moreover, several recent studies using mice deficient in genes related to lipid metabolism, have described that the accumulation of excess lipid droplets in Sertoli cells resulted in impaired spermatogenesis (Coussens et al., 2008). Therefore, a balance of lipid metabolism in Sertoli cells is essential for normal spermatogenesis (Selva et al., 2004).

Ratchford et al. have hypothesized that abnormalities in oocyte metabolism, such as that observed in diabetes, could potentially preprogramme the oocyte for unfavorable outcomes after fertilization (Ratchford et al., 2007). Furthermore, Wang et al. (2009) concluded that maternal diabetes results in numerous oocyte deficiencies. Glucose metabolism is essential for successful oocyte maturation and the recommencement of meiosis (Downs and Mastropolo, 1994). It is well known that mitochondria can influence the developmental competence of the oocyte (Thouas et al., 2004). Certainly mitochondria play a key role in cellular energy generation, the control of cell death (Perez et al., 2000) and the dynamic process of meiosis including DNA reorganization (Wang et al., 2009). In the case of diabetes, mitochondria are abnormally distributed around the spindle or in the oocyte cytoplasm (Wang et al., 2009). Ratchford et al. observed that under hyperglycaemic conditions, phosphorylated ACC, a downstream target of AMPK and phosphorylated AMPK were both decreased in diabetic oocytes, demonstrating decreased AMPK activity (Ratchford et al., 2007). Diabetic oocytes were also metabolically perturbed leading to altered AMPK activity. Interestingly, increasing AMPK with AICAR in these oocytes during the preovulatory phase corrected the metabolic and meiotic perturbations observed. For these crucial activities in oocyte maturation, mitochondrial redistribution, activity or dysfunction have been suggested as markers of oocyte quality and are strongly related to fertilization rates and embryo development (Van Blerkom, 2004; Wang et al., 2009).

During the last decade a variety of natural ligands and synthetic ligands have been shown to activate AMPK including resveratrol (Baur et al., 2006), sulforaphane (Choi et al., 2014), niacin (Thirunavukkarasu et al., 2006), berberine (Brusg et al., 2006), metformin (Zhou et al., 2001), and thiazolidinediones (Fryer et al., 2002). Some of these compounds have non-linear dose-response characteristics, such as that of hormesis and have the ability to inhibit the mitochondrial complex I at elevated concentrations that mimick diet restriction (Gems and Partridge, 2008). The hypothesis of hormesis lends weight to differences in phenotype associated with differences of metformin concentration. High metformin concentrations (approximately 5 mM) is enough to inhibit the respiratory chain complex 1 in mitochondria leading to an increase in the AMP/ATP ratio (El-Mir et al., 2000; Owen et al., 2000) and different metformin concentrations induce increases in oxidant defenses as well as an extension of lifespan (Onken and Driscoll, 2010; Martin-Montalvo et al., 2013). The difference in species sensitivity has been already observed as mouse tissue is 10 fold less sensitive than human tissue (Tartarin et al., 2012b).

Metformin is a good example for mimicking diet restriction, because in mouse liver, metformin has been shown to induce a similar transcription pattern to diet restriction especially (Dhahbi et al., 2005). However, similar effects have been described in *C. elegans* where metformin administration increases the lifespan and produces several diet restriction-like phenotypes such as reduction in fecundity and a decrease in fat storage in animals which are fed *ad-libitum* (Onken and Driscoll, 2010). In drosophila, metformin exposure for 7 days at 25 and 50 mM concentration increases significantly the number of eggs laid in contrast to untreated controls. But after 14 days of treatment, egg-laying in females on 25 mM metformin was similar to controls and at 50 mM of metformin the females laid significantly fewer eggs (Onken and Driscoll, 2010). Interestingly in flies, metformin targets AMPK and inhibits the TOR pathway (Kalender et al., 2010; Slack et al., 2012). From the reports to date, we can conclude that effects on fertility (increases or reductions in the number of egg laid depending the time and concentration of metformin treatment) remains partially understood and controversial (He and Wondisford, 2015).

SIRT1 is widely regarded as a critical regulator of energy homeostasis and is implicated in a wide variety of cellular processes including metabolic diseases, cancer, aging, and reproduction (Bordone and Guarente, 2005; Brooks and Gu, 2009; Haigis and Sinclair, 2010). Furthermore it is known to interact with AMPK (Fulco et al., 2008; Narala et al., 2008; Canto and Auwerx, 2009). We have recently provided evidence in the oocyte that α1AMPK could be involved in chromatin remodeling, because we observed an increase in acetylation of H3 histone in oocytes from α1AMPK knockout oocytes (Bertoldo et al., 2015). This was correlated, as expected with a reduction in histone deacetylase SIRT1 expression *in vivo*. *In vitro* Sirt1 has the ability to deacetylate histone substrates in a NAD^+-dependent manner (Vaquero et al., 2004b) and hyperacetylation occurs when SIRT1 is knocked down (Vaquero et al., 2004b). Male mice deficient in SIRT1 present with altered germ cell maturation and increased DNA damage in germ cells (Coussens et al., 2008). Together, these data suggest that AMPK can modify oocyte proteins and histone acetylation status. These observations could be linked to other reports such as those relating to the aorta and heart tissue where a decrease in AMPK and SIRT1 expression is associated with increased H3 acetylation (Bendale et al., 2013). Interestingly, acetylation of histones H3 and H4 appear to be linked to an overexpression of connexin 43 in a prostate cell line (Ogawa et al., 2005; Hernandez et al., 2006), and PGC1α and p53 can modify their accessibility (Vaquero et al., 2004a; Wakeling et al., 2009; Nelson et al., 2012), possibly suggesting some level of control of intercellular communication and apoptosis. Interestingly, inadequate histone deacetylation causes changes in gene expression, which can lead to embryopathy in mice (Akiyama et al., 2006).

Conclusion

The involvement of AMPK in fertility control is conserved throughout several animal species from the oyster, *C. elegans*, drosophila, birds and mammals. Its expression is present in different compartments of the ovary and testis and through the different stages of maturation of germ cells, germline stem cells to oocytes and spermatozoa. Apart from its classical functions on metabolism, proliferation and anti-inflammatory effects observed in the gonad, AMPK is also able to modulate steroidogenesis, and to impact morphology and normal nuclear maturation of germ cells though interaction of germ cells with their nurse somatic cells. Some mechanisms elucidated are directly linked with mitochondrial function and junctional proteins. Despite the possibility of different sub-unit combinations of AMPK, absence of only α1AMPK leads to moderate failure of fertility in both sexes.

References

Abdou, H. S., Bergeron, F., and Tremblay, J. J. (2014). A cell-autonomous molecular cascade initiated by AMP-activated protein kinase represses steroidogenesis. *Mol. Cell. Biol.* 34, 4257–4271. doi: 10.1128/MCB.00734-14

Akiyama, T., Nagata, M., and Aoki, F. (2006). Inadequate histone deacetylation during oocyte meiosis causes aneauploidy and embryo death in mice. *Proc. Natl. Acad. Sci. U.S.A.* 103, 7339–7344. doi: 10.1073/pnas.0510946103

Alesutan, I., Sopjani, M., Munoz, C., Fraser, S., Kemp, B. E., Foller, M., et al. (2011). Inhibition of connexin 26 by the AMP-activated protein kinase. *J. Membr. Biol.* 240, 151–158. doi: 10.1007/s00232-011-9353-y

Arrantes-Oliveira, N., Apfeld, J., Dillin, A., and Kenyon, C. (2002). Regulation of life-span by germ-lne stem cells in *Caenorhabditis elegans*. *Science* 295, 502–505. doi: 10.1126/science.1065768

Attia, S. M., Helal, G. K., and Alhaider, A. A. (2009). Assessment of genomic instability in mormal and diabetic rats treated with metformin. *Chem. Biol. Interact.* 180, 296–304. doi: 10.1016/j.cbi.2009.03.001

Baur, J. A., Pearson, K. J., Price, N. L., Jamieson, H. A., Lerin, C., Prabhu, V. V., et al. (2006). Resveratrol improves health and survival of mice on a high-calorie diet. *Nature* 444, 337–342. doi: 10.1038/nature05354

Bendale, D. S., Karpe, P. A., Chhabra, R., Shete, S. P., Shah, H., and Tikoo, K. (2013). 17-β Estradiol prevents cardiovascular dysfunction in post-menopausal metabolic syndrome by involving SIRT1/AMPK/H3 acetylation. *Br. J. Pharmacol.* 170, 779–795. doi: 10.1111/bph.12290

Bertoldo, M. J., Guibert, E., Faure, M., Rame, C., Foretz, M., Viollet, B., et al. (2015). Specific deletion of AMP-activated protein kinase (α1AMPK) in murine oocytes alters junctional protein expression and mitochindrial physiology. *PLoS ONE* 10:e0119680 doi: 10.1371/journal.pone.0119680

Bertoldo, M. J., Guibert, E., Tartarin, P., Guillory, V., and Froment, P. (2014a). Effect of metformin on the fertilizing ability of mouse spermatozoa. *Cryobiology* 68, 262–268. doi: 10.1016/j.cryobiol.2014.02.006

Bertoldo, M. J., Guibert, E., Tartarin, P., Guillou, F., Foretz, M., Viollet, B., et al. (2013). L'AMPK, une protéine impliquée dans les interactions entre les cellules nourricières et les cellules germinales. *Ann. Endocrinol.* 74, 266. doi: 10.1016/j.ando.2013.07.097

Bertoldo, M. J., Locatelli, Y., O'neill, C., and Mermillod, P. (2014b). Impacts of and interactions between environmental stress and epigenetic programming during early embryo development. *Reprod. Fertil. Dev.* doi: 10.1071/RD14049. [Epub ahead of print].

Bessone, S., Vidal, F., Le Bouc, Y., Epelbaum, J., Bluet-Pajot, M. T., and Darmon, M. (1999). EMK protein kinase-null mice: dwarfism and hypofertility associated with alterations in the somatotrope and prolactin pathways. *Dev. Biol.* 214, 87–101. doi: 10.1006/dbio.1999.9379

Biggers, J. D., Whittingham, D. G., and Donahue, R. P. (1967). The pattern of energy metabolism in the mouse oocyte and zygote. *Proc. Natl. Acad. Sci. U.S.A.* 58, 560–567. doi: 10.1073/pnas.58.2.560

Bilodeau-Goeseels, S. (2011). Cows are not mice: the role of cyclic AMP, phosphodiesterases, and adenosine monophosphate-activated protein kinase in the maintenance of meiotic arrest in bovine oocytes. *Mol. Reprod. Dev.* 78, 734–743. doi: 10.1002/mrd.21337

Bilodeau-Goeseels, S., Sasseville, M., Guillemette, C., and Richard, F. J. (2007). Effects of adenosine monophosphate-activated kinase activators on bovine oocyte nuclear maturation *in vitro*. *Mol. Reprod. Dev.* 74, 1021–1034. doi: 10.1002/mrd.20574

Bordone, L., and Guarente, L. (2005). Calorie restriction, SIRT1 and metabolism: understanding longevity. *Nat. Rev. Mol. Cell Biol.* 6, 298–305. doi: 10.1038/nrm1616

Brooks, C. L., and Gu, W. (2009). How does SIRT1 affect metabolism, senescence and cancer? *Nat. Rev. Cancer* 9, 123–128. doi: 10.1038/nrc2562

Brusg, J. M., Ancellin, N., Grondin, P., Guillard, R., Martin, S., Saintillan, Y., et al. (2006). Inhibition of lipid synthesis through activation of AMP kinase: an additional mechanism for the hypolipidemic effects of berberine. *J. Lipid Res.* 47, 1281–1288. doi: 10.1194/jlr.M600020-JLR200

Canto, C., and Auwerx, J. (2009). PGC-1alpha, SIRT1 and AMPK, an energy sensing network that controls energy expenditure. *Curr. Opin. Lipidol.* 20, 98–105. doi: 10.1097/MOL.0b013e328328d0a4

Chen, H., Ruan, Y. C., Xu, W. M., Chen, J., and Chan, H. C. (2012). Regulation of male fertility by CFTR and implications in male infertility. *Hum. Reprod. Update* 18, 703–713. doi: 10.1093/humupd/dms027

Chen, J., and Downs, S. M. (2008). AMP-activated protein kinase is involved in hormone-induced mouse oocyte meiotic maturation *in vitro*. *Dev. Biol.* 313, 47–57. doi: 10.1016/j.ydbio.2007.09.043

Chen, J., Hudson, E., Chi, M. M., Chang, A. S., Moley, K. H., Hardie, D. G., et al. (2006). AMPK regulation of mouse oocyte meiotic resumption *in vitro*. *Dev. Biol.* 291, 227–238. doi: 10.1016/j.ydbio.2005.11.039

Choi, K. M., Lee, Y. S., Kim, W., Kim, S. J., Shin, K. O., Yu, J. Y., et al. (2014). Sulforaphane attenuates obesity by inhibiting adipogenesis and activating the AMPK pathway in obese mice. *J. Nutr. Biochem.* 25, 201–207. doi: 10.1016/j.jnutbio.2013.10.007

Cordova, A., Strobel, P., Vallejo, A., Valenzuela, P., Ulloa, O., Burgoa, R. A., et al. (2014). Use of hypometabolic TRIS extenders and high cooling rate refrigeration for cryopreservation of stallion sperm: presence and sensitivity of 5' AMP-activated protein kinase (AMPK). *Cryobiology* 69, 473–481. doi: 10.1016/j.cryobiol.2014.10.008

Coussens, M., Maresh, J. G., Yanagimachi, R., Maeda, G., and Allsopp, R. (2008). Sirt1 deficiency attenuates spermatogenesis and germ cell function. *PLoS ONE* 3:e1571. doi: 10.1371/journal.pone.0001571

Creighton, J., Jian, M., Sayner, S., Alexeyev, M., and Insel, P. A. (2011). Adenosine monophosphate-activated kinase alpha1 promotes endothelial barrier repair. *FASEB J.* 25, 3356–3365. doi: 10.1096/fj.10-179218

Dhahbi, J. M., Mote, P. L., Fahy, G. M., and Spindler, S. R. (2005). Identification of potential caloric restriction mimetics by mircroarray profiling. *Physiol. Genomics* 23, 343–350. doi: 10.1152/physiolgenomics.00069.2005

Downs, S. M. (2011). Mouse versus rat: profound differences in meiotic regulation at the level of the isolated oocyte. *Mol. Reprod. Dev.* 78, 778–794. doi: 10.1002/mrd.21377

Downs, S. M., and Chen, J. (2006). Induction of meiotic maturation in mouse oocytes by adenosine analogs. *Mol. Reprod. Dev.* 73, 1159–1168. doi: 10.1002/mrd.20439

Downs, S. M., Hudson, E. R., and Hardie, D. G. (2002). A potential role for AMP-activated protein kinase in meiotic induction in mouse oocytes. *Dev. Biol.* 245, 200–212. doi: 10.1006/dbio.2002.0613

Downs, S. M., Humpherson, P. G., Martin, K. L., and Leese, H. J. (1996). Glucose utilization during gonadotropin-induced meiotic maturation in cumulus-cell enclosed mouse oocytes. *Mol. Reprod. Dev.* 44, 121–131.

Downs, S. M., and Mastropolo, A. M. (1994). The participation of energy substrates in the control og meiotic maturation in murine oocytes. *Dev. Biol.* 162, 154–168. doi: 10.1006/dbio.1994.1075

Downs, S. M., Ya, R., and Davis, C. C. (2010). Role of AMPK throughout meiotic maturation in the mouse oocyte: evidence for promotion of polar body formation and suppression of premature activation. *Mol. Reprod. Dev.* 77, 888–899. doi: 10.1002/mrd.21229

Drummond-Barbosa, D., and Spradling, A. C. (2001). Stem cells and their progeny respond to nutritional changes during Drosophila oogenesis. *Dev. Biol.* 231, 265–278. doi: 10.1006/dbio.2000.0135

Dupont, J., Reverchon, M., Cloix, L., Froment, P., and Rame, C. (2012). Involvement of adipokines, AMPK, PI3K and the PPAR signaling pathways in ovarian follicle development and cancer. *Int. J. Dev. Biol.* 56, 959–967. doi: 10.1387/ijdb.120134jd

El-Mir, M. Y., Nogueira, V., Fontaine, E., Averet, N., Rigoulet, M., and Leverve, X. (2000). Dimethylbiguanide inhibits cell respiration via an indirect effect targeted on the respiratory chain complex I. *J. Biol. Chem.* 275, 223–228. doi: 10.1074/jbc.275.1.223

Faubert, B., Boily, G., Izreig, S., Griss, T., Samborska, B., Dong, Z., et al. (2013). AMPK is a negative regulator of the Warburg effect and suppresses tumor growth *in vivo*. *Cell Metab.* 17, 113–124. doi: 10.1016/j.cmet.2012.12.001

Fryer, L. G., Parbu-Patel, A., and Carling, D. (2002). The Anti-diabetic drugs rosiglitazone and metformin stimulate AMP-activated protein kinase through distinct signaling pathways. *J. Biol. Chem.* 277, 25226–25232. doi: 10.1074/jbc.M202489200

Fukuyama, M., Sakuma, K., Park, R., Kasuga, H., Nagaya, R., Atsumi, Y., et al. (2012). *C. elegans* AMPKs promote survival and arrest germline development during nutrient stress. *Biol. Open* 1, 929–936. doi: 10.1242/bio.2012836

Fulco, M., Cen, Y., Zhao, P., Hoffman, E. P., McBurney, M. W., Sauve, A. A., et al. (2008). Glucose restriction inhibits skeletal myoblast differentiation by activating SIRT1 through AMPK-mediated regulation of Nampt. *Dev. Cell* 14, 661–673. doi: 10.1016/j.devcel.2008.02.004

Galardo, M. N., Riera, M. F., Pellizzari, E. H., Cigorraga, S. B., and Meroni, S. B. (2007). The AMP-activated protein kinase activator, 5-aminoimidazole-4-carboxamide-1-b-D-ribonucleoside, regulates lactate production in rat Sertoli cells. *J. Mol. Endocrinol.* 39, 279–288. doi: 10.1677/JME-07-0054

Galardo, M. N., Riera, M. F., Pellizzari, E. H., Sobarzo, C., Scarcelli, R., Denduchis, B., et al. (2010). Adenosine regulates Sertoli cell function by activating AMPK. *Mol. Cell. Endocrinol.* 330, 49–58. doi: 10.1016/j.mce.2010.08.007

Garcez, M. E., dos Santos Branco, C., Lara, L. V., Pasqualotto, F. F., and Salvador, M. (2010). Effects of resveratrol supplementation on cryopreservation medium of human semen. *Fertil. Steril.* 94, 2118–2121. doi: 10.1016/j.fertnstert.2010.01.058

Gems, D., and Partridge, L. (2008). Stress-response hormesis and aging: "that which does not kill us makes us stronger." *Cell Metab.* 7, 200–203. doi: 10.1016/j.cmet.2008.01.001

Gharibi, S. H., Hajian, M., Ostadhosseini, S., Forouzanfar, M., and Nasr-Esfahani, M. H. (2013). Effect of phosphodiesterase type 3 inhibitor on nuclear maturation and *in vitro* development of ovine oocytes. *Theriogenology* 80, 302–312. doi: 10.1016/j.theriogenology.2013.04.012

Ghillebert, R., Swinnen, E., Wen, J., Vandesteene, L., Ramon, M., Norga, K., et al. (2011). The AMPK/SNF1/SnRK1 fuel gauge and energy regulator: structure, function and regulation. *FEBS J.* 278, 3978–3990. doi: 10.1111/j.1742-4658.2011.08315.x

Gilchrist, R. B. (2011). Recent insights into oocyte-follicle cell interactions provide opportunities for the development of new approaches to *in vitro* maturation. *Reprod. Fertil. Dev.* 23, 23–31. doi: 10.1071/RD10225

Gilchrist, R. B., Ritter, L. J., and Arsmstrong, D. T. (2004). Oocyte-somatic cell interactions during follicle development in mammals. *Anim. Reprod. Sci.* 82–83, 431–446. doi: 10.1016/j.anireprosci.2004.05.017

Guévelou, E., Huvet, A., Galindo-Sanchez, C. E., Milan, M., Quillien, V., Daniel, J.-Y., et al. (2013). Sex-specific regulation of AMP-activated protein kinase (AMP) in the Pacific Oyster *Crassostrea gigas*. *Biol. Reprod.* 89, 1–15. doi: 10.1095/biolreprod.113.109728

Haigis, M. C., and Sinclair, D. A. (2010). Mammalian sirtuins: biological insights and disease relevance. *Annu. Rev. Pathol.* 5, 253–295. doi: 10.1146/annurev.pathol.4.110807.092250

Ham, S., Meachem, S. J., Choong, C. S., Charles, A. K., Baynam, G. S., Jones, T. W., et al. (2013). Overexpression of aromatase associated with loss of heterozygosity of the STK11 gene accounts for prepubertal gynecomastia in boys with Peutz-Jeghers syndrome. *J. Clin. Endocrinol. Metab.* 98, E1979–E1987. doi: 10.1210/jc.2013-2291

Hardie, D. G. (2011). AMP-activated protein kinase: an energy sensor that regulates all aspects of cell function. *Genes Dev.* 25, 1895–1908. doi: 10.1101/gad.17420111

Hardie, D. G. (2015). AMPK: positive and negative regulation, and its role in whole-body energy homeostasis. *Curr. Opin. Cell Biol.* 33, 1–7. doi: 10.1016/j.ceb.2014.09.004

Hardie, D. G., Scott, J. W., Pan, D. A., and Hudson, E. R. (2003). Management of cellular energy by the AMP-activated protein kinase system. *FEBS Lett.* 546, 113–120. doi: 10.1016/S0014-5793(03)00560-X

Harper, K. M., and Brackett, B. G. (1993). Bovine blastocyst development after *in vitro* maturation in a defined medium with epidermal growth factor and low concentrations of gonadotropins. *Biol. Reprod.* 48, 409–416. doi: 10.1095/biolreprod48.2.409

Hawley, S. A., Pan, D. A., Musatrd, K. J., Ross, L., Bain, J., Edelman, A. M., et al. (2005). Calmodulin-dependent protein kinase kinase-beta is an alternative upstrream kinase for AMP-activated protein kinase. *Cell Metab.* 2, 9–19. doi: 10.1016/j.cmet.2005.05.009

He, L., and Wondisford, F. E. (2015). Metformin: concentrations matter. *Cell Metab.* 21, 159–162. doi: 10.1016/j.cmet.2015.01.003

Hernandez, M., Shao, Q., Yang, X. J., Luh, S. P., Kandouz, M., Batist, G., et al. (2006). A histone deacetylation-dependent mechanism for transcriptional repression of the gap junction gene cx43 in prostate cancer cells. *Prostate* 66, 1151–1161. doi: 10.1002/pros.20451

Hirsch, A., Hahn, D., Kempna, P., Hofer, G., Mullis, P. E., Nuoffer, J. M., et al. (2012). Role of AMP-activated protein kinase on steroid hormone biosynthesis in adrenal NCI-H295R cells. *PLoS ONE* 7:e30956. doi: 10.1371/journal.pone.0030956

Hormon, S., Browne, G., Krause, U., Patel, J., Vertommen, D., Bertrand, L., et al. (2002). Activation of AMP-activated protein kinase leads to the phosphorylation of elongation factor 2 and an inhibition of protein synthesis. *Curr. Biol.* 12, 1419–1423. doi: 10.1016/S0960-9822(02)01077-1

Hurtado de Llera, A., Martin-Hidago, D., Gil, M. C., Garcia-Marin, L. J., and Bragado, M. J. (2012a). AMP-activated kinase AMPK is expressed in boar spermatozoa and regulates motility. *PLoS ONE* 7:e38840. doi: 10.1371/journal.pone.0038840

Hurtado de Llera, A., Martin-Hidago, D., Gil, M. C., Garcia-Marin, L. J., and Bragado, M. J. (2012b). The AMPK activator metformin inhibits one of the main functions of boar spermatozoa, motility. *FEBS J.* 279(Suppl. 1), 52–576.

Hurtado de Llera, A., Martin-Hidago, D., Rodriguez-Gil, J. E., Gil, M. C., Garcia-Marin, L. J., and Bragado, M. J. (2013). AMP-activated kinase, AMPK, is involved in the maintenance of plasma membrane organization in boar. *Biochim. Biophys. Acta* 1928, 2143–2151. doi: 10.1016/j.bbamem.2013.05.026

Hurtado de Llera, A., Martin-Hidalgo, D., Gil, M. C., Garcia-Marin, L. J., and Bragado, M. J. (2015). AMPK up-activation reduces motility and regulates other functions of boar spermatozoa. *Mol. Hum. Reprod.* 21, 31–45. doi: 10.1093/molehr/gau091

Jaleel, M., McBride, A., Lizcano, J. M., Deak, M., Toth, R., Morrice, N. A., et al. (2005). Identification of the sucrose non-fermenting realted kinase SNRK, as a novel LKB1 substrate. *FEBS Lett.* 579, 1417–1423. doi: 10.1016/j.febslet.2005.01.042

Joseph, B. K., Liu, H. Y., Francisco, J., Pandya, D., Donigan, M., Gallo-Ebert, C., et al. (2015). Inhibition of AMP kinase by the protein phosphatase 2A heterotrimer, PP2APpp2r2d. *J. Biol. Chem.* 290, 10588–10598. doi: 10.1074/jbc.M114.626259

Kalender, A., Selvaraj, A., Gulati, P., Brule, S., Viollet, B., Kemp, B. E., et al. (2010). Metformin, independent of AMPK, inhibits mTORC1 in a rag GTPase-dependent manner. *Cell Metab.* 11, 390–401. doi: 10.1016/j.cmet.2010.03.014

Kayampilly, P. P., and Menon, K. M. (2009). Follicle-stimulating hormone inhibits adenosine 5'-monophosphate-activated protein kinase activation and promotes cell proliferation of primary granulosa cells in culture through an Akt-dependent pathway. *Endocrinology* 150, 929–935. doi: 10.1210/en.2008-1032

Kayampilly, P. P., and Menon, K. M. (2012). AMPK activation by dihydrotestosterone reduces FSH-stimulated cell proliferation in rat granulosa cells by inhibiting ERK signaling pathway. *Endocrinology* 153, 2831–2838. doi: 10.1210/en.2011-1967

Kerr, G. E., Young, J. C., Horvay, K., Abud, H. E., and Loveland, K. L. (2013). Regulated Wnt/Beta-catenin signaling sustains adult spermatogenesis in mice. *Biol. Reprod.* 90:3. doi: 10.1095/biolreprod.112.105809

Kierszenbaum, A. L., and Tres, L. L. (2004). The acrosome-acroplaxome-manchette complex and the shaping of the spermatid head. *Arch. Histol. Cytol.* 67, 271–284. doi: 10.1679/aohc.67.271

Kleymenova, E., Swanson, C., Boekelheide, K., and Gaido, K. W. (2005). Exposure *in utero* to di(*n*-butyl) phthalate alters the vimentin cytoskeleton of fetal rat Sertoli cells and disrupts Sertoli cell-gonocyte contact. *Biol. Reprod.* 73, 482–490. doi: 10.1095/biolreprod.104.037184

Kojima, Y., Miyoshi, H., Clevers, H. C., Oshima, M., Aoki, M., and Taketo, M. M. (2007). Suppression of tubulin polymerization by the LKB1-microtubule-associated protein/microtubule affinity-regulating kinase signaling. *J. Biol. Chem.* 282, 23532–23540. doi: 10.1074/jbc.M700590200

Kopera, I. A., Bilinska, B., Cheng, C. Y., and Mruk, D. D. (2010). Sertoli-germ cell junctions in the testis: a review of recent data. *Philos. Trans. R. Soc. Lond. B Biol. Sci.* 365, 1593–15605. doi: 10.1098/rstb.2009.0251

Lafever, L., and Drummond-Barbosa, D. (2005). Direct control of germline stem cell division and cyst growth by neural insulin in Drosophila. *Science* 309, 1071–1073. doi: 10.1126/science.1111410

Lafever, L., Feokitistov, A., Hsu, H. J., and Drummond-Barbosa, D. (2010). Specific roles of target of rapmycin in the control of stem cells and their progeny in the Drosophila ovary. *Development* 137, 2117–2126. doi: 10.1242/dev.050351

La Marca, A., Eqbe, T. O., Morqante, G., Paglia, T., Cianci, A., and De Leo, V. (2000). Metformin treatment reduces ovarian cytochrome P-450c17alpha response to human chorionic gonadotrophin in women with insulin resistance-related polycystic ovary syndrome. *Hum. Reprod.* 15, 21–23. doi: 10.1093/humrep/15.1.21

Larosa, C., and Downs, S. M. (2007). Meiotic inductionb by heat stress in mouse oocytes: involvement of AMP-activated protein kinase and MAPK family members. *Biol. Reprod.* 76, 476–486. doi: 10.1095/biolreprod.106.057422

Lee, H., Cho, J. S., Lambacher, N., Lee, J., Lee, S. J., Lee, T. H., et al. (2008). The *Caenorhabditis elegans* AMP-activated protein kinase AAK-2 is phosphorylated by LKB1 and is required for resistance to oxidative stress and for normal motility and foraging behavior. *J. Biol. Chem.* 283, 14988–14993. doi: 10.1074/jbc.M709115200

Lee, N. P. Y., Mruk, D., Wong, C., and Cheng, C. Y. (2005). Regulation of Sertoli-Germ cell adherens junction dynamics in the testis via the nitric oxide synthase (NOS)/cGMP/protein kinase G (PRKG)/ β-catenin (CATNB) signaling pathway: an *in vitro* and *in vivo* study. *Biol. Reprod.* 73, 458–471. doi: 10.1095/biolreprod.105.040766

Leese, H. J., and Barton, A. M. (1984). Pyruvate and glucose uptake by mouse ova and preimplantation embryos. *J. Reprod. Fertil.* 72, 9–13. doi: 10.1530/jrf.0.0720009

Lewis, S. E., Boyle, P. M., McKinney, K. A., Young, I. S., and Thompson, W. (1995). Total antioxidant capacity of seminal plasma is different in fertile and infertile men. *Fertil. Steril.* 64, 868–870.

Li, R., and Albertini, D. F. (2013). The road to maturation: somatic cell interaction and self-organization of the mammalian oocyte. *Nat. Rev. Mol. Cell Biol.* 14, 141–152. doi: 10.1038/nrm3531

Liang, H., Yoo, S. E., Na, R., Walter, C. A., Richardson, A., and Ran, Q. (2009). Short form glutathione peroxidase 4 is the essential isoform required for survival and somatic mitochondrial functions. *J. Biol. Chem.* 284, 30836–30844. doi: 10.1074/jbc.M109.032839

Lonergan, P., Carolan, C., Van Langendonckt, A., Donnay, I., Khatir, H., and Mermillod, P. (1996). Role of epidermal growth factor in bovine oocyte maturation and preimplantation embryo development *in vitro*. *Biol. Reprod.* 54, 1420–1429. doi: 10.1095/biolreprod54.6.1420

Lu, J., Wu, D. M., Zheng, Y. L., Hu, B., Zhang, Z. F., Shan, Q., et al. (2010). Quercetin activates AMP-activated protein kinase by reducing PP2C expression protecting old mouse brain against high cholesterol-induced neurotoxicity. *J. Pathol.* 222, 199–212. doi: 10.1002/path.2754

Lui, W. Y., and Lee, W. M. (2005). cAMP perturbs inter-Sertoli tight junction permeability barrier *in vitro* via its effect on proteasome-sensitive ubiquitination of occludin. *J. Cell. Physiol.* 203, 564–572. doi: 10.1002/jcp.20254

Macaulay, A. D., Gilbert, I., Caballero, J., Barreto, R., Fournier, E., Tossou, P., et al. (2014). The gametic synapse: RNA transfer to the bovine oocyte. *Biol. Reprod.* 91, 90. doi: 10.1095/biolreprod.114.119867

Machell, N. H., and Farookhi, R. (2003). E- and N-cadherin expression and distribution during luteinization in the rat ovary. *Reproduction* 125, 791–800. doi: 10.1530/rep.0.1250791

Martin-Hidago, D., Hurtado de Llera, A., Yeste, M., Cruz Gil, M., Bragado, M. J., and Garcia-Marin, L. J. (2013). Adenosine monophosphate-activated kinase, AMPK, is involved in the maintenance of the quality of extended boar semen during long-term storage. *Theriogenology* 80, 285–294. doi: 10.1016/j.theriogenology.2013.02.015

Martin-Montalvo, A., Mercken, E. M., Mitchell, S. J., Palacios, H. H., Mote, P. L., Scheibye-Knudsen, M., et al. (2013). Metformin improves healthspan and lifespan in mice. *Nat. Commun.* 4:2192. doi: 10.1038/ncomms3192

Mayes, M. A., Laforest, M. F., Guillemette, C., Gilchrist, R. B., and Richard, F. J. (2007). Adenosine 5'-monophosphate kinase-activated protein kinase (PRKA) activators delay meiotic resumption in porcine oocytes. *Biol. Reprod.* 76, 589–597. doi: 10.1095/biolreprod.106.057828

Mueller, S., Rosenquist, T. A., Takai, Y., Bronson, R. A., and Wimmer, E. (2003). Loss of nectin-2 at Sertoli-spermatid junctions leads to male infertility and correlates with severe spermatozoan head and midpiece malformation, impaired binding to the zona pellucida, and oocyte penetration. *Biol. Reprod.* 69, 1330–1340. doi: 10.1095/biolreprod.102.014670

Nakada, K., Sato, A., Yoshida, K., Morita, T., Tanaka, H., Inoue, S., et al. (2006). Mitochondria-related male infertility. *Proc. Natl. Acad. Sci. U.S.A.* 103, 15148–15153. doi: 10.1073/pnas.0604641103

Narala, S. R., Allsopp, R. C., Wells, T. B., Zhang, G., Prasad, P., Coussens, M. J., et al. (2008). SIRT1 acts as a nutrient-sensitive growth suppressor and its loss is associated with increased AMPK and telomerase activity. *Mol. Biol. Cell* 19, 1210–1219. doi: 10.1091/mbc.E07-09-0965

Nelson, L. E., Valentine, R. J., Cacicedo, J. M., Gauthier, M.-S., Ido, Y., and Ruderman, N. B. (2012). A novel inverse relationship between metformin-triggered AMPK-SIRT1 signaling and p53 protein abundance in high glucose-exposed HepG2 cells. *Am. J. Physiol. Cell Physiol.* 303, C4–C13. doi: 10.1152/ajpcell.00296.2011

Nguyen, T. M. D., Alves, S., Grasseau, I., Metayer-Coustard, S., Praud, C., Froment, P., et al. (2014). Central role of 5'-AMP-activated protein kinase in chicken sperm functions. *Biol. Reprod.* 91, 1–15. doi: 10.1095/biolreprod.114.121855

Ogawa, T., Hayashi, T., Tokunou, M., Nakachi, K., Trosko, J. E., Chang, C. C., et al. (2005). Suberoylanilide hydroxamic acid enhances gap junctional intercellular communication via acetylation of histone containing connexin 43 gene locus. *Cancer Res.* 65, 9771–9778. doi: 10.1158/0008-5472.CAN-05-0227

Onken, B., and Driscoll, M. (2010). Metformin induces a dietary restriction-like state and oxidative stress response to extend *C. elegans* healthspan via AMPK, LKB1, and SKN-1. *PLoS ONE* 5:e8758. doi: 10.1371/journal.pone.0008758

Owen, M. R., Doran, E., and Halestrap, A. P. (2000). Evidence that metformin exerts its anti-diabetic effects through inhibition of complex 1 of the mitochondrial respiratory chain. *Biochem. J.* 348, 607–614. doi: 10.1042/0264-6021:3480607

Pellatt, L. J., Rice, S., and Mason, H. D. (2011). Phosphorylation and activation of AMP-activated protein kinase (AMPK) by metformin in the human ovary requires insulin. *Endocrinology* 152, 1112–1118. doi: 10.1210/en.2009-1429

Pelliccione, F., Micillo, A., Cordeschi, G., D'angeli, A., Necozione, S., Gandini, L., et al. (2011). Altered ultrastructure of mitochondrial membranes is strongly associated with unexplained asthenozoospermia. *Fertil. Steril.* 95, 641–646. doi: 10.1016/j.fertnstert.2010.07.1086

Peluso, J. J. (2006). N-cadherin mediated cell contact inhibits germinal vesicle brakdown in mouse oocytes maintained *in vitro*. *Reproduction* 131, 429–437. doi: 10.1530/rep.1.00863

Perez, G. I., Trbovich, A. M., Gosden, R. G., and Tilly, J. L. (2000). Mitochondria and the death of oocytes. *Nature* 403, 500–501. doi: 10.1038/35000651

Pikiou, O., Vasilaki, A., Leondaritis, G., Vamvakopoulos, N., and Messinis, I. E. (2015). Effects of metformin of fertilisation of bovine oocytes and early embryo development: possible involvement of AMPK3-mediated TSC2 activation. *Zygote* 23, 58–67. doi: 10.1017/S0967199413000300

Proud, C. G. (2004). Role of mTOR signalling in the control of translation initiation and elongation of nutrients. *Curr. Top. Microbiol. Immunol.* 279, 215–244. doi: 10.1007/978-3-642-18930-2_13

Ratchford, A. M., Chang, A. S., Chi, M. M.-Y., Sheridan, R., and Moley, K. H. (2007). Maternal diabetes adversely affects AMP-activated protein kinase activity and cellular metabolism in murine oocytes. *Am. J. Physiol. Endocrinol. Metab.* 293, E1198–E1206. doi: 10.1152/ajpendo.00097.2007

Ratchford, A. M., Esguerra, C. R., and Moley, K. H. (2008). Decreased oocyte-granulosa cell gap junction communication and connexin expression in a Type 1 diabetic mouse model. *Mol. Endocrinol.* 22, 2643–2654. doi: 10.1210/me.2007-0495

Rice, S., Elia, S., Jawad, Z., Pellatt, L., and Mason, H. D. (2013). Metformin inhibits follicle-stimulating hormone (FSH) action in human granulosa cell: relevance to polycystic ovary syndrome. *J. Clin. Endocrinol. Metab.* 98, E1491–E1500. doi: 10.1210/jc.2013-1865

Richardson, M. C., Ingamells, S., Simonis, C. D., Cameron, I. T., Sreekumar, R., Vijendren, A., et al. (2009). Stimulation of lactate production in human granulosa cells by metformin and potential involvement of adenosine 5' monophosphate-activated protein kinase. *J. Clin. Endocrinol. Metab.* 94, 670–677. doi: 10.1210/jc.2008-2025

Rider, M. H., Hussain, N., Horman, S., Dilworth, S. M., and Storey, K. B. (2006). Stress-induced activation of the AMP-activated protein kinase in the freeze tolerant frog *Rana sylvatica*. *Cryobiology* 53, 297–309. doi: 10.1016/j.cryobiol.2006.08.001

Riera, M. F., Regueira, M., Galardo, M. N., Pellizzari, E. H., Meroni, S. B., and Cigorraga, S. B. (2012). Signal transduction pathways in FSH regulation of rat Sertoli cell proliferation. *Am. J. Physiol. Endocrinol. Metab.* 302, E914–E923. doi: 10.1152/ajpendo.00477.2011

Ritter, L. J., Sugimura, S., and Gilchrist, R. B. (2015). Oocyte induction of EGF responsiveness in somatic cells is associated with the acquisition of porcine oocyte developmental competence. *Endocrinology* 156, 2299–2312. doi: 10.1210/en.2014-1884

Roberts, R., Franks, S., and Hardy, K. (2002). Culture environment modulates maturation and metabolism of human oocytes. *Hum. Reprod.* 17, 2950–2956. doi: 10.1093/humrep/17.11.2950

Rufas, O., Fisch, B., Ziv, S., and Shalgi, R. (2000). Expression of cadherin adhesion molecules on human gametes. *Mol. Hum. Reprod.* 6, 163–169. doi: 10.1093/molehr/6.2.163

Saether, T., Tran, T. N., Rootwelt, H., Christophersen, B. O., and Haugen, T. B. (2003). Expression and regulation of delta5-desaturase, delta6-desaturase, stearoyl-coenzyme A (CoA) desaturase 1, and stearoyl-CoA desaturase 2 in rat testis. *Biol. Reprod.* 69, 117–124. doi: 10.1095/biolreprod.102.014035

Santiquet, N., Sasseville, M., Laforest, M., Guillemette, C., Gilchrist, R. B., and Richard, F. J. (2014). Activation of 5′ adenosine monophosphate-activated protein kinase blocks cumulus cell expansion through inhibition of protein synthesis during *in vitro* maturation in swine. *Biol. Reprod.* 91, 1–12. doi: 10.1095/biolreprod.113.116764

Schneider, M., Forster, H., Boersma, A., Seiler, A., Wehnes, H., Sinowatz, F., et al. (2009). Mitochondrial glutathione peroxidase 4 disruption causes male infertility. *FASEB J.* 23, 3233–3242. doi: 10.1096/fj.09-132795

Scobey, M. J., Bertera, S., Somers, J. P., Watkins, S. C., Zeleznik, A. J., and Walker, W. H. (2001). Delivery of a cylic adenosine 3′,5′-monophosphate response element-binding protein (CREB) mutant to seminiferous tubules results in impaired spermatogenesis. *Endocrinology* 142, 948–954. doi: 10.1210/endo.142.2.7948

Selva, D. M., Hirsch-Reinshagen, V., Burgess, B., Zhou, S., Chan, J., McIsaac, S., et al. (2004). The ATP-binding cassette transporter 1 mediates lipid efflux from Sertoli cells and influences male fertility. *J. Lipid Res.* 45, 1040–1050. doi: 10.1194/jlr.M400007-JLR200

Shyh-Chang, N., Daley, G. Q., and Cantley, L. C. (2013). Stem cell metabolism in tissue development and aging. *Development* 140, 2535–2547. doi: 10.1242/dev.091777

Simon, A. M., Goodenough, D. A., Li, E., and Paul, D. L. (1997). Female fertility in mice lacking connexin 37. *Nature* 385, 525–529. doi: 10.1038/385525a0

Slack, C., Foley, A., and Partridge, L. (2012). Activation of AMPK by the putative dietary restriction mimetic metformin is insufficient to extend lifespan in Drosophila. *PLoS ONE* 7:e47699. doi: 10.1371/journal.pone.0047699

Stricker, S. A. (2011). Potential upstream regulators and downstream targets of AMP-activated kinase signaling during oocyte maturation in a marine worm. *Reproduction* 142, 29–39. doi: 10.1530/REP-10-0509

Stricker, S. A., Cline, C., and Goodrich, D. (2013). Oocyte maturation and fertilization in marine nemertean worms: using similar sorts of signaling pathways as in mammals, but often with differing results. *Biol. Bull.* 224, 137–155.

Stricker, S. A., Swiderek, L., and Nguyen, T. (2010). Stimulators of AMP-activated kinase (AMPK) inhibit seawater - but not cAMP-induced oocyte maturation in a marine worm: implications for interactions between cAMP and AMPK signaling. *Mol. Reprod. Dev.* 77, 497–510. doi: 10.1002/mrd.21177

Surace, E. I., Strickland, A., Hess, R. A., Gutmann, D. H., and Naughton, C. K. (2006). Tslc1 (nectin-like molecule-2) is essential for spermatozoa motility and male fertility. *J. Androl.* 27, 816–825. doi: 10.2164/jandrol.106.000398

Sutton, M. L., Cetica, P. D., Beconi, M. T., Kind, M. L., Gilchrist, R. B., and Thompson, J. G. (2003a). Influence of oocyte-secreted factors and culture duration on the metabolic activity of bovine cumulus cell complexes. *Reproduction* 126, 27–43. doi: 10.1530/rep.0.1260027

Sutton, M. L., Gilchrist, R. B., and Thompson, J. G. (2003b). Effects of *in-vivo* and *in-vitro* environments on the metabolism of the cumulus-oocyte complex and its influence on oocyte developmental capacity. *Hum. Reprod. Update* 9, 35–48. doi: 10.1093/humupd/dmg009

Svechnikov, K., Spatafora, C., Svechnikova, I., Tringali, C., and Soder, O. (2009). Effects of resveratrol analogs on steroidogenesis and mitochondrial function in rat Leydig cells *in vitro*. *J. Appl. Toxicol.* 29, 673–680. doi: 10.1002/jat.1456

Tanwar, P. S., Kaneko-Tarui, T., Zhang, L., Rani, P., Taketo, M. M., and Teixeira, J. (2010). Constitutive WNT/Beta-catenin signaling in murine Sertoli cells disrupts their differentiation and ability to support spermatogenesis. *Biol. Reprod.* 82, 422–432. doi: 10.1095/biolreprod.109.079335

Tanwar, P. S., Kaneko-Tarui, T., Zhang, L., and Teixeira, J. M. (2012). Altered LKB1/AMPK/TSC1/TSC2/mTOR signaling causes disruption of Sertoli cell polarity and spermatogenesis. *Hum. Mol. Genet.* 21, 4394–4405. doi: 10.1093/hmg/dds272

Tartarin, P., Guibert, E., Touré, A., Ouiste, C., Leclerc, J., Sanz, N., et al. (2012a). Inactivation of AMPKα1 induces asthenozoospermia and alters spermatozoa morphology. *Endocrinology* 153, 3468–3481. doi: 10.1210/en.2011-1911

Tartarin, P., Moison, D., Guibert, E., Dupont, J., Habert, R., Rouiller-Fabre, V., et al. (2012b). Metformin exposure affects human and mouse fetal testicular cells. *Hum. Reprod.* 27, 3304–3314. doi: 10.1093/humrep/des264

Thirunavukkarasu, M., Penumathsa, S., Juhasz, B., Zhan, L., Bagchi, M., Yasmin, T., et al. (2006). Enhanced cardiovascular function and energy level by a novel chromium (III)-supplement. *Biofactors* 27, 53–67. doi: 10.1002/biof.5520270106

Thomas, R. E., Armstrong, D. T., and Gilchrist, R. B. (2004). Bovine cumulus cell-oocyte gap junctional communication during *in vitro* maturation in response to manipulation of cell-specific cyclic adenosine 3′,5′-monophosophate levels. *Biol. Reprod.* 70, 548–556. doi: 10.1095/biolreprod.103.021204

Thouas, G. A., Trounson, A. O., Wolvetang, E. J., and Jones, G. M. (2004). Mitochondrial dysfunction in mouse oocytes results in preimplantation embryo arrest *in vitro*. *Biol. Reprod.* 71, 1936–1942. doi: 10.1095/biolreprod.104.033589

Tosca, L., Chabrolle, C., Uzbekova, S., and Dupont, J. (2007a). Effect of metformin on bovine granulosa cell steroidogenesis: possible involvement of adenosine 5' monophosphate-activated protein kinase (AMPK). *Biol. Reprod.* 76, 368–378. doi: 10.1095/biolreprod.106.055749

Tosca, L., Crochet, S., Ferré, P., Foufelle, F., Tesseraud, S., and Dupont, J. (2006a). AMP-activated protein kinase activation modulates progesterone secretion in granulosa cells from hen preovulatory follicles. *J. Endocrinol.* 190, 85–97. doi: 10.1677/joe.1.06828

Tosca, L., Froment, P., Solnais, P., Foufelle, F., and Dupont, J. (2005). Adenosine 5′-monophosphate-activated protein kinase regulates progesterone secretion in rat granulosa cells. *Endocrinology* 146, 4500–4513. doi: 10.1210/en.2005-0301

Tosca, L., Rame, C., Chabrolle, C., Tesseraud, S., and Dupont, J. (2010). Metformin decreases IGF1-induced cel proliferation and protein synthesis through AMP-activated protein kinase in cultured bovine granulosa cells *Reproduction* 139, 409–418. doi: 10.1530/REP-09-0351

Tosca, L., Solnais, P., Ferre, P., Foufelle, F., and Dupont, J. (2006b). Metformin-induced stimulation of adenosine 5′ monophosphate-activated protein kinase (PRKA) impairs progesterone secretion in rat granulosa cells. *Biol. Reprod.* 75, 342–351. doi: 10.1095/biolreprod.106.050831

Tosca, L., Uzbekova, S., Chabrolle, C., and Dupont, J. (2007b). Possible role of 5′ AMP-activated protein kinase in the metformin-mediated arrest of bovine oocytes at the germinal vesicle stage during *in vitro* maturation. *Biol. Reprod.* 77, 452–465. doi: 10.1095/biolreprod.107.060848

Towler, M. C., Fogarty, S., Hawley, S. A., Pan, D. A., Martin, D. M., Morrice, N. A., et al. (2008). A novel short splice variant of the tumour suppressor LKB1 is required for spermiogenesis. *Biochem. J.* 416, 1–14. doi: 10.1042/BJ20081447

Ulbright, T. M., Amin, M. B., and Young, R. H. (2007). Intratubular large cell hyalinizing sertoli cell neoplasia of the testis: a report of 8 cases of a distinctive lesion of the Peutz-Jeghers syndrome. *Am. J. Surg. Pathol.* 31, 827–835. doi: 10.1097/PAS.0b013e3180309e33

Van Blerkom, J. (2004). Mitochondria in human oogenesis and preimplantation embryogenesis: engines of metabolism, ionic ergulation and developmental competence. *Reproduction* 128, 269–280. doi: 10.1530/rep.1.00240

Vaquero, A., Scher, M., Lee, D., Erdjument-Bromage, H., Tempst, P., and Reinberg, D. (2004a). Human SirT1 interacts with histone H1 and promotes formation of facultative heterochromatin. *Mol. Cell* 16, 93–105. doi: 10.1016/j.molcel.2004.08.031

Vaquero, A., Scher, M., Lee, D., Erdument-Bromage, H., Tempst, P., and Reinberg, D. (2004b). Human SirT1 interacts with histone H1 and promotes formation of facultative heterochromatin. *Mol. Cell* 16, 93–105. doi: 10.1016/j.molcel.2004.08.031

Vasangkar, D., and Downs, S. M. (2013). A requirement for fatty acid oxidation in the hormone-induced meiotic maturation of mouse oocytes. *Biol. Reprod.* 89, 43. doi: 10.1095/biolreprod.113.109058

Wakeling, L. A., Ions, L. J., and Ford, D. (2009). Could Sirt1-mediated epigenetic effects contribute to the longevity response to dietary restriction and be mimicked by other dietary interventions? *Age* 31, 327–341. doi: 10.1007/s11357-009-9104-5

Wang, Q., Ratchford, A. M., Chi, M. M.-Y., Schoeller, E., Frolova, A., Schedl, T., et al. (2009). Maternal diabetes causes mitochondrial dysfunction and meiotic defects in murine oocytes. *Mol. Endocrinol.* 23, 1603–1612. doi: 10.1210/me.2009-0033

Winterhager, E., and Kidder, G. M. (2015). Gap junction connexins in female reproductive organs: implications for women's reproductive health. *Hum. Reprod. Update* 21, 340–352. doi: 10.1093/humupd/dmv007

Woods, A., Johnstone, S. R., Dickerson, K., Leiper, F. C., Fryer, L. G., Neumann, D., et al. (2003). LKB1 is the upstream kinase in the AMP-activated protein kinase cascade. *Curr. Biol.* 13, 2004–2008. doi: 10.1016/j.cub.2003.10.031

Ya, R., and Downs, S. M. (2014). Perturbing microtubule integrity blocks AMP-activated protein kinase-induced meiotic resumption in cultured mouse oocytes. *Zygote* 22, 91–102. doi: 10.1017/S0967199412000457

Zhou, G., Myers, R., Li, Y., Chen, Y., Shen, X., Fenyk-Melody, J., et al. (2001). Role of AMP-activated protein kinase in mechanism of metformin action. *J. Clin. Invest.* 108, 1167–1174. doi: 10.1172/JCI13505

Ziv, S., Rufas, O., and Shalgi, R. (2002). Cadherin expression during gamete maturation and fertilzation in the rat. *Mol. Reprod. Dev.* 62, 547–556. doi: 10.1002/mrd.10149

21

The "ram effect": New insights into neural modulation of the gonadotropic axis by male odors and socio-sexual interactions

Claude Fabre-Nys[1], Keith M. Kendrick[2] and Rex J. Scaramuzzi[3]*

[1] UMR 7247 Physiologie de la Reproduction et des Comportements, Centre National de la Recherche Scientifique, Institut National de la Recherche Agronomique, Institut Français du Cheval et de L'équitation, Université de Tours, Nouzilly, France,
[2] Key Laboratory for Neuroinformation, University of Electronic Science and Technology of China, Chengdu, China,
[3] Department of Comparative Biological Sciences, Royal Veterinary College, South Mimms, UK

Edited by:
Hubert Vaudry, University of Rouen, France

Reviewed by:
Berta Levavi-Sivan, The Hebrew University, Israel
Ruud Buijs, Universidad Autónoma de México, Mexico
Graeme Bruce Martin, University of Western Australia, Australia

***Correspondence:**
Claude Fabre-Nys, Physiologie de la Reproduction et des Comportements, Centre INRA Val de Loire, 37380, Nouzilly, France
claude.fabre@tours.inra.fr

Reproduction in mammals is controlled by the hypothalamo-pituitary-gonadal (HPG) axis under the influence of external and internal factors such as photoperiod, stress, nutrition, and social interactions. Sheep are seasonal breeders and stop mating when day length is increasing (anestrus). However, interactions with a sexually active ram during this period can override the steroid negative feedback responsible for the anoestrus state, stimulate luteinizing hormone (LH) secretion and eventually reinstate cyclicity. This is known as the "ram effect" and research into the mechanisms underlying it is shedding new light on HPG axis regulation. The first step in the ram effect is increased LH pulsatile secretion in anestrus ewes exposed to a sexually active male or only to its fleece, the latter finding indicating a "pheromone-like" effect. Estradiol secretion increases in all ewes and this eventually induces a LH surge and ovulation, just as during the breeding season. An exception is a minority of ewes that exhibit a precocious LH surge (within 4 h) with no prior increase in estradiol. The main olfactory system and the cortical nucleus of the amygdala are critical brain structures in mediating the ram effect since it is blocked by their inactivation. Sexual experience is also important since activation (increased c-fos expression) in these and other regions is greatly reduced in sexually naïve ewes. In adult ewes kisspeptin neurons in both arcuate and preoptic regions and some preoptic GnRH neurons are activated 2 h after exposure to a ram. Exposure to rams also activates noradrenergic neurons in the locus coeruleus and A1 nucleus and increased noradrenalin release occurs in the posterior preoptic area. Pharmacological modulation of this system modifies LH secretion in response to the male or his odor. Together these results show that the ram effect can be a fruitful model to promote both a better understanding of the neural and hormonal regulation of the HPG axis in general and also the specific mechanisms by which male cues can overcome negative steroid feedback and trigger LH release and ovulatory cycles.

Keywords: ram effect, odor, LH, estradiol, main olfactory system, experience, noradrenaline, kisspeptin

Introduction

Reproduction is essential for the survival and evolution of species and in most vertebrates it is controlled by similar networks of hormonal signals. The key regulator of the network is the hypothalamic neuropeptide, gonadotrophin releasing hormone (GnRH), which controls the release of the pituitary hormones, luteinizing hormone (LH), and follicle stimulating hormone (FSH). These latter hormones then stimulate the gonads to produce functional gametes and secrete estradiol, progesterone and testosterone that sustain reproductive function and auto-regulate the activity of the gonadotrophic axis by modulating the secretion of GnRH, LH, and FSH through positive and negative feedback systems. The mechanisms involved in the regulation of this network, often referred to as the hypothalamo-pituitary gonadal axis (HPG), have been the object of abundant research for several decades (Knobil, 1981; Karsch, 1984) but a central question which remained unresolved was how sex steroids modulate the activity of GnRH neurons while the latter lack receptors for steroids involved in feedback action (Herbison, 1998). However, the discovery of kisspeptin-containing neurons as being the most potent secretagogues of GnRH (Messager et al., 2005), and the recent observation that, in mice, all kisspeptin neurons projecting on GnRH neurons have estradiol receptors (Kumar et al., 2015) make them the most probable target of steroid action (Clarkson and Herbison, 2009) and has opened up a new era in this field of research.

The HPG axis is also modulated by many internal and external factors such as nutrition, stress, immunological status, physical, and social environment (Signoret, 1980; Tomaszewska-Zaremba and Herman, 2009; Dobson et al., 2012; Follett, 2014; Roa and Tena-Sempere, 2014) but the mechanisms involved are largely unclear. The effects of the social environment are particularly intriguing because they are very diverse. In mammals they can inhibit reproduction such as in naked mole rat social groups in which reproduction is restricted to a few individuals (Goldman et al., 2006). This is also the case in marmoset family groups where the presence of the mother inhibits reproduction of her daughters (Abbott et al., 1981) or in mice where overcrowding can block reproduction (Whitten, 1959). In contrast, the presence of a sexual partner in many mammalian species can stimulate reproduction (Signoret, 1980; Vandenbergh, 2006) and may even be necessary for females to ovulate, such as in the cat, rabbit, and camel (Bakker and Baum, 2000). In sheep contact with a sexual partner has profound effects on reproductive events at all stages of reproductive life; it hastens puberty (Dyrmundsson and Lees, 1972), induces ovulation during seasonal anestrus (see review by Ungerfeld, 2007a,b) or lactational anestrus (Mauléon and Dauzier, 1965), and modifies the timing of the LH surge during the breeding season (Lindsay et al., 1975). The most spectacular and best known effect is the induction of ovulation in sexually quiescent females by exposure to a sexually active male, a phenomenon known as the "ram effect" in sheep (Martin et al., 1986; Ungerfeld, 2007a). This effect of a male has also been described in goats (Chemineau, 1983; Walkden-Brown et al., 1999) and in several wild ungulates (Skinner et al., 2002; Shipka et al., 2002). The "ram effect" was discovered in 1944 (Underwood et al., 1944) but studies on the mechanisms involved only started in the 80's when reliable LH assays became readily available and when the sheep, because of their size, availability and economic importance became a widely used model for the study of the HPG axis (Karsch et al., 1997). The object of this review is to summarize what we have learned in the last few decades about the mechanisms involved in the "ram effect" and to discuss how this knowledge could help us to understand the regulation of the HPG axis more generally.

Description of the "Ram Effect"

Sheep are seasonal breeders. Ewes have regular 17 days oestrous cycles when day length is decreasing (the breeding season) and give birth in the spring when the environmental conditions are most favorable for the survival of their young. As day length increases ewes stop cycling (anestrus) but the introduction of a sexually active ram into a group of seasonally anoestrous animals will induce a pulse of LH (the short-term LH response **Figure 1A**) within minutes, whereas FSH does not undergo such a rapid change (Martin et al., 1980; Poindron et al., 1980). Exposure to a ram, or his odor, does not induce marked behavioral changes in ewes, but seems to focus their attention and induce urination (Gelez et al., 2004a). If contact with the male is maintained, the increase in pulsatile LH secretion initiates a sequence of physiological events that in some ewes will culminate in a LH surge 6–54 h later (Oldham et al., 1978; Chanvallon et al., 2011). Ovulation nearly always follows the LH surge (100% cases in Chanvallon et al., 2011; 97% in Scaramuzzi et al., 2014) but is described as "silent" because it is not associated with estrous behavior. Some females will then have a normal estrous cycle with a luteal phase lasting approximately 10 days and display estrous behavior 17–20 days after the introduction of rams (**Figure 1B**). In others, the corpus luteum from this first "silent" ovulation does not develop normally and regresses after a few days with a resultant short cycle; the ewe starts a new cycle but without a display of estrus (Oldham and Martin, 1978). Sexual behavior in these females only appears 22–28 days after the introduction of ram at the time of the third ovulation (**Figure 1B**). If ewes are mated at the time of the male induced estrus, a synchronized pattern of lambing occurs with two peaks 164 and 172 days afterwards. This singular pattern of births (**Figure 1C**) is the origin of the discovery of this phenomenon (Underwood et al., 1944) and could be used a convenient tool to identify those breeds responding to the "ram effect."

Nearly all adult ewes have a short-term LH response after exposure to a sexually active ram during anestrus (93% in Chanvallon et al., 2011; 92% in Scaramuzzi et al., 2014). However, the intensity of this short term response varies and LH pulsatility after the "ram effect" is lower in ewes with low as opposed to high body condition (Scaramuzzi et al., 2014). An analysis of the LH response to a bolus of GnRH (75 ng) given to the same animals the day before they were exposed to the "ram effect" indicated that at least part of this variability was due to altered sensitivity of the pituitary. This was due to ewes with a low body condition having LH pulses of a lower amplitude in response to the GnRH

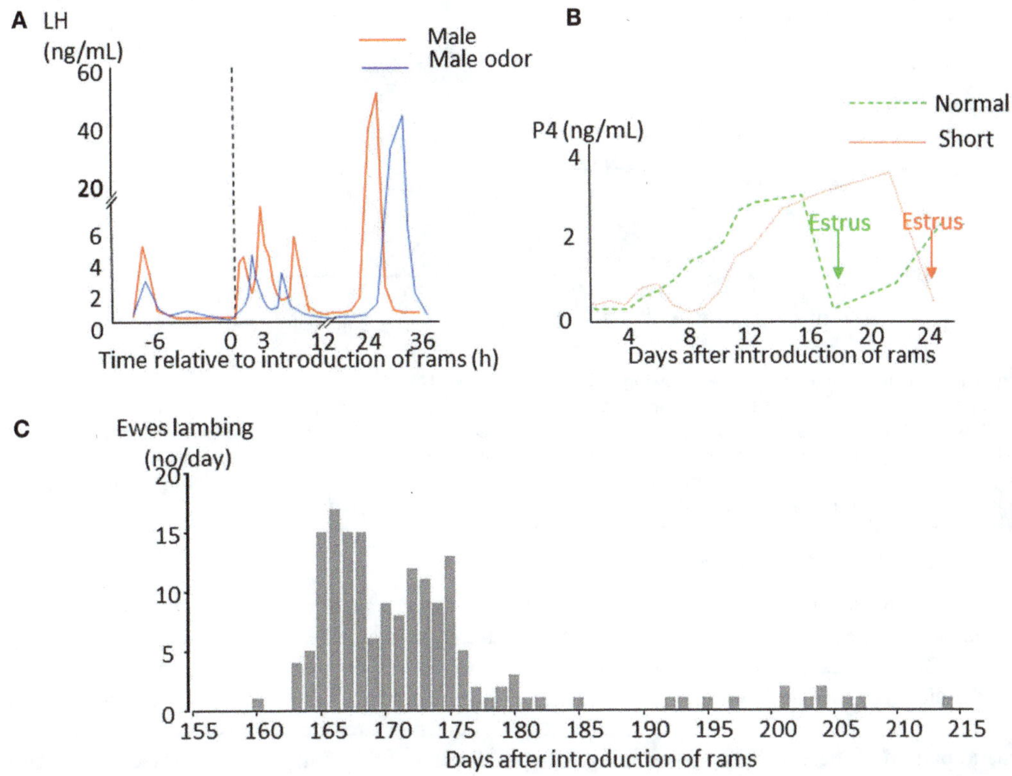

FIGURE 1 | Schematic representation of the effects of the introduction of sexually active rams to anestrus ewes. (A) Changes in LH plasma concentrations in ewes exposed to a sexually active ram (red line) or to its fleece (blue line). **(B)** Changes in progesterone plasma concentrations indicating formation of a corpus luteum. In ewes presenting a luteal phase lasting around 10 days (normal cycle green line), estrus (green arrow) is displayed 16–19 days after male introduction before the second ovulation. In ewes with a short luteal phase (short cycle red line), estrus (red arrow) appears 21–26 days after ram introduction before the third ovulation. **(C)** Example of distribution of lambing in a flock of anestrus Mérinos d'Arles ewes exposed to the ram during the middle of anestrus. The ewes lambing during the first wave around 165 days after male introduction are those that first presented a normal cycle, those lambing in the second wave are those that first presented a short cycle. The ewes lambing later than 180 days are generally ones that did not became pregnant at their first mating.

bolus than those with a high body condition (Scaramuzzi et al., 2014).

A short-term LH response to the presence of a ram is not restricted to the anestrus period and is observed in some cycling ewes during the luteal phase (Hawken et al., 2007; Chanvallon et al., 2010a) although less frequently than in anestrous ones. This is rather surprising because progesterone is known to have a strong inhibitory action on LH secretion (Goodman and Karsch, 1980; Goodman et al., 2002) and suggests that the network by which male cues stimulate LH secretion is at least partially different from that involved in ovarian steroid feedback. Interestingly the intensity of short-term LH secretion is a parameter that can predict the occurrence of ovulation since LH pulse frequency after the introduction of rams is higher in ewes that subsequently ovulate than in ones that do not (Chanvallon et al., 2011).

In contrast to the high incidence of short-term LH responses to cues from the ram, the frequency of actual LH surges and resultant ovulations is much more variable ranging from 0 to 100%. This is dependent upon many factors, but especially on the breed, age, experience, nutritional state of the animals and time of the year (Oldham et al., 1978; Chanvallon et al., 2010a,b, 2011; Johnson et al., 2011), suggesting that the induction of the LH surge is the major cause of variability in response to the "ram effect."

Role of Estradiol

In sheep, as in all mammalian species, the LH surge is stimulated by an increase in secretion of the hypothalamic neuropeptide, GnRH induced by an increase in circulating estradiol (Hauger et al., 1977; Karsch et al., 1979; Goodman, 1994) during the follicular phase. This phenomenon referred to as "estradiol positive feedback," lasts 12–24 h depending on the breed (Land et al., 1976; Cahill et al., 1981; Ben Saïd et al., 2007). It is widely assumed that the LH surge following the "ram effect" is induced by the same "estradiol positive feedback" mechanism (Martin et al., 1986). However, partly because of the difficulty in measuring the very low concentrations of circulating estradiol present during anestrus there has been very little experimental support for this hypothesis (Knight et al., 1978; Johnson et al., 2011). In a recent study we showed that, in all ewes the introduction of rams is followed by an increase in the circulating concentration of estradiol (**Figure 2A**, Fabre-Nys et al., 2015). In most anestrus ewes, the LH surge induced by the "ram effect" was preceded

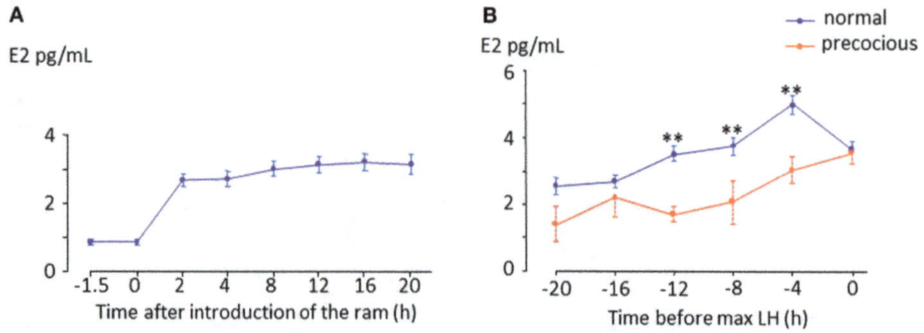

FIGURE 2 | Changes in plasma in anestrus ewes following the introduction of a ram. (A) Data are means ± SEM of estradiol concentrations in 67 ewes of different breeds (Ile de France, Mérinos d'Arles, Mouton Vendéens and Romane) from the study by Chanvallon et al. (2011) after ram introduction at time 0. **(B)** Means ± SEM estradiol concentrations in the hours preceding a male induced-LH surge; blue line = ewes presenting a surge 8–56 h after male introduction (normal, $n = 44$ ewes of the four breeds above), dotted red line = ewes presenting a LH surge within 4 h after male introduction (precocious, $n = 19$ Ile de France and Mérinos d'Arles ewes). ** indicate significant within time differences between the two groups at $p < 0.001$.

by increases in the circulating concentration of estradiol at least three-fold above the basal concentration for 14.5 ± 0.86 h (min 6 h; max 36 h, **Figure 2B**). Similar to the breeding season, the concentration of estradiol decreased at the time of the LH surge (**Figure 2B**).

The duration and pattern of these increases in estradiol concentrations varies among breeds. This variability in a highly seasonal breed, the Mouton Vendéen, is due to the low sensitivity of the ovary that releases very little amount of steroids in response to stimulation by a ram. The granulosa cells of these ewes in culture, also have a low response to *in vitro* stimulation by IGF-I and FSH and reduced expression of StAR (Fabre-Nys et al., 2015). In other breeds such as the Romane the frequency and latency of the LH surge is variable, although the quantities of estradiol secreted after the "ram effect" do not differ from those in breeds such as the Mérinos d'Arles and Ile de France that respond well to it. In these breeds the variability in response seems to be due to fluctuating sensitivity of the hypothalamo-hypophyseal complex to estradiol feedback.

In some ewes LH surges are induced immediately after exposure to a ram and these "precocious" LH surges are not preceded by increased concentrations of estradiol (Fabre-Nys et al., 2013; **Figure 2B**). Contrary to the spontaneous LH surges that occur in ewes during the breeding season, these "precocious" LH surges cannot be the result of classical "estradiol positive feedback." Indeed the important question raised here is whether the mechanism of induction of these male-induced LH surges shares any similarities with that in spontaneous ovulators (Fabre-Nys et al., 2013).

The Stimuli Involved

The ram emits a considerable range of different sensory stimuli that could be responsible for evoking a reproductive neuroendocrine response in ewes, but olfactory stimuli clearly play a dominant role. Direct physical contact with a ram is not necessary (Watson and Radford, 1960) and a complete reproductive neuroendocrine response can be induced by exposure to ram fleece (i.e., ram odor) alone (Knight and Lynch, 1980). However, fewer ewes ovulate when exposed only to ram odor (Pearce and Oldham, 1988) and additionally the frequency of short-term LH pulses is lower and they appear later (Gelez et al., 2004a). The active compounds involved are present in the fleece from all parts of the coat and in the anteorbital glands but are absent from urine (Cohen-Tannoudji et al., 1994). They are also androgen-dependant since ewes do not ovulate when exposed to a castrated ram (Fulkerson et al., 1981). A mixture of compounds is clearly involved because the biological activity of fleece requires the combined extracts of both the neutral and acidic fractions (Knight and Lynch, 1980; Cohen-Tannoudji et al., 1994). Those from the neutral fraction have been identified as 1,2-hexanedecanediol and 1,2-octanedecanediol, but those of the acidic fraction have not yet been identified (Cohen-Tannoudji et al., 1994).

The olfactory stimuli which generate the "ram effect" are not strictly species specific since hair from male goats stimulates LH pulsatile secretion (Over et al., 1990) and induces ovulation in ewes (Birch et al., 1989). A recent study showed that an acidic fraction of male goat hair that stimulated multiunit activity of the mediobasal hypothalamus of ovariectomized Shiba goats also stimulated pulsatile LH secretion in St Croix ewes (Ohara et al., 2014). The same group has also used this approach to show that 4-ethyloctanol is of key importance for activating the GnRH pulse generator in goats (Murata et al., 2014). This could therefore represent a very interesting way to approach the chemical identification of all the odorant compounds responsible for influencing the HPG axis.

However, the complete identification of all the active components of ram odor, might not be so simple a task because it appears that ewes need to "learn" to recognize them (see section below) and they can be trained to show an LH response to other odors. For example, ewes can show an increase in LH pulsatility in response to the odor of lavender if it has been associated with rams (Gelez et al., 2004a). This means that some odorant compounds may be common to both rams and bucks, some common to all rams but others may be specific to individual rams. Sheep can distinguish between odor cues from different individuals (Baldwin and Meese, 1977) and the presence of such individual olfactory signatures is important for mate selection in rodents (Brennan and Kendrick, 2006). In sheep it may help ewes identify specific rams and explain the increased response to newly introduced, "novel" ones (Jorre de St. Jorre et al., 2012).

Non-olfactory stimuli are also involved since short-term LH responses can be observed in anosmic ewes exposed to sexually active rams (Cohen-Tannoudji et al., 1986) indicating that other sensory inputs can substitute for male odor. The intensity of male sexual behavior is also important with males exhibiting high libido appearing to be more effective than males with low libido in inducing ovulation in some studies (Signoret et al., 1982; Perkins and Fitzgerald, 1994), although not in others (Fisher et al., 1994).Visual cues alone from rams alone have very limited effects with exposure of ewes to projected images of rams only inducing small increases in LH secretion (Hawken et al., 2009a). Auditory cues also seem to have very limited effects (Hawken et al., 2009a) which is not that surprising because not all rams vocalize when courting ewes.

Factors Affecting Female Sensitivity to Male Stimuli

Breed and Time of Anestrus

The proportion of ewes ovulating in response to the "ram effect" varies with breed and time of year, the latter being highest in late anestrus (Ungerfeld, 2007b; Chanvallon et al., 2011). Sheep breeds also vary greatly in their sensitivity to photoperiodic cues (Malpaux, 2006).

Breeds are considered less seasonal if a high proportion of females are spontaneously cyclic during anestrus. This parameter is usually regarded as a sign of a "shallow" anestrus and is linked to a higher frequency of pulsatile LH secretion indicative of a lower response to the negative feedback of estradiol (Goodman et al., 1982). According to Lindsay and Signoret (1980) there is a positive correlation between the proportion of ewes in a flock that cycle spontaneously in anoestrus and that which ovulate after the "ram effect." However, this theory has been challenged recently. In Limousine ewes, a moderately seasonal breed, Tournadre et al. (2002) found that the proportion of anestrus ewes ovulating was higher when there were fewer cyclic ewes in the flock. In another study comparing the responses of four French breeds of sheep Chanvallon et al. (2011) found that there was no link between the proportion of ewes ovulating after the "ram effect" and that of cyclic ewes present in the test flock. In some breeds, such as the Ile de France, ewes always show a high ovulatory response even if few females are cyclic in the flock, whereas the less seasonal Romane breed has highly variable ovulatory responses at the beginning of anestrus. This suggests the existence of a "sensitivity to socio-sexual stimulation" factor that in some conditions can override sensitivity to estradiol negative feedback.

Experience and Age

Young and sexually naïve ewes have a generally poorer ovarian response to the "ram effect" than adult, experienced ones (Oldham et al., 1984; Thimonier et al., 2000; Chanvallon et al., 2010a) even though they show good short-term LH responses (Gelez et al., 2004a). Pre-exposure of young ewes to rams several months before the "ram effect" increased the proportion of ewes ovulating in one study (Murtagh et al., 1984) but failed to do so in another (Chanvallon et al., 2010b), and had no effect on the short-term LH response (Gelez et al., 2004a). Pre-exposure to rams however increased the short-term LH response when the stimulus at the time of the ram effect was the odor of the fleece of the male (Gelez et al., 2004a). This effect involved some "learning" of male characteristics. If during the pre-exposure, the male had been scented with lavender some ewes showed a short-term LH response to lavender, whereas ewes exposed to an unscented ram or to unfamiliar ewes scented with lavender did not (Gelez et al., 2004a). However, the conditions required for the ewes to learn the necessary male characteristics and the mechanisms involved are currently unclear (Chanvallon et al., 2010b). They are likely to occur at the level of brain areas known to undergo structural changes associated with olfactory learning involved in social recognition such as the hippocampus, amygdala and olfactory bulb (Brennan and Keverne, 1997; Sanchez-Andrade and Kendrick, 2009). Additionally, recent studies have reported plasticity changes in pituitary gonadotrope cells with increases in cell numbers and connectivity being found after puberty and lactation (Budry et al., 2011; Alim et al., 2012; Hodson et al., 2012). Thus plasticity changes in the pituitary itself might also contribute to the effect of sexual experience on the response to the "ram effect." Clearly more research is needed to improve our understanding of these conditions and to provide more information on the circuits that enhance the ability of the HPG axis to respond to environmental cues. This would also provide information of potential economic value to farmers wanting to improve the responses of their flocks to the "ram effect."

Stress

Stress can affect reproduction in many different ways (Rivier and Rivest, 1991; Ferin, 1993; Dobson et al., 2012). The abrupt change in the socio-sexual environment at the time of the "ram effect may be stressful and especially so for young sexually naïve ewes. However, this area of research has received very little attention. To examine the potential role of socio-sexual stress on modifying responses to the "ram effect" both adult sexually experienced and young sexually naïve Merino ewes genetically selected for "calm" or "nervous" temperaments over 15 generations (Murphy et al., 1994) were compared after "ram effect" (Chanvallon et al., 2010a). The hypothesis was that having a "calm" temperament would help young sexually naïve ewes cope with this novel and potentially stressful situation and so improve their response to the "ram effect." The neuroendocrine responses of all ewes were quantitatively the same although the adult experienced ewes had a faster neuro-endocrine response compared to young sexually naïve ewes independent of their temperament. Contrary to our expectation, fewer "calm" sexually naïve ewes ovulated after the ram effect; 18% compared 62% for "nervous" ewes and 100% in adults of either temperament. Being "nervous" seems to have helped the young sexually naïve ewes respond to the "ram effect," possibly because they were more alert and attentive toward the male. In another experiment exposure to a series of different acute stressors for the 2 days before and after the "ram effect" which increased cortisol levels decreased the proportion of young sexually naïve Ile de France ewes ovulating (Chanvallon et al., 2010b), although the short-term LH responses were not affected. The causes of these breed differences is unknown but in several species (rat, mice, pig, quail, human) the response to stress has a genetic component (Eley and Plomin, 1997; Mormede et al., 2011) and this may also apply to sheep.

Neural Circuitry Involved in the Ram Effect

Socio-sexual cues, similar to other factors that modulate reproduction (nutrition, stress, photoperiod), act on central nervous system networks that ultimately converge on the GnRH neurons and in this way modulate the activity of the HPG axis. According to Herbison (2006) the activity of each GnRH neuron could be affected by approximately 5 million neurons, so it seems a big challenge to understand how information derived from external cues such as the "ram effect" can have such a specific effect.

Most work has focussed on establishing the neural circuitry within the hypothalamus and preoptic regions which is critical for the male effect. In sheep, as in most mammals, GnRH is released in a pulsatile fashion with each pulse of GnRH inducing a pulse of LH which is the parameter generally analyzed in neuroendocrine studies. This pulsatile secretion of GnRH is regulated by gonadal steroids at the level of the mediobasal hypothalamus (Knobil, 1981; Karsch, 1984; Maeda et al., 2010; MBH) by mechanisms that are not yet clear (Tsutsumi and Webster, 2009). Studies from a Japanese group have correlated, multiunit electrical activity of neurons in the MBH with the LH response to male goat odor in ovariectomized females (Mori et al., 1991; Hamada et al., 1996; Murata et al., 2014) and this area of the brain is also thought to be central to the male effect in sheep (De Bond et al., 2013; Ohara et al., 2014).

By contrast, the surge mode of GnRH secretion that is responsible for the preovulatory LH surge has for a long time, been considered in rodents and sheep to emanate from the preoptic area (Herbison, 2006). In rodents only a subset of GnRH neurons located in the preoptic area around the organum vasculosum lateral terminalis (OVLT) are activated during the preovulatory LH surge (Lee et al., 1992). In sheep the GnRH neurons activated during the LH surge are not preferentially localized but are scattered throughout the entire distributed field of GnRH neurons (Moenter et al., 1993). Localized implantation of estradiol has also shown that the MBH is the critical area for estradiol positive feedback in the ewe (Blache et al., 1991; Caraty et al., 1998).

The precise neural networks linking the various cues associated with the "ram effect" to the GnRH neurons are not completely established. The focus to date has mainly been on how male odor cues can influence their activity since it is clear that olfactory cues are of the great importance (Swaney and Keverne, 2009; Baum and Cherry, 2015). However, there may be some species differences particular with regard to the involvement of the main and accessory olfactory systems.

In rodents, in which most studies have been carried out, the active chemosensory cues from sexual partners are mainly detected and processed by the accessory olfactory system. Chemosensory cues from the male are detected by receptors in the vomeronasal organ and transmitted to the hypothalamus via the accessory olfactory bulb (AOB), with only one relay in the medial nucleus of the amygdala (Buck, 2000; Swann et al., 2009). Removal of the vomeronasal organs or lesioning of the accessory olfactory bulbs results in the disappearance of the effect of the partner (Beltramino and Taleisnik, 1983). However, this strict relationship between the accessory olfactory system and partner cues in rodents has been challenged by Yoon et al. (2005) who used transgenic mice to demonstrate the presence of direct projections from the main olfactory bulbs to GnRH neurons but none from the accessory olfactory system.

While much less research has been carried out in non-rodent mammals effects of olfactory cues from sexual partners appear to primarily involve air-born odors. Thus in the pig, rabbit and ferret it is the main and not the accessory olfactory system that seems to be involved in the processing of partner odor (Hudson and Distel, 1986; Dorries et al., 1997; Kelliher et al., 1999). The predominant role of the main olfactory system in processing olfactory cues from rams has been confirmed by the effects of lesions or inactivation. Destruction of the olfactory epithelium by intranasal administration of zinc sulfate or inactivation of the cortical nucleus of the amygdala by local administration of lidocaïne completely blocked the short-term LH response to ram odor (Gelez and Fabre-Nys, 2004; Gelez et al., 2004b). By contrast electro- cauterization of the vomeronasal organ, sectioning of the vomeronasal nerve or inactivation of the medial nucleus of the amygdala had no inhibitory effects, again suggesting that the accessory olfactory system is not necessary for the effect of male cues (Cohen-Tannoudji et al., 1989; Gelez et al., 2004b).

Another approach that has been used to reveal the neural circuitry involved in processing male odor cues has been by through quantifying the expression of Fos protein in neurons as a molecular marker of cerebral activation (Hoffman et al., 1993). Using this approach we have shown that in adult experienced ewes male cues activate both the main and the accessory olfactory systems, although effects are much stronger within the main system (Gelez and Fabre-Nys, 2006). These findings are illustrated in **Figure 3**. In the main olfactory bulb, the cortical nucleus of the amygdala and the hippocampal dentate gyrus activation is relatively selective since Fos expression was increased to a greater extent after exposure to ram fleece than after exposure to female fleece (**Figure 3A**). In the piriform and entorhinal cortices, that are relays of the main olfactory system (Kevetter and Winans, 1981; Jansen et al., 1998), male and female odors induced higher Fos expression than the control situation, suggestive of a more general response to socio-sexual stimulation. In the accessory olfactory bulb on the other hand while Fos expression was higher after exposure to male odor than after the control situation it showed a similar response to female odor, indicating that the accessory olfactory system may respond more generally to social odors rather than in selective detection of those associated with males. These results are however challenged by a recent study which found Fos activation in the accessory but not the main olfactory system of St Croix ewes in response to extracts of hair from male goats that induce an increase in LH secretion (Ohara et al., 2014).

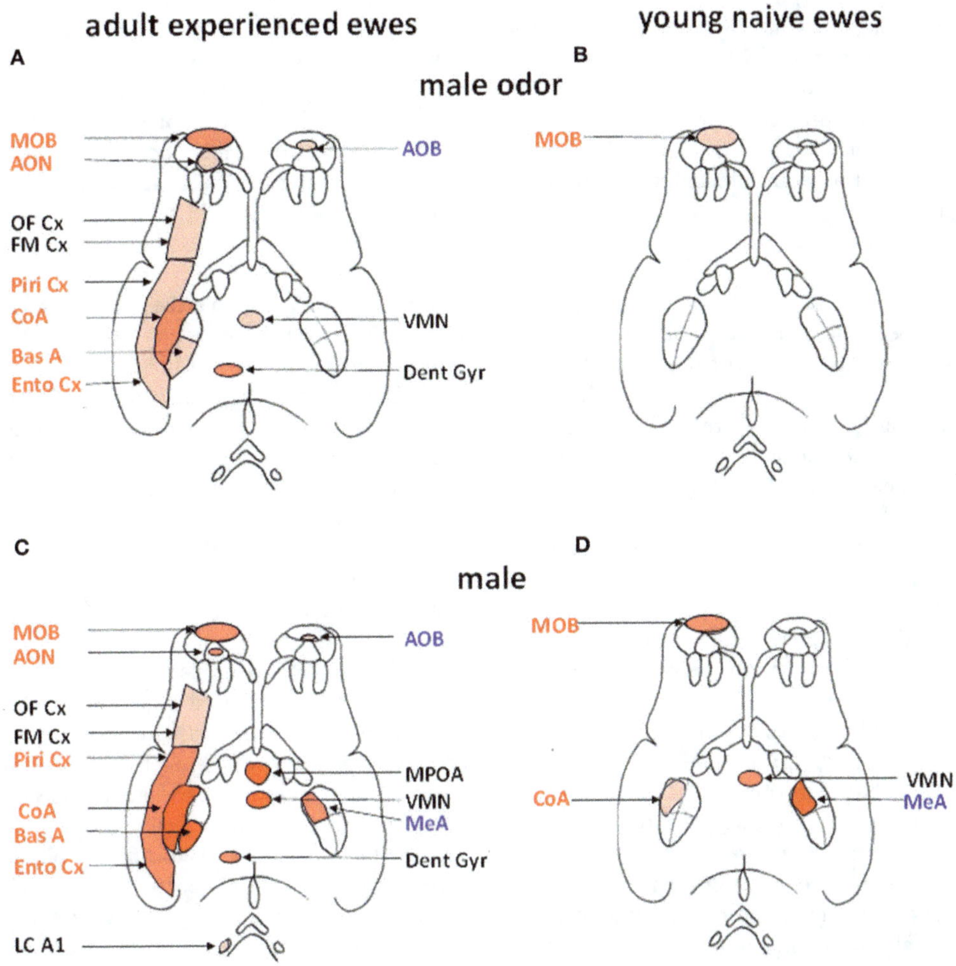

FIGURE 3 | Schematic representation of the brain regions activated (Fos immunoreactive, Fos IR) after exposure to male fleece (A, B) or to male odor (C, D) in adult ewes (A, C) or young naïve ewes (B, D). Regions belonging to the main olfactory system are shown in red on the left side of each panel and those belonging to the accessory olfactory system in blue on right side (adapted from Jansen et al., 1998). Within each of the four diagrams, regions shown in red are those in which the density of Fos IR cells is significantly greater than in ewes exposed to ram fleece. Regions shown in dark pink are those in which the density of Fos IR cells in treated ewes is significantly greater than in ewes exposed to the fleece of an unfamiliar ewe. Regions shown in pale pink are those in which the density of Fos IR cells is significantly higher than in ewes exposed to the test pen only. AOB, accessory olfactory bulb; AON, accessory olfactory nucleus; BasA, basal nucleus of the amygdale; CoA, cortical nucleus of the amygdala; Dent Gyr, dentate gyrus; Ento Cx, entorhinal cortex; FM Cx, frontomedial cortex; LC A1, locus coeruleus complex and A1 nucleus; MeA, medial nucleus of the amygdala; MPOA, medial preoptic area; OF Cx, orbitofrontal cortex; Piri Cx, piriform cortex; VMN, ventromedial nucleus of the hypothalamus.

However, the physiological relevance of these intriguing results remains to be established. Interestingly male odors also activate a number of other brain regions known to have more generalized roles in cognitive, emotional and reproductive functions including the basal amygdala, frontomedial cortex and ventromedial nucleus of the hypothalamus. Thus male odors may potentially influence a range of female behavioral responses as well as the gonadotropic axis.

Specific activation of the hippocampal dentate gyrus by male odor together with the olfactory bulb (Gelez and Fabre-Nys, 2006) is indicative of either formation and/or recall of a social recognition memory since both regions are known to play a key role in this respect (Brennan and Kendrick, 2006; Sanchez-Andrade and Kendrick, 2009). Contact with a ram has also been reported to stimulate greater cellular proliferation in ewes compared to when they are left alone (Hawken et al., 2009b). The main source of axons to the dentate gyrus is the perforant path that arises from the entorhinal cortex and intrinsic connections with the rest of the hippocampus (Treves et al., 2008). Thus differential processing of odor cues from individual rams by olfactory and hippocampal regions may in turn impact on the ultimate effects that their individual cues have, or simply whether they are familiar or not, on the subsequent activitation of GnRH neurons.

We have also found that experience modifies the extent of activation within the olfactory system in response to male odor cues. Thus, exposure to rams has very limited effects in young and sexually naïve ewes by comparison with experienced ones

(Chanvallon and Fabre-Nys, 2009). In these inexperienced ewes the only region more strongly activated by male than by female odors is the first relay of olfactory inputs, the main olfactory bulb (**Figure 3B**). Thus in the absence of any previous experience with rams, the link between their specific olfactory cues and limbic and hypothalamic regions mediating effects on GnRH neurons and reproduction are absent or weak, although the animals are capable of discriminating their odors.

As discussed above, actual contact with rams is generally more potent than simple exposure to their fleece in inducing the "ram-effect." In support of this it has been found that such direct contact with a ram does indeed induce greater activation in many brain regions in contrast to exposure to male odor alone, or female odor, or control situations. Regions showing such enhanced activation include the preoptic area (MPOA), the ventromedial nucleus (VMN), the medial (MeA), cortical (CoA) and basal nuclei of the amygdala (**Figure 3C**). Importantly, destruction of the olfactory epithelium or its inactivation by lidocaine fail to prevent an increase in LH pulsatility when adult ewes are exposed to direct contact with a ram (Gelez et al., 2004b). Thus it would appear that male cues involving other sensory modalities must be contributing in some way. However, to date we have found no evidence for activation in the visual association cortex of anestrus animals in response to visual cues from rams (Gelez and Fabre-Nys, 2006) in agreement with the limited effect of exposure to images of rams on LH secretion in anestrus ewes (Hawken et al., 2009a). This is in contrast to the situation in estrus when association visual cortex is activated (Ohkura et al., 1997) and visual cues from ram faces can induce neurochemical changes in the MBH (Fabre-Nys et al., 1997). Similarly we have found no evidence for activation in auditory brain regions.

The enhanced neural activation pattern seen in response to actual male cues as opposed to odor cues alone also shows an impact of experience. Thus in young and sexually naïve ewes Fos expression changes were only detected in the main olfactory bulb, the cortical and medial nuclei of the amygdala and the ventromedial nucleus of the hypothalamus (**Figure 3D**) (Chanvallon and Fabre-Nys, 2009). This is more extensive than seen in response to male fleece, where only activation in the olfactory bulb was found. Indeed, the most notable difference between responses to the ram, as opposed to only its fleece, in naïve animals was in the strength of olfactory bulb activation. An important role of experience may therefore be to enhance the response of the olfactory bulb to male cues resulting in a more extensive pattern of activation in cortical, limbic and hypothalamic regions. This experience-dependent increased activation in the olfactory bulb may reflect learning of odor (Shea et al., 2008; Sanchez-Andrade and Kendrick, 2009; Tong et al., 2014) and other characteristics of rams and strengthened interactions with other downstream projection regions.

An increasing amount of research has focussed on hypothalamic and preoptic region circuitry involved in translating the information from male cues conveyed by projections from olfactory and limbic regions. Direct contact with a ram or exposure to ram odor increases the percentage of GnRH cells expressing Fos in the POA and OVLT of adult experienced ewes (Gelez and Fabre-Nys, 2006) but not in young naïve ones (Chanvallon and Fabre-Nys, 2009). This is clearly consistent with the different responses to the "ram effect" observed in experienced and sexually naïve ewes. Although increased Fos expression also occurs in the hypothalamic ventromedial nucleus after exposure to either the ram or its odor, inactivation of this structure has no effect on the LH response to either ram odor or the ram itself. This suggests that this region, which is also activated in naïve ewes, may play a more general function in responding to cues from the ram, possibly related to increased attention (Gelez and Fabre-Nys, 2004).

An important question is therefore whether information from male odor and other cues is relayed directly to GnRH neurons, or by a more indirect route? In mice there is a direct connection between the main olfactory bulb and GnRH neurons (Yoon et al., 2005), so it is possible that part of the activation of GnRH neurons observed in ewes is due to such a direct connection, although this has yet to be established. On the other hand, in recent years many studies have shown that kisspeptin neurons have a major role in the control of GnRH secretion, and provide an important link between the GnRH neurons and sex steroids. Kisspeptin neurons may also mediate the effects of many other factors which influence the HPG axis (see review by Pinilla et al., 2012).

So are kisspeptin neurons the target for olfactory and limbic system projections involved in processing male cues important for mediating the "ram effect?" In sheep, as in other species, there are two populations of kisspeptin neurons, one in the preoptic area and another in the arcuate nucleus (Franceschini et al., 2006; Mikkelsen and Simonneaux, 2009). It was first considered that the two populations had different physiological roles (see review by Lehman et al., 2010); the preoptic area population of kisspeptin neurons in the LH surge and the arcuate population in the control of the pulsatile secretion of GnRH. However, a recent study has shown that in sheep the arcuate population of kisspeptin also has a role the LH surge (Merkley et al., 2012).

A potential direct functional role for kisspeptin neurons in mediating the "ram effect" is indicated by the finding that intracerebroventricular (ICV) administration of a kisspeptin antagonist (P271) 1 h before the introduction of rams prevents the increase in pulsatile LH secretion in response to them (De Bond et al., 2013). Furthermore, an increased proportion of kisspeptin neurons express Fos after ewes are exposed to a ram as opposed to an unfamiliar ewe (Ghenim et al., 2012), or not exposed to any other sheep (De Bond et al., 2013). Both populations of kisspeptin neurons seem to be involved and exposure to a ram for 2 h (Ghenim et al., 2012) or 3 h (De Bond et al., 2013) results in a 10 fold increase in the proportion of kisspeptin neurons expressing Fos in the arcuate nucleus. We also found an increase in the preoptic area although it was less marked (38%) than in the arcuate population, with 71% of the kisspeptin neurons expressing Fos-IR after 2 h of contact with a ram (Ghenim et al., 2012). De Bond et al. (2013) on the other hand failed to detect any preoptic changes. The recruitment of kisspeptin neurons in both locations is rapid and does not change significantly when the duration of exposure to rams is extended to 12 h. This suggests that the kisspeptin neurons become involved very soon after the first contact between the sexual partners. The involvement of kisspeptin neurons may also last for some time because Fos protein normally disappears a few hours after transient stimulation (Hoffman et al., 1993), whereas in our experiment 38% of kisspeptin neurons in the arcuate population and 67% in the preoptic area population still contained Fos-IR in ewes exposed to the ram for 12 h (Ghenim et al., 2012).

Thus while the precise neural circuitry involved in mediating the ram effect requires further confirmation, a working hypothesis at this stage is that odor cues from males are processed primarily by a core circuit involving the main olfactory bulb and cortical amygdala and influence both preoptic and hypothalamic kisspeptin neurons which in turn then activate GnRH neurons (see Kendrick, 2014). Kisspeptin and/or GnRH neurons may also be more indirectly influenced by other cortical, limbic and hypothalamic regions responding to olfactory or other cues produced by the male.

Classical Neurotransmitters Involved

The classical neurotransmitter systems via which socio-sexual stimulation modulates GnRH neurons are only poorly understood. The best documented is the noradrenergic system which is involved in male-stimulated ovulation in rabbits and ferrets (Wersinger and Baum, 1997; Yang et al., 1996, 1997). In rabbits for example there is a parallel increase in noradrenalin (NA) and GnRH in the MBH within 10 min of mating (Kaynard et al., 1990). Furthermore, ICV infusions of the α1 adrenergic receptor antagonist prazosin, or administering it directly into the arcuate median eminence, either suppressed or reduced the post-coital GnRH and LH surge surges (Yang et al., 1998).

In sheep, when anestrus ewes are exposed to rams the rapid increase in LH is paralleled by a nearly10-fold increase in NA concentrations in the posterior part of the medial preoptic area (MPOA, **Figure 4**), suggesting that evoked NA release in this region may be influencing GnRH neurons to promote subsequent LH release (Fabre-Nys et al., 2005, Supplementary Material). However, interestingly when estrus ewes are exposed to a ram, or just to a picture of its face, increased NA release is observed in the MBH rather than the MPOA (Fabre-Nys et al., 1994, 1997), although the onset of increased concentrations together with their amplitude and duration are very similar in the two contexts. These findings overlap to some extent with those in the rabbit where post-coital GnRH surges in females are also associated with increased NA release in the MBH but not in the anterior hypothalamus (Kaynard et al., 1990). Thus there may be some subtle differences in the ways that male cues alter LH release when animals are in anestrus as opposed to estrus, possibly associated with differing reproductive hormone profiles.

Direct manipulation of the noradrenergic system in the posterior MPOA during the ram effect using localized retrodialysis infusions has further confirmed its role in the response to male cues (Fabre-Nys and Scaramuzzi, 2014, Supplemetary Material). Infusion of NA into the posterior preoptic area increased the proportion of ewes responding to a handful of ram fleece that by itself had a sub-threshold stimulating effect (10/11 vs. 5/10 animals). The frequency of LH pulses was also increased following NA infusions whereas the ram odor alone had no significant effects in

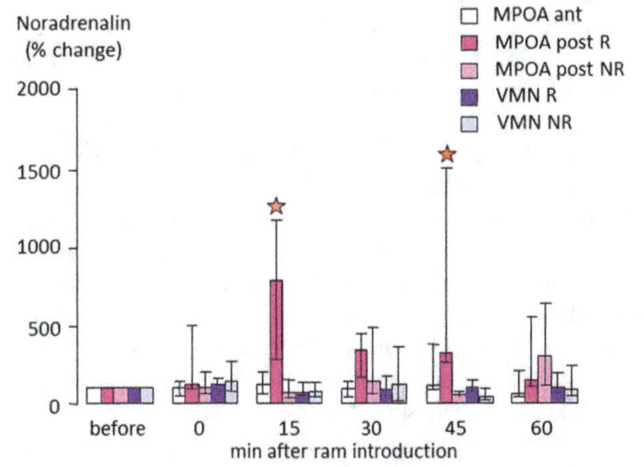

FIGURE 4 | Changes in extracellular noradrenaline concentration in the anterior (ant) or posterior part (post) of the medial preoptic area (MPOA) or in the ventromedial nucleus (VMN) of anestrus ewes that either responded (R) or did not respond by an increase in LH pulsatile secretion when exposed to a ram (NR). Samples were collected by microdialysis every 15 min and measured by electrochemical detection as in Fabre-Nys et al. (1994). Data are presented as percentage changes compared to the mean concentration during the three samples before male introduction. Data were compared using Friedman analysis of variance followed (when $p < 0.05$) by Dunn's multiple comparisons test a red star indicates that the post-treatment mean is different from the pretreatment mean ($p < 0.05$) and a pink star that it tended to be different ($p = 0.054$).

control ewes. Infusion of the α1 antagonist Prazosin in the posterior MPOA did not affect the proportion of ewes responding to the "ram effect" (7/11 vs. 8/11), and LH pulse frequency was increased both in control and Prazosin-treated ewes. However, the frequency and the amplitude of LH pulses following the "ram effect" were significantly reduced following Prazosin compared to the controls. These findings are somewhat similar to those in the rabbit where Prazosin infusions into the arcuate median eminence region only attenuated post-coital GnRH and LH surges, whereas ICV infusions completely suppressed them (Yang et al., 1998). Thus it is possible that NA is acting at multiple sites via the α1 receptor to influence LH secretion and ovulation both in the context of male-induced ovulation in female rabbits, and the ram effect in anestrus ewes.

In sheep, as in other species, noradrenergic neurons have their cell bodies within the pons and medulla of the brainstem (Tillet and Thibault, 1989) and some of them project to the MPOA and the MBH (Tillet et al., 1993). The proportion of tyrosine hydroxylase (TH), the rate limiting enzyme for the synthesis of NA, immunoreactive cells that were also immunoreactive for Fos in the A1 and in the locus coeruleus (LC) complex (A6–A7) is higher in ewes exposed to a ram than in controls (Fabre-Nys and Scaramuzzi, 2014, Supplementary Material). This suggests that noradrenergic afferents are involved in the response to male cues in anestrus ewes, in a similar way to that observed in rabbits and ferrets after mating (Kaynard et al., 1990; Wersinger and Baum, 1997; Yang et al., 1997, 1998). The noradrenergic projection from the LC to the olfactory bulb has been shown to be important in olfactory recognition memory (Brennan and Kendrick, 2006;

Sanchez-Andrade and Kendrick, 2009) and may also play a role in increasing sensitivity of the olfactory bulb to weak odors (Jiang et al., 1996). Furthermore, in the context of maternal ewes recognizing their lambs there is an experience dependent enhancement of olfactory bulb NA release (Lévy et al., 1993). Locus coeruleus stimulation has also been shown to augment MPOA stimulated GnRH release in rodents (Gitler and Barraclough, 1987). Thus in the context of odor stimuli from rams the LC noradrenergic projections to the olfactory bulb and to the MPOA may play a key role both in experience dependent perception and recognition of these odors at the level of the olfactory bulb and in facilitating GnRH release at the level of the MPOA. Importantly, since the LC is also associated more generally with relaying arousal and autonomic changes to widespread regions of the forebrain (Sara and Bouret, 2012), it is in a position to signal more general responses to the actual presence of a ram beyond those relating to specific odor molecules from its wool alone. Thus the LC projections may play a role in mediating more general influences of male cues on both reproductive and odor processing functions.

An important unanswered question at this stage is clearly how altered noradrenergic signaling modulates the activity of GnRH neurons (Herbison, 1997; Goodman et al., 2002; Clarke et al., 2006; Szawka et al., 2013). If inputs to the hypothalamic and preoptic area conveying information about ram cues involve noradrenergic signaling then one might expect from our above discussion of the potential neural circuitry mediating the ram effect that there would be some interaction with kisspeptin neurons. While this has not been shown directly a recent report on *Kiss1* knockout rats has shown that they fail to show LH release in response to either noradrenergic or glutamatergic stimulation (Uenoyama et al., 2015). Thus noradrenergic involvement in the ram effect might indeed be partly via an interaction with kisspeptin signaling, although further studies are clearly required to establish this.

Potential Scenarios of Events during the Ram Effect

The results obtained so far allow us to suggest a model of the sequence of events when anestrus ewes are exposed to a sexually active rams (**Figure 5**).

Step 1: The ram using principally odor cues and socio-sexual behavior patterns activates the main olfactory bulb and to a lesser extent the accessory olfactory system, of the courted ewe. This activation is transmitted along relays in the amygdala and the associated cortices (piriform, entorhinal cortices) and also to several cortical areas that have broader "cognitive "functions in terms of associative learning (orbitofrontal and frontomedian cortices) and to the noradrenergic system. Activation of these structures depends on the ewe's previous experience with rams and the olfactory bulb and dentate gyrus probably have an important role in learning or remembering both male cues in general and also those of specific individuals.

Step 2: The brain regions that have been activated by ram cues in turn stimulate the GnRH network at least partly via activation of kisspeptin neurons. Factors such as stress or nutrition might also interact at this level to modulate the activation of the GnRH network.

Step 3: Activated GnRH neurons secrete GnRH that induces short-term pulsatile secretion of LH. Most ewes will show this response but the frequency and amplitudes of the pulses can be modulated by several environmental factors; stress, nutrition, photoperiod and socio-sexual experience, and also by variation in the sensitivity of the gonadotrophic axis to estradiol feedback. The increased pulsatile secretion of LH stimulates ovarian follicles to secrete estradiol. In some ewes there are no follicles mature enough to respond to LH and so they will not secrete sufficient estradiol to induce a LH surge. In these ewes the action of the "ram effect" will be arrested at this stage.

Step 3b: In some ewes exposure to a ram immediately induces a LH surge ("precocious" LH surges) without the need for a period of increased pulsatile secretion of LH. We suggest that NA is involved in the induction of "precocious" LH surges. Ewes with higher activity of the noradrenergic system or a higher sensitivity to noradrenergic inputs may be more likely to have "precocious" LH surges.

Step 4: Estradiol secreted by responsive follicles stimulates preovulatory secretion of GnRH and LH surges as occurs in cyclic animals, leading to a LH surge and ovulation. Differences in sensitivity to estradiol result in ewes displaying different latencies in terms of the onset of their LH surge.

What the Ram Effect Could Tell Us About the HPG Axis

In many species, social interactions are major contributors to the adaptation of reproduction to a changing environment. This is the case for sheep and many other ungulate species in which the introduction of a male into a group of females in a reproductively quiescent state will reinstate cyclicity. These socio-sexual effects act by the modulation of GnRH secretion. In this last section we will propose a few questions that could be addressed either directly or indirectly using the "ram effect" as the experimental model in a new and fruitful way.

Pulsatile Secretion of GnRH

A Japanese group has already shown in very elegant studies in goats that the effects of male stimuli in goats can help unravel the details of pulsatile GnRH secretion (Hamada et al., 1996; Ichimaru et al., 2008). Their techniques have been developed using a miniature Shiba goat. However, the sheep is a species in which it is possible to study GnRH secretion directly by sampling hypothalamo-pituitary portal blood (Caraty and Locatelli, 1988). Because of the over-riding significance of ovarian steroids in the control of pulsatile GnRH secretion most studies have focused on this. The "ram effect" modulates pulsatile LH secretion and so probably also the pulsatile secretion of GnRH, although this has never been tested.

The "ram effect" is most potent when ewes are anestrus and more sensitive to the influence of negative estradiol feedback (Goodman et al., 1981, 2002). Furthermore, rams can also influence reproductive neuro-endocrine function in ewes during the

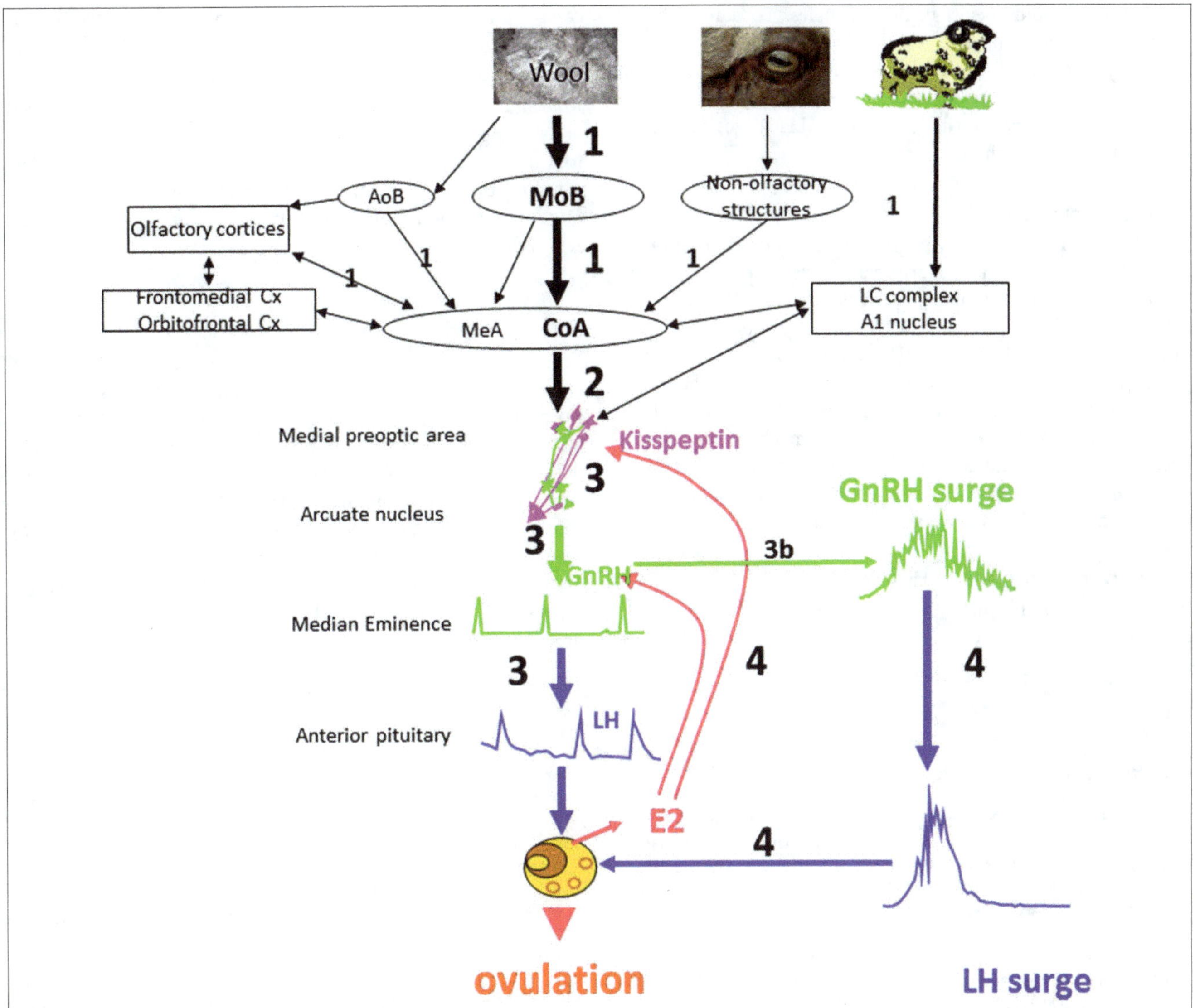

FIGURE 5 | Schematic illustration of a proposed model for the sequence of neuroendocrine events in ewes following the "ram effect". The numbers indicate the chronology of events and their size the relative importance of a specific step. In a small proportion of ewes the step 3 leads directly to a LH surge (step 3b) without the need for estradiol positive feedback. MOB, main olfactory bulb; AOB, accessory olfactory bulb; CoA, corticomedial nucleus of the amygdala; Cx, cortex; MeA, medial nucleus of the amygdala; LC, locus coeruleus complex.

luteal phase when some progesterone is present, although this steroid is known to have a very strong negative feedback effect on GnRH pulsatile secretion (Goodman, 1996; Goodman et al., 2011). So clearly exposure to male cues can in some situations override the negative feedback effect of steroids. The mechanisms involved are currently unknown but it would be interesting to test if the control of GnRH secretion by ram cues is through a different neural network to that involved in negative feedback. Experiments in mice have identified a direct link between male odor and GnRH neurons (Boehm et al., 2005; Yoon et al., 2005), although demonstrating such a direct link in ewes may be difficult. Furthermore, considering the number of brain regions that are activated when ewes are exposed to rams it is very likely that many more of them could have direct or indirect links with the medial preoptic area and the GnRH neuronal network than are known currently. Studies on the "ram effect" could help discover these unknown connections.

The LH Surge

The induction of a LH surge by exposure of anestrus ewes to a ram is nearly always due to an increase in estradiol secretion. The mechanism involved is most likely the same as the one that induces the preovulatory LH surge in spontaneous ovulators. However, in a few ewes the LH surge is induced immediately after rams are introduced suggesting a different mechanism and one closer to that in induced ovulators (Fabre-Nys et al., 2013). Several authors have suggested that the dualistic theory of spontaneous or induced ovulation is an over simplification and that both systems could coexist in most females. To date very few attempts have been made to test this hypothesis and to unravel the two types of neural circuitry that would be required to explain the duality of induced and spontaneous ovulation. The identification of factors associated with "precocious" LH surges could help identify these neural circuits.

Role of Noradrenalin

Noradrenalin is clearly involved in the male induced LH surge in induced ovulators but has a more "permissive" role in the control of GnRH secretion in spontaneous ovulators. Direct connections between GnRH neurons and NA terminals have been described in many species and since GnRH neurons possess noradrenergic receptors the action of NA on them could be direct. However NA is released in a variety of circumstances and mediates changes both in attention and general arousal. The mechanisms of these effects are not clear and the hypothesis that some of these actions could take place though the kisspeptin neurons has not been tested, although this would be an interesting possibility.

Study of the Impact of Environmental Factors

A number of environmental factors (e.g., nutrition or stress) can modulate the response to the "ram effect" and in many cases the target of this modulation is the pulsatile secretion of GnRH. Indeed, some factors are known to have direct modulatory effects on the GnRH network (Chand and Lovejoy, 2011; Roa and Tena-Sempere, 2014) and the mechanisms involved are starting to be understood, although, exactly how these factors interact with the effect of the male is not known. Understanding these interactions would help provide a more thorough understanding of the impact of environmental factors on reproduction.

Effect of Experience

Young ewes that are sexually naive have weaker physiological responses to the ram or to ram odor and the socio-sexual cues from the ram are less able to activate brain regions than in sexually experienced ewes. The physiological response of sexually naïve ewes to the ram is enhanced if the ewes have had previous contact with sexually mature rams so that they could "learn" their characteristics. In a physiological sense, exactly what is meant by "learned" and how can sexual experience modulate the GnRH network? To our knowledge, this has never been studied, but the "ram effect" would certainly be a useful and potentially fruitful model to address this question.

References

Abbott, D. H., McNeilly, A. S., Lunn, S. F., Hulme, M. J., and Burden, F. J. (1981). Inhibition of ovarian function in subordinate female marmoset monkeys (*Callithrix jacchus jacchus*). *J. Reprod. Fertil.* 63, 335–345.

Alim, Z., Hartshorn, C., Mai, O., Stitt, I., Clay, C., Tobet, S., et al. (2012). Gonadotrope plasticity at cellular and population levels. *Endocrinology* 153, 4729–4739. doi: 10.1210/en.2012-1360

Bakker, J., and Baum, M. J. (2000). Neuroendocrine regulation of GnRH release in induced ovulators. *Front. Neuroendocrinol.* 21:220-62. doi: 10.1006/frne.2000.0198

Baldwin, B. A., and Meese, G. B. (1977). The ability of sheep to distinguish between conspecifics by means of olfaction. *Physiol. Behav.* 18, 803–808.

Baum, M. J., and Cherry, J. A. (2015). Processing by the main olfactory system of chemosignals that facilitate mammalian reproduction. *Horm. Behav.* 68, 53–64. doi: 10.1016/j.yhbeh.2014.06.003

Beltramino, C., and Taleisnik, S. (1983). Release of LH in the female rat by olfactory stimuli. Effect of the removal of the vomeronasal organs or lesioning of the accessory olfactory bulbs. *Neuroendocrinology* 36, 53–58.

Ben Saïd, S., Lomet, D., Chesneau, D., Lardic, L., Canepa, S., Guillaume, D., et al. (2007). Differential estradiol requirement for the induction of estrus behavior and the luteinizing hormone surge in two breeds of sheep. *Biol. Reprod.* 76, 673–680. doi: 10.1095/biolreprod.106.057406

Birch, E. J., Knight, T. W., and Shaw, G. J. (1989). Separation of male goat pheromones responsible for stimulating ovulatory activity in ewes. *N. Z. J. Agric. Res.* 32, 337–341. doi: 10.1080/00288233.1989.10421750

Blache, D., Fabre-Nys, C. J., and Venier, G. (1991). Ventromedial hypothalamus as a target for oestradiol action on proceptivity, receptivity and luteinizing hormone surge of the ewe. *Brain Res.* 546, 241–249.

Boehm, U., Zou, Z., and Buck, L. B. (2005). Feedback loops link odor and pheromone signaling with reproduction. *Cell* 123, 683–695. doi: 10.1016/j.cell.2005.09.027

Brennan, P. A., and Keverne, E. B. (1997). Neural mechanisms of mammalian olfactory learning. *Prog. Neurobiol.* 51, 457–481.

Brennan, P. A., and Kendrick, K. M. (2006). Mammalian social odours: attraction and individual recognition. *Philos. Trans. R. Soc. Lond. B. Biol. Sci.* 361, 2061–2078. doi: 10.1098/rstb.2006.1931

Buck, L. B. (2000). The molecular architecture of odor and pheromone sensing in mammals. *Cell* 100, 611–618. doi: 10.1016/S0092-8674(00)80698-4

Budry, L., Lafont, C., El Yandouzi, T., Chauvet, N., Conéjero, G., Drouin, J., et al. (2011). Related pituitary cell lineages develop into interdigitated 3D cell networks. *Proc. Natl. Acad. Sci. U.S.A.* 108, 12515–12520. doi: 10.1073/pnas.1105929108

Cahill, L. P., Saumande, J., Ravault, J. P., Blanc, M., Thimonier, J., Mariana, J. C., et al. (1981). Hormonal and follicular relationships in ewes of high and low ovulation rates. *J. Reprod. Fert.* 62, 141–150.

Caraty, A., Fabre-Nys, C., Delaleu, B., Locatelli, A., Bruneau, G., Karsch, F. J., et al. (1998). Evidence that the mediobasal hypothalamus is the primary site of action of estradiol in inducing the preovulatory gonadotropin releasing hormone surge in the ewe. *Endocrinology* 139, 1752–1760.

Caraty, A., and Locatelli, A. (1988). Effect of time after castration on secretion of LHRH and LH in the ram. *J. Reprod. Fert.* 82, 263–269.

Chand, D., and Lovejoy, D. A. (2011). Stress and reproduction: controversies and challenges. *Gen. Comp. Endocrinol.* 171, 253–257. doi: 10.1016/j.ygcen.2011.02.022

Chanvallon, A., Blache, D., Chadwick, A., Esmaili, T., Hawken, P. A. R., Martin, G. B., et al. (2010a). Sexual experience and temperament affect the response of Merino ewes to the ram effect during the anoestrous season. *Anim. Reprod. Sci.* 119, 205–211. doi: 10.1016/j.anireprosci.2010.02.003

Chanvallon, A., and Fabre-Nys, C. (2009). In sexually naive anestrous ewes, male odour is unable to induce a complete activation of olfactory systems. *Behav. Brain Res.* 205, 272–279. doi: 10.1016/j.bbr.2009.08.013

Chanvallon, A., Sagot, L., Pottier, E., Debus, N., Francois, D., Fassier, T., et al. (2011). New insights into the influence of breed and time of the year on the response of ewes to the 'ram effect'. *Animal* 5, 1594–1604. doi: 10.1017/S1751731111000668

Chanvallon, A., Scaramuzzi, R. J., and Fabre-Nys, C. (2010b). Early sexual experience and stressful conditions affect the response of young ewes to the male. *Physiol. Behav.* 99, 457–465. doi: 10.1016/j.physbeh.2009.12.014

Chemineau, P. (1983). Effect on oestrus and ovulation of exposing creole goats to the male at three times of the year. *J. Reprod. Fertil.* 67, 65–72.

Clarke, I. J., Scott, C. J., Pereira, A., and Pompolo, S. (2006). The role of noradrenaline in the generation of the preovulatory LH surge in the ewe. *Domest. Anim. Endocrinol.* 30, 260–275. doi: 10.1016/j.domaniend.2005.07.006

Clarkson, J., and Herbison, A. E. (2009). Oestrogen, kisspeptin, GPR54 and the pre-ovulatory luteinising hormone surge. *J. Neuroendocrinol.* 21, 305–311. doi: 10.1111/j.1365-2826.2009.01835.x

Cohen-Tannoudji, J., Einhorn, J., and Signoret, J. P. (1994). Ram sexual pheromone: first approach of chemical identification. *Physiol. Behav.* 56, 955–961.

Cohen-Tannoudji, J., Lavenet, C., Locatelli, A., Tillet, Y., and Signoret, J. P. (1989). Non-involvement of the accessory olfactory system in the LH response of anoestrous ewes to male odour. *J. Reprod. Fertil.* 86, 135–144. doi: 10.1530/jrf.0.0860135

Cohen-Tannoudji, J., Locatelli, A., and Signoret, J. P. (1986). Non-pheromonal stimulation by the male of LH release in the anoestrous ewe. *Physiol. Behav.* 36, 921–924.

De Bond, J. A., Li, Q., Millar, R. P., Clarke, I. J., and Smith, J. T. (2013). Kisspeptin signaling is required for the luteinizing hormone response in anestrous ewes following the introduction of males. *PLoS ONE* 8:e57972. doi: 10.1371/journal.pone.0057972

Dobson, H., Fergani, C., Routly, J. E., and Smith, R. F. (2012). Effects of stress on reproduction in ewes. *Anim. Reprod. Sci.* 130, 135–140. doi: 10.1016/j.anireprosci.2012.01.006

Dorries, K. M., Adkins-Regan, E., and Halpern, B. P. (1997). Sensitivity and behavioral responses to the pheromone, androstenone, are not mediated by the vomeronasal organ in domestic pigs. *Brain Behav. Evol.* 49, 53–62.

Dyrmundsson, O. R., and Lees, J. L. (1972). Effect of rams on the onset breeding activity in the clun forest ewe lamb. *J. Agric. Sci. Camb.* 79, 269–271.

Eley, T. C., and Plomin, R. (1997). Genetic analyses of emotionality. *Curr. Opin. Neurobiol.* 7, 279–284.

Fabre-Nys, C., Archer, E., De la Riva, C., Gelez, H., Kendrick, K. M., and Petitbarat, M. (2005). Norepinephrine is also implicated in the “ram effect.” *Horm. Behav.* 48, 99.

Fabre-Nys, C., Blache, D., Hinton, M. R., Goode, J. A., and Kendrick, K. M. (1994). Microdialysis measurement of neurochemical changes in the mediobasal hypothalamus of ovariectomized ewes during oestrus. *Brain Res.* 649, 282–296.

Fabre-Nys, C., Chanvallon, A., Debus, N., François, D., and Bouvier, F., et al., (2015). Plasma and ovarian oestradiol and the variability in the LH surge induced in ewes by the ram effect. *Reproduction* 149.

Fabre-Nys, C., Chanvallon, C., Dupont, J., and Scaramuzzi, R. (2013). “Oestradiol and the LH surge induced after the ram effect or how a sheep can be turned into a rabbit,” in *Proc. 39th Conf. Soc. Neuroendocr. Fes*, 78.

Fabre-Nys, C., Ohkura, S., and Kendrick, K. M. (1997). Male faces and odours evoke differential patterns of neurochemical release in the mediobasal hypothalamus of the ewe during oestrus: an insight into sexual motivation? *Eur. J. Neurosci.* 9, 1666–1677.

Fabre-Nys, C., and Scaramuzzi, R. (2014). “The “ram effect”: a model for new insights into how the activity of the gonadotropic axis can be modulated by socio-sexual interactions,” in *Proc. Int. conf. Neuroendocr.* (Sydney), abstract N°250.

Ferin, M. (1993). Neuropeptides, the stress response, and the hypothalamo-pituitary-gonadal axis in the female rhesus monkey. *Ann. N.Y. Acad. Sci.* 697, 106–116.

Fisher, J., Martin, G., Oldham, C., and Shepherd, K. (1994). Do differences in nutrition or serving capacity affect the ability of rams to elicit the “ram effect”? *Proc. Austr. Soc. Anim. Prod.* 20, 426.

Follett, B. K. (2014). “Seasonal changes in the neuroendocrine system”: some reflections. *Front. Neuroendocrinol.* doi: 10.1016/j.yfrne.2014.11.003. [Epub ahead of print].

Franceschini, I., Lomet, D., Cateau, M., Delsol, G., Tillet, Y., and Caraty, A. (2006). Kisspeptin immunoreactive cells of the ovine preoptic area and arcuate nucleus co-express estrogen receptor alpha. *Neurosci. Lett.* 401, 225–230. doi: 10.1016/j.neulet.2006.03.039

Fulkerson, W. J., Adams, N. R., and Gheradi, P. B. (1981). Ability of castrate male sheep treated with oestrogen of testosterone to induce and detect oestrus in ewes. *Appl. Anim. Ethol.* 7, 57–66.

Gelez, H., Archer, E., Chesneau, D., Campan, R., and Fabre-Nys, C. (2004a). Importance of learning in the response of ewes to male odor. *Chem. Senses* 29, 555–563. doi: 10.1093/chemse/bjh054

Gelez, H., Archer, E., Chesneau, D., Magallon, T., and Fabre-Nys, C. (2004b). Inactivation of the olfactory amygdala prevents the endocrine response to male odour in anoestrus ewes. *Eur. J. Neurosci.* 19, 1581–1590. doi: 10.1111/j.1460-9568.2004.03261.x

Gelez, H., and Fabre-Nys, C. (2004). The “male effect” in sheep and goats: a review of the respective roles of the two olfactory systems. *Horm. Behav.* 46, 257–271. doi: 10.1016/j.yhbeh.2004.05.002

Gelez, H., and Fabre-Nys, C. (2006). Neural pathways involved in the endocrine response of anestrous ewes to the male or its odor. *Neuroscience* 140, 791–800. doi: 10.1016/j.neuroscience.2006.02.066

Ghenim, M., Dufourny, L., and Fabre-Nys, C. (2012). “Kisspeptin neurons are activated during the male effect in sheep,” in *2nd World Conference Kisspeptin Signaling in the Brain* (Tokyo), 122.

Gitler, M. S., and Barraclough, C. A. (1987). Locus coeruleus (LC) stimulation augments LHRH release induced by medial preoptic stimulation. Evidence that the major LC stimulatory component enters contralaterally into the hypothalamus. *Brain Res.* 422, 1–10.

Goldman, S. L., Forger, N. G., and Goldman, B. D. (2006). Influence of gonadal sex hormones on behavioral components of the reproductive hierarchy in naked mole-rats. *Horm. Behav.* 50, 77–84. doi: 10.1016/j.yhbeh.2006.01.013

Goodman, R., Bittman, E. L., Foster, D. L., and Karsch, F. J. (1982).Alterations in the control of luteinizing hormone pulse frequency underlie the seasonal variation in estradiol negative feedback in the ewe. *Biol. Reprod.* 27, 580–589. doi: 10.1095/biolreprod27.3.580

Goodman, R. L. (1994). “Neuroendocrine control of the ovine estrous cycle,” in *The Physiology of Reproduction, 2nd Edn.*, Vol. 2, eds E. Knobil and J. D. Neill (New York, NY: Raven Press), 659–709.

Goodman, R. L. (1996). Neural systems mediating the negative feedback actions of estradiol and progesterone in the ewe. *Acta Neurobiol. Exp. (Wars.)* 56, 727–741.

Goodman, R. L., Gibson, M., Skinner, D. C., and Lehman, M. N. (2002). Neuroendocrine control of pulsatile GnRH secretion during the ovarian cycle: evidence from the ewe. *Reprod. Suppl.* 59, 41–56.

Goodman, R. L., Holaskova, I., Nestor, C. C., Connors, J. M., Billings, H. J., Valent, M., et al. (2011). Evidence that the arcuate nucleus is an important site of progesterone negative feedback in the ewe. *Endocrinology* 152, 3451–3460. doi: 10.1210/en.2011-0195

Goodman, R. L., and Karsch, F. J. (1980). Pulsatile secretion of luteinizing hormone: differential suppression by ovarian steroids. *Endocrinology* 107, 1286–1290. doi: 10.1210/endo-107-5-1286

Goodman, R. L., Legan, S. J., Ryan, K. D., Foster, D. L., and Karsch, F. J. (1981). Importance of variations in behavioural and feedback actions of oestradiol to the control of seasonal breeding in the ewe. *J. Endocrinol.* 89, 229–240. doi: 10.1677/joe.0.0890229

Hamada, T., Nakajima, M., Takeuchi, Y., and Mori, Y. (1996). Pheromone-induced stimulation of hypothalamic gonadotropin-releasing hormone pulse generator in ovariectomized, estrogen-primed goats. *Neuroendocrinology* 64, 313–319. doi: 10.1159/000127134 doi: 10.1159/000127134

Hauger, R. L., Karsch, F. J., and Foster, D. L. (1977). A new concept for control of the estrous cycle of the ewe based on the temporal relationships between luteinizing hormone, estradiol and progesterone in peripheral serum and evidence that progesterone inhibits tonic LH secretion. *Endocrinology* 101, 807–817. doi: 10.1210/endo-101-3-807

Hawken, P. A., Beard, A. P., Esmaili, T., Kadokawa, H., Evans, A. C., Blache, D., et al. (2007).The introduction of rams induces an increase in pulsatile LH secretion in cyclic ewes during the breeding season. *Theriogenology* 68, 56–66. Erratum in: *Theriogenology* 68:820. doi: 10.1016/j.theriogenology.2007.03.023

Hawken, P. A., Esmaili, T., Scanlan, V., Blache, D., and Martin, G. B. (2009a). Can audio-visual or visual stimuli from a prospective mate stimulate a reproductive neuroendocrine response in sheep? *Animal* 3, 690–696. doi: 10.1017/S1751731109003954

Hawken, P. A., Jorre, T. J., Rodger, J., Esmaili, T., Blache, D., and Martin, G. B. (2009b). Rapid induction of cell proliferation in the adult female ungulate brain (*Ovis aries*) associated with activation of the reproductive axis by exposure to unfamiliar males. *Biol. Reprod.* 80, 1146–1151. doi: 10.1095/biolreprod.108.075341

Herbison, A. E. (1997). Noradrenergic regulation of cyclic GnRH secretion. *Rev. Reprod.* 2, 1–6. doi: 10.1530/ror.0.0020001

Herbison, A. E. (1998). Multimodal influence of estrogen upon gonadotropin-releasing hormone neurons. *Endocr. Rev.* 19, 302–330. doi: 10.1210/edrv.19.3.0332

Herbison, A. E. (2006). "Physiology of the gonadotropin-releasing hormone neuronal network" in *Physiology of Reproduction*, ed J. D. Neill (New York, NY: Elsevier), 1415–1482.

Hodson, D. J., Schaeffer, M., Romanò, N., Fontanaud, P., Lafont, C., Birkenstock, J., et al. (2012). Existence of long-lasting experience-dependent plasticity in endocrine cell networks. *Nat. Commun.* 3, 605. doi: 10.1038/ncomms1612

Hoffman, G. E., Smith, M. S., and Verbalis, J. G. (1993). c-Fos and related immediate early gene products as markers of activity in neuroendocrine systems. *Front. Neuroendocrinol.* 14, 173–213. doi: 10.1006/frne.1993.1006

Hudson, R., and Distel, H. (1986). Pheromonal release of suckling in rabbit does not depend on the vomeronasal organ. *Physiol. Behav.* 37, 123–128. doi: 10.1016/0031-9384(86)90394-X

Ichimaru, T., Mogi, K., Ohkura, S., Mori, Y., and Okamura, H. (2008). Exposure to ram wool stimulates gonadotropin-releasing hormone pulse generator activity in the female goat. *Anim. Reprod. Sci.* 106, 361–368. doi: 10.1016/j.anireprosci.2007.05.012

Jansen, H. T., Iwamoto, G. A., and Jackson, G. L. (1998). Central connections of the ovine olfactory bulb formation identified using wheat germ agglutinin-conjugated horseradish peroxidase. *Brain Res. Bull.* 45, 27–39. doi: 10.1016/S0361-9230(97)00279-7

Jiang, M., Griff, E. R., Ennis, M., Zimmer, L. A., and Shipley, M. T. (1996). Activation of locus coeruleus enhances the responses of olfactory bulb mitral cells to weak olfactory nerve input. *J. Neurosci.* 16, 6319–6329.

Johnson, L., Fabre-Nys, C., Chanvallon, A., François, D., Fassier, T., Menassol, J. B., et al. (2011). The effect of short-term nutritional supplementation and body condition score on the ovarian responses of anoestrus ewes to the "ram effect." *J. Vet. Sci. Technol.* S2:001. doi: 10.4172/2157-7579.S2-001

Jorre de St. Jorre, T., Hawken, P. A., and Martin, G. B. (2012). Role of male novelty and familiarity in male-induced LH secretion in female sheep. *Reprod. Fertil. Dev.* 24, 523–530. doi: 10.1071/RD11085

Karsch, F. J. (1984). "The hypothalamus and anterior pituitary gland," *in Reproduction in Mammals,* Vol. 3, eds C. R. Austin, and R. V. Short (Cambridge: Cambridge University Press). 1–20. doi: 10.1017/CBO9781139167727.004

Karsch, F. J., Bowen, J. M., Caraty, A., Evans, N. P., and Moenter, S. M. (1997). Gonadotropin-releasing hormone requirements for ovulation. *Biol. Reprod.* 56, 303–309. doi: 10.1095/biolreprod56.2.303

Karsch, F. J., Foster, D. L., Legan, S. J., Ryan, K. D., and Peter, G. K. (1979). Control of the preovulatory endocrine events in the ewe, interrelationship of estradiol, progesterone, and luteinizing hormone. *Endocrinology* 105, 421–426. doi: 10.1210/endo-105-2-421

Kaynard, A. H., Pau, F., K.-Y., Hess. D. L., and Spies, H. G. (1990). Gonadotropin-releasing hormone and norepinephrine release from the rabbit mediobasal and anterior hypothalamus during the mating-induced luteinizing hormone surge. *Endocrinology* 127, 1176–1185. doi: 10.1210/endo-127-3-1176

Kelliher, K. R., Liu, Y. C., Baum, M. J., and Sachs, B. D. (1999). Neuronal Fos activation in olfactory bulb and forebrain of male rats having erections in the presence of inaccessible estrous females. *Neuroscience* 92, 1025–1033. doi: 10.1016/S0306-4522(99)00050-0

Kendrick, K. M. (2014). Pheromones: the scent of a male. *Curr. Biol.* 24, R228–R230. doi: 10.1016/j.cub.2014.02.019

Kevetter, G. A., and Winans, S. S. (1981). Connections of the corticomedial amygdala in the golden hamster: II. Efferents of the "olfactory amygdala." *J. Comp. Neurol.* 197, 99–111. doi: 10.1002/cne.901970108

Knight, T. W., and Lynch, P. R. (1980). Source of ram pheromones that stimulate ovulation in the ewe. *Anim. Reprod. Sci.* 3, 133–136. doi: 10.1016/0378-4320(80)90040-8

Knight, T. W., Petersen, A. J., and Payne, E. (1978). The ovarian and hormonal response of the ewe to stimulation by the ram early in the breeding season. *Theriogenology* 10, 343–348. doi: 10.1016/0093-691X(78)90038-9

Knobil, E. (1981). Patterns of hypophysiotropic signals and gonadotropin secretion in the rhesus monkey. *Biol. Reprod.* 24, 44–49. doi: 10.1095/biolreprod24.1.44

Kumar, D., Candlish, M., Periasamy, V., Avcu, N., Mayer, C., and Boehm, U. (2015). Specialized subpopulations of kisspeptin neurons communicate with GnRH neurons in female mice. *Endocrinology* 156, 32–38. doi: 10.1210/en.2014-1671

Land, R. B., Wheeler, A. G., and Carr, W. R. (1976). Seasonal variation in the oestrogen induced LH discharge on ovariectomized Finnish Landrace and Scottish Blackface ewes. *Ann. Biol. Anim. Bioch. Biophys.* 16, 521–528. doi: 10.1051/rnd:19760402

Lee, W. S., Smith, M. S., and Hoffman, G. E. (1992). cFos activity identifies recruitment of luteinizing hormone-releasing hormone neurons during the ascending phase of the proestrous luteinizing hormone surge. *J. Neuroendocrinol.* 4, 161–166. doi: 10.1111/j.1365-2826.1992.tb00154.x

Lehman, M. N., Merkley, C. M., Coolen, L. M., and Goodman, R. L. (2010). Anatomy of the kisspeptin neural network in mammals. *Brain Res.* 1364, 90–102. doi: 10.1016/j.brainres.2010.09.020

Lévy, F., Guevara-Guzman, R., Hinton, M. R., Kendrick, K. M., and Keverne, E. B. (1993). Effects of parturition and maternal experience on noradrenaline and acetylcholine release in the olfactory bulb in sheep. *Behav. Neurosci.* 107, 662–668. doi: 10.1037/0735-7044.107.4.662

Lindsay, D. R., Cognie, Y., Pelletier, J., and Signoret, J. P. (1975). Influence of the presence of rams on the timing of ovulation and discharge of LH in ewes. *Physiol. Behav.* 15, 423–426. doi: 10.1016/0031-9384(75)90253-X

Lindsay, D. R., and Signoret, J. P. (1980). Influence of behaviour on reproduction. *Proc. Intern. Cong. Anim. Reprod. Artif. Insem.* 1, 83–92.

Maeda, K., Ohkura, S., Uenoyama, Y., Wakabayashi, Y., Oka, Y., and Tsukamura, H., et al. (2010). Neurobiological mechanisms underlying GnRH pulse generation by the hypothalamus. *Brain. Res.* 1364, 103–115. doi: 10.1016/j.brainres.2010.10.026

Malpaux, B. (2006). "Seasonal regulation of reproduction," in *Physiology of Reproduction*, ed J. D. Neill (St. Louis, MO: Elsevier), 2231–2282.

Martin, G. B., Oldham, C. M., and Lindsay, D. R. (1980). Increased plasma LH levels in seasonally anovular Merino ewes following the introduction of rams. *Anim. Reprod. Sci.* 3, 125–132. doi: 10.1016/0378-4320(80)90039-1

Martin, G. B., Oldham, C. M., Cognié, Y., and Pearce, D.L. (1986). The physiological responses of anovulatory ewes to the introduction of rams – a review. *Livest. Prod. Sci.* 15, 219–247. doi: 10.1016/0301-6226(86)90031-X

Mauléon, P., and Dauzier, L. (1965). Variations de durée de l'anoestrus de lactation chez les brebis de race Ile-de-France. *Ann. Biol. Anim. Biochem. Biophys.* 5, 131–143 doi: 10.1051/rnd:19650109

Merkley, C. M., Porter, K. L., Coolen, L. M., Hileman, S. M., Billings, H. J., Drews, S., et al. (2012). KNDy (kisspeptin/neurokinin B/dynorphin) neurons are activated during both pulsatile and surge secretion of LH in the ewe. *Endocrinology* 153, 5406–5414. doi: 10.1210/en.2012-1357

Messager, S., Chatzidaki, E. E., Ma, D., Hendrick, A. G., Zahn, D., Dixon, J., et al. (2005). Kisspeptin directly stimulates gonadotropin-releasing hormone release via G protein-coupled receptor 54. *Proc. Natl. Acad. Sci. U.S.A.* 102, 1761–1766. doi: 10.1073/pnas.0409330102

Mikkelsen, J. D., and Simonneaux, V. (2009). The neuroanatomy of the kisspeptin system in the mammalian brain. *Peptides* 30, 26–33. doi: 10.1016/j.peptides.2008.09.004

Moenter, S. M., Karsch, F. J., and Lehman, M. N. (1993). Fos expression during the estradiol-induced gonadotropin-releasing hormone (GnRH) surge of the ewe: induction in GnRH and other neurons. *Endocrinology* 133, 896–903. doi: 10.1210/en.133.2.896

Mori, Y., Nishihara, M., Tanaka, T., Shimizu, T., Takeuchi, Y., and Hoshino, K. (1991). Chronic recording of electrophysiological manifestation of the hypothalamic gonadotropin-releasing hormone pulse generator in the goat. *Neuroendocrinology* 53, 392–395. doi: 10.1159/000125746

Mormede, P., Foury, A., Barat, P., Corcuff, J. B., Terenina, E., Marissal-Arvy, N., et al. (2011). Molecular genetics of hypothalamic-pituitary-adrenal axis activity and function. *Ann. N.Y. Acad. Sci.* 1220, 127–136. doi: 10.1111/j.1749-6632.2010.05902.x

Murata, K., Tamogami, S., Itou, M., Ohkubo, Y., Wakabayashi, Y., Watanabe, H., et al. (2014). Identification of an olfactory signal molecule that activates the central regulator of reproduction in goats. *Curr. Biol.* 24, 681–686. doi: 10.1016/j.cub.2014.01.073

Murphy, P. M., Purvis, I. W., Lindsay, D. R., Le Neindre, P., Orgeur, P., and Poindron, P. (1994). Measures of temperament are highly repeatable in Merino sheep and some are related to maternal behaviour. *Proc. Aust. Soc. Anim. Prod.* 20, 247–250.

Murtagh, J. J., Gray, S. J., Lindsay, D. R., and Oldham, C. M. (1984). The influence of the ram effect in 10–11 month old Merino ewes on subsequent performance when introduced to rams again at 15 months. *Proc. Aust. Soc. Anim. Prod.* 15, 490–493.

Ohara, H., Mogi, K., Ichimaru, T., Ohkura, S., Takeuchi, Y., Mori, Y., et al. (2014). Effects of exposure to male goat hair extracts on luteinizing hormone secretion and neuronal activation in seasonally anestrous ewes. *J. Vet. Med. Sci.* 76, 1329–1337. doi: 10.1292/jvms.14-0260

Ohkura, S., Fabre-Nys, C., Broad, K. D., and Kendrick, K. M. (1997). Sex hormones enhance the impact of male sensory cues on both primary and association cortical components of visual and olfactory processing pathways as well as in limbic and hypothalamic regions in female sheep. *Neuroscience* 80, 285–297. doi: 10.1016/S0306-4522(97)00103-6

Oldham, C. M., and Martin, G. B. (1978). Stimulation of the seasonally anovular Merinos ewes by rams. II. Premature regression of ram-induced corpora lutea. *Anim. Reprod. Sci.* 1, 291–295. doi: 10.1016/0378-4320(79)90014-9

Oldham, C. M., Martin, G. B., and Knight, T. W. (1978). Stimulation of the seasonally anovular Merinos ewes by rams. I. Time from introduction of the rams to the preovulatory surge and ovulation. *Anim. Reprod. Sci.* 1, 283–290. doi: 10.1016/0378-4320(79)90013-7

Oldham, C. M., Pearce, D. T., and Gray, S. T. (1984). Progesterone priming and age of ewe affect the life-span of corpora lutea in the seasonally anovulatory Merino ewe by the 'ram effect'. *J. Reprod. Fertil.* 75, 29–33. doi: 10.1530/jrf.0.0750029

Over, R., Cohen-Tannoudji, J., Dehnhard, M., Claus, R., and Signoret, J. P. (1990). Effect of pheromones from male goats on LH-secretion in anoestrous ewes. *Physiol. Behav.* 48, 665–668. doi: 10.1016/0031-9384(90)90208-L

Pearce, G. P., and Oldham, C. M. (1988). Importance of non-olfactory ram stimuli in mediating ram-induced ovulation in the ewe. *J. Reprod. Fertil.* 84, 333–339. doi: 10.1530/jrf.0.0840333

Perkins, A., and Fitzgerald, J. A. (1994).The behavioral component of the ram effect: the influence of ram sexual behavior on the induction of estrus in anovulatory ewes. *J. Anim. Sci.* 72, 51–55.

Pinilla, L., Aguilar, E., Dieguez, C., Millar, R. P., and Tena-Sempere, M. (2012). Kisspeptins and reproduction: physiological roles and regulatory mechanisms. *Physiol. Rev.* 92, 1235–1316. doi: 10.1152/physrev.00037.2010

Poindron, P., Cognie, Y., Gayerie, F., Orgeur, P., Oldham, C. M., and Ravault, J. P. (1980). Changes in gonadotrophins and prolactin levels in isolated (seasonally or lactationally) anovular ewes associated with ovulation caused by the introduction of rams. *Physiol. Behav.* 25, 225–236. doi: 10.1016/0031-9384(80)90210-3

Rivier, C., and Rivest, S. (1991). Effect of stress on the activity of the hypothalamic-pituitary-gonadal axis: peripheral and central mechanisms. *Biol. Reprod.* 45, 523–532. doi: 10.1095/biolreprod45.4.523

Roa, J., and Tena-Sempere, M. (2014). Connecting metabolism and reproduction: Roles of central energy sensors and key molecular mediators. *Mol. Cell. Endocrinol.* 307, 4–14. doi: 10.1016/j.mce.2014.09.027

Sanchez-Andrade, G., and Kendrick, K. M. (2009). The main olfactory system and social learning in mammals. *Behav. Brain Res.* 200, 323–335. doi: 10.1016/j.bbr.2008.12.021

Sara, S. J., and Bouret, S. (2012). Orienting and reorienting: the locus coeruleus mediates cognition through arousal. *Neuron* 76, 130–141. doi: 10.1016/j.neuron.2012.09.011

Scaramuzzi, R. J., Oujagir, L., Menassol, J. B., Freret, S., Piezel, A., Brown, H. M., et al. (2014). The pattern of LH secretion and the ovarian response to the 'ram effect' in the anoestrous ewe is influenced by body condition but not by short-term nutritional supplementation. *Reprod. Fert. Dev.* 28, 1154–1165. doi: 10.1071/RD13139

Shea, S. D., Katz, L. C., and Mooney, R. (2008). Noradrenergic induction of odor-specific neural habituation and olfactory memories. *J. Neurosci.* 28, 10711–10719. doi: 10.1523/JNEUROSCI.3853-08.2008

Shipka, M. P., Rowell, J. E., and Ford, S. P. (2002). Reindeer bull introduction affects the onset of the breeding season. *Anim. Reprod. Sci.* 72, 27–35. doi: 10.1016/S0378-4320(02)00072-6

Signoret, J. P. (1980). Effet de la présence du male sur les mécanismes de reproduction chez la femelle des mammifères. *Reprod. Nut. Dev.* 20, 457–468 doi: 10.1051/rnd:19800305

Signoret, J. P., Fulkerson, W. J., and Lindsay, D. R. (1982). Effectiveness of testosterone treated wethers and ewes as teasers. *Appl. Anim. Eth.* 9, 37–45. doi: 10.1016/0304-3762(82)90164-X

Skinner, D. C., Cilliers, S. D., and Skinner, J. D. (2002). Effect of ram introduction on the oestrous cycle of springbok ewes (*Antidorcas marsupialis*). *Reproduction* 124, 509–513 doi: 10.1530/rep.0.1240509

Swaney, W. T., and Keverne, E. B. (2009).The evolution of pheromonal communication. *Behav. Brain. Res.* 200, 239–247. doi: 10.1016/j.bbr.2008.09.039

Swann, J., Fabre-Nys, C., and Barton, R. (2009). "Hormonal and pheromonal modulation of the extended amygdala: implications for social behaviour," in *Hormones, Brain and Behavior*, eds D. W. Pfaff, A. P. Arnold, S. E. Fahrbach, A. M. Etgen, and R. T. Rubin (San Diego, CA: Academic Press), 441–472. doi: 10.1016/B978-008088783-8.00012-7

Szawka, R. E., Poletini, M. O., Leite, C. M., Bernuci, M. P., Kalil, B., Mendonça, L. B., et al. (2013). Release of norepinephrine in the preoptic area activates anteroventral periventricular nucleus neurons and stimulates the surge of luteinizing hormone. *Endocrinology* 154, 363–374. doi: 10.1210/en.2012-1302

Thimonier, J., Cognié, Y., Lassoued, N., and Khaldi, G. (2000). L'effet mâle chez les ovins: une technique actuelle de maîtrise de la reproduction. *INRA Prod. Anim.* 13, 223–231.

Tillet, Y., Batailler, M., and Thibault, J. (1993). Neuronal projections to the medial preoptic area of the sheep, with special reference to monoaminergic afferents, immunohistochemical and retrograde tract tracing studies. *J. Comp. Neurol.* 330, 195–220. doi: 10.1002/cne.903300205

Tillet, Y., and Thibault, J. (1989). Catecholamine-containing neurons in the sheep brainstem and diencephalon, immunohistochemical study with tyrosine hydroxylase (TH) and dopamine-beta-hydroxylase (DBH) antibodies. *J. Comp. Neurol.* 290, 69–104. doi: 10.1002/cne.902900106

Tomaszewska-Zaremba, D., and Herman, A. (2009). The role of immunological system in the regulation of gonadoliberin and gonadotropin secretion. *Reprod. Biol.* 9, 11–23. doi: 10.1016/S1642-431X(12)60091-6

Tong, M. T., Peace, S. T., and Cleland, T. A. (2014). Properties and mechanisms of olfactory learning and memory. *Front. Behav. Neurosci.* 8:238. doi: 10.3389/fnbeh.2014.00238. eCollection.

Tournadre, H., Bocquier, F., Petit, M., Thimonier, J., and Benoit, M. (2002). "Efficacité de l'effet bélier chez la brebis limousine à différents moments de l'anoestrus saisonnier et selon la durée de l'intervalle tarissement-mise en lutte," in *Proceedings of the 9th Rencontres Recherches Ruminants* (Paris), 143–146.

Treves, A., Tashiro, A., Witter, M. P., and Moser, E. I. (2008). What is the mammalian dentate gyrus good for? *Neuroscience* 154, 1155–1172. doi: 10.1016/j.neuroscience.2008.04.073

Tsutsumi, R., and Webster, N. J. (2009). GnRH pulsatility, the pituitary response and reproductive dysfunction. *Endocr. J.* 56, 729–737. doi: 10.1507/endocrj.K09E-185

Uenoyama, Y., Nakamura, S., Hayakawa, Y., Ikegami, K., Watanabe, Y., Deura, C., et al. (2015). Lack of pulse and surge modes and glutamatergic stimulation of LH release in *Kiss1* knockout rats. *J. Neuroendocrinol.* 27, 187–197. doi: 10.1111/jne.12257

Underwood, E. J., Shier, F. L., and Davenport, N. (1944). Studies in sheep husbandry in WA. The breeding season of Merino, crossbreed and British breed ewes in agricultural districts. *J. Agric. West. Aust.* 11, 135–143.

Ungerfeld, R. (2007a). Socio-sexual signalling and gonadal function, opportunities for reproductive management in domestic ruminants. *Soc. Reprod. Fertil. Suppl.* 64, 207–221. doi: 10.5661/RDR-VI-207

Ungerfeld, R. (2007b). "Social factors and ovarian function," in *Novel Concepts in Ovarian Endocrinology*, ed A. González-Bulnes (Nottingham: Research Signpost), 169–221.

Vandenbergh, J. G. (2006). "Pheromones and Mammalian Reproduction," in *Physiology of Reproduction*, ed J. D. Neill (St Diego, CA: Elsevier), 2041–2058.

Walkden-Brown, S. W., Martin, G. B., and Restall, B. J. (1999). Role of male-female interaction in regulating reproduction in sheep and goats. *J. Reprod. Fertil. Suppl.* 54, 243–257.

Watson, R. H., and Radford, H. M. (1960). The influence of rams on the onset of oestrus in Merino ewes in the spring. *Aust. J. Agric. Res.* 11, 65–71.

Wersinger, S. R., and Baum, M. J. (1997). Sexually dimorphic activation of midbrain tyrosine hydroxylase neurons after mating or exposure to chemosensory cues in the ferret. *Biol. Reprod.* 56, 1407–1414.

Whitten, W. K. (1959). Occurrence of anoestrus in mice caged in groups. *J. Endocrinol.* 18, 102–107.

Yang, S. P., Pau, K. Y., Airhart, N., and Spies, H. G. (1998). Attenuation of gonadotropin-releasing hormone reflex to coitus by alpha1-adrenergic receptor blockade in the rabbit. *Proc. Soc. Exp. Biol. Med.* 218, 204–209.

Yang, S. P., Pau, K. Y. F., Hess, D. L., and Spies, H. G. (1996). Sexual dimorphism in secretion of hypothalamic gonadotropin-releasing hormone and norepinephrine after coitus in rabbits. *Endocrinology* 137, 2683–2693.

Yang, S. P., Pau, K. Y., and Spies, H. G. (1997). Tyrosine hydroxylase and norepinephrine transporter mRNA levels increase in locus coeruleus after coitus in rabbits. *J. Mol. Endocr.* 19, 311–319.

Yoon, H., Enquist, L. W., and Dulac, C. (2005). Olfactory inputs to hypothalamic neurons controlling reproduction and fertility. *Cell* 123, 669–682. doi: 10.1016/j.cell.2005.08.039

Permissions

All chapters in this book were first published in TCEN, by Frontiers; hereby published with permission under the Creative Commons Attribution License or equivalent. Every chapter published in this book has been scrutinized by our experts. Their significance has been extensively debated. The topics covered herein carry significant findings which will fuel the growth of the discipline. They may even be implemented as practical applications or may be referred to as a beginning point for another development.

The contributors of this book come from diverse backgrounds, making this book a truly international effort. This book will bring forth new frontiers with its revolutionizing research information and detailed analysis of the nascent developments around the world.

We would like to thank all the contributing authors for lending their expertise to make the book truly unique. They have played a crucial role in the development of this book. Without their invaluable contributions this book wouldn't have been possible. They have made vital efforts to compile up to date information on the varied aspects of this subject to make this book a valuable addition to the collection of many professionals and students.

This book was conceptualized with the vision of imparting up-to-date information and advanced data in this field. To ensure the same, a matchless editorial board was set up. Every individual on the board went through rigorous rounds of assessment to prove their worth. After which they invested a large part of their time researching and compiling the most relevant data for our readers.

The editorial board has been involved in producing this book since its inception. They have spent rigorous hours researching and exploring the diverse topics which have resulted in the successful publishing of this book. They have passed on their knowledge of decades through this book. To expedite this challenging task, the publisher supported the team at every step. A small team of assistant editors was also appointed to further simplify the editing procedure and attain best results for the readers.

Apart from the editorial board, the designing team has also invested a significant amount of their time in understanding the subject and creating the most relevant covers. They scrutinized every image to scout for the most suitable representation of the subject and create an appropriate cover for the book.

The publishing team has been an ardent support to the editorial, designing and production team. Their endless efforts to recruit the best for this project, has resulted in the accomplishment of this book. They are a veteran in the field of academics and their pool of knowledge is as vast as their experience in printing. Their expertise and guidance has proved useful at every step. Their uncompromising quality standards have made this book an exceptional effort. Their encouragement from time to time has been an inspiration for everyone.

The publisher and the editorial board hope that this book will prove to be a valuable piece of knowledge for researchers, students, practitioners and scholars across the globe.

List of Contributors

Nobuyuki Itoh
Medical Innovation Center, Kyoto University Graduate School of Medicine, Kyoto, Japan

Hiroya Ohta and Morichika Konishi
Department of Microbial Chemistry, Kobe Pharmaceutical University, Kobe, Japan

Gilmer Vanegas, Frédéric Lancien, Nagi Mimassi and Jean-Claude Le Mével
Institut National de la Santé et de la Recherche Médicale UMR1101, Laboratoire de Neurophysiologie, SFR ScInBioS, Université de Brest, Brest, France

Jérôme Leprince and Hubert Vaudry
Institut National de la Santé et de la Recherche Médicale U982, UA Centre National de la Recherche Scientifique, Différenciation et Communication Neuronale et Neuroendocrine, Université de Rouen, Mont-Saint-Aignan, France

Rosa Lauretta and Marialuisa Appetecchia
Endocrinology Unit, IRCCS Regina Elena National Cancer Institute, Rome, Italy

Andrea Sansone, Massimiliano Sansone and Francesco Romanelli
Section of Medical Pathophysiology, Food Science and Endocrinology, Department of Experimental Medicine, Sapienza Università di Roma, Rome, Italy

Jean-Paul V.Paluzzi
Department of Biology, York University, Toronto, ON, Canada

Garima Bhatt
Department of Biology, York University, Toronto, ON, Canada
Department of Biology, University of Toronto Mississauga, Mississauga, ON, Canada

Chang-Hui J. Wang, Meet Zandawala, Angela B. Lange and Ian Orchard
Department of Biology, University of Toronto Mississauga, Mississauga, ON, Canada

Marcos Antonio Fernandez
Marine Ecotoxicology Laboratory, Chemical Oceanography Department, Faculty of Oceanography, Rio de Janeiro State University, Rio de Janeiro, Brazil

Els Lismont, Rut Vleugels, Liesbeth Badisco, Pieter Van Wielendaele, Cynthia Lenaerts, Sven Zels, Jozef Vanden Broeck and Heleen Verlinden
Molecular Developmental Physiology and Signal Transduction, KU Leuven, Leuven, Belgium

Elisabeth Marchal
Molecular Developmental Physiology and Signal Transduction, KU Leuven, Leuven, Belgium
Department of Cell and Systems Biology, University of Toronto, Toronto, ON, Canada

Stephen S. Tobe
Department of Cell and Systems Biology, University of Toronto, Toronto, ON, Canada

Rossella Cannarella, Rosita A. Condorelli, Federica Barbagallo, Sandro La Vignera and Aldo E. Calogero
Department of Clinical and Experimental Medicine, University of Catania, Catania, Italy

Valérie Simonneaux
Institut des Neurosciences Cellulaires et Intégratives, CNRS (UPR 3212), Strasbourg, France

Thibault Bahougne
Institut des Neurosciences Cellulaires et Intégratives, CNRS (UPR 3212), Strasbourg, France
Service d'Endocrinologie et Diabète, Hôpital Civil, Hôpitaux Universitaires de Strasbourg, Strasbourg, France

Thomas Knigge
Normandy University, FR CNRS 3730 SCALE, UMR-I 02 INERIS-URCA-ULH Environmental Stress and Aquatic Biomonitoring (SEBIO), Universite´ Le Havre Normandie, Le Havre, France

Gerald A. LeBlanc
Department of Biological Sciences, North Carolina State University, Raleigh, NC, United States

Alex T. Ford
School of Biological Sciences, Institute of Marine Sciences, University of Portsmouth, Portsmouth, United Kingdom

Marta C. Romano, Carolina Miranda-Brito and Ricardo A. Valdez
Departamento de Fisiología, Biofísica y Neurociencias, CINVESTAV del IPN, Mexico city, Mexico

Pedro Jiménez
Centro de Investigación en Reproducción Animal, CINVESTAV-UAT, Tlaxcala, Mexico

Tomás Reinert
Postgraduate Program in Medical Sciences, Universidade Federal Do Rio Grande Do Sul (UFRGS), Porto Alegre, Brazil
Centro de Pesquisa da Serra Gaucha (CEPESG), Caxias Do Sul, Brazil
Latin American Cooperative Oncology Group (LACOG), Porto Alegre, Brazil

Susana Ramalho, Vivian Castro Antunes de Vasconcelos, Leonardo Roberto Silva, Ana Elisa Ribeiro da Silva, Cesar Cabello, Camila Annicchino de Andrade and Maria Beatriz de Paula Leite Kraft
Department of Obstetrics and Gynecology, Faculty of Medical Sciences, State University of Campinas (UNICAMP), Campinas, Brazil

Guilherme Portela Coelho and Jovana Mandelli
Diagnose Patologia e Biologia Molecular, Caxias Do Sul, Brazil

Monique Binotto
Centro de Pesquisa da Serra Gaucha (CEPESG), Caxias Do Sul, Brazil

Geisilene Russano de Paiva Silva
Laboratory of Molecular and Investigative Pathology - LAPE, Faculty of Medical Sciences, State University of Campinas (UNICAMP), Campinas, Brazil

José Bines
Instituto Nacional Do Câncer (INCA - HCIII), Rio de Janeiro, Brazil

Carlos H. Barrios
Latin American Cooperative Oncology Group (LACOG), Porto Alegre, Brazil

Matthew J. Ellis
Lester and Sue Smith Breast Cancer Center, Baylor College of Medicine, Houston, TX, United States

Marcia Silveira Graudenz
Postgraduate Program in Medical Sciences, Universidade Federal Do Rio Grande Do Sul (UFRGS), Porto Alegre, Brazil

Sourav Mukherjee and Saumen Kumar Maitra
Department of Zoology, Visva-Bharati University, Santiniketan, India

Keith M. Welker and June Gruber
Department of Psychology and Neuroscience, University of Colorado Boulder, Boulder, CO, USA

Pranjal H. Mehta
Department of Psychology, University of Oregon, Eugene, OR, USA

Putul Banerjee and Keerikkattil P. Joy
Department of Zoology, Centre of Advanced Study, Banaras Hindu University, Varanasi, India

Radha Chaube
Zoology Department, Mahila Mahavidhylaya, Banaras Hindu University

David S. Jackson, Shwetha Ramachandrappa, Adrian J. Clark and Li F. Chan
Centre for Endocrinology, William Harvey Research Institute, Barts and the London School of Medicine and Dentistry, Queen Mary University of London, London, UK

Ibtissam Chakir
Laboratory of Biology and Health, Faculty of Science, Abdelmalek Essaâdi University, Tetouan, Morocco
Regulation of Circadian Clocks Team, Institute for Cellular and Integrative Neurosciences, UPR3212, Centre National de la Recherche Scientifique and University of Strasbourg, Strasbourg, France

Stéphanie Dumont, Paul Pévet, Etienne Challet and Patrick Vuillez
Regulation of Circadian Clocks Team, Institute for Cellular and Integrative Neurosciences, UPR3212, Centre National de la Recherche Scientifique and University of Strasbourg, Strasbourg, France

Ali Ouarour
Laboratory of Biology and Health, Faculty of Science, Abdelmalek Essaâdi University, Tetouan, Morocco

Ningyi Zhang, Haoyan Wang, Liyuan Zhang and Tianyi Zang
School of Computer Science and Technology, Harbin Institute of Technology, Harbin, China

Chen Xu
Center for Bioinformatics, Harbin Institute of Technology, Harbin, China

Marina Grimaldi, Abdelhay Boulahtouf, Erwan Thouennon and Patrick Balaguer
Institut de Recherche en Cancérologie de Montpellier, Montpellier, France
Institut National de la Santé et de la Recherche Médicale U1194, Montpellier, France
Université Montpellier, Montpellier, France
Institut Reìgional du Cancer de Montpellier, Montpellier, France

Vanessa Delfosse and William Bourguet
Institut National de la Santé et de la Recherche Médicale U1054, Montpellier, France
Centre National de la Recherche Scientifique UMR5048, Centre de Biochimie Structurale, Université Montpellier, Montpellier, France

Thierry D. Charlier
Institut de Recherche en Santé, Environnement et Travail, University of Rennes 1, Rennes, France
Department of Biological Sciences, Ohio University, Athens, OH, USA

Charlotte A. Cornil and Jacques Balthazart
GIGA Neuroscience, University of Liège, Liege, Belgium

Christine Patte-Mensah, Laurence Meyer and A. Guy Mensah-Nyagan
INSERM1119, University of Strasbourg, Strasbourg, France

Michael J. Bertoldo
Discipline of Obstetrics and Gynaecology, School of Women's and Children's Health, University of New South Wales, Sydney, NSW, Australia

Melanie Faure, Joëlle Dupont and Pascal Froment
Unité de Physiologie de la Reproduction et des Comportements, Institut National de la Recherche Agronomique, UMR85, Nouzilly, France

Fabre-Nys
UMR 7247 Physiologie de la Reproduction et des Comportements, Centre National de la Recherche Scientifique, Institut National de la Recherche Agronomique, Institut Français du Cheval et de L'équitation, Université de Tours, Nouzilly, France

Keith M. Kendrick
Key Laboratory for Neuroinformation, University of Electronic Science and Technology of China, Chengdu, China

Rex J. Scaramuzzi
Department of Comparative Biological Sciences, Royal Veterinary College, South Mimms, UK

Index

www.ingramcontent.com/pod-product-compliance
Lightning Source LLC
LaVergne TN
LVHW081021210926
848485LV00004B/918